HEALTH SYSTEMS POLICY, FINANCE, AND ORGANIZATION

HEALTH SYSTEMS POLICY, FINANCE, AND ORGANIZATION

EDITOR-IN-CHIEF

GUY CARRIN
World Health Organization
Geneva
Switzerland

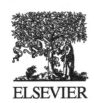

Amsterdam • Boston • Heidelberg • London • New York • Oxford
Paris • San Diego • San Francisco • Singapore • Sydney • Tokyo
Academic Press is an imprint of Elsevier

ACADEMIC PRESS

Academic Press is an imprint of Elsevier
Linacre House, Jordan Hill, Oxford OX2 8DP, UK
525 B Street, Suite 1900, San Diego, CA 92101-4495, USA

Copyright © 2009 Elsevier Inc. All rights reserved

The following article is a US government work in the public domain and is not subject to copyright:

Economic Models of Hospital Behavior

The following articles are © 2008 World Health Organization:

Cost-influenced Treatment Decisions and Cost Effectiveness Analysis
Health Care Costs, Structures and Trends

No part of this publication may be reproduced, stored in a retrieval system or transmitted in any form or by any means electronic, mechanical, photocopying, recording or otherwise without the prior written permission of the publisher

Guy Carrin and Kent Buse are associated with the WHO and UNAIDS, respectively. They, and not their respective organizations, share the responsibility with Harald Kristian Heggenhougen and Stella Quah, for the selection of the papers from the International Encyclopedia of Public Health (San Diego: Elsevier and Academic Press, 2008) for this particular volume. All views expressed in those papers are the responsibility of the respective authors.

Permissions may be sought directly from Elsevier's Science & Technology Rights Department in Oxford, UK: phone (+44) (0) 1865 843830; fax (+44) (0) 1865 853333; email: permissions@elsevier.com. Alternatively you can submit your request online by visiting the Elsevier web site at (http://elsevier.com/locate/permissions), and selecting *Obtaining permission to use Elsevier material*

Notice
No responsibility is assumed by the publisher for any injury and/or damage to persons or property as a matter of products liability, negligence or otherwise, or from any use or operation of any methods, products, instructions or ideas contained in the material herein. Because of rapid advances in the medical sciences, in particular, independent verification of diagnoses and drug dosages should be made

British Library Cataloguing in Publication Data
A catalogue record for this book is available from the British Library

Library of Congress Catalog Number: 2009927178

ISBN: 978-0-12-375087-7

For information on all Elsevier publications
visit our website at books.elsevier.com

PRINTED AND BOUND IN USA
09 10 11 12 13   10 9 8 7 6 5 4 3 2 1

Working together to grow
libraries in developing countries

www.elsevier.com | www.bookaid.org | www.sabre.org

ELSEVIER   BOOK AID International   Sabre Foundation

EDITORIAL BOARD

Editor-in-Chief

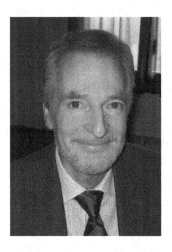

Guy Carrin is senior health economist and coordinator in the Department of Health Systems Financing at the World Health Organization in Geneva, Switzerland. He is also part-time professor of health economics at the University of Antwerp (Belgium). He published extensively in the areas of social security, macroeconomic modelling, and health economics. In the field of health economics, he is the author of *"Economic Evaluation of Health Care in Developing Countries"* and *"Strategies for Health Care Finance in Developing Countries"*. He is co-editor of *"Macroeconomic Environment and Health"* and *"Health Financing for Poor People"* and of a special issue of *Social Science and Medicine* on *"The Economics of Health Insurance in Low and Middle-income Countries"*.

He holds a M.A. and Ph.D. in economics from the University of New Hampshire (USA) and the University of Leuven (Belgium), respectively. He was Canada Council fellow at the University of Toronto (Canada), econometrician at the Institut d'Economie Quantitative in Tunis (Tunisia), researcher at the Center for Operations Research and Econometrics in Leuven, Takemi Fellow in International Health at the Harvard School of Public Health, economic adviser to the Minister of Public Health of the Federal Government of Belgium and adjunct-professor of public health at Boston University. He was also the Section Editor for economics and finance in the *International Encyclopedia of Public Health*.

Co-Editors

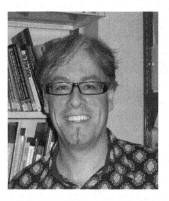

Kent Buse is a political economist with expertise in health policy analysis. He is currently senior adviser in the office of the Executive Director of UNAIDS, Geneva, Switzerland. He has previously taught at Yale University and at the London School of Hygiene and Tropical Medicine. He has worked and consulted for a range of organizations including the World Bank, UNAIDS, the Global Fund, UNICEF, DFID, WHO, UNFPA as well as for national governments and major public–private health partnerships (e.g., PMNCH, GAIN, the Global Fund, GAVI) at headquarters and field levels. He holds a PhD in policy analysis and an M.Sc (Econ) in health policy, planning, and financing. His text book *Making Health Policy* (Open University Press) has been widely adopted around the world and was short-listed for the Baxter award. He has co-edited *Making Sense of Global Health Governance: A policy perspective* (Palgrave Macmillan), *Health Policy in Globalizing World* (Cambridge) and is the Policy Section editor of the *International Encyclopedia of Public Health*.

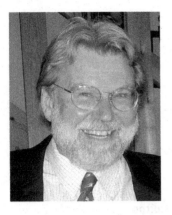

Harald Kristian (Kris) Heggenhougen received his B.A. in English and American Literature from Bowdoin College, Maine, USA, an M.A. in Sociology and his Ph.D in Anthropology from the New School for Social Research, New York City. He was a Professor (now retired), Department of International Health, Boston University School of Public Health, (and Department of Anthropology at BU, Boston USA (1999–2008)) where he will continue as an Adjunct Professor. He is also an Adjunct Professor at the Centre for International Health, University of Bergen, Norway and a Lecturer in the Department of Global Health and Social Medicine, Harvard Medical School. He has carried out extensive health and behavior/medical anthropological research for several years each in Guatemala, Malaysia and Tanzania and since starting out in Norway he has lived and worked for at least three years on each of five continents and speaks a number of languages. Prior to his professorship at Boston University he was for ten years (1990–1999) an Associate Professor at Harvard Medical School and at Harvard School of Public Health, and for ten years prior to that was a Senior Lecturer at the London School of Hygiene and Tropical Medicine (1979–1999).

He is a fellow of the American Public Health Association, the American Anthropological Association (and other associations) and was for six years the Senior Editor for Medical Anthropology of the journal *Social Science and Medicine*. From 1999 to 2008 he was a member of the Committee on Social, Economic and Behavioural Research of TDR/WHO, and he was also a consultant to WHO's EPI (immunization) program in the 1980s. In addition to his academic activities, over the past 30 years he has carried out consultancy work with UK, Scandinavian and other development agencies in a range of countries from Bhutan to Bolivia.

His most recent book (co-edited with J. Lugalla) is *Social Change and Health in Tanzania* (2005). Some of his other books include *The Behavioural and Social Aspects of Malaria and Its Control* (2003), co-authored with V. Hackethal and P. Vivek, *Reaching New Highs: Alternative Therapies for Drug Addicts* (1997) and (with P. Vaughan, E. Muhondwa and J. Rutabanzibwa-Ngaiza *Community Health Workers—The Tanzanian Experience* (1987).

Among numerous book chapters is one based on his talk at the 8th World Federation of Public Health Associations meeting in Arusha, Tanzania, "A Return to Arusha – Structural Adjustment, Indeed! Violence, Globalization, Health and Human Rights" which appeared in *Health in Transition: Opportunities and Challenges* (1999).

His research interests include health and development; social change and health; the alternative therapies for drug addiction; adolescent health and sexuality, including the health and welfare of orphans (affected by AIDS); the New Public Health, and the interaction of health, human rights, inequity and poverty. He was also the Editor-in-Chief of the *International Encyclopedia of Public Health*.

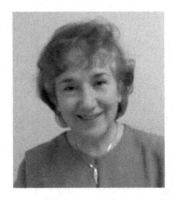

Stella Quah (Ph.D) is Professor of Sociology at the National University of Singapore. She began conducting sociological research on health behaviour in Singapore in 1972, initially at the Department of Community Medicine and Public Health and later on at the Department of Sociology of the National University of Singapore (formerly known as the University of Singapore). She was awarded a Fulbright-Hays scholarship from 1969 to 1971. Her research and professional activities include sabbaticals as Research Associate and Visiting Scholar at the Institute of Governmental Studies, University of California Berkeley (1986–87); the Center for International Studies at the Massachusetts Institute of Technology and the Department of Sociology at Harvard University (1993–94); the Harvard-Yenching Institute, Harvard University (1997); the Stanford Program in International Legal Studies, Stanford University (1997); the National Centre for Development Studies, Australian National University (2002); and the Walter H. Shorenstein Asia-Pacific Research Center, Spogli Institute for International Studies, Stanford University (2006). She was elected Vice-President for Research of the International Sociological Association (ISA) and Chairperson of the ISA Research Council for the session 1994–1998; and served as Associate Editor of *International Sociology* (1998–2004). As part of her professional activities, Stella Quah serves in institutional review boards; is member of the *Society for Comparative Research* (US); and is member of international Editorial and Advisory Boards of several referee journals. She has published extensively on medical sociology, public policy and family sociology. Among her most recent publications are *Crisis Preparedness: Asia and the Global Governance of Epidemics*, Ed., (Stanford, CA: Stanford University Shorenstein APARC & Brookings Institution, 2007); "Public image and governance of epidemics: Comparing HIV/AIDS and SARS," *Health Policy*, volume 80, 253–272, 2007; "Crisis Prevention and Management during SARS Outbreak, Singapore", *Emerging Infectious Diseases*, Vol. 10, No. 2 (February), 364–368, 2004, with Lee Hin Peng; "Traditional Healing Systems and the Ethos of Science," *Social Science and Medicine*, 57, 10, pp. 1997–2012, 2003; the *International Handbook of Sociology* (London: Sage, 2000) edited with Arnaud Sales; and *Families in Asia: Home and Kin* (London: Routledge, 2009). She was also the Associate Editor-in-Chief of the *International Encyclopedia of Public Health*.

CONTENTS

Editorial Board	v–vii
Contents	ix–x
Contributors	xi–xiii
Preface	xv–xvii

PART I: HEALTH POLICY AND PUBLIC HEALTH

Health Policy: Overview	C Paton	3
Agenda Setting in Public Health Policy	J Shiffman	17
Politics, and Public Health Policy Reform	A Glassman and K Buse	23
Evidence-Based Public Health Policy	V Lin	30
Planning, for Public Health Policy	A T Green and T N Mirzoev	39
The State in Public Health, Role of	A Alvarez-Rosete	51
Alma-Ata and Primary Health Care: An Evolving Story	J H Bryant and J B Richmond	59
Health Issues of the UN Millennium Development Goals	M Claeson and P Folger	82
Health Inequalities	P Braveman	89
Resource Allocation: Justice and Resource Allocation in Public Health	R Rhodes	97
Human Rights Approach to Public Health Policy	D Tarantola and S Gruskin	105
Interest Groups and Civil Society, in Public Health Policy	N Mays	115
People's Health Movement	R Narayan and C Schuftan	123
Global Health Initiatives and Public Health Policy	R Brugha	128
Corruption and the Consequences for Public Health	T Vian	137

PART II: HEALTH FINANCING

Health Care Financing and the Health System	C Normand and S Thomas	149
Health Care Costs, Structures and Trends	T Tan-Torres Edejer, C Garg, P Hernandez, N Van de Maele, and C Indikadahena	164
Determinants of National Health Expenditure	A K Nandakumar and M E Farag	171
International Perspectives on Resource Allocation	D K Martin and S R Benatar	180
Cost-Influenced Treatment Decisions and Cost Effectiveness Analysis	D B Evans	186
Decision Analytic Modeling	P Muennig	190

Health Finance, Equity in *D De Graeve and K Xu*	195
Governance Issues in Health Financing *M Lewis and P Musgrove*	204
Universal Coverage in Developing Countries, Transition to *T Ensor*	211
Insurance Plans and Programs: An Overview *S Greß and J Wasem*	223
Community Health Insurance in Developing Countries *B Criel, M-P Waelkens, W Soors, N Devadasan, and C Atim*	236
The Demand for Health Care *G Mwabu*	245
Long Term Care, Organization and Financing *M Knapp and A Somani*	250
Innovative Financing of Health Promotion *V Tangcharoensathien, P Prakongsai, W Patcharanarumol, S Limwattananon, and S Buasai*	259

PART III: ORGANIZATION OF HEALTH SERVICES

Health System Organization Models (Including Targets and Goals for Health Systems) *F C J Stevens and J van der Zee*	275
Primary Health Care *D Sanders, N Schaay, and S Mohamed*	284
Demand and Supply of Human Resources for Health *G Dussault and M Vujicic*	296
The Private Sector in Health Care Provision, The Role of *A Harding and D Montagu*	303
Competition in Health Care *P H Song, J D Barlow, E E Seiber, and A S McAlearney*	309
Public/Private Mix in Health Systems *C R Keane and M C Weerasinghe*	314
Provider Payment Methods and Incentives *R P Ellis and M M Miller*	322
Managed Care *S Glied and K Janus*	329
Economic Models of Hospital Behavior *X Liu and A Mills*	336
Essential Drugs Policy *H Haak*	342
Long Term Care in Health Services *J Brodsky and A M Clarfield*	351
Long Term Care for Aging Populations *E Stallard*	357
Patient Empowerment in Health Care *J F P Bridges, S Loukanova, and P Carrera*	370
Community Health Workers *S B Rifkin*	381

PART IV: KEY FEATURES OF HEALTH SYSTEMS AROUND THE WORLD

National Health Systems: Overview *N Goodwin*	393
Urban Health Systems: Overview *D C Ompad, S Galea, and D Vlahov*	408
Comparative Health Systems *H Wang*	415
The Health Care of Indigenous Peoples/Nations *G Bodeker*	422
Index	429

CONTRIBUTORS

Contributors' affiliations are those applicable at the time of submitting their chapters for the International Encyclopedia of Public Health, edited by H K Heggenhougen & S R Quah (San Diego: Elsevier and Academic Press, 2008)

A Alvarez-Rosete
Health Policy Researcher, London, UK

C Atim
PATH Malaria Vaccine Initiative, France

J D Barlow
The Ohio State University, Columbus, OH, USA

S R Benatar
University of Cape Town, Cape Town, South Africa

G Bodeker
University of Oxford, Oxford, UK; Columbia University, New York, NY, USA

P Braveman
University of California, San Francisco, CA, USA

J F P Bridges
Johns Hopkins Bloomberg School of Public Health, Baltimore, MD, USA

J Brodsky
Myers-JDC-Brookdale Institute, Jerusalem, Israel

R Brugha
Royal College of Surgeons in Ireland, Dublin, Ireland

J H Bryant
Johns Hopkins School of Public Health, Baltimore, MD, USA

S Buasai
Thai Health Promotion Foundation, Thailand

K Buse
Overseas Development Institute, London, UK

P Carrera
Management Center Innsbruck, Innsbruck, Austria

M Claeson
The World Bank, Washington, DC, USA

A M Clarfield
Ben-Gurion University, Beersheba, Israel

B Criel
Public Health Department, Prince Leopold Institute of Tropical Medicine, Antwerp, Belgium

D De Graeve
University of Antwerp, Antwerp, Belgium

N Devadasan
Institute of Public Health, Bangalore, India

G Dussault
New University of Lisbon, Lisbon, Portugal

R P Ellis
Boston University, Boston, MA, USA

T Ensor
Oxford Policy Management, York, UK

D B Evans
World Health Organization, Geneva, Switzerland

M E Farag
Brandeis University, Waltham, MA, USA

P Folger
The World Bank, Washington, DC, USA

S Galea
University of Michigan School of Public Health, Ann Arbor, MI, USA

C Garg
World Health Organization, Geneva, Switzerland

A Glassman
The Brookings Institution, Washington, DC, USA

S Glied
Columbia University, New York, NY, USA

N Goodwin
King's Fund, London, UK

S Greß
University of Applied Sciences, Fulda, Germany

A T Green
University of Leeds, Leeds, UK

S Gruskin
Harvard School of Public Health, Boston, MA, USA

H Haak
Consultants for Health and Development, Leiden, The Netherlands

Contributors

A Harding
Center for Global Development, Washington, DC, USA

P Hernandez
World Health Organization, Geneva, Switzerland

C Indikadahena
World Health Organization, Geneva, Switzerland

K Janus
Columbia University, New York, NY, USA

C R Keane
University of Pittsburgh, Pittsburgh, PA, USA

M Knapp
London School of Economics and Political Science, London, UK

M Lewis
World Bank, Washington, DC, USA

S Limwattananon
Khon Kaen University, Thailand

V Lin
La Trobe University, Bundoora, Victoria, Australia

X Liu
National Institutes of Health, Bethesda, MD, USA

S Loukanova
University of Heidelberg, Heidelberg, Germany

D K Martin
University of Toronto, Toronto, Ontario, Canada

N Mays
London School of Hygiene and Tropical Medicine, London, UK

A S McAlearney
The Ohio State University, Columbus, OH, USA

M M Miller
Boston University, Boston, MA, USA

A Mills
London School of Hygiene and Tropical Medicine, London, UK

T N Mirzoev
University of Leeds, Leeds, UK

S Mohamed
School of Public Health, University of the Western Cape, South Africa

D Montagu
Institute for Global Health, University of California, San Francisco, CA, USA

P Muennig
Columbia University, New York, NY, USA

P Musgrove
Health Affairs, Bethesda, MD, USA

G Mwabu
University of Nairobi, Nairobi, Kenya

A K Nandakumar
Brandeis University, Waltham, MA, USA

R Narayan
Bangalore, India

C Normand
University of Dublin Trinity College, Dublin, Ireland

D C Ompad
Center for Urban Epidemiologic Studies, New York Academy of Medicine, New York, NY, USA

W Patcharanarumol
International Health Policy Program, Thailand

C Paton
Keele University, Newcastle-under-Lyme, UK

P Prakongsai
International Health Policy Program, Thailand

R Rhodes
Mount Sinai School of Medicine, New York, NY, USA

J B Richmond
Harvard Medical School, Boston, MA, USA

S B Rifkin
London School of Economics and Political Science, London, UK

D Sanders
School of Public Health, University of the Western Cape, South Africa

N Schaay
School of Public Health, University of the Western Cape, South Africa

C Schuftan
Ho Chi Minh City, Vietnam

E E Seiber
The Ohio State University, Columbus, OH, USA

J Shiffman
Maxwell School of Syracuse University, Syracuse, NY, USA

A Somani
London School of Economics and Political Science, London, UK

P H Song
The Ohio State University, Columbus, OH, USA

W Soors
Public Health Department, Prince Leopold Institute of Tropical Medicine, Antwerp, Belgium

E Stallard
Duke University, Durham, NC, USA

F C J Stevens
University of Maastricht, Maastricht, The Netherlands

V Tangcharoensathien
International Health Policy Program, Thailand

T Tan-Torres Edejer
World Health Organization, Geneva, Switzerland

D Tarantola
School of Public Health and Community Medicine, Sydney, NSW, Australia

S Thomas
University of Dublin Trinity College, Dublin, Ireland

N Van de Maele
World Health Organization, Geneva, Switzerland

T Vian
Boston University School of Public Health, Boston, MA, USA

D Vlahov
Mailman School of Public Health, Columbia University, New York, NY, USA

M Vujicic
World Bank, Washington, DC, USA

M-P Waelkens
Public Health Department, Prince Leopold Institute of Tropical Medicine, Antwerp, Belgium

H Wang
Yale University School of Public Health, New Haven, CT, USA

J Wasem
University of Duisburg Essen, Essen, Germany

M C Weerasinghe
University of Colombo, Colombo, Sri Lanka

K Xu
World Health Organization, Geneva, Switzerland

J van der Zee
NIVEL, Netherlands Institute for Health Services Research, Utrecht, The Netherlands

PREFACE

This volume compiles selected chapters from the International Encyclopedia of Public Health[1], dealing with three crucial features of the development of health systems: policy, finance, and organization. It offers readers of various professional backgrounds a systematic approach to health systems analysis and development seen from these three perspectives. Therefore, professionals and students in public health, health economics, health management and other health-related fields will jointly have access to a wide range of papers addressing the public health aspects of health policies, key issues in health finance and the organization of health services. In addition, they will be introduced to selected reviews of health systems from across the world. In doing so, we intend to convey that these three perspectives are heavily intertwined, enabling readers to consider them simultaneously for analysis and policy design in health systems.

The development and functioning of health systems depend on the nature and quality of governance exercised by Government. Governance, how a society or sector steers itself, involves a broad range of activities: from the manner in which professional associations, civil society, and representatives from the private sector or international sphere are involved in decision-making to the manner in which strategic information is filtered and used to make policy on public health issues. Governance provides the general frame of reference for the series of policy papers presented in *Part I*. In his overview of health policy, Paton sets out the parameters of public policy, introduces key definitions, identifies factors which account for policy change, and, importantly in relation to this volume, explains how policy affects health systems. Policy making is often portrayed as four stages in a cycle: agenda setting, formulation, implementation and evaluation. Shiffman presents the key models, which explain why certain issues become part of the Government agenda while others fail to do so.

Glassman and Buse demonstrate that politics plays a central role in each stage of the policy process. They introduce the major theoretical approaches to understanding health politics and argue that such analysis should be more routinely used to improve the feasibility of policy reform. Despite its inherently political nature, there has been a long-standing desire for scientific evidence to serve as the basis of policy. Lin presents the key explanations of how and why evidence is used in the policy process and what researchers and policy makers can do to improve its practice. Planning may be understood as the continuation of policy making in that it involves a translation of policy outputs into implementation strategies. Green and Mirzoev discuss a conceptual framework for making sense of this intricate process. Increasingly, a range of actors are involved in health policy making. Yet, as Alvarez-Rosete explains, the Government remains the central player. Its challenge is to identify new tools to do so effectively despite increasing complexity.

International and transnational influences are now part of everyday life and are a major source of the rising complexity of national policy making. External forces on policy emanate from diverse sources including intergovernmental regulation and commercial interests. The following two chapters describe the development and impact of two international efforts to guide health policy development in low and middle income countries. Bryant and Richmond trace the development and influence of the Primary Health Care movement on health policies over the past three decades. Efforts to support countries to implement policies to achieve the Millennium Development Goals are described by Claeson and Folger.

Braveman explores one common aim of social policy – to address health inequalities – by examining its conceptualization, underpinning values and the way it is measured. Rhodes uses two dramatic examples of resource allocation in the U.S.A. to demonstrate that it is difficult to achieve 'justice' in public health policy because of the lack of an agreed governing principle. Nevertheless, Tarantola and Gruskin argue that a human rights approach to public health policy can provide a framework to guide policy towards the goals of Primary Health Care. Whether or not such a framework serves in practice to guide policy depends on the balance of power among actors and their underlying interests as

---

[1] H.K.Heggenhougen & S.R.Quah (eds.), *International Encyclopedia of Public Health* (San Diego: Elsevier and Academic Press, 2008).

analyzed by Mays. The specific contributions of civil society in steering global and national health policy development are further explored by Narayan and Schuftan. The manner and extent to which novel collaborative 'global health initiatives' impact on national health policies and systems in low income countries is critically analyzed by Brugha. Vian draws Part I to a close by discussing the types of corruption and their effects on health systems (and hence public health outcomes) and what policy makers can do to prevent it.

Good governance is a prerequisite for adequate implementation of health policies. An equally critical prerequisite is the establishment of sound health financing. Key features of health financing are addressed in *Part II*. First, Normand and Weber study how health financing is embedded within the overall health system and stress the relationship between health financing mechanisms and overall health policy objectives. A specific health accounting framework is presented by Tan-Torres et al. who demonstrate the utility of data on levels and sources of expenditure for the design of health financing policy. Nandakumar and Farag then propose a framework to study the main determinants of health expenditure, including such factors as governance, the needs of the population, income, supply of health services, and technology.

Apart from a general concern to secure appropriate funding for health care, good health financing also demands the best possible allocation of the available resources. Martin and Benatar provide insights into resource allocation at the global level, health system level as well as the institutional and clinical levels. A further focus is on tools such as cost-effectiveness analysis and decision-analytic modelling that help analysts and decision-makers in resource allocation decisions. Evans reasons that cost-effectiveness analysis contributes to guiding decision-makers as to how available resources could lead to better health and also focuses on a number of methodological issues that prevent this tool from being applied more widely. Muennig explains that decision analysis is a formalized approach that is closely linked to cost-effectiveness analysis and that assists in selecting the best option among alternatives in the event of uncertainty.

For health expenditure to benefit the greatest number of people, equity criteria also need to be considered. De Graeve and Xu present quantitative methodologies for the study of equity in health finance, enabling researchers and policy makers to better assess the equity impact of alternative health financing policies. While concepts and tools to reach targets such as efficiency and equity are widely available, it is nevertheless a challenge for policy-makers to effectively make use of them. The general significance of governance in health financing is underlined by Lewis and Musgrove who demonstrate how health outcomes can be enhanced by skilful governance practices.

In the area of health systems finance, greater attention ought to be paid to establishing or reforming organizational mechanisms as these are practical and critical vehicles for reaching health policy objectives. Universal coverage of health services continues to be part of health policy debates in many countries, in particular, the developing ones. Ensor discusses the various options for the transition to universal coverage and provides evidence related to OECD countries and to patterns of transition in the developing world. Health insurance belongs to those options, and a global overview of its key characteristics is provided by Gress and Wasem. They take into account both private and social health insurance, and address the impact of health insurance on health outcomes. Furthermore, community health insurance is examined by Criel et al. who identify lessons from experiences in various parts of the world.

Mwabu presents an economic model of people's demand for health care, the insights from which are useful for designing policies towards health improvement. Changes in morbidity and mortality patterns have also brought about new needs and demands—such as for long-term care. Knapp and Somani study the various forms of provision of long-term care and argue that its adequate financing is a new challenge for the health system. Health services are, however, not only concerned with curative care. Health promotion (and prevention) ought also to be regarded as an integral part of the health system, for which innovative financing methods are assessed by Tangcharoensathien et al.

A country's structure and quantity of health services stem from its health policies and its basic health financing provisions. The next important step is to look into how health services will be organized. *Part III* includes papers that address the organization of the inputs for health services and of the subsequent provision of health care to the population. It opens with Stevens and Zee's comprehensive overview of the concept of health systems and its application in comparative research. They address the definition of health systems and organize their discussion around these important questions: why do health care systems differ, how can they be classified, and what innovations can we expect in the future. Then Sanders, Schaay, and Mohamed analyze critically the concept of primary health care from its infancy to the formulation and pursuit of the primary health care approach informed by the premise of social justice.

Economic aspects of the functioning of the labor market in health systems are highlighted by Dussault and Vujicic. Harding and Montagu contribute another dimension to the analysis of health care services in their review of the role of the private sector in health care provision. The related aspect of competition in health care involving providers, insurers, and pharmaceutical companies, is examined by Song and colleagues. Keane and Weerasinghe scrutinize the partnership between public and private health care systems and highlight the difficulties of its implementation. One of the obstacles is agreeing on the optimum way to pay health care providers across sectors, which is the theme addressed by

Ellis and Miller. A solution first tested in the United States is discussed by Glied and Janus. These authors argue that managed care addresses not only individual patients' costs but also population expenditure for health care.

The role of hospitals in regulation and payment is discussed by Liu and Mills. Haak then addresses the essential drug policy and provides a comprehensive discussion of people's access to medicines. Long-term care is examined from two perspectives: Brodsky and Clarfield study long-term care for the chronically ill and disabled; and Stallard focuses on long-term care for the aged including nursing care, hospice care, home health care and other health care services especially designed for the elderly.

The last two chapters in Part III deal with two important and unique aspects of health system development: the concept of patient empowerment in health care by Bridges, Loukanova, and Carrera, and the role of community health workers in the provision of health care by Rifkin.

The final *Part IV* of this book contains four overview chapters focusing on key features of health systems around the world. A major point made by Goodwin is the need for effective stewardship of a nation's health system, which would manage the relationships between government, insurance providers, health and medical providers, and the public. Thus the most effective health systems are those most "carefully and responsibly managed."

Half the world's population is now urban, and this proportion is expected to increase, especially in low and middle income countries. With this in mind, Ompad et al. state that it is imperative to give attention to urban health if we expect to maintain and improve current and future public health. Especially important in this regard is that urban populations are made up of a minority of the very rich and a majority of the poor and disenfranchised. The urban health systems chapter discusses this and other public health challenges of urbanization, including demographic trends, the state of urban health in different parts of the world and provides an outline of current urban health policy options.

Wang then makes the point that most nations' health systems are constantly undergoing reforms and system improvement, and that a major reason for the rapid growth of comparative health systems as a field of study is that it can guide such reforms. However, the author also warns that comparisons should be made with caution, since there are many factors which differ in different settings—including the criteria that the health of a population is not only influenced by the quality of its nation's health system—making comparisons difficult.

Finally, Bodeker discusses the plight of the 300 million of the world's most marginalized (indigenous) populations who suffer the highest burden of health challenges. It is argued that these populations should have equal access to quality national health systems, as well as to indigenous systems, but it is here also clear that health status is determined by a range of different factors, and thus attention would need to be given to issues of equity and human rights both inside and outside health systems.

In this volume, we offer a broad look at health systems analysis, with the intention to support professionals and students from various academic backgrounds to look beyond their own specific disciplines. Moreover, we felt that such a comprehensive approach would facilitate the understanding of complex health system issues and would contribute to better policy-making as well.

Our sincere thanks go to the authors for their contributions, without which we could not have presented this volume. Last but not least, we are indebted to Dr J. Scott Bentley, Executive Editor at Elsevier Inc., who enthusiastically supported this project from the start, and encouraged us all along.

Guy Carrin
Kent Buse
Harald Kristian Heggenhougen
and
Stella Quah

HEALTH POLICY AND PUBLIC HEALTH

Health Policy: Overview

C Paton, Keele University, Newcastle-under-Lyme, UK

© 2008 Elsevier Inc. All rights reserved.

Introduction

This article provides an overview of health policy, a basis for understanding what it is, and key definitions relevant to the subject; the various factors that can be used to explain policy making; how policy is or is not rationalized in practice; how health policy affects health systems, exemplified by analyzing how they are financed and governed; and the politics of health policy in the world today. A conclusion is then provided.

Clearly health policy is – both in theory and in practice – an application of public policy more generally. It is therefore important to set it in the context of public policy and politics. It is equally important to appreciate that a global review of health policy with potential reference and relevance worldwide must concentrate on generic factors, yet with selective illustrations: principles of analysis, generic global trends, and illustrations of policy making and actual policy in different parts of the world.

Key Definitions

Health

It is crucial to define policy but also to give a brief account of how health is being defined and treated. Doing the latter first, health is defined, in the spirit of this Encyclopedia, in terms of its public aspect: The health of the public and therefore the responsibility and role of government and other agencies to meet public objectives for the public health. Public health is sometimes defined in a more specific way, that is, the particular set of programs and activities that seek to make an impact upon the promotion of better health, the prevention of ill health, and also environmental health.

Rather than the latter definition, this article refers to health policy in the broadest sense – affecting the health of the public – ranging, for example, from the effect of policy upon individuals' access to care, on the one hand, to policy made overtly in pursuit of social goals for both the health-care system and health outcomes for the population, on the other hand. Its focus is upon policy, policy making, and the implementation of policy, but it is as well to be clear at the outset as to policy's scope in terms of health. Policy can be negative as well as positive; for example, different health and health-care systems may affect health care for – and the health of – individuals, groups, and the whole population by what it omits as well as what it provides. With this in mind, let us turn to policy as the basis for understanding health policy.

Policy

A pragmatic definition of public policy would be what the government does (just as the British Cabinet Minister in the post-war government, Herbert Morrison, defined socialism as what Labour governments do!). This puts the emphasis as much upon public as upon policy: On its own, policy can be used in relation to any organization, public or private (e.g., it is the policy of the firm to specialize in luxury goods). But we need to go beyond such a pragmatic definition in order to unpack and examine the concept.

Politics, Policy, and Administration

Our concern here is indeed with public policy (as the means to understanding health policy). Policy comes from the Greek *polis*, which meant a city or more relevantly city-state and also gave rise to the term polity, i.e., political unit of self-government or the political part of a society, i.e., (in classical terms) the state. Policy came to mean the statecraft of the (modern) state. Etymologically it is bound up intricately with politics. But this is not just of historical curiosity. For public policy is embedded in politics – the politics embodied by the government, the politics of those who advise the government, the political ideologies that shape one's political ideas, the political structures required to pass legislation, and the administrative, managerial, and social structures and personnel required to implement policy (that is, to produce social outcomes from policy outputs).

In the French language, for example, *la politique* can mean either politics or policy; the two are not distinguished (Hill, 1997). In traditional British language referring to the traditional British approach to statecraft, on the other hand, the word was often missing: There was politics, on the one hand, and administration, on the other hand. Hence the salience of the academic subdiscipline, public administration, which persists to this day, even in an age when the real world rather disparages administration, turning first to management and then to leadership. It persists no doubt in part because of convention (see for example the spread from the United States to the rest of the world of MPAs – Masters degrees in Public Administration – even when the subject matter is modern business, management, and leadership). But it may also persist because there is a healthy scepticism in certain parts of academe about whether or not we should merge (private sector-derived) concepts of management and leadership with the overall terrain of government and its output – which may well be called public administration with some degree of accuracy (Hood and Scott, 2000).

Between these two extremes (French and British) above, there is the domain of public policy, which is different from politics (although intertwined with it) and also different from administration with the connotation of the civil service that takes politics/policy, codifies it, and translates it into systems capable of being implemented in the field. This domain recognizes policy's intimate relations to other domains but still thinks it worthwhile to give it a domain of its own. That is my perspective, broadly, in this article.

Public Policy

Going beyond the pragmatic definition of public policy as what the government does, it can be defined as the outputs from a process geared to making laws, enactments, and even regulations that are intended to affect society, i.e., produce social outputs and outcomes as a result of the outputs from the political system that we may call policy. Note that, in some countries, systems, and cultures, policy even by this definition may not be handled primarily by the politicians, but this is in itself a (political) characteristic of the political system.

On this approach to the process, the inputs are various (Paton, 2006a). They range from ideas and ideologies, through the political culture, through political movements or parties, through the effect of political institutions and structures generally, through social movements, interests, and pressure groups, through dominant modes of behavior (whether rational or otherwise), to the administrative or bureaucratic culture. Below, I examine the key factors involved.

Meanwhile, selectively, the following section defines some more terms.

General Terms

- Environment/context: The external climate and actual constraints, or pressures, which influence policy. For example: In the economic environment of global capitalism, it is difficult for individual countries to create or maintain progressive taxation systems with high tax rates, and the prospects for expanding public health-care systems are therefore diminished.
- Actors/agents/stakeholders: All those individuals, groups, interests, agencies, and organizations that are involved with, concerned with, or affected by, a specific policy (see Kingdon, 1984; Buse et al., 2005).
- Agenda: The terms of debate on which an issue is developed in the policy process, or the prioritizing of one issue rather than another – or none – in the political process, or in an agent's schedule (see Kingdon, 1984).
- Problem: Seemingly straightforward (for example, "the primary problem with the British NHS in the 1990s was long waiting times") but useful when considering how agendas are formed (e.g., is there agreement as to what the problem(s) is/are), and how politics, problems, and policies interact (John, 1999; Paton, 2006a).
- Power: The ability of Actor A to win in an overt political battle (Dahl, 1980) (in our case, in the health policy arena) with B; or the ability of A to prevent B from raising an issue (effectively) within the political process (Bachrach and Baratz, 1970); or the ability of A to prevent B from even being aware he has a grievance or should have a grievance (see Crenson, 1971; Lukes, 1974); or the effect of the dominant (or prevailing, or pervasive) discourse upon the perception of issues (in the poststructuralist sense, in terms of the effects of language upon concepts and thought) (Peck and Coyle, 2002: 214–219). Note that the last definition de-centers the actor – power is less a conscious attempt to win, by an agent, than an effect.

Practical Terms for the (Health) Policy World

- Regulation: A framework of rules (e.g., a legally backed code) or practices (e.g., by an inspecting agency) that define permitted activity, or type and mode of activity, in a field, as opposed to planning or management, which intervene directly rather than set a framework for self-action. For example, the new regulation in health care sets out the rules for markets or quasi-markets, in formerly directly managed health-care systems. Day and Klein (1987) argued that a regulator is external (so that, for example, a higher tier within a public health-care system does not regulate but instructs or manages).
- Strategy: Often contrasted with (on the one hand) tactics, it refers to the means of achieving a direction of travel or goal (as in military strategy), e.g., "the strategy for involving the public more in decision-making is to set up local self-governing units in the healthcare system"; contrasted (on the other hand) with an operational focus on keeping things running, as in "the Health Authority's Director of Strategy will ensure that our plans are consistent with our goal of improving access to the under-served; whereas the Director of Operations will seek to increase throughput in the wards to meet government targets."
- Governance: Within public services such as health care, the adoption of an appropriate structure and culture of oversight of the organization (as in corporate

governance, which seeks to assure that the organization is run and controlled ethically, soundly, sustainably and appropriately; or clinical governance, which is the corporate governance of the clinical process in particular).

Explaining Public Policy

Through one interpretation, actors (e.g., policy makers) are rational. This might be in the sense of either maximizing their utility (the neoclassical microeconomic viewpoint) or planning a coherent – perhaps evidence-based – route to achievement of objectives, i.e., the tailoring of means to ends.

This latter view is found in political and administrative science, e.g., in Allison (1971). The question is begged as to whether such rationality commands consensus (the unitarist view, or Allison's Model 1 when applied to policy making within the portals of central government) or whether different interests, elites, structural interests, or economic classes – either in government or across the wider polity and society – have different objectives (respectively, the pluralist, elitist, corporatist, or Marxist views) (Paton, 2006a). These different objectives might be rational on the terms of the individuals and groups who have them, and they may be pursued rationally in terms of the instrumental tailoring of means to needs. Yet the overall effect is not consensual pursuit of universally acknowledged rational outcomes. Instead there may be pluralism, with compromise as the basis for outcome – leading, perhaps, to incremental, small-scale policy changes overall even when each group or interest seeks radical, large-scale change. (Compromise is a very different thing from consensus, although there may be eventual consensus upon the need for, and nature of, compromise.) Or indeed there may be domination by an elite or ruling class, which creates a dominant agenda. This may look like rationalism, not least in terms of the passage of comprehensive policy rather than cautious adjustment, but is a very different thing, once again.

One may also consider actors seeking to achieve their chosen outputs and outcomes (as defined above), but tailoring their behavior in line with the incentives created or enhanced by the institutions' way of working. This is institutional rational choice (Dunleavy, 1989).

But perhaps the culture created or encouraged by structures, and the behavior they encourage, takes on a life of its own: There is a mobilization of bias (Schattschneider, 1960; Paton, 1990) in policy. This may be due to the effect of external structures upon people's expectations and ways of thinking (i.e., cognitive structures) rather than (just) upon the calculations of autonomous rational actors whose thought processes and agency are unaffected by structures.

Indeed there is a difficulty with assuming that humans have an unchanging, rational, or maximizing nature – what Archer calls Modernist Man (Archer, 2000). While it has the merit of preventing the agent from being (implausibly) completely subsumed by society, it begs the question as to where this intrinsic nature comes from. Not only are the assumptions behind rational man questionable (an ontological matter), but their origin is too (an epistemological matter).

Structuralism (Peck and Coyle, 2002: 211–214) arguably solves the dualism by going too far in the other direction. It either removes man's autonomy, positing that deep cognitive or real (natural or social) structures dominate agency. Poststructuralism posits that structures are linguistically determined but variable, indeed arbitrary (Peck and Coyle, 2002: 214–219). On this approach, varying discourses and perspectives that are thus based are constitutive of the individual. The paradox is that the agent is no longer determined by deep or unchanging structures but that there seems no basis for agency other than by changing language. On this basis, agents *qua* policy makers are neither rational nor irrational: There is no objective basis for evaluating their actions.

Other approaches point to the actor's autonomy being limited but not eradicated. In public administration, this might provide a useful reminder of the role of cultures, ideologies, and ideas in policy studies.

Particular structures of relevance to health policy are political institutions, governmental and administrative structures, and specific health agencies. We may wish to define culture separately from structure, or to interpret cultures, habits, and beliefs (including ideologies and ideas) as structures for the present purpose – identifying external factors when seeking to explain or influence policy.

The literature concerning the factors that influence, shape, and even cause public policy is now immense. It is necessary to walk the tightrope between theory, on the one hand, and plausible explanation of what is actually happening in the real world, on the other hand. Rhodes (in Stoker, 2000) stated memorably that social science can cope with a lot of hindsight, a little insight, and almost no foresight! Thus it is with explanations of public policy.

The policy process (Hill, 1997) is a phrase that characterizes the story of how policies develop, are implemented, in often unpredictable or even perverse ways, and are amended, in a process that is less linear than (variously) wave-like, stew-like, cyclical, and even circular. It should also be understood to encapsulate how politics both shapes and is shaped by policy and the social outcomes that result from policy outputs.

Explanatory Factors (Illustrated for Health)

The key factors used in political science and public administration to explain outputs and outcomes in public policy are:

1. Political economy (generally, and also embracing regime or regulation theory) (Aglietta, 1979; Jessop, 2002): Political economy can be defined as the way in which wealth is produced and distributed. It is a crucial backdrop to understanding the underlying pressures and constraints upon health policy. The global capitalist economy puts significant pressures upon public health systems, as well as (for some countries) generating wealth and income that can be used for both private and public purchasing of health care. Additionally, effects upon health outside the health-care system altogether can affect health both positively and negatively. How public policy generally and health policy in particular interact in this environment is crucial.

For most but not all countries of the world, current international political economy as opposed to purely national political economy is more important than during the period from 1945 to 1975, which was an era of expansion of economies and of the welfare state in what was then called the industrialized West; expansion which had knock-on effects elsewhere around the globe. Subsequent retrenchment, plus a (related) change in dominant type of political economy (or regime), has had significant effects on health-care systems.

The first wave of global health sector reform in the 1940s and 1950s (WHO, 2000a) consisted in the establishment of national health-care systems in many countries. The second wave (1960s and 1970s) consisted in primary health care as a strategy for affordable universal coverage (given already-experienced cost pressures) in developing countries. The third wave – moving into the 1980s and beyond – consisted in a move away from statist public systems to either public or mixed systems relying more on market, quasi-market, or new public management mechanisms (WHO, 2000a).

2. Socioeconomic factors. These are distinguished from (1), although they are related in that they refer to data and demographics, such as the level of wealth of a country and the distribution of wealth and income. Health and welfare expenditure, for example, has been correlated to the former (see Wilensky, 1974; Maxwell, 1982).

3. Institutionalist, new institutionalist, and structural explanations, which give primacy to the effect of political institutions (and the behavior and incentives that they create) in explaining policy outputs (Dowding, 1990; Paton 1990). In health policy, policy may result both from the way institutions operate and also how they create a dependency that constrains future policy or directs it in a particular way.

4. Institution-based rational choice. Individuals may act in groups or share interests which influence their behavior, yet have goals and objectives that are determined independently of political structures (institutions) and of cultural factors (for example, a putative dominant ideology). Nevertheless, their behavior is influenced by institutions and the incentives to which the latter give rise, as they seek to achieve their objectives in the most rational manner. This is a version of institutional rational choice (which, as Dowding (1990) points out, need not be methodologically individualist).

Original or pure rational choice theory as applied to politics was individualist. Public choice theory was based on the view that both individuals and agencies (collectivities of individuals) are selfish maximizers. The implications were that bureaus and bureaucracies would seek to maximize their budget beyond the point of efficiency or effectiveness. For example, the chiefs of a health department – or publicly funded hospital system – would use the political process (perhaps in coalition with politicians, civil servants, and doctors, all building their empires) to expand.

This was one of the rationales for the purchaser/provider split (Osborne and Gaebler, 1993), which has featured significantly in both the theory and practice of health sector reform since the late 1980s and 1990s. The trend started in developed countries, particularly the UK and New Zealand (Paton et al., 2000). Countries with public or publicly regulated insurance in central Europe systems, such as the Bismarckian systems of social insurance (Paton et al., 2000), always had financier/provider splits in the tautologous sense that payers and insurers were separate entities from providers. But this is merely the traditional system that operated through guilds (self-governing providers, professions, and payers regulated by the state) relating to each other without much competition. It is not the same thing as a deliberately created quasi-market or new public management reform.

The latter has also been used to reform Bismarckian systems by instigating competition between payers and insurers (whether public or private) for subscribers. Providers of services would have to justify their product (effectiveness) and their costs (efficiency) through tendering competitively in order to win a contract, or at least, if competition was not possible, through setting out clearly their services in response to a specification that might be contestable in the longer run if it was unacceptable in cost or quality.

The trouble with this was that purchasing authorities and agencies would also be selfish maximizers if the theory were right. Who would control them? The answer – especially in health care – has often been a system regulator (Saltman et al., 2002). But the same applies to the regulator! So we are driven back to government, as the regulator of regulators. And who controls government? The answer is (idealistically) the people or (realistically) special interests or the ruling class. There is no technical solution – such as purchaser/provider splits – to what is in essence a political problem.

5. Issues of power, of how power is distributed in society and within the political system, and how it influences public policy. For example, is power distributed

pluralistically, or are decisions taken by – or in the interests of – the ruling elite or a ruling class? Here, it is important to distinguish instrumentalism (arguing that, if politics and policy benefit a group, elite, or class, how this occurs must be actually demonstrated) and functionalism (which implies that means that are functional for ends somehow are realized).

An example of using functionalism to defend Marxism, for example, was found in Cohen (1978) A strong variant of functionalism is evolutionism, which draws an analogy with Darwinism in natural science to imply that the policies that come to dominate are those best suited to surviving in their (political) environment (John, 1999).

Functionalism implies that policies develop because they are functional for the external environment, whereas evolutionism implies that policies develop if the external environment is functional for them. Neither stance is satisfactory, as the how is missing. And evolutionism in particular – in social science and policy studies – is either tautologous or vacuous. This is because, unlike in the natural world, the environment is human-made and mutable and can be made functional for policies. Anything can therefore be explained in this manner.

The classic example of power in health policy has concerned the medical profession and its relationship both with other actors in health-care systems (especially managers) and with the state.

Network theory, whether sociological, political, or managerial, has had prominence recently. To some it is descriptive rather than analytical (Dowding, 1995), although if integrated with power studies (i.e., networks explained in terms of power and influence) it can be useful (Marsh, 1998). At its best, it has the potential to explore how regimes at various levels of government (international, national, and local) are responsible for investment and consumption, and therefore to link political economy with institutional and behavioral analysis.

For example, the corporatist approach – which depicts iron triangles of business, government, and labor in policy decision making (see for example Cawson, 1986) – was extended to depict how national government organizes investment and local government organizes consumption. More recently, in the global and European era, local and regional government and governance are responsible for investment to a greater extent, with national government ironically increasingly controlling or circumscribing consumption. This is related to a (concealed) change in power relations in the economy, with corporatist trilateralism replaced with the bilateralism of business and the state.

6. Ideas and ideologies, which are important, but often linked to wider social factors (and political economy), and in complicated ways. An approach emphasizing the primacy of ideas may sound rational. On the other hand, an approach emphasizing ideology may be ambiguous. Ideology can suggest moral goals and a program to achieve them, or it can suggest false consciousness of agents who are cultural dupes. In health, the primary care movement is sometimes seen as ideologically motivated. Equally Navarro (1978) has argued that high-technology medicine is a means of buying off workers given the disadvantages of (and lack of effective public health in) capitalist society.

A Synthesis

Clearly, different factors can be combined in explaining public (and health) policy. Different typologies are available to aid with this task (see **Tables 1** and **2**)

Two examples are provided:

1. Policy may be made for health, or it may be made with other factors in mind (e.g., trade, the economy). We can call these, respectively, internal and external policy.

Table 1 Power

	Pluralism	*Elitism/ruling class*
Internal	Pluralist conflict within health systems over priorities	Domination of power and resources by the medical profession or business
External	Pluralist conflict within local communities or districts over control of health agencies for political purposes	Use of the health system to benefit the capitalist economy, as in promotion or private provision not for health system reasons but to support or subsidize corporations

Table 2 Type and degree of rationality

	Unitarist	*Pluralist*
Rationalist	Government pursuing system-wide reform on the basis of agreed objectives	Each interest group or stakeholder pursues its goals rationally, but the overall result has to be a compromise
Incrementalist	Government gradually amending policy on the basis of agreed objectives (perhaps with a conservative bias by civil servants)	Disjointed incrementalism, where mutual adjustment (and its direction) depends upon the resolution of different agendas on the part of different actors behaving incrementally

Additionally, power may be distributed widely in making – or implementing – policy, or it may be concentrated. We can call these, respectively, pluralism and elitism (or ruling class theory).

Table 1 shows four possibilities, with four health examples. The aim is not to develop grand theory but to provide a checklist or an *aide mémoire* when examining empirical possibilities.

2. Policy may be made from a zero base on the basis of seeking means to achieve ends on which there is agreement (either within government or in wider society). This can be called rationalism. Alternatively, it might be made incrementally, on the basis of minor adjustments to previous policy (see the second paragraph in 'Explaining public policy' above).

Additionally, policy may be made consensually (or with only one viewpoint featuring, not the same thing), which variants can all be termed unitarism. This in turn can be contrasted with pluralism (defined as in Example 1). This time, the latter refers more to the breadth of influence upon central government than to the nature of social power more generally.

Table 2 shows four possibilities. As with Table 1, it illustrates and clarifies rather than helps decide, which must be done on a context-specific basis, i.e., empirically rather than *a priori*.

Explaining Implementation

A framework for explaining implementation can begin simply, analyzing inputs, outputs, and outcomes. Inputs draw on aspects of the explanatory factors described above, translated into concrete terms. It is helpful to categorize these as ideas, institutions, and political behavior (e.g., by political parties). At root the structure versus agency debate in social science (Archer, 2000) is at the heart of the issue: Individuals operating in (structural) contexts, individually or collectively, help to determine outputs and outcomes.

While ideas versus institutions has long been a talking point in policy analysis (King, 1973; Heidenheimer *et al.*, 1975), these inputs produce outputs in the form of public policy. Implementation concerns the process by which such outputs (e.g., laws; an organization's objectives) are translated into social outcomes. For example, health policy may concern the creation of a publicly funded national health service (NHS). The effect of the NHS upon access to services and health inequalities (for example) occurs as a result of how, where, and when the policy is implemented.

It is possible to have good policy but bad implementation and vice versa (Paton, 2007: Chapter 5). The former may occur when policy is designed (and enacted) rationally, but without taking into account opposition that later is mobilized effectively during the implementation phase. The latter may occur when policy is enacted after significant, possibly debilitating, compromise, but then implemented in a straightforward manner, as all opposition has already been taken into account.

Regulation is a means of seeking to achieve goals and objectives though a process of implementation, which occurs through self-modification of behavior in response to external rules rather than by direct command and control. Clearly, this is a pertinent issue in health policy, where international trends overtly embrace the new governance through regulation rather than direct control. The recent reorganization of the UK Department of Health (Greer, 2007) (which administers the English NHS but not those of Scotland, Wales, and Northern Ireland) reflects the creation of many quangos (external public agencies) allegedly to replace direct control by government.

There are, broadly, three systems of governance for implementing health policy. Firstly, there is what economists call by the catch-all term of hierarchy (i.e. one word as an alternative to markets) but which may be better described, on examination, as classical bureaucracy or – not the same thing – planning. This is sometimes described as command and control. Often this has pejorative overtones, but it need not: Bureaucracy has advantages in both normative and practical terms. These may include equity, consistency, and transparency (normative) as well as an ability to rationalize systems, reduce inappropriate discretion, and minimize unintended outcomes from local action (practical). Furthermore, the term hierarchy may be inappropriate to describe planning, in health care at least: The latter may eschew the market (see below), but allow considerable devolution of responsibility in meeting goals (Paton, *et al.*, 1998; Paton, 2007).

Secondly, there is the market. Many countries have recently sought to use both market incentives within the public sector (Paton *et al.*, 2000) and private provision to reshape their health-care systems.

Thirdly, there is guild self-regulation. This approach has historically existed in central Europe and also some countries in Latin America as the basis by which the government guarantees access (national health insurance) but providers, payers, and professionals self-regulate to a large extent, often in the context of a corporatism in which quasi-official, nongovernment agencies manage agreement about pay, the prices of services, and market entry.

It has been argued that providers (especially professionals) have knavish as well as knightly tendencies and that guild self-regulation requires both an assumption of altruism (Le Grand, 2003) and the assumption that providers respond to the correct signals in supplying services. Generally policy advocates such as Le Grand (2003) suggest the market as the answer. Yet it is vital to examine what happens when politics meets economics in market-driven health systems, which notoriously produce perverse results (Paton, 2007).

Furthermore, hierarchy, or command, need not be based on the assumption that providers (and managers in health care) only behave in a self-interested (knavish) manner. Planning approaches in health care, with official targets, may be a means of coordinating altruistic public service as well as providing material incentives for compliance.

Clinical networks, bringing together professionals from different institutions, may (for example) require both (internal) coordination and (external) compatibility with wider policy and managerial objectives. To replace these with atomized market incentives may encourage knavish behavior rather than channel it.

In terms of global health policy, we have the paradox that the ideology of the market sometimes continues to be on the ascendant but that its effects upon implementation are complex and often perverse (Segall, 2000; Blas, 2005).

Policy in Practice

The seemingly random interplay of ideas, groups organized around ideas, interests or advocacy (combining both values and interests; Hann, 1995), and opportunities for policy decisions leads us to the garbage can approach (Cohen *et al.*, 1972). Policy now seems an arbitrary mess. And it may be, at one level or for some of the time. Agendas are successful, in this approach, not because of rationality but because of time or timing and chance (Kingdon, 1984). Policy, politics, and problems are separate streams rather than components of a rational process, and only when they flow together is policy created. This might, for example, be when politicians seize an answer (i.e., a policy) because it is available, trendy, and (coincidentally rather than logically) seemingly an answer to a problem that is perceived to be pressing.

The question then arises: If policies emerge haphazardly, one after another, how is policy rationalized, if indeed it is, to ensure that the aims of the state are realized or that policy outputs, at least to a minimal extent, achieve the social outcomes required for both the legitimacy of the state and the requisite stability of institutions? This is a more fundamental question than one about the aims of government. Clearly individual governments' aims simply may not be realized. Nor should one assume that there is some teleology or functionalism favoring the aims of the state.

My argument is a different one, which can be illustrated from health policy. An institution such as the British NHS is only politically legitimate and economically viable if it satisfies several conditions: Investment in cadres of domestic workers occupying salient niches in the international economy; acceptability to the demanding middle classes, in terms of both quality and financial outlay (i.e., comparable to what they would pay if only insuring themselves); and fulfillment of its egalitarian founding mission at least to the extent that it seems worth the moral bother of protecting in the first place.

How can action by the state or its agents seek to fulfill these conditions? How in other words does the political realm ensure the compatibility of social institutions (such as the NHS) with economic reproduction? This is the crucial question for the sustainability of public health systems in the era of global capitalism.

There is no inevitability here. The state may act effectively to square the circle – not just of competing social demands in the conventional sense, but of the competing agendas listed two paragraphs above. If it does not or cannot – for example, if a country's public health service does not satisfy employers' needs and demands for healthy employees – employers will seek to finance their own occupational health. If doctors fail to cooperate at least adequately to prioritize the outputs and outcomes that the state requires, then either they will be coerced into doing so within the NHS or they will be disciplined by market forces outside the NHS, as corporations take responsibility for health care on a sectional basis (perhaps taking advantage of European Union law).

What this does, then, is give governments that are sympathetic to preserving at least publicly financed health care an interest in ensuring that the state coordinates policy at the end of the day, so that a complex amalgam of aims can be furthered. There is in practice a major conflict between the garbage can that produces continual waves of incompatible, media-driven policy, mostly in the developed world (Paton, 2006) or policy distorted by the predatory state (Martinussen, 1994), mostly in the developing world, on the one hand; and the need for effective coordination, on the other hand.

The latter means tight control of resources given the ambitiousness and complexity of aims, which means political centralism against all prevailing rhetoric. Most devolution and decentralization in state-dominated health systems is devolution of responsibility for functions, not devolution of power. Again, we can see that, in order to explain public policy outputs, we have to consider, respectively, the backdrop of political economy; social power; the structure of the state and political institutions; and how individuals, groups, interests, and classes behave in the context of the structures they must use.

For example, Allison's (1971) Model 1 posits a unified executive pursuing the national good, having been developed empirically to explain the U.S. government's behavior during the Cuban missile crisis. It is therefore a kind of grounded theory that is context-specific, and therefore the model may be less suitable for wider explanation of social decision making, interest-group politics, and power.

The challenge is to incorporate different explanatory factors at different levels of analysis. These levels can be considered to be a hierarchy in that there is a move from the underlying to the immediate in terms of their causal nature as regards policy outputs, but this is heuristic rather than wholly empirical. It is important not to be too rigid about (for example) what is undoubtedly a two-way relationship between political structure and social power: The latter will exert itself, except in exceptional circumstances, through different forms of structure, it is true; but the former's mode of channeling power may alter the nature of that power in so doing.

For example, the medical profession was powerful, as a stratum within a social and economic elite in the 30 postwar years of the last century, in both the United Kingdom and the United States. It was capable of exerting its power through the then very different political institutions of the United Kingdom and the United States. In the centralized, executive-heavy UK with (then) a political culture of insider networks that were relatively invisible (like all effective power!), an implicit bargain was made through informal channels between the state and the profession (Klein, 1990), which meant a symbiotic relationship in governing the NHS. In the United States, with its decentralized interest-group politics as the stuff of the system, the profession preserved its power using different institutions in different ways, primarily by blocking reform (in the way that the insurance industry did with the Clinton Plan in the 1990s (Mann and Ornstein, 1995; Paton, 1996), by which time it had replaced the now toothless tiger of the American Medical Association (AMA) as the lobby feared by reforming legislators).

The question that arises is: Is power economically rooted at base, with the decline in the AMA's – and the wider medical profession's – power caused by a surplus of doctors, on the one hand, by comparison with the 1950s and 1960s (when access to health care was extended by government, and the medical profession's fears of socialization were shown to be ideological rather than economic), and by new corporate approaches to purchasing and organizing health care for their workers, on the other hand?

There is clearly truth in this. Yet it is not the whole story. The centralist UK political system was capable of more systematic reform – including the creation of the NHS itself – than in the United States, when the UK state was governed by a strong political party with clear and comprehensive aims, in other words, majority rule rather than the passage of policy by the painstaking assemblage of winning coalitions in the legislature. The latter creates a mobilization of bias (Schattschneider, 1960) away from comprehensive or rationalist reform as opposed to incremental reform, which in turn alters mindsets and limit ambitions. That is, structures can have cultural and ideological effects.

It is important to study an issue such as health policy over a long enough period (subjectively, about 20–30 years, in today's world) to allow different eras to register and therefore the changing salience of different explanatory factors in public policy. In a nutshell, the 1970s was the era of political structures, as the prevailing political economy was nationally based; the 2000s are the era of political economy, as capitalist globalism reduces the salience of nations and their institutions.

In other words, political economy is at the top of the hierarchy of salient factors in delimiting and explaining public policy. It sets the background, environment, and constraints. Depicting a regime in political economy shows how the state and other elements of the polity come together to steer the economy in a particular way. It is Marxist, in that it prioritizes economic production, situates political viability and legitimacy in terms of the political economy and has crisis as the motivation to move from one type of regime to another (for example, from the Keynesian national welfare state to the Schumpeterian workfare state, in the language of Jessop (2002)). It is, however, post-Marxist or non-Marxist in that regimes vary within capitalism, that is, a regime is less than a mode of production in the Marxist sense.

Institutions and political structures shape behavior, partly by channeling rational behavior (i.e., institutional rational choice) but also by changing cultures and expectations, which feed into future ideas for policy, reform, or whatever, as outlined above. For example, in the United States, the failure of successive attempts at federal health reform, foundering on the rocks of established structures and interests inhabiting them, has lowered expectations for future action on the part of many reformers even without them realizing.

Power is exerted, that is, through institutions overtly and covertly, but the latter equates neither to Lukes' (1974) nor to the poststructuralist vision of dialogues that are enclosed and arbitrary. Loss of ambition in reform ideas is a fatalism, in this sense, rather than a false consciousness, perhaps because elites are systematically lucky (in Dowding's (1990) arresting oxymoron). In the end, it is just that, an oxymoron, because – with reflexivity of actors and even of passive public(s) – those who are systematically lucky are likely to go beyond luck, i.e., to build on it in a deliberate strategy to maximize their instrumental power.

Political structures and institutions vary between countries (as well as sub- and supranational levels). Thus executives vary in structure, scope, salience, and power, within the political system in general and state in particular. Regimes are more than governments and less than state systems. In health policy, regimes embody the prevailing orthodoxy in ideas (or ideology) as adapted to, and amended by, political institutions and social structures.

Policy for Financing Health Care and Structuring Health Systems

We can illustrate how health policy reflects a variety of different influences by examining how health systems may be financed and governed.

Financing Options

The main options for financing health care (ranged along a continuum from private to public) are as follows:

1. private payment (out of pocket), including partial private payment, i.e., co-payments (coinsurance or deductibles) (coinsurance means the consumer paying a proportion of the cost, e.g., 20%; a deductible means the consumer paying a fixed amount on each claim, e.g., £50);
2. voluntary private insurance, including partial versions (e.g., supplementary and complementary insurance, to be discussed below);
3. statutory private insurance regulated by the state (including partial versions such as substitutive insurance, meaning – in this option – mandatory private contributions by certain categories of citizen (generally the better-off) toward core rather than supplementary or optional health services. That is, everyone is covered, but the better-off pay a form of insurance that is obligatory;
4. community pooling;
5. public/social insurance;
6. hypothecated (earmarked) health taxation;
7. general taxation.

Assessment of Options Against Criteria

A specific policy analysis would assess options, one by one, against identified criteria and (perhaps) incorporate a weighting procedure to rank the options. From the viewpoint of understanding how policy is actually made, however, this would only be part of the picture.

It might constitute an attempt at rational policy making, that is, an attempt to provide a basis for scientific consensus among the key actors holding power in either the policy process generally or government in particular. Alternatively, it might seek to build in to the criteria for judging options (or even, to the options themselves) pragmatic or political factors (such as the political feasibility of an option in a particular political context).

Either way, it is important to be explicit about the range of factors likely to affect a policy's success as regards both enactment and implementation (i.e., outputs and outcome, respectively), as explored in the sections titled 'Explaining public policy' and 'Policy in practice'. Otherwise, there is a divorce in the policy dialogue between what might be termed technocrats (such as economists), on the one hand, and political scientists on the other. The divorce between such worlds is often responsible for extremes of optimism and disillusionment, respectively, in assessing policy *ex ante* and *ex post*, as with recent health reform programs in England, for example.

Governance

There are fundamentally three categories of system:

1. statist systems;
2. market systems (whether private, public, or mixed);
3. self-governing systems (with varying degrees of state regulation) (Arts and Gelissen, 2002), in which either guilds or organized functional interests or networks (of providers, financiers, and employees) organize the delivery of care.

Statist systems have replaced the market with public planning, whether it is dominated by politics, the public, or experts. Market systems rely on either private markets that have evolved historically or on the creation of market structures and incentives within (formerly) publicly planned systems. Self-governing systems are systems where central state control is limited or weak or both, but where guild-like relationships rather than market relationships between key actors predominate. For example, physicians' associations, insurers' associations, and the state will thrash out deals in a corporatist manner, with corporatism meaning (in this context) the institutionalization of major social interests into a reasonably stable decision-making machinery overseen by – but not dominated by – the state.

Clearly most advanced health-care systems are hybrids in varying degrees. The question is whether the degree of hybridity is dysfunctional or not, i.e., whether cultures and incentives are adequately aligned throughout the system.

Using the language of incentives, it is important to distinguish between macro and micro incentives. Statist systems, for example, are generally good (often too good!) at macro cost control; their record in terms of micro-level allocations (e.g., to providers or clinical teams) to achieve objectives is variable (a statement that should be taken at face-value; some are good at it; others are not). Those systems that allow meso-level planning authorities, such as regions, to avoid the excesses of both central control and local capture by unrepresentative interests, often have the capacity to square the circle in terms of incentives, as long as attention is paid to steering the system to achieve desired outcomes.

While all systems are likely to be hybrids, it is important to ensure that the dominant incentives, geared to achieving the most important objectives agreed by government on behalf of society, are not stymied by cross-cutting policies with separate incentives. This has been an occupational hazard of (for example) England in recent years, arguably, with four different policy streams vying for dominance: The purchaser/provider split inherited from the 1990s' old market and deepened by the creation of Primary Care Trusts; local collaboration as an alleged third-way alternative to state control and markets; central control through myriads of targets; and the new market of patient choice implemented alongside payment by results (Paton, 2005a, 2005b).

In consequence, in considering structures, attention ought to be paid to the central structure, i.e., how the political level is and is not distinguished in terms of governance from the top management, i.e., health executive level. There is no one answer (again, as the United Kingdom and especially England's *volte faces* on whether or not health ought to be managed strategically at arm's length from government or not probably show). Nevertheless, the question ought to be considered in terms of roles and functions of the different levels within a coherent governance structure: Is the system capable of articulating consistent policy?

The Politics of Policy Analysis and Policy Outcomes

Policy studies have evolved the term path dependency to illustrate how historical choices create paths that constrain (although do not necessarily determine) future options. This is sometimes allied with the concept of the new institutionalism, which is actually just a way of emphasizing that agency, ideas, and ideologies are only part of the picture.

For example, policy debates vary from country to country – say, in terms of how to reform health services or with regard to the best type of health-care systems – for reasons that do not involve only the cultural relativism of ideas. There are relatively universal typologies of health-care systems, analyzed along dimensions such as how universal coverage is, how comprehensive services are, and how payment is made. Yet these debates are handled very differently, with different results, in domestic policy communities in different countries, even when these countries might seem fairly similar in global terms (e.g., France, Germany, Switzerland, Sweden, and the countries of the UK). Political institutions and their normal functioning constrain and direct policy (Paton, 1990).

The field of policy studies also analyzes how different policy communities and networks (both insider and outsider) influence policy. Even in an era of globalization and (in particular) global capitalism, "global policy debates arrive at local conclusions." This observation was made by political scientist Hugh Hedo in commenting on a book by Scott Greer (2004), which explores how – even within the United Kingdom – territorial politics and local policy advocacy after devolution have produced diversity within the UK's National Health Services. This is such that one can now talk about four distinctive NHSs (England, Scotland, Wales, and Northern Ireland).

To make an analogous observation, a rational approach to policy analysis may seek to combine (for example) universalism, comprehensiveness, and prepayment (whether by tax or insurance) in different ways. In the abstract, there may be little to choose, for example, between a rationally designed NHS and a rationally designed social insurance system.

Yet the proof of the pudding is in the political digestion. How viable a system is in practice depends not just on technical factors such as efficiency (which are rarely only technical, in any case), but also upon how the politics of both policy design and policy implementation play out. It could be argued, for example, that England's confused and overloaded health reform agenda is destabilizing its NHS, unlike, say, in Finland. Or that France's social insurance system is being adapted to reap the benefits of an NHS-type system. Globalization constrains, but policy and implementation are affected by politics and political structures. As a result, whether or not a system is viable in the global era depends upon practice as well as theory. For example, is an NHS capable of spending money efficiently and effectively enough to make the requisite taxation rates for a comprehensive service viable? The answer, in theory, is yes. The answer, in practice, is we do not know until we have examined if and how different policy objectives, and policy strands, are rendered compatible (Paton, 2006).

The Politics of Health Policy in the World Today

In order to analyze health policy, it is necessary to analyze politics in health, a better phrase than the politics of health. That is, while there may be certain respects in which the politics of health is unique to health, it is generally true that the effect of general political factors upon health, health-care systems, and the delivery of health care is more significant. In other words, political economy (both national and international), political structures, and political systems condition health-care systems and indeed the prospects for health.

Control and conflict over resources for both health and health care put health at the center of politics. Consider also the role of the state. Moran (1999) has talked of the health-care state, with echoes of the welfare state, and the implication both that the state affects health care (and health) and that health-care systems in turn affect the state and political life more generally. The traditional concerns of political science – ranging from normative political theory (concerning the nature of the good society and the role of the state) to both analytical political theory and public administration analyzing the nature of, distribution, uses, and consequences of power – are fairly and squarely replicated in analyzing the field of health and health care.

Political history is also important. The twentieth century saw the expansion of health systems, often (especially in the developed world, including the communist block, but also in much of South America) into universal systems (i.e., open to all) if not always fully comprehensive (i.e., covering people for everything). (The United States was a notable exception.) This in itself reflected the politics of the twentieth century in which (from a Western perspective) *laissez-faire* gave way to the interventionism of either social democracy or at least increased government activism. While this may seem like a characterization of the developed world, in the developing world, the expansion of schemes of health insurance in South America and the export to colonies and ex-colonies in Africa and Asia of health-care systems from the developed world make it a broader picture.

Health Sector Reform

The logic of globalization has been transmitted directly to the world of health policy (even if the detail that emerges is politically conditioned). For example, a think tank of leading businessmen from multinational corporations in Europe in the mid-1980s, setting out just this rationale (Warner, 1994), had as one of its members a certain Dekker, from the Phillips group in the Netherlands, who also chaired the Dutch health reform committee leading to the Dekker plan of 1987 (which was partially implemented over the 1990s albeit in a restricted form).

The Dutch model of managed competition became the prototype for reform of Bismarckian social insurance schemes in Europe and beyond (including South America), as well as for the failed Clinton Plan in the US (Paton, 1996). The UK model of internal markets and purchaser/provider splits in tax-funded health systems became the prototype for reform of NHS and government systems both in developed and developing worlds. It was devised by right-wing political advisers and politicians who advocated commercialization in the public sector. This model (shared with health sector reform in New Zealand) even became the prototype, somewhat incredibly, for health system reform in the poorest countries of Asia and Africa. Later in the 1990s and early 2000s, the World Bank sought to broaden the framework by which reform ideas and criteria were assessed, but the watchwords were still competition, market forces, and privatization.

The World Health Organization has sought a broader basis for evaluating (and therefore, implicitly, exporting) health system reform. The WHO (2000b) has sought to evaluate health systems around the world by a variety of criteria, including quality, cost-effectiveness, acceptability to citizens, and good governance. The World Bank's approach, as stated, is heavily influenced by the neoliberal economic agenda applied to health and welfare, an agenda itself influenced by public choice theory (Dunleavy, 1989), especially purchaser/provider splits between buyers and sellers of health services, managed competition, and quasi-commercial providers.

The assumption is that publicly funded health care has to be delivered more efficiently, or cheaply, and has to be more carefully targeted. In Western countries such as the Netherlands, the latter could be done by advocating publicly funded universal access for a restricted basket of services (i.e., universality but not comprehensiveness).

In the developing world from the 1980s onward, usually under the aegis of multilateral agencies such as the World Bank and bilateral aid departments such as Britain's Overseas Development Administration (which became the Department for International Development in 1997), Western policies promoting market forces in health care have been advocated and partially implemented. In other developing countries, the watchword has been decentralization, but the political intention has frequently been both to limit the role of the state in health care and to make communities more responsible for their own health (which sounds culturally progressive but is likely to be fiscally regressive).

As for the whole world, the key question for developing countries is: How is better health (care) to be financed? The options range from private payment through private insurance, through community self-help or cooperative activity, through public insurance, to national systems financed from government revenues, whether operated from the political center or from devolved, decentralized or deconcentrated agencies. (The last refers to field agencies of the central government.) In developing countries, the infrastructure for modern tax-based or national insurance systems often does not exist.

Moreover, the decline of tax and spend in the developing as well as developed world means that third-way solutions (meaning neither traditional state or fully public services nor unregulated markets) are also sought in the third world, irrespective of the names or slogans used. In health, the poorest countries have focused upon building social capital (as in the West): Communities, with aid from bilateral and multilateral agencies as well as nongovernmental organizations (NGOs), have sought to create mutual or cooperative local (informed) insurance schemes.

The priorities for investment in health are often set through a mixture of expert-based needs assessment and local choice via rapid appraisal of local people's needs. Not surprisingly, this offer leads to a focus upon the key determinants of public health such as sanitation, immunization, reproductive and sexual health (embracing maternal and child health), and so on.

Regarding access to more expensive and acute or secondary health services, the key issues are the availability of pharmaceuticals at affordable prices (with both state and market solutions such as parallel imports being attempted); the provision of integrated primary and secondary care, often through actually siting primary care facilities at hospitals; and the charging policy of public hospitals (i.e., should they be free, should they implement user charges, and if so, how can equity be protected?).

Politics is important in all of these areas. For example, if the private sector in hospital provision is encouraged, it may undermine public hospitals' ability to raise revenue from user charges for better-off patients.

The Changing Capitalist State and Health System Reform

Paradoxically, the capacity of the health-care state (Paton et al., 2000) is increasing in proportion to the complexity of social regulation, while the state's autonomy from economic interests is diminishing. Either the new managerialism (i.e., business systems to replace public administration (Exworthy and Halford, 1999) or direct politicization of public sector targets (Paton, 2006)) is used is to seek to tailor health services to both economist needs and economically filtered social needs. Use of the central state to extract maximum additional surplus value for private business from health-care provision can reach its apotheosis in the NHS model. Two paradoxes therefore arise. Firstly, the most progressive and egalitarian model for health services (the NHS model) is also the most easily subverted. (The central state can be used and abused.) Secondly, where the NHS model is off the political agenda (as in the United States) because of a pro-business ideology, the surrogate policy for taming health care in the interests of business (i.e., managed care) is much less cost-effective.

Consider the hypothesis that state-funded health services (such as the NHS) are a cheap means of investment in the workforce and the economy. If firms derive extra profit (surplus value) as a result of healthier workers that is due to social spending, then that extra profit can be thought of as the total extra income minus the costs of the social spending (e.g., corporate tax used to contribute to the NHS) that firms make. The residual – the extra profit – is composed of two elements: The contribution that workers make to their own health-care costs and social expenses (e.g., through tax), which increases their productivity and firms' profits; and the exploitation, i.e., surplus value extracted from, for example, health-care workers. This latter element, if it exists, derives from the incomes of health-care workers being less than the value they create, i.e., the classic Marxist definition of surplus value.

It might be objected that governments do not plot such a scenario or situation. But sociopolitical pressures help to produce such an underlying reality. The changing socioeconomic structure of Western societies, and the international class structure produced under global capitalism, leads to pressures on publicly financed health systems. This is *inter alia* because more inequality and more complex differentiation of social structures leads to different ability and willingness to pay tax and/or progressive social contributions on the part of different strata. Either private financing of (say) health care will increase or public services will have to please affluent consumers and satisfy corporate expectations for their employees, as well as investing in health on behalf of the economy's needs. The latter may not be equitable, if equity means equal access to services on the basis of equal need. Put bluntly, health-care consumption demands by the richer and investment in the health of skilled, scarce employees, will conflict with egalitarianism in health services.

Greater social inequality plus the absence of a left-of-center electoral majority thus puts pressure on egalitarian policy and institutions such as an NHS available to all irrespective of ability to pay. Attempts to defend such a service tend to be forced onto the terrain of economic justifications, to the argument that international competitive advantage requires a healthy workforce. But the workforce is not the same as the whole of society. Nor is a post-Fordist workforce (i.e., a national class structure shaped by international capitalism) an undifferentiated structure: Some workers are more equal than others when it comes to prioritizing health for economic reasons. It is here that arguments about social capital are sometimes used: A healthy workforce requires a healthy civil society. But this in turn may be a zero-sum game between regions and communities.

At this point, it is worth bringing in the classic Marxist dispute about the nature of the state: Is it a (crude) committee of the bourgeoisie and does it manage the long-term viability of capitalism; or is it an area of hegemonic struggle. In health and health care, what would the rational capitalist state do?

If the state is the rationalizing executive board of the capitalist class, one can imagine the board's secret minutes saying, it makes economic sense for us for the state to fund and provide health care. That way, we will pay less than if we directly provide health benefits for our workforce, company by company or industry by industry. It makes sense because taxation is less progressive than it used to be (so workers pay more; we pay less); the state can force hospitals and other providers to do more for less, i.e., exploit the health workforce to produce additional surplus value for most of us; and the said public services can invest in the productive using allegedly technocratic means of rationing.

At this point, however, if the country's health-care providers were private, for-profit concerns, they might object, on the grounds that the broader interests of (the majority of) capitalists went against their interests, namely, to derive as much profit as possible from a generously funded health system (broadly, the U.S. position). Equally corporate insurers in the United States resist a single-payer or statist model. Note that such a situation does not pertain in the United Kingdom, with the commercial sector in health care being less economically and therefore politically salient and essentially content with marginal income from the NHS (important as that is in its own terms). Additionally, leaving investment in the workforce to individual firms means a system whereby there is a problem of collective action: Firms will not do it for fear of simply fattening up workers who then move to another firm; or rather, they will only do it in order to recruit and retain the most valuable workers. Again, this is broadly the U.S. situation.

On the other hand, if the state finances and provides a common basket of health services for all (the European model), mechanisms will have to be put in place to limit that basket and to increase productivity in its production. This will mean that wider benefits will be sought privately by individuals or employers. This, very broadly, is the agenda driving European health system reform.

If the state is more than a committee of capitalists (whether with or without the health-care industry) then ironically the hard-nosed longer-term agenda of competitiveness may be easier to implement; hence the continuing viability of the British NHS on economic as opposed to ethical lines, rather than the messy and expensive U.S. system. (Note how New Labour – in defending the NHS – points to how European social insurance taxes business directly.)

The choice between state health care to promote selective investment rather than equitable consumption is glossed over in the rhetoric of the third way, whereby the former becomes social investment and the latter is downplayed either as old tax and spend or as failing adequately to emphasize health promotion, and so on.

Overall, the state in the developed world balances the claims of individual firms, the overall capitalist system and particular laborist or welfarist claims. But in today's international capitalism, securing inward investment is the crucial imperative. Health policy is not determined by political economy, but it is influenced and constrained by it. This occurs in two ways: It affects the money available and its distribution, and policy regimes (associated with regimes in political economy) influence governments and policy makers, with policy transfer across ministries.

Conclusion

This article has defined and explored public policy, applying general concepts to ensure that health policy is not treated in too exceptional or parochial a manner. It has gone on to explore some of the complexities in making (and understanding) policy and in implementation.

Policy analysis can be defined in two ways. The first is the systematic but normative examination of situations and options in order to generate choice of policy. The second is the academic analysis of how policies originate and where they come from; who and what shapes them; how power is exerted; and what the consequences or outcomes are.

There is often confusion between those two domains both in theory and in practice, perhaps based on the fact that the two meanings are linked psychologically if not logically. Analysts and advocates who wish to find an analytical basis for policy choice (first domain) often have a subconscious picture of the policy process as rational. That is, they assume there is some basis through which evidence can create consensus as a direction or a decision.

Yet the reality is often that interests, ideologies, or both determine policy choice. These choices (by individuals, groups, or classes) may be rational in that the means are chosen (the policies) for the ends or goals. It is just that there is no scientific basis for adjudicating among ends, especially now that teleologies such as Marxism do not hold sway and would-be universal values such as capitalist liberalism are revealed to be partisan rather than universal.

That is, health policy, like public policy generally, is made as a result of the interplay of powerful actors influencing politicians to make decisions (politics), on the basis of policies that are available and currently salient, either because they are trendy or because they are seen as convenient solutions to those problems that currently dominate agendas. Rationality, in the sense of evidence-based tailoring of means to ends, is only consensual if the key decision makers agree as to ends. This may occur if there is wide and genuine social consensus, or – a very different state of affairs – if those who disagree are excluded from a powerful role in the policy process.

In health policy, as in other spheres, we see – locally, nationally, and globally – that orthodoxies wax and wane over decades. (For example, in what used to be called Western countries, the era of public administration gave way to the new public management in the 1980s, 1990s, and beyond, with the latter subsequently being influenced in a harder market direction by both globalization *per se* and the mission of supranational block such as the European Union.) We may call these orthodoxies policy regimes. They are regimes because they combine elements of the dominant political economy and the (usually related) current political orthodoxies i.e., they are more than just a policy yet less than an evidence-based certainty.

See also: Agenda Setting in Public Health Policy; The State in Public Health, The Role of.

Citations

Aglietta M (1979) *The Theory of Capitalist Regulation*. London: New Left Books.
Allison G (1971) *Essence of Decision*. Boston, MA: Little, Brown.
Altenstetter C and Björkman J (eds.) (1997) *Health Policy Reform, National Variations and Globalization*. London: Macmillan.
Archer M (2000) *Being Human: The Problem of Agency*. Cambridge, UK: Cambridge University Press.
Arts W and Gelissen J (2002) Three worlds of welfare capitalism or more? A state of the art report. *Journal of European Social Policy* 12: 137–158.
Bachrach P and Baratz M (1970) *Power and Poverty*. New York: Oxford University Press.
Bell D (1960) *The End of Ideology*. Glencoe, IL: Free Press.
Blas E (2005) *1990–2000: A Decade of Health Sector Reform in Developing Countries*. Göteborg, Sweden: Nordic School of Public Health.
Buse K, Mays N, and Walt G (2005) *Making Health Policy*. Buckingham, UK: Open University Press.
Cawson A (1986) *Corporatism and Political Theory*. Oxford, UK: Basil Blackwell.
Cohen G (1978) *Karl Marx's Theory of History: A Defence*. Oxford, UK: Clarendon.
Cohen M, March JG, and Olsen JP (1972) A garbage can model for rational choice. *Administrative Science Quarterly* 1: 1–25.
Crenson M (1971) *The Un-politics of Air Pollution*. Baltimore, MD: Johns Hopkins University Press.
Dahl R (1980) *Dilemmas of Pluralist Democracy*. New Haven: Yale University Press.
Day P and Klein R (1987) *Accountabilities. Five Public Services*. London: Tavistock.
Dowding K (1990) *Power and Rational Choice*. London: Edward Elgar.
Dowding K (1995) Model or metaphor? A critical review of the policy networks approach. *Political Studies* XLIII: 136–158.
Dunleavy P (1989) *Democracy, Bureaucracy and Public Choice*. London: Harvester Wheatsheaf.
Exworthy M and Halford A (eds.) (1999) *Professionals and the New Managerialism in the Public Sector*. Buckingham, UK: Open University Press.
Greer S (2004) *Territorial Politics and Health Policy*. Manchester, UK: Manchester University Press.
Greer S (2007) *The UK Department of Health: From Whitehall to Department to Delivery to What?*. London: Nuffield Trust.
Hann A (1995) Sharpening up Sabatier. *Politics* 15: 19–26.
Heidenheimer A, Heclo H, Adams C, et al. (1975) *Comparing Public Policy*. London: Macmillan.
Hill M (1997) *The Policy Process in the Modern State*. London: Harvester Wheatsheaf.
Hood C and Scott C (2000) *Regulating Government in a 'Managerial' Age: Towards a Cross-National Perspective*. London: Centre for Analysis of Risk and Regulation, London School of Economics.
Jessop B (2002) *The Future of the Capitalist State*. Cambridge, UK: Polity.
John P (1999) *Analysing Public Policy*. London: Pinter.
King A (1973) Ideas, institutions and the policies of governments. *British Journal of Political Science* 3: 291–313.
Kingdon J (1984) *Agendas, Alternatives and Public Policies*. Boston, MA: Little, Brown.
Klein R (1990) The State and the Profession: The Politics of the Double Bed. *British Medical Journal* 301: 700–702.
Le Grand J (2003) *Motivation, Agency and Public Policy*. Oxford, UK: Oxford University Press.
Lukes S (1974) *Power: A Radical View*. London: Macmillan.
Mann T and Ornstein NJ (1995) *Intensive Care: How Congress Shapes Health Policy*. Washington, DC: Brookings Institute.
Marsh D (ed.) (1998) *Comparing Policy Networks*. Buckingham, UK: Open University Press.
Martinussen J (1994) *Samfund, stat og marked*. Copenhagen, Denmark: Mellemfolkeligt Samvirke.
Maxwell R (1982) *Health and Wealth*. London: Kings Fund.
Moran M (1999) *Governing the Health Care State*. Manchester, UK: Manchester University Press.
Navarro V (1978) *Class Struggle, the State and Medicine*. London: Martin Robertson.
Osborne D and Gaebler T (1993) *Reinventing Government*. New York: Plume.
Paton C (1990) *US Health Politics : Public Policy and Political Theory*. Aldershot, UK: Avebury.
Paton C (1996) The Clinton Plan. In: Bailey C, Cain B, Peele G, and Peters BG (eds.) *Developments in American Politics*. London: Macmillan.
Paton C (2005a) Open Letter to Patricia Hewitt. *Health Service Journal*, pp. 21. May 19.
Paton C (2005b) The State of the Health Care System. In: Dawson S and Sausman C (eds.) *Future Health Organisations and Systems*. Basingstoke, UK: Palgrave.
Paton C (2006) *New Labour's State of Health: Political Economy, Public Policy and the NHS*. Aldershot, UK: Avebury.
Paton C (2007) Visible hand or invisible fist? Choice in the English NHS. *Journal of Health Economics, Policy and Law* 2(3).
Paton C, Birch K, Hunt K, et al. (1998) *Competition and Planning in the NHS, The Consequences of the Reforms*. 2nd edn. Cheltenham, UK: Stanley Thornes.
Paton C, et al. (2000) *The Impact of Market Forces Upon Health Systems*. Dublin, Ireland: European Health Management Association.
Peck J and Coyle M (2002) *Literary Terms and Criticism*. London: Palgrave.
Saltman R, Busse R, and Mossialos E (eds.) (2002) *Regulating Entrepreneurial Behaviour in European Health Care Systems*. Buckingham, UK: Open University Press.
Schattschneider EE (1995) *The Semi-Sovereign People: A Realist's View of Democracy*. London: Holt.
Segall M (2000) From co-operation to competition in national health systems – and back? Impact on professional ethics and quality of care. *International Journal of Health Planning and Management* 15: 61–79.
Stoker G (ed.) (2000) *The New Politics of Local Governance*. London: Macmillan.
Taylor-Gooby P (1985) *Public Opinion, Ideology and State Welfare*. London: Routledge.
Warner M (1994) In: Lee K (ed.) *Health Care Systems: Can They Deliver?* Keele, UK: Keele University Press.
Wilensky H (1974) *The Welfare State and Equality*. Berkeley, CA: University of California Press.
World Health Organization (2000a) *The World Health Report*. Geneva, Switzerland: World Health Organization.
World Health Organization (2000b) *The World Health Report 2000 Health Systems: Improving Performance*. Geneva, Switzerland: World Health Organization.

Futher Reading

Braverman H (1998) *Labour and Monopoly Capital*. New York: Monthly Review Press.
Department of Health (2002) *The NHS Plan: Next Steps for Investment, Next Steps for Reform*. London: Department of Health.
Galbraith JK (1992) *The Culture of Contentment*. London: Sinclair-Stevenson.
Gough I (1979) *The Political Economy of the Welfare State*. London: Macmillan.
Gray J (1998) *False Dawn: The Delusions of Global Capitalism*. London: Granta.
Jessop B (1994) The transition to post-Fordism and the Schumpeterian workfare state. In: Burrows R and Loader B (eds.) *Towards a Post-Fordist Welfare State?* London: Routledge.
Lowi T (1964) American business, public policy, case studies and political theory. *World Politics* XVI: 677–715.
O'Connor J (1973) *The Fiscal Crisis of the State*. New York: Harper and Row.

Paton C (1995) Present dangers and future threats: Some perverse incentives in the NHS reforms. *British Medical Journal* 310: 1245–1248.

Paton C (2000) *World, Class, Britain: Political Economy, Political Theory and Public Policy*. London: Macmillan.

Paton C (2001) The state in health: Global capitalism, conspiracy, cock-up and competitive change in the NHS. *Public Policy and Administration* 16(4): 61–83.

Poulantzas N (1973) *Political Power and Social Classes*. London: New Left Books.

Price D, Pollock A, and Shaoul J (1999) How the World Trade Organization is shaping domestic policies in healthcare. *Lancet* 354: 1889–1892.

Skocpol T (1997) Boomerang: *Health Care Reform and the Turn Against Government*. 2nd edn. New York: W.W. Norton.

Stockman D (1986) *The Triumph of Politics*. New York: Harper and Row.

Agenda Setting in Public Health Policy

J Shiffman, Maxwell School of Syracuse University, Syracuse, NY, USA

© 2008 Elsevier Inc. All rights reserved.

Introduction

Definitions

The public policy process, in simplified form, can be understood as a sequence of four phases: agenda setting, formulation, implementation, and evaluation. Agenda setting is the first phase, the issue-sorting stage, during which some concerns rise to the attention of policy makers while others receive minimal attention or are neglected completely. The importance of this phase lies in the fact that there are thousands of issues that might occupy the attention of policy makers, but in practice only a handful actually do gain their consideration.

Research in this field investigates how issues emerge on the policy agenda, defined (Kingdon, 1984, p. 3) as 'the list of subjects or problems to which governmental officials, and people outside of government closely associated with those officials, are paying some serious attention at any given time.' Kingdon (p. 4) distinguishes between the governmental agenda, the list of subjects that are getting attention, and the decision agenda, the subset of issues on the governmental agenda that are 'up for an active decision.'

Agenda Setting and Priority Setting

The subject of public policy agenda setting has inspired considerable research, but little of that is in the field of public health. There has been much greater attention in public health scholarship to a concept that is related to but distinct from agenda setting: priority setting. While those investigating priority setting in health have studied how scarce resources are allocated among health causes, their predominant concern has been how scarce resources should be allocated, a normative issue. Often they are motivated by uneasiness that resources and attention are not fairly distributed. For instance, the Global Forum for Health Research monitors resource commitments for health research. It is committed to redressing what it calls 'the 10/90' gap – a concern that only 10% of the world's research funds are being applied to conditions of the developing world that account for 90% of the world's health problems (Global Forum for Health Research, 2004).

An assumption in much, if not all, of this research tradition is that there are objective facts about the world – such as the burden caused by a particular disease and the cost-effectiveness of an intervention – that can be used to make rational decisions on health resource allocation. As Reichenbach notes (2002), one example of priority-setting research is cost-effectiveness analysis, which seeks to evaluate alternative interventions based on how much health improvement can be purchased per monetary unit. A second example is the disability-adjusted life year (DALY), a measure of the number of years of healthy life lost due to individual conditions, enabling comparisons across diseases. Its developers have used DALYs to identify the ten diseases posing the greatest burden globally: perinatal conditions, lower respiratory infections, ischemic heart disease, cerebrovascular disease, HIV/AIDS, diarrheal diseases, unipolar major depression, malaria, chronic obstructive pulmonary disease, and tuberculosis (Lopez *et al.*, 2006). Researchers have also combined studies of DALYs with cost-effectiveness analysis to inform a disease control priority project that offers recommendations concerning which interventions should be prioritized globally (Jamison *et al.*, 2006).

In contrast to priority-setting research, inquiry on agenda setting is concerned primarily with explaining how attention and resources actually are allocated (although agenda-setting researchers often are motivated by normative concerns). Central to their inquiry is an interest in power. They investigate matters such as which actors are able to put issues on the agenda, how they come to hold this capacity, and how this influence alters agendas away from what might be considered a 'rational' allocation of resources. Reichenbach (2002), for instance, demonstrates that despite epidemiological evidence that cervical cancer presents a higher burden than breast cancer in Ghana, the latter received greater political priority. This outcome was due in part due to local politics as well as to the influence of international women's groups from North America, along with the higher incidence of breast than cervical cancer among wealthier Ghanaian women.

Another difference from priority-setting research is that many individuals investigating agenda setting are influenced by a tradition called social constructionism, which views issues not as problems objectively 'out there' waiting to be discovered, but rather as created in the process of social interactions. This idea is similar to the observation that drives agenda-setting research: There are thousands of conditions in society causing harm that may become social priorities, including drug addiction, HIV/AIDS, road traffic injuries, and homelessness. In practice, however, only a handful of these conditions become widely embraced social priorities (Hilgartner and Bosk, 1988). Thus, we cannot explain how some problems become prominent and others are neglected by appeal to material facts alone: We must also consider social processes, such as how problems are defined and framed, who holds the power to define them, and how interest groups mobilize to advance their agendas.

Actors in and Models of Public Policy Agenda Setting

Actors in Agenda Setting

Many individuals and institutions are involved in shaping health policy agendas, including political officials, civil society organizations, United Nations agencies, and philanthropic foundations (**Table 1**). Kingdon (1984) distinguishes between visible and hidden participants. Senior political and administrative officials including prime ministers, legislators, ministers of finance, and leaders of international donor agencies are likely to be more visible, moving large problems and issues on to the agenda, such as lack of health-care access for the poor and the reform of national health sectors. Specialists including scientists, doctors, academics, and career civil servants may play less visible but nevertheless crucial roles, proposing policy alternatives that can address these problems, hoping to convince political leaders to take the issue seriously. However, this distinction is not clear-cut, and there are many instances where specialists – often as part of large policy networks – take on visible roles, contributing to the emergence of broad issues on to national and international health agendas.

Walt (2001) notes a transformation in the relationships among international actors involved in health that has influenced agenda-setting processes. After World War II, a system of vertical representation emerged globally, as

Table 1 Actors in public health policy agenda setting

Type of actor	Primary sectors	Examples
Political officials	Public	President; prime minister; parliamentarian
Senior public servants	Public	Minister of health; minister of finance
Mid-level public servants	Public	Chief of Maternal and Child Health Division in Ministry of Health; head of state-level family planning bureau
Domestic nongovernmental organizations	Nongovernmental	Women's health advocacy groups; national family planning associations; Catholic Church
Medical associations	Nongovernmental	American Medical Association; British Medical Association
Academics	Nongovernmental; international	Think-tank policy analysts; scientists and social scientists at universities
Philanthropic foundations	Nongovernmental; international	Bill and Melinda Gates Foundation; Wellcome Trust; MacArthur Foundation; Rockefeller Foundation; Robert Wood Johnson Foundation
Medical journals and the media	Private	*New England Journal of Medicine; Lancet; Journal of the American Medical Association; New York Times; Guardian;* CNN
For-profit companies	Private	Pharmaceutical companies (Merck; Bristol-Myers Squibb); health insurance companies
United Nations agencies	International	World Health Organization; UNICEF; United Nations Population Fund (UNFPA)
International financial institutions	International	World Bank; Inter-American Development Bank; African Development Bank; IMF
Bilateral donors	International	United States Agency for International Development (USAID); United Kingdom's Department for International Development (DFID)
International nongovernmental organizations	International	International Planned Parenthood Federation; Doctors Without Borders; Oxfam
Public–private partnerships	Mixed	Global Fund to Fight AIDS, Tuberculosis and Malaria; Global Alliance for Vaccines and Immunizations (GAVI)

states cooperated in international health through the United Nations system and particularly the World Health Organization. Over time a complex array of actors became involved in health, and the role of the UN system diminished. She argues that the global health system is now best characterized as one of horizontal participation, with partnerships (and conflicts) among a broad array of actors. A particularly notable development since the 1980s is the growing role of the World Bank in global health, and the tensions this emergence has caused between this institution and the World Health Organization, which originally had the mandate for global health coordination (Buse and Gwin, 1998). Another prominent development is the increasing role of private actors in global health, including philanthropic foundations (particularly the Bill and Melinda Gates Foundation) and a proliferation of public–private partnerships that link pharmaceutical companies, foundations, international agencies, nongovernmental organizations, and donor governments in cause-specific initiatives, such as the Global Fund to Fight AIDS, Tuberculosis and Malaria (GFATM), and the Global Alliance for Vaccines and Immunizations (GAVI).

Early Models of Agenda Setting

Researchers have developed a number of public policy agenda-setting models that consider actors, processes, and contexts (**Table 2**). Early frameworks include the rationality and incrementalist models, and a model invoking the concepts of legitimacy, feasibility, and support. Newer frameworks include the streams and punctuated equilibria models. Public health policy researchers have employed these in order to investigate health policy agenda-setting processes. In recent years a body of work on international relations has come to influence thinking on health policy agenda setting, and it is worth considering ideas from this field as well.

The rationality model was founded on a presumption that policy makers define carefully the nature of the problems they face, propose alternative solutions, evaluate these solutions on the basis of a set of uniform and objective criteria, and select and implement the best solutions. It continues to be employed by many economics-oriented policy analyses that use cost–benefit calculations to select among competing alternatives. As noted above, in health policy the desire to inject rationality into resource allocation decisions is the impetus behind the development of the disability-adjusted life year and underpins much analysis in the cost-effectiveness tradition.

Many scholars who have studied the political dynamics of policy making believe that the rationality model does not capture how agendas are formed in practice, questioning the presumption that actors deliberate in a logical, linear fashion (Lindblom, 1959; Buse et al., 2005). Among the points they raise are that actors have limited information, are not able to imagine all the alternatives, even if cognizant of multiple alternatives are not likely to consider each systematically, hold ambiguous goals, and change these goals as they act. An alternative understanding of the agenda-setting process, termed incrementalism, emerged that takes into account a number of these critiques (Kingdon, 1984). Drawing in part from research on public budgetary processes, scholars have postulated that policy makers are inclined to take the status quo as given and carry out only small changes at a time, making the policy-making process less complex, more manageable, and more politically feasible than a comprehensive rational deliberative process would entail (Lindblom, 1959; Wildavsky, 1979). Applying this idea to health, we observe that one of the most reliable predictors of the size of a national health budget, as well as its subcomponents such as hospital construction and maternal and child health, is the previous year's budget, evidence that policy makers alter their priorities slowly.

Hall and colleagues produced one of the earliest works that considers the role of power in public policy agenda setting (1975). They argue that an issue is more likely to reach the policy agenda if it is strong on three dimensions: legitimacy, feasibility, and support. Legitimacy refers to the extent to which the issue is perceived to justify government action. For instance, the control of tobacco use in the United States formerly had little legitimacy, defined

Table 2 Models of public policy agenda setting

Model	View of how an issue emerges on the policy agenda	Key developers
Rationality	Through careful consideration of multiple possibilities	Numerous microeconomists
Incrementalism	Slowly, as policy makers for a variety of reasons make only small changes at a time	Lindblom (1959); Wildavsky (1979)
Legitimacy, feasibility, support	When policy makers consider the issue to be appropriate for government action, easy to carry out, and supported by the public	Hall, Land, Parker, and Webb (1975)
Streams	Usually unpredictably; at random junctures, the problem itself, solutions to it, and political developments converge to place it there	Kingdon (1984)
Punctuated equilibria	In a burst, as new actors with new understandings of the issue take it up and break existing policy monopolies	Baumgartner and Jones (1993)

in these terms, but this situation has changed. Feasibility refers to the ease with which the problem can be addressed, and is shaped by factors such as the availability of a technical solution and the strength of the health system that must carry out the policy. For instance, the development of a vaccine for polio made control of this disease much more feasible. Support refers to the degree to which interest groups embrace the issue and the public backs the government that is to address it. Health-care reform in the United States failed under the Clinton administration in part because organized medical interests mobilized to oppose its enactment.

Newer Models of Agenda Setting

In the most influential model of the public policy agenda-setting process, Kingdon (1984) challenges traditional models of agenda setting that conceptualize it as a predictable, linear process. He argues that agenda setting has a random character in which problems, policies, and politics flow along in independent streams. The problems stream is the flow of broad conditions facing societies, some of which become identified as issues that require public attention. The policy stream refers to the set of alternatives that researchers and others propose to address national problems. This stream contains ideas and technical proposals on how problems may be solved. Finally, there is a politics stream. Political transitions, global political events, national mood, and social pressure are among the constituent elements of the politics stream. At particular junctures in history the streams combine, and in their confluence windows of opportunity emerge and governments decide to act. The opening of these windows usually cannot be anticipated. Prior to the combining there may be considerable activity in any given stream, but it is not until all three streams flow together that an issue emerges on the policy agenda.

Several scholars have adapted ideas from Kingdon's model to explain how particular health issues have emerged on policy agendas. Reich argues that five political streams – organizational, symbolic, economic, scientific, and politician politics – all favored child over adult health through the 1990s, explaining the higher position of the former on the international health agenda (Reich, 1995). By organizational politics he means efforts by organizations such as the WHO and World Bank to use their resources to enhance their authority. Symbolic politics concerns how actors use imagery to advance their positions – for instance UNICEF's effective use of the tragedy of child ill health to mobilize social institutions and raise funds. Economic politics concerns the ability of for-profit organizations to advance their interests, such as the power that the tobacco industry has wielded to block efforts to control this substance. Scientific politics concerns the influence of financial support and other political factors on public health research agendas. These four streams shape the cost–benefit calculations of national politicians – the politicians' stream – concerning which problems to place on national policy agendas. Ogden et al. have also drawn on Kingdon's ideas in their research on tuberculosis (Ogden et al., 2003). They demonstrate that the emergence of the HIV/AIDS epidemic contributed to the opening of global policy windows, facilitating advocacy networks to promote directly observed treatment, short-course (DOTS) as a treatment of choice for tuberculosis.

Baumgartner and Jones (1993) have developed another model that challenges the rationality and incrementalist frameworks. Their punctuated equilibria model postulates periods of stability with minimal or incremental change, disrupted by bursts of rapid transformation. Central to their model are the concepts of the policy image and the policy venue. The policy image is the way in which a given problem and set of solutions are conceptualized. One image may predominate over a long period of time, but may be challenged at particular moments as new understandings of the problem and alternatives come to the fore. The policy venue is the set of actors or institutions that make decisions concerning a particular set of issues. These actors may hold monopoly power but will eventually face competition as new actors with alternative policy images gain prominence. When a particular policy venue and image hold sway over an extended period of time, the policy process will be stable and incremental. When new actors and images emerge, rapid bursts of change are possible. Thus, the policy process is constituted both by stability and change, rather than one or the other alone, and cannot be characterized exclusively in terms of incrementalism or rationality.

For instance, Baumgartner and Jones show that little changed in U.S. tobacco policy in the first half of the twentieth century as the subject generated little coverage in the U.S. media, government supported the industry through agricultural subsidies, and the product was seen positively as an important engine for economic growth. Beginning in the 1960s, however, health officials mobilized, health warnings came to dominate media coverage, and the industry was unable to counter a rapid shift in the policy image that focused on the adverse effects of tobacco on health. Shiffman et al. (2002) have used the punctuated equilibria model to examine the ebbs and flows in global attention for polio, tuberculosis, and malaria control. They argue that priority for each of these three diseases rose surprisingly and rapidly at different historical junctures, in ways not explainable by the rationality and incrementalist models of the agenda-setting process. In each case the rise of attention conformed to a punctuated equilibria dynamic, in which new actors became involved with the issue, creating new images of the nature of the problem and of its solutions.

International Influences

These five models were developed based on analyses of national political systems. Increasingly, agenda-setting researchers have come to understand that policy agendas are set not by national actors and processes alone, but also by forces from outside the borders of individual nation-states. International organizations, officials from other countries, donor agencies, and philanthropic foundations, among other transnational actors, have considerable influence over domestic health priorities, particularly those of poor countries that are reliant upon external sources for health funding and technical advice. A body of research from the political science subfield of international relations offers a set of concepts useful for understanding the agenda-setting power of these actors.

Policy Networks

Scholars are giving increasing attention to the role of policy networks as actors in the international system. These vary both in form and level of institutionalization. Two of the more widely researched forms are epistemic communities and transnational advocacy networks. Haas (1992) and colleagues coined the term 'epistemic communities' to refer to groups of professionals who by virtue of their knowledge-based authority and shared beliefs about causal processes are able to influence national policies. The community of scientists concerned about global warming is one example of an epistemic community. It has been able to influence ozone protection policy successfully. Keck and Sikkink (1998) have examined transnational advocacy networks. These differ from epistemic communities in that their members consist of multiple organizational types, from labor unions to churches, and are linked not by expertise but by shared commitment to particular causes. In the early 1990s a transnational advocacy network formed for reproductive health, linking domestic women's groups, international nongovernmental organizations, and governments across northern and southern countries. This network was able to dominate the agenda at the United Nations' Third International Conference on Population and Development in Cairo in 1994, mounting a significant challenge to the population control paradigm that had been ascendant for decades. The influence of this network is the major reason that reproductive health is now on the global health agenda.

Policy Transfer

While attention has been paid to the emergence and forms of these health networks, there has been less research on the means by which they influence national priorities. One concept of value on this subject is that of 'policy transfer,' which concerns the use of knowledge about policies or administrative arrangements in one time or place to develop such arrangements in another time or place (Dolowitz and March, 1996). Research by Ogden et al. (2003) on the emergence of standards for the treatment of tuberculosis, noted above, concerns an example of an international network promoting policy transfer. Stone (1999) notes that scholars employ multiple terms to speak of the concept of policy transfer, including 'lesson-drawing,' 'emulation,' 'external inducement,' 'convergence,' and 'diffusion.' She identifies three modes of transfer. Policy may be transferred voluntarily if elites in one country value ideas from elsewhere and import these of their own accord. Policies may be transferred with compulsion if powerful organizations such as the World Bank threaten to withhold lending to countries that do not embrace particular practices. Policies may be transferred via structural forces when policy-making elites play no active role and ideas enter national systems through processes scholars often refer to as 'convergence.'

Constructivist theory from political science offers a useful framework for thinking about how policy transfer may occur in certain instances. Constructivism works from the premise that nation-states, like individuals, are not isolated entities. They exist within societies of other nation-states and are socialized into commonly shared norms by their encounters with international actors such as the policy networks just discussed (Finnemore, 1996). Mainstream international relations scholars traditionally have downplayed this form of transnational influence as they have sought to understand the behavior of nation-states in the international arena by looking inside states, taking state preferences as given (Finnemore, 1996). Constructivist theorists argue that on any given policy issue, a state may not initially know what it wants but come to hold certain preferences as a result of interactions in international society with other state and nonstate actors. For instance, a state originally may not prioritize a health cause such as polio eradication, but it may come to adopt the cause because domestic health officials learn at international gatherings that other countries are pursuing this goal and they are likely to be left behind. Thus, constructivists argue, state preferences cannot be taken as given (Finnemore, 1996), but rather should be conceived of as created in the process of transnational interactions.

International organizations are critical global actors in frameworks influenced by constructivism. Organizations such as the WHO, UNICEF, the World Bank, and the United Nations Population Fund are created by a global community of nation-states with a view to serving their jointly and individually held interests. However, these organizations may acquire the power to act as independent, autonomous agents, shaping the policy preferences of the nation-states that created them (Abbot and Snidal,

1998). Thus, UNICEF pushes nation-states to prioritize child health and UNFPA to prioritize reproductive health, even as some of the nation-states that created these organizations may object to their initiatives. International health policy networks, which link these actors with other kinds of organizations, may play similar roles in shaping national policy preferences.

Future Research

Public policy agenda setting is a well-developed field of inquiry. Few public health scholars have paid attention to the subject or its constructs, however, and as a result we have accumulated little systematic knowledge on health policy agenda setting.

We do understand a few facets of the process. It is clear that the emergence of health issues onto policy agendas does not conform closely to criteria that many observers would call rational or equitable. The diseases of rich people are more likely to appear on health agendas than those of the poor. The health problems of wealthy countries attract more research funding than the conditions that afflict less-developed nations. In many countries, hospitals and other tertiary care facilities that serve curative functions, often directed toward members of wealthier socioeconomic classes, command larger percentages of national health budgets than do local-level primary health-care facilities that might address the health problems of the poor.

At a general level we understand why such imbalances exist: The distribution of power and wealth within and across societies heavily shape which health conditions are identified as problems, which health problems receive attention, and which health causes receive public and private resources. The problem lies in understanding the specific dynamics of these processes. What influence does the public framing of a health issue have on its likelihood of appearing on a national agenda? Under what conditions do policy monopolies – networks of actors that hold the power to control and define health issues in ways advantageous to themselves – fall? Why do some health causes such as HIV/AIDS control rise to global prominence while other high-burden diseases such as malaria struggle for attention? How is the global health agenda formed? These constitute some of the central questions for future research on agenda setting in public health policy.

Conclusion

It is useful to consider explicitly how health agendas are formed, both nationally and globally. Doing so reminds us that resources are scarce, not all needs can be met, and factors beyond rational deliberation and careful consideration of evidence shape the process. The five models discussed in this chapter – rationality; incrementalism; legitimacy, feasibility, support; streams; punctuated equilibria – offer alternative understandings of the agenda-setting process. Ideas from each may help in advancing our limited knowledge of how health agendas are formed, and what actors may do to alter health policy priorities.

See also: Health Policy: Overview; The State in Public Health, The Role of.

Citations

Abbott KW and Snidal D (1998) Why states act through formal international organizations. *Journal of Conflict Resolution* 42: 3–32.

Baumgartner FR and Jones BD (1993) *Agendas and Instability in American Politics*. Chicago, IL: University of Chicago Press.

Buse K and Gwin C (1998) The World Bank and global cooperation in health: The case of Bangladesh. *Lancet* 351: 665–669.

Buse K, Mays N, and Walt G (2005) *Making Health Policy*. Maidenhead, UK: Open University Press.

Dolowitz D and March D (1996) Who learns from whom: A review of the policy transfer literature. *Political Studies* 44: 343–357.

Finnemore M (1996) *National Interests in International Society*. Ithaca, NY: Cornell University Press.

Global Forum for Health Research (2004) *Monitoring Financial Flows for Health Research, 2004*. Geneva, Switzerland: Global Forum for Health Research.

Haas PM (1992) Introduction: Epistemic communities and international policy coordination. *International Organization* 46: 1–35.

Hall P, Land H, Parker R, and Webb A (1975) *Change, Choice and Conflict in Social Policy*. London: Heinemann.

Hilgartner S and Bosk CL (1988) The rise and fall of social problems: A public arenas model. *American Journal of Sociology* 94: 53–78.

Jamison DT, Breman JG, Measham AR, et al. (2006) *Disease Control Priorities in Developing Countries*. 2nd edn. Washington, DC: International Bank for Reconstruction and Development.

Keck ME and Sikkink K (1998) *Activists Beyond Borders: Advocacy Networks in International Politics*. Ithaca, NY: Cornell University Press.

Kingdon JW (1984) *Agendas, Alternatives and Public Policies*. Boston, MA: Little, Brown and Company.

Lindblom CE (1959) The science of muddling through. *Public Administration Review* 14: 79–88.

Lopez AD, Mathers CD, Ezzati M, Jamison DT, and Murray CJL (2006) Global and regional burden of disease and risk factors, 2001: Systematic analysis of population health data. *Lancet* 367: 1747–1757.

Ogden J, Walt G, and Lush L (2003) The politics of 'branding' in policy transfer: The case of DOTS for tuberculosis control. *Social Science and Medicine* 57: 179–188.

Reich MR (1995) The politics of agenda setting in international health: Child health versus adult health in developing countries. *Journal of International Development* 7: 489–502.

Reichenbach L (2002) The politics of priority setting for reproductive health: Breast and cervical cancer in Ghana. *Reproductive Health Matters* 10: 47–58.

Shiffman J, Beer T, and Wu Y (2002) The emergence of global disease control priorities. *Health Policy and Planning* 17: 225–234.

Stone D (1999) Learning lessons and transferring policy across time, space and disciplines. *Politics* 19: 51–59.

Walt G (2001) Global cooperation in international public health. In: Milsen M, Black R and Mills A (eds.) *International Public Health: Diseases, Programs, Systems and Policies*, pp. 667–697. Gaithersburg, MD: Aspen Publishers.

Wildavsky A (1979) *The Politics of the Budgetary Process*, 3rd edn. Boston, MA: Little, Brown and Company.

Further Reading

Cobb RW and Elder CD (1983) *Participation in American Politics: The Dynamics of Agenda-Building.* Baltimore, MD: Johns Hopkins University Press.

Lewis JM and Considine M (1999) Medicine, economics and agenda-setting. *Social Science and Medicine* 48: 393–405.

Oliver TR (2006) The politics of public health policy. *Annual Review of Public Health* 27: 195–233.

Reich MR (2001) *Toxic Politics: Responding to Chemical Disasters.* Ithaca, NY: Cornell University Press.

Sabatier P (1998) The advocacy coalition framework: Revisions and relevance for Europe. *Journal of European Public Policy* 5: 98–130.

Shiffman J (2007) Generating political priority for maternal mortality reduction in 5 developing countries. *American Journal of Public Health* 97: 796–803.

Shiffman J and Smith S (2007) Generation of polical priority for global health initiatives. A framework and case study of maternal mortality. *Lancet* 370: 1370–1379.

Stone DA (1989) Causal stories and the formation of policy agendas. *Political Science Quarterly* 104: 281–300.

Politics, and Public Health Policy Reform

A Glassman, The Brookings Institution, Washington, DC, USA
K Buse, Overseas Development Institute, London, UK

© 2008 Elsevier Inc. All rights reserved.

Introduction

Politics – defined classically as who gets what, when and how by Lasswell (1936) – affects the origins, formulation, and implementation of public policy in the health sector (Reich, 1995). Politics dictates, for example, who is entitled to services, which are the priority areas, who will provide services, who will be subsidized, and how the budget ought to be allocated and spent (Gonzalez-Rossetti and Munar, 2003). Because vested interests are usually affected by reforms (for example, health-care workers unions) and beneficiaries are dispersed and unorganized (for example, the poor and sick), there are inherent political difficulties associated with the definition and negotiation of the costs and benefits of reforms. Further, the implementation of reforms is often associated with new administrations or political crises, while reforms can also affect the stability of political administrations.

In spite of its acknowledged importance, there is also broad agreement that politics and political issues are rarely analyzed and frequently ignored at all stages of the policy identification, development, and implementation process in the health sector, particularly in the interactions between international donor agencies, recipient developing country governments, and their domestic political context (Buse *et al.*, 2006). There is ample documentation that politics frequently trumps evidence as a driver of policy priorities and reforms (e.g., Gilson *et al.*, 2003) and there are calls for both prospective and retrospective analyses of the politics of public health policy to improve the probability of policy implementation and impact and to understand more fully the political environments in which reforms operate (Walt and Gilson, 1994; Reich, 1995).

This article will review the major theoretical treatments of politics in the health sector in developing countries and provide examples of common issues that have emerged in the study of the politics of public health policy reform. The article does not purport to cover all of the many ways that politics affects public health policies and, in particular, omits the social medicine literature that centers on the role that politics and political regimes play as a determinant of health status. Although there is clearly overlap, the focus is rather on the analysis of politics of public health policy making and implementation in developing countries and how these analyses have been used to improve the feasibility and durability of pro-public health policies. The article presents an overview of the theoretical approaches to understanding the political dimensions of public health policy making, before setting out a number of common features of health sector politics. This discussion provides the backdrop to a discussion of approaches to managing the politics of sector reform.

Major Theoretical Treatments

There are three major literatures that comprise the bulk of theoretical frameworks and models used in the analysis of political aspects of public health policy. A first approach builds on the political science literature. A second literature relates to the politics of health reforms in developed countries. A final group of work deals with policy reform in developing countries mainly focused on structural adjustment reforms implemented in the 1980s and 1990s. Drawing on all three sources, Reich defines three models of policy change, reflected in most of the literature since its publication in 1995.

The political will or technocratic model assumes that decisions by political leaders or a reform champion are necessary and sufficient for policy change and that these leaders are rational actors maximizing the public interest (Alesina, 1992). Reform can occur from outside the political system – for example, via an international agency project – when will is sufficiently strong. While this model has shown its limitations when applied to the realities of the policy process in most contexts (IDB, 2006), it is a policy-making model that is frequently referenced in the public health literature as the mechanism via which to effect change in the sector (see **Table 1** for two prominent examples). The enduring appeal of this myth, which has not been directly addressed in the literature, may reflect the common finding that champions are necessary (although not sufficient) for priorities to land on the agenda and reach implementation.

The political factions or partisan or pluralist model assumes that politicians seek to serve the desires of different groups, including interest groups, bureaucratic agencies, and political parties. This model encompasses the interest group approach to policy-making, with its emphasis on the political competition of groups and ideas (Kingdon, 1984), as well as the bureaucratic politics approach, with its emphasis on how government organizations and employees seek to protect and promote their own narrow sectarian interests. Reform occurs when incentives and benefits to preferred constituencies are sufficiently large.

A variant on the model was developed by González-Rossetti (2005) building on the neoinstitutional school of thought from the discipline of political science; her approach goes beyond interest groups to analyze the formal and informal rules of the game that govern the interaction of social actors and the role of mediation played by the state in the reform process, positing that these factors determine the feasibility of reform (North, 1990). Rules of the game governing the status quo in a developing country's health system may include, for example, clientelistic hiring practices in public health facilities or extensive discretionary spending on health by entities other than the Ministry of Health.

The political survival model assumes public officials seek to protect their individual interests to maintain or expand their existing control over resources. The model reflects the principles of the public choice school, arguing that politicians operate opportunistically to maximize their own power, reflected in pre-election spending sprees, for example. Reform occurs when personal benefits are sufficient to overcome personal costs.

Reich concludes that the models co-exist in most countries' reform processes, are not exhaustive, and have advantages and disadvantages as tools to generate insights on policy-making. Recent work by Spiller and Tommasi (2003) outside the health sector helps to understand the more nuanced, process-focused view of policy making and policy outcomes that is evolving in the literature. The policy-making process itself encompasses the entire process of negotiation, approval, and implementation in which different political actors and institutions interact in formal (i.e., parliaments) and informal (i.e., back rooms) settings. The behavior of the political actors and institutions depend on the preferences and incentives faced by each, the expectations each have of the others' behavior and the rules of the game governing their interactions. These processes, like policies themselves, are complex. There are multiple actors, with differing attributes, time horizons, and incentives, interacting in different contexts, under different rules.

There are other theories, particularly used in policy analysis, which provide insights into understanding of politics in the health sector. These include the stagist model of the policy making, Kingdon's streams approach to understanding agenda setting (Kingdon, 1984), the street-level bureaucrat model concerning implementation (Lipsky, 1980), a number of variants of models that focus their analysis of the role of networks in modern policy making, as well as the so-called punctuated equilibrium model, which explains why periods of policy stability are periodically beset by reform.

In relation to the stagist model, analysts have studied the different stages of the policy-making process, used mainly retrospectively to assess health policy reforms. Gonzalez-Rossetti (2005) focuses on six reform moments: Problem definition, policy formulation, policy legislation, policy regulation, policy implementation, and policy consolidation. Nelson sets out sequential policy tasks: Getting on the agenda, reaching agreement with the executive, winning legislative approval, and implementation (Nelson, 1999). In reality, policy may not be linear as implied, and the stages may overlap and never proceed from one to the next, but the stages model helps to

Table 1 Examples of the political will model used in the literature

"Broad reforms in the health sector are possible when there is sufficient political will and when changes to the health sector are designed and implemented by capable planners and managers."
World Bank (1993) *World Development Report 1993: Investing in Health.* New York: Oxford University Press.
"With political will and financial support, most countries could meet the Millennium Development Goals."
Costello and Osrin arguing for a global fund for maternal, neonatal and child survival; Costello A and Osrin D (2005) The case for a new Global Fund for maternal, neonatal, and child survival. *Lancet* 366: 603–605.

unravel the complexity of the politics of different phases of the life course of a given policy reform.

Still others have zeroed in on one stage of policy-making, for example, agenda-setting. The focus of Shiffman's work on generating political will for safe motherhood in Indonesia, Honduras, and other countries, which identified a series of international and domestic factors determining the priority of safe motherhood issues (Shiffman, 2007). International factors determining agenda setting included the promotion of global norms and the provision of financial and technical resources to support adoption and implementation of those norms in-country. Domestic factors included the extent of cohesion among advocacy groups, the existence of political champions, the availability of data necessary to establish the problem, the occurrence of a focusing event, the availability of feasible and affordable policy solutions, the stage of the electoral cycle, and the priority given to competing health priorities.

The politics of the implementation phase have received considerable attention, often drawing on Lipsky's insights into the considerable discretion and influence enjoyed by front-line providers of services (the street-level bureaucrats) to shape policy in relation to their values, interests and/or working routines (Lipsky, 1980). For example, in examining the influence of nurses and clinic coordinators on the implementation of South Africa's free health-care policy, Walt and Gilson (2004) focused on understanding frontline staff experiences, paying particular attention to the personal and professional consequences of the policy, the factors that influenced their responses to the policy, and what they perceived as the barriers to effective implementation. Results revealed that nurses were asked to implement a policy about which they had not been consulted, and whose consequences for their routines were largely ignored. These features of the policy process as well as nurses' values, including their perceptions of deserving or undeserving patients, had significant implications for the manner in which the free health-care policy was implemented in practice.

As the number and types of actors involved in health sector decision making has multiplied (for reasons explored in the Interest groups section), greater attention has been paid to network analysis as a tool for describing systems of interactions and interconnectedness between groups of actors. In particular, they seek to understand the extent to which variations in the number and type of participants, features of their interactions (formal and informal), the openness of the network, and relationships to other networks account for specific policy outcomes. Lee and Goodman, for example, examined a small group of internationally networked policy elites that effectively propagated the worldwide health-care financing reforms of the 1980s and 1990s (Lee and Goodman, 2002). Sabatier has focused on competition among advocacy coalitions (whose membership comprises government officials and non-state actors that shared policy goals) to dominate policy subsystems (e.g., AIDS policy). And while most would acknowledge that the role of government remains central to policy making, network analysis attempts to make sense of how the increasingly complex and mutually dependent relationships of politicians and bureaucrats with non-state actors influence policy decisions.

Baumgartner and Jones' (1991) punctuated equilibrium theory attempts to explain why policy making is characterized by periods of stability with minimal or incremental policy change, disrupted by bursts of rapid transformation – drawing attention not only to competition between networks but also between policy images and the policy venues. The policy image is the way in which a given problem and solutions are conceptualized. One image may prevail over a long period of time, but may be challenged at particular moments as new understandings of the problem and alternatives emerge. The policy venue is the set of actors or institutions that make decisions concerning a particular set of issues. These actors may hold monopoly power but will eventually face competition as new actors with alternative policy images come to the fore. When a particular policy venue and image hold sway over an extended period of time, the policy process will be stable and incremental. When new actors and images emerge, rapid bursts of change are possible.

Given the place of ideas, evidence and argument in policy making – a process described by some as an exercise in persuasion – it is not surprising that politics plays a role in attempting to shape understandings, values, and beliefs, giving rise to the use of discourse analysis in public health policy. Connelly and Macleod (2003), for example, argue that the media in South Africa has constructed the HIV/AIDS problem in military terms, thus making the solution more amenable to conventional national responses, and at the same time reinforcing gender stereotypes.

Approaches to Understanding the Politics of the Health Sector

While there have been many calls for greater attention to the analysis of the political dimensions of health sector reform, there has been very little guidance on how best to do so. Primary data sources for most analyses rely on in-depth interviews and document review to draw up stakeholder maps and assess power and position or to design actor management strategies (for example, Thomas and Gilson, 2004). The case study approach, often using a tracer policy or set of policies, is most common and has well-known constraints associated with such comparative methods (Reich, 1995). Alternative approaches are identified by Reich (1995), but to date have not been implemented. Although few in number, there have been some useful linked comparative case studies, for example on the politics of family planning policy (Lee et al., 1998) or of aid coordination and policy-making more generally (Walt et al., 1999).

Common Issues Identified in Political Analyses in the Health Sector

The major theoretical treatment section adopts elements of the theoretical frameworks described above to illustrate and organize some of the common themes identified in the literature as characteristic of health politics in developing countries.

Context and Institutions

The nature of the sector itself creates political challenges; Nelson (1999) refers to these as "the special politics of social service reforms." Gonzalez and Munar have highlighted the particular problems of policy reform in the health sector where the state is the central provider and where a main role of the state is as an employer (Gonzalez and Munar, 2003). This direct employment and provision role has led to clientelistic practices – provision of jobs, wages, subsidies, and benefits to provider groups and other discretionary practices in exchange for political or other support – and has played a historical role in creating political stability for fragile governments. The common content of reforms – merit-based selection and reward of employees, public–private mix based on best price and supply, standard and transparent criteria to determine entitlements to public goods and services, transparent budget allocation criteria – directly undermine the stability that may be associated with the status quo created by the clientelistic model. The political cost–benefit of the reform is thus affected and conditions the extent that decision makers pursue them in any serious way. Despite resistance, new public management reforms have been adopted in some countries.

There is also the common observation that there is not a single dominant technical consensus model guiding health reforms, as opposed to macroeconomic reforms (Nelson, 1999). This lack of consensus can itself exacerbate the political difficulty of moving reforms forward, since there are few precedents, solid evidence of impact is scarce, and choices are often difficult to explain to the public at large.

Another particular feature of the health sector has to do with the "crucial role of motivations and capacities of individual service providers in the quality of outputs" (Nelson, 1999). The principal–agent dilemma – that interests of the principal (payer) and the agent (providers) may not be aligned – is particularly acute in the sector. A payer – a Ministry of Health – may be most concerned to maximize health for funds invested, while a provider may wish to maximize her own income. It is thus particularly difficult to mobilize providers behind reforms. In a study of public hospital reforms, for example, Over and Watanabe (2003) find that hospital staff and the professional unions that represent them fear potential job losses due to reforms of almost any type.

The institutional and more general governance setting can also be critical in how political events play out around a given policy. A social security reform in Mexico (1994–2000) analyzed by Gonzalez-Rossetti (2005) found that, given the country's strong presidentialist system, the executive branch had a great deal of autonomy in policy making, so set the agenda and moved quickly through problem identification and policy design. Problems came later in implementation after the closed policy development process; unions resisted and implementation failed.

In India, the persistent gap between promised pro-poor policies such as the National Rural Health Mission (an initiative to deliver primary care to the poor intended to increase the national health budget by 1% of GDP) and budget allocation and execution is attributed in part to the practices of the Indian civil service, where frequent rotation among ministries is common, driven by political party affiliation, and expertise in a particular area, such as health, is infrequent, leading to poor follow-up and little ownership.

Interest Groups

Governments often consult external groups to see what they think about issues and to obtain information. In turn, groups attempt to influence ministers and civil servants. If governments make policies that are strongly disliked by the public or particular groups, they know that these may well be resisted with the result that their policies may not be implemented. In most countries, there are a growing number of groups outside government, referred to as interest or pressure groups, which want to influence government thinking on policy or the provision of services in a direction favorable to their point of view, social group, or material position. They use a range of tactics to get their voices heard, including building relationships with those in power, mobilizing the media, setting up formal discussions, or providing the political opposition with criticisms of government policy. Although the existence of interest groups indicates that political power is not the monopoly of any one group, it is clear that some interest groups are far more influential than others. In the health field, the medical profession is still the most significant interest group outside government in most countries.

Design trade-offs made as concessions to political interest groups affect the ability of policies to achieve their originally stated objectives. For example, a common contribution and financial risk pool across a new social health insurance scheme and any existing private insurers in South Africa was lost during negotiations, thus compromising the equity-improvement objective of the planned reform (McIntyre et al., 2003). Dung (1996) analyzed actor perceptions during four stages of policy development in Vietnam (policy formulation, approval, implementation, and impact) and shows how the technical objectives of efficiency, equity, and quality within a policy on private sector health provision decrease in perceived value over the policy-making process as more political interest groups – public sector providers – become involved in setting policy.

Related to the above, the opposition of providers' unions and associations is a political issue in health reform worldwide. The ample literature on the role of political ideologies (socialism versus capitalism) on health status is front and center in the analysis of politics since it is so frequently cited as a characteristic of the positions of certain stakeholders in the health sector. Medical worker unions or provider associations (Dung, 1996) frequently take the position that neoliberal and privatizing reforms, regardless of their supposed or actual impact on the health systems' objectives, are likely to threaten public health worker jobs and compromise access by the poor, while reformers (usually technocrats) attempt to document how reforms will increase access for the poor or improve efficiency.

An evaluation of a pilot of hospital autonomy/purchaser–provider split/contracting out in Panama found very positive outcomes for both patients and hospital performance indicators in the intervention hospital versus two control hospitals, but attributed lack of further uptake of the model to "an environment dominated by interest groups" (Bitran, 2005). Resistance related to job security issues was observed from both medical and nonmedical staff in the nonreforming Ministry and social security hospitals.

Three further groups merit some attention in the politics of health reform in low- and middle-income countries. First, financial donors and providers of technical cooperation can and have influenced health policy, by privileging some ideas and activities over others in their funding decisions and by providing tacit support to some individuals and programs at the expense of others. Second, a range of industries, most prominently the pharmaceutical industry, play active roles supporting and resisting policy affecting their interests. Notwithstanding the comments that follow on the limited role of civil society in health policy processes, which arises in part from the institutional context in which many operate as well as from limited capacity, it is apparent that across a range of health policy issues (from essential medicines to breast milk substitutes to tobacco control), civil society organizations have set agendas and influenced policy formulation and implementation. The success of domestic nongovernment organizations can be linked on one hand to international cause groups as well as links they have to decision makers through the various networks in which they participate.

Limited Public Participation in Policy Reform

Unlike the literature on developed countries, which shows that strong and sustained public sentiment can affect agenda-setting, interest group leverage over government officials and policy makers' formulation of policy (Jacobs, 1994), little attention has been paid to the role of public perceptions in shaping politician behaviors with respect to health reform in developing countries. This is perhaps due to the still limited role of and attention paid by civil society in developing countries to the details of health policy, the limited availability of detailed information on the sources and uses of public spending for health, and the near-total absence of detailed opinion polling on health issues in developing countries. Even where opinion polling is becoming more routine, as in Latin America via the *Latinobarometro* surveys, the health data are not detailed and little used to influence policy.

Timing

Unlike economic and fiscal stabilization reforms, so called stroke-of-the-pen reforms in health sector take time, giving opportunity for opposition to be mobilized (Nelson, 1999). Further, there are political windows of opportunity where reform is feasible – at the beginning of political mandates, when a policy maker has a strong and narrow political coalition and when benefits outweigh costs for a government or a politician. These moments are critical, but can have an impact on the durability of a reform during implementation.

Reform Champions

Nelson synthesizes insights and commonly recommended strategies made in the 1990s to improve the feasibility of reform in the literature (Nelson, 1999). Only limited and relatively uncontroversial reforms can be realized by a single champion (the political will model above). Leadership vacuums similarly have led to lack of success in reform (Glassman et al., 1999).

Since major reforms are usually controversial both inside and outside of government, internal change teams can be useful to generate consensus amongst official groups and conduct outreach to stakeholders. Gonzalez-Rossetti's analysis of Colombia credits the technocratic change team, led by a charismatic and exceptionally able minister, with passing a comprehensive health insurance scheme whose implementation has been more or less sustained over the past decade (Gonzalez-Rossetti, 2000).

Creating Political Feasibility

The main purpose of many of the analyses is to prospectively analyze political barriers necessary to reform success. Reich followed his earlier work with an applied political analysis tool called *PolicyMaker*, which focused mainly on how to prospectively design and implement a policy so as to maximize its chances of approval and implementation (Reich and Cooper, 1996). The tool facilitates the definition of the policy, the analysis of the costs and benefits facing stakeholders and institutions (party, parliament, bureaucracy, civil society, etc.), the influence and commitment of these stakeholders to the reform, the impact of these positions on the feasibility of the reform under consideration, and the design of political strategies to deal with opposition. The method has been applied prospectively in the Dominican Republic (Glassman *et al.*, 1999) and elsewhere.

Assessment of political feasibility requires stakeholder analysis – stakeholders in this case are the political actors, or players, affected by or affecting a given policy. Players can be organizations or individuals, but should be weighted differently according to their power resources. Players in health reform politics usually include:

- Public sector organizations such as ministries of health, ministries of finance, social security institutes, regulatory agencies, teaching hospitals, national laboratories, public universities, and others;
- Public sector individuals such as ministers permanent secretaries (PS), heads of programs, hospital directors, state and local government leaders, and legislative leaders;
- Private sector institutions such as private providers, pharmacies, wholesalers, drugs manufacturers and their associations, insurance companies, and private universities;
- Labor organizations such as medical worker unions, community health agent groups, civil service unions, as well as professional associations;
- Civil society organizations such as nongovernmental foundations, faith-based or other philanthropic groups, and sometimes watchdog groups focused on particular health issues;
- Media organizations such as television, print, and the Internet.

There are usually a large number of unmobilized, potentially supportive players in the political environment that can be involved in reforms to outweigh opponents. In the case of the Dominican Republic (Glassman *et al.*, 1999), for example, nurses' unions, private health management organizations, business associations, nongovernmental associations, churches, and universities, had only limited voice in public debates on health policy. Those groups and individuals that stand to benefit most can also be organized, as would be the case for example, of hospital directors if hospital autonomy is the reform under consideration. Reformers can tap these potential sources of support. Thomas and Gilson (2004) review the development of a health insurance policy in South Africa (1994–99) and also make recommendations in this regard. Involving friends in planning can help to better sequence actions and political strategies.

Leadership can also be prepared better. Technocratic reform models frequently fail if the reform champion is not also a skilled politician backed by powerful constituents and defined rules of the game. The Dominican Republic analysis by Glassman *et al.* (1999) found that in spite of millions of dollars of investment in the technical preparation of reforms, there was no bureaucratic or legislative process agreed or in place that would allow for the legal adoption of the new proposals. Leadership capacity is also deeply affected by the system of government, the credibility of government, political timing and the political effects of the technical content of reforms.

Closely linked to mobilizing support networks and building capacity is the acquisition of financial and media resources to move agendas ahead. These resources practically speaking constitute the power to move reforms. Frequently, developing country reforms receive funding to carry out small-scale studies and other technical assistance, but have no recourse to the soft monies that allow for the polling, policy option appraisal, convening, communications, media, and materials positioning that is so much a part of reforms in developed countries. The United States-based Kaiser Family Foundation, for example, uses many of these policy influence tools to neutrally set out facts, respond to myths perpetuated in the media, and give voice to unorganized beneficiaries through opinion polls. Such strategies and institutions might be built in developing countries with good results for pro-poor reforms.

Framing the reform and the perceptions of the reform must be a major piece of any controversial policy change, as the discourse theory points out. Reforms require new ideas and language that can change the political discourse. In Mexico, for example, where public expenditure had been regressively distributed, the Minister reframed a reform that would reallocate funds from wealthy to poor areas from a health issue to a poverty issue, which had more resonance within the Executive and the Legislature (Frenk *et al.*, 2006).

Conclusion

Politics is a reality for health policy makers, a reality which is too often ignored by public health advocates and researchers alike. The limited literature on the politics of the health sector points to the attenuation of much reform due to the specific constellation of interests and distribution of costs and benefits, with the former often concentrated and falling on well-organized interest groups while the latter are distributed widely across the poor and largely unorganized potential beneficiaries. Despite the gloomy prospective for pro-poor, evidence-informed health sector reform, success is possible, if more attention is paid to managing the politics of the process.

See also: Agenda Setting in Public Health Policy; Interest Groups and Civil Society, in Public Health Policy; The State in Public Health, The Role of.

Citations

Alesina A (1992) Political models of macroeconomic policy and fiscal reform. World Bank Policy Research Working Papers. WPS 970, September 1992.

Baumgartner FR and Jones BD (1991) *Agendas and Instability in American Politics*. Chicago, IL: The University of Chicago Press.

Bitran R, Má C, and Gómez P (2005) The San Miguelito Hospital Reform in Panama, Chapter 3. In: La Forgia GM (ed.) *Health System Innovations in Central America: Lessons and Impact of New Approaches*. World Bank Working Paper No. 57. Washington, DC: The World Bank.

Buse K, Martin-Hilber A, Widyantoro N, and Hawkes SJ (2006) Management of the politics of evidence-based sexual and reproductive health policy. *The Lancet* 368: 2101–2103.

Connelly M and Macleod C (2003) Waging war: Discourses of HIV/AIDS in South African media. *African Journal of Aids Research* 2(1): 1–11.

Costello A and Osrin D (2005) The case for a new Global Fund for maternal, neonatal, and child survival. *Lancet* 366: 603–605.

Dung PH (1996) The political process and the private health sector's role in Vietnam. *International Journal of Health Planning and Management* 11: 217–230.

Frenk J (2006) Bridging the divide: Global lessons from evidence-based health policy in Mexico. *Lancet* 368: 954–961.

Gilson L, Doherty J, Lake S, McIntyre D, Mwikisa C, and Thomas S (2003) The SAZA study: implementing health financing reform in South Africa and Zambia. *Health Policy Plan* 31–46.

Glassman A, Reich MR, Laserson K, and Rojas F (1999) Political analysis of health reform in the Dominican Republic. *Health Policy Plan* 14: 115–126.

Gonzalez-Rossetti A (2000) Enhancing the political feasibility of reform: the Colombia case. LAC HSR Working Paper. Washington, DC: Pan American Health Organization.

Gonzalez A and Munar W (2003) *The Political Economy of Social Sector Reforms*. Region II, Economic and Sector Study Series. Washington, DC: Inter American Development Bank, December.

Gonzalez-Rossetti A (2005) La factibilidad política de las reformas del sector social en América Latina. Serie Estudios y Perspectivas 39. Proyecto CEPAL/GTZ "Equidad II", CEPAL/Mexico.

IDB (2006) *The Politics of Public Policy*. Washington, DC: Inter-American Development Bank and Harvard University.

Jacobs LR (1994) The politics of American ambivalence toward government. In: Morone JA and Belkin GS (eds.) *The Politics of Health Care Reform: Lessons from the Past, Prospects for the Future*. Durham and London: Duke University Press.

Kingdon JW (1984) *Agendas, Alternatives and Public Policies*. Boston and Toronto: Little, Brown and Company.

Lasswell HD (1936) *Who Gets What, When, How*. New York: McGraw-Hill.

Lee K and Goodman C (2002) "Global policy networks: The propagation of health care financing reforms from the 1980s" In: Lee K, Buse K, and Fustukian S (eds.) *Health Policy in a Globalising World*. Cambridge, UK: Cambridge University Press.

Lee K, Lush L, Walt G, and Cleland J (1998) Family planning policies and programmes in eight low-income countries: a comparative policy analysis. *Social Science and Medicine*. 47(7): 949–959.

Lipsky M (1980) *Street-level Bureaucracy: Dilemmas of the Individual in Public Services*. New York: Russell Sage Foundation.

McIntyre D, Doherty J, and Gilson L (2003) A tale of two visions: the changing fortunes of Social Health Insurance in South Africa. *Health Policy Plan* 18: 47–58.

Nelson JM (1999) Reforming health and education: the World Bank, the IDB, and complex institutional change. Policy Essay No. 26. Washington, DC: Overseas Development Council.

North DC (1990) *Institutions, Institutional Change and Economic Performance*. Cambridge, UK: Cambridge University Press.

Over M and Watanabe N (2003) Evaluating the Impact of Organizational Reforms in Hospitals. In: Preker A and Harding A (eds.) *Innovations in Health Service Delivery: The Corporatization of Public Hospitals*. Human Development Network; Health, Nutrition and Population Series. Washington, DC: the World Bank.

Reich MR (1995) The politics of health sector reform in developing countries: Three cases of pharmaceutical policy. In: Berman P (ed.) *Health Sector Reform in Developing Countries: Making Health Development Sustainable*. Boston, MA: Harvard University Press.

Reich MR and Cooper D (1996) Policy Maker: Computer assisted political analysis. Available at http://erc.msh.org/mainpage.cfm?file=6.50.htm&module=toolkit&language=English.

Shiffman J (2007) Generating political priority for maternal mortality reduction in 5 developing countries. *American Journal of Public Health* 97: 796–803.

Spiller PT and Tommasi M (2003) The institutional foundations of public policy: A transactions approach with application to Argentina. *Journal of Law, Economics and Organization* 19(2): 281–306.

Thomas S and Gilson L (2004) Actor management in the development of health financing reform: health insurance in South Africa, 1994–1999. *Health Policy Plan* 19: 279–291.

Walt G, Pavignani E, Gilson L, and Buse K (1999) Health sector development: from aid coordination to resource management. *Health Policy and Planning* 14(3): 207–218.

Walt G and Gilson L (1994) Reforming the health sector in developing countries: the central role of policy analysis. *Health Policy Plan* 353–370.

World Bank (1993) *World Development Report 1993: Investing in Health*. New York: Oxford University Press.

Further Reading

Buse K, Mays N, and Walt G (2005) *Making Health Policy*. Milton Keynes, UK: Open University Press.

Reich MR (2002) The politics of reforming health policies. *Promotion and Education* 9(4): 138–142.

Relevant Websites

http://www.latinobarometro.org – Latinobarómetro.
http://www.kaiserfamilyfoundation.org – The Henry J. Kaiser Family Foundation.

Evidence-Based Public Health Policy

V Lin, La Trobe University, Bundoora, Victoria, Australia

© 2008 Elsevier Inc. All rights reserved.

Why the Interest in Evidence-Based Public Health Policy?

The desire for scientific evidence as the basis for public health policy is not new (Terris, 1980). There has been, however, sharply increased interest in evidence-based policy making since the 1990s. This trend could be seen to have arisen from multiple sources. The language of evidence-based public health and evidence-based health policy derives from the advent of the evidence-based medicine (EBM) movement. However, the idea that policies should be based on knowledge of what works has a history steeped in the rise of social programs and their evaluation in the 1960s, as well as public sector management reforms of the 1990s that make demands for value-for-money.

There are many reasons put forth by analysts about why the notion of evidence-based policy making has become popular. Ham *et al.* (1995) suggest that if medicine should be evidence-based, then so too should health policy. The UK government broadly adopted this thinking across public policy, with their *Modernising Government White Paper* (United Kingdom Cabinet Office 1999a), which argued for a more professional approach to policy making. Mounting pressures for transparency, accountability, and efficiency, in all areas of public health, has increased the demand for use of evidence (Cookson, 2005), but there are other benefits to be gained as well. Use of evidence in policy making helps to shift away from expert opinion and increase legal accountability, thus minimizing the dominance of competing interest groups in policy making (Rodwin, 2001). Basing policy on what has been proven to work (rather than speculation, guesswork, or intuition) also reduces the risks associated with policy making (Rix and Matete, 2005).

In relation to health care and health policy, the pace of technological change in medicine has meant that decisions are increasingly being made involving higher costs and more at stake with each decision. Political factors also shape the decision-making process. Gelijns *et al.* (2005) have suggested that rigorous clinical and economic evidence can help depoliticize difficult policy decisions. Gray (2001) similarly argues that public decision-making processes will increasingly require decision making in health care to be explicitly evidence-based. The idea that healthcare practice should be standardized, equal, accountable, and cost-effective is also consistent with principles of social justice. Furthermore, an ethical position would suggest that if health-care resources are limited, then there is an obligation on the part of decision makers to ensure resource allocation is based on the best evidence possible.

While there is much agreement about the ideals of and rationale for evidence-based policy making, how to make it a reality is much more challenging. These perspectives and debates are explained in this article, starting with some definitions.

What Is Meant by Evidence-Based Public Health Policy?

Definitions of EBM have been adapted to public health as "the development, implementation, and evaluation of effective programs and policies in public health through application of principles of scientific reasoning including systematic uses of data and information systems and appropriate use of program planning models" (Brownson *et al.*, 1999: 87). More recently, Kohatsu (2004: 419) has further broadened the definition of evidence-based public health as "the process of integrating science-based interventions with community preferences to improve the health of populations."

By extension, evidence-based health policy would focus on public policy decisions about groups of people, rather than decisions about individual patients (Cookson, 2005), with such decisions drawing from the best available knowledge throughout the process by which governments translate their political vision into programs and actions to deliver outcomes (United Kingdom Cabinet Office, 1999b). If a distinction is to be made between health policy and public health policy, one might suggest that the former is focused on the health-care system while the latter is concerned with systems which produce health. In other words, public health policy making takes into consideration how other public policies influence all the determinants of health, and not just the delivery of health services.

If evidence-based public health policy is meant to draw from the best knowledge available, then the first two points of contention are (1) what is the nature of that knowledge, or evidence and (2) should policy be based solely on this evidence? Given the array of possible definitions of evidence to be found in any English dictionary (i.e., ranging from known fact, to support for belief, to testimony – see Davies *et al.*, 2000; Lin, 2003a), it is not surprising that the notion of evidence-based policy making should be contested.

Essentially, there are two views about the role of scientific evidence in informing public health policy (Lomas *et al.*, 2005): (1) that science can reveal universal truths and offers context-free guidance, and (2) that scientific evidence has little meaning or importance for decision making until it is adapted to the circumstances of its application. Furthermore, the notion of colloquial evidence has also emerged (Lomas *et al.*, 2005; CHSRF, 2006), recognizing that nonscientific evidence such as expert and professional opinion, political judgment, values, habits and traditions, resources, and outputs by lobbyists and pressure groups, can be incorporated with scientific evidence to provide contextual information and fill information gaps.

For policy making, there is further recognition of the importance of context as well as what might be a range of information that might constitute evidence. The UK Cabinet Office (1999b) states that "good quality policy making depends on high quality information derived from a variety of sources – expert knowledge; existing domestic and international research; existing statistics; stakeholder consultation; evaluation of previous policies; new research, if appropriate; or secondary sources, including the internet." They also suggest that costings of policy options and results of economic or statistical modeling are also likely to be important types of evidence that inform policy decision.

Much of the discourse about evidence-based medicine, public health, policy, and so on, presumes that evidence is context-free, value-free, and interest-neutral. Gelijns *et al.* (2005), however, argue that policy making necessarily has to wrestle with conflicts of value, and is therefore, inherently political. Gray (2005) not only recognizes the existence of social and political influences in health care, but agrees that value-based decision making may also be important. Increasingly, the language is shifting to evidence-informed health care (and health policy) in order to recognize that decision making is informed by research, but not driven by it.

What Evidence Is Required for Public Health Policy?

The process of evidence-based clinical practice includes decision making. This process is suggested by the Sicily Statement to be (Dawes *et al.*, 2005):

- translation of uncertainty to an answerable question;
- systematic retrieval of the best evidence available;
- critical appraisal of evidence for validity, clinical relevance, and applicability;
- application of results in practice;
- evaluation of performance.

In theory, this same rational, technical model would apply to public health policy making. That is, a policy question would be defined, which would lead to the systematic retrieval and appraisal for the best evidence possible; this would lead, in turn, to the adoption of evidence-based policy. In this construction of evidence-based health policy, evidence means knowledge derived from rigorous research (Gray, 2001). Obstacles for the realization of this rational model might be that research lacks relevance, is of poor quality, results are not published or are difficult to find. When a decision maker requires knowledge, solutions to these obstacles or evidence gaps need to be found throughout the research process – from commencement of research, right through to its publication, critical appraisal, critical evaluation, and practical implementation of findings (Gray, 2001).

However, whether evidence-based public health policy is possible depends both on the range of evidence available and the nature of the decision-making process, including factors that influence decision making. If the information desired for decision making is not available, then it is unrealistic to expect decisions to be based on systematic reviews (Anderson *et al.*, 2005). There are many reasons for these gaps in information: The research or evaluation may not have been undertaken, the research may not be of interest to research funders, the results of evaluation have not been released, published, or is not readily located, and so on. Furthermore, what is published is likely to be skewed toward developed countries because of the availability of research funding, orientation of research funding bodies, interest of scientific journals, and the nature of peer reviewing processes adopted by research funders and journal editors. These factors act as filters that lead to the underrepresentation of some forms of evidence (Kavanagh *et al.*, 2002).

Health and medical research is typically focused on either describing the nature and magnitude of specific health problems, or on the effectiveness of particular clinical interventions. From the perspective of public health policy, there may be a range of other questions for which policy makers want answers, but for which evidence is not available, such as the conditional effectiveness and the return on investment for policy measures, the feasibility and acceptability of policy proposals, and the possible distributional impact of different policy options.

In other words, it is likely that evidence will be needed from economic, social, political, and cultural perspectives, and not just from the perspective of health and medicine. A wide range of disciplines, from epidemiology to anthropology to management sciences, will all contribute to policy making. Certainly, evidence will be needed that offers possible solutions rather than simply describing the problem. For example, Millward *et al.* (2003) reviewed the evidence related to effectiveness of interventions related to reducing health inequalities and found only 0.4% of published scientific papers discussed interventions that might reduce inequalities. The precise nature of causal pathways and how different interventions might work in different population groups were underinvestigated. Lavis (2002) investigated what information decision makers did want in the policy domains that might alter health inequalities (i.e., tax transfer, labor market, social services) and found their interests to be in finding what the effective policy interventions and their trade-offs are (including the health consequences of policy alternatives). His findings suggest that decision makers are interested in actionable policies based on causal links. This implies that evaluation research, as research that may be more predictive of future policy impact, may be more valued by policy makers.

It is clear that different types of research will be needed to influence policy making, as seen in **Table 1**.

Lin and Fawkes (2005), in looking at health promotion effectiveness, point to a long pathway between the availability of good-quality evidence to the successful implementation of that evidence. They suggest that evidence only provides a theoretical understanding about effectiveness, and achievement of effectiveness *in situ* depends on adequate infrastructure and capacity (such as a skilled workforce, sufficient financing, and policy and management support), as well as an appropriate scale of intervention (including adequate population coverage and targeting). The problem of adequate infrastructure and capacity may be a particularly important barrier to implementing evidence-based public health policy in developing countries.

By the logic outlined by Lin and Fawkes (2005), the mere assessment of evidence on intervention (or policy) effectiveness would require an understanding of the implementation conditions for various policy regimes or program delivery. Process evaluation becomes as important as summative evaluation (that is, evaluation of outcomes, outputs, and efficacy upon completion of active intervention) for policies and programs, as the evidence derived from process evaluation would inform how new policies and programs could be successfully implemented.

How Does Evidence Get Taken up in the Policy Process?

Conventional wisdom supposes that evidence is created by researchers and then transferred to decision makers. Lomas (2000) depicts this assumption as policy makers coming to the retail store where researchers have filled the shelves with all possible relevant studies that might be useful. This notion that evidence is readily transferred to policy makers is likely to be based on an assumption that policy making occurs through a relatively linear process, as well as an assumption that research dissemination is a linear process. This rational, technical perspective is also used to characterize the policy-making process as a set of sequential steps, frequently as a cycle of activities. For example, see **Figure 1**.

Within such a framework, knowledge derived from research and evaluation can be fed into decision making at different points in time, just as information obtained through consultation and other sources can be incorporated. In theory, formative evaluation (concerned with the process of program development and delivery) becomes particularly important during the implementation stage, while summative evaluation contributes to the reformulation of the policy.

This rational or instrumental model of policy making also recognizes that there are formal institutions of policy making, such as parliament and government departments, along with formal processes for policy deliberation within each of these organizations. This rational model of policy making and research transfer is consistent with the engineering model (or knowledge-driven model) of research utilization, that is, basic research leads to applied research, which in turn leads to product development, and then finally to application (Short, 1997; Nutley and Webb, 2000; Lin, 2003a).

In reality, both policy making and research transfer into decision making are more complex processes.

Table 1 Examples of research paradigms for generating policy-relevant evidence

Research paradigm	Description	Links to policy
Applied	Seeks to apply information learned from basic research to develop practical use	Clarify immediate societal problem
Descriptive	Explore in-depth information and phenomenon in order to gain fuller understanding	Clarify problem, context, and response to possible interventions
Evaluative	Assess processes and outcomes of interventions or of prevailing practices and current policies	Clarify effects of policy
Community	Collaborative research effort between researchers and stakeholders, particularly the affected communities	Focus on stakeholders' concerns in order to target better possible solutions
Systems	Examines the organization, financing, staffing, governance, and delivery of services	Suggest ways to improve quality, performance, efficiency, and effectiveness of service delivery

Adapted from Potter M, Quill B, Aglipay G, et al. (2006) Demonstrating excellence in practice-based research for public health. *Public Health Report* 121: 1–16.

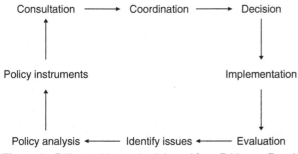

Figure 1 Policy-making cycle. Adapted from Bridgman P and Davis G (2004) *The Australian Policy Handbook*, 3rd edn. Crows Nest NSW: Allen and Unwin.

Multiple meanings can be attributed to research utilization. Writers such as Weiss (1979) and Short (1997) suggest that a range of models of research utilization exist in addition to the rational model described (**Table 2**).

These models might describe the relationship between research evidence and policy making, but there remains another question of the role evidence plays in policy formulation, and by implication, what are other influences on the decision-making process, including whose evidence counts? A number of theories are pertinent (**Table 3**).

Bowen and Zwi (2005) propose that many different forms of evidence are taken up and utilized in a nonlinear or diffuse manner, in evidence-informed policy and practice pathways, which may have three progressions: (1) sourcing the evidence, whereby knowledge, research, ideas, interests, politics, and economics influence the extent to which evidence is adopted or rejected; (2) using the evidence, where evidence is introduced, interpreted, applied, and then either used or rejected; and (3) implementing the evidence, where individual, organizational, and system-level actions are taken. The policy advocate's skills, experience, and networks may be critical in determining the pathway by which evidence travels.

However, despite all the theoretical explanations of how evidence may be taken up into policy, the possibility of serendipity should not be ruled out (Lin, 2003a). Being at the right place, at the right time, in the company of the right people may be a predesigned course of action; it can also be pure circumstance and accidental.

Given the complex factors that influence policy making and the uptake of research in that process, there are likely to be a number of conditions that have to be met if research evidence is to be taken up in public health policy (Buse *et al.*, 2005: 160):

- The existence of comprehensive, authoritative statements based on systematic reviews of research evidence.
- The usefulness of such statements to provide direct guidance to decision making in specific circumstances.

Table 2 Models of research utilization relevant for policy making. The relationship between research evidence and policy making

Model	Description
Rational	Basic research leads to applied research, which in turn leads to product development, and then finally to application
Problem solving	The results of a specific study are applied to a pending decision
Political	Research is used to support a predetermined policy position
Tactical	Research is used as a delaying tactic in order to avoid responsibility for unpopular policies
Interactive	Researchers are one set of participants among many, with policies also being informed by politics, experience, insights, and judgment calls
Enlightenment	Research diffuses through multiple channels over time and provides new ways of thinking, so that policy reflects the indirect influence of research, rather than being the direct outcome of particular research findings
Materialist	Policies are informed more by economic imperatives than by scientific truths or moral stance
Elective affinity	Policy makers are more likely to respond to research findings if they have participated in the research process, and where the beliefs and values of the policy audience coincide with research findings

Adapted in part from Weiss C (1979) The many meanings of research utilization. *Public Administration Review* 39: 426–31 and Short S (1997) Elective affinities: Research and health policy development. In: Gardner H (ed.) *Health Policy in Australia*. Melbourne: Oxford University Press.

- Knowledge and acceptance of such statements by all relevant players.
- Adequate resources to act upon the statements of evidence.
- Appropriate and sufficient incentives to apply the evidence.
- Concurrent absence of disincentives to apply the evidence.
- Control over the implementation chain to ensure compliance with direction and with the evidence base.

These conditions are not easily met. As Pawson (2002) observes, the policy cycle is generally quicker than the research cycle, resulting in the need for policy makers to turn to systematic reviews to gather evidence in the form of results from previous inquiries. In concert with the EBM movement, the use of systematic reviews is increasing in health policy and practice, particularly since the establishment of the Cochrane Collaboration in the early 1990s. While systematic reviews are mostly focused on evidence of effectiveness, the call by policy makers for a

Table 3 Theories of the role of evidence in policy formation

Theory	Originator	Description
Old institutionalism	e.g., Woodrow Wilson, Herbert Simon	There are formal processes for policy making and institutions and actors designated to play. Therefore, research is necessarily filtered by the formal policy processes and the political and organizational context of decision making within these bodies
Garbage-can model	Cohen, March, and Olsen (1972)	Within policy-making organizations, there are a myriad of policy problems looking for solutions, as well as policy ideas looking for problems for which they can provide the solution
Organizational epistemology	Dery (1984)	Policy-making bodies (i.e., government bureaucracies) may adopt and lock into preferred positions. In these instances, systematic bias occurs in policy making through search for and use of data that supports predetermined organizational imperatives
Advocacy coalition	Sabatier and Jenkins-Smith (1993)	Policy making does not happen within a closed organizational system. There are advocates for different policy solutions who work within the bureaucracy as well as outside. These advocacy coalitions work across government and civil society, with shared values and common ways of framing problems and solutions. Research thus influences policy through beliefs of advocacy coalitions
Agenda-setting	Kingdon (1984)	Many policy problems persist without solutions. Many policy ideas persist without being taken up in decisions. Policy making relies on political will, but that policy will be focused on matters other than long-standing policy problems or policy solutions. Thus, policy making occurs only when these three streams (policy problems, policy solutions, and political will) come together

wider range of evidence means that the methodologies used for the synthesis of diverse sources of evidence are being widened and are continually in a process of development (Popay, 2006).

Why Does Evidence Not Always Get Taken Up (or Why Are Public Health Policies Not Always Evidence-Based)?

The history of public health policy points to examples of evidence-based policy as well as numerous instances where policies do not seem to be evidence-based. It could be argued, for instance, that the ill effects of tobacco on smoking were known in the 1950s, but policy action was relatively minimal until the 1980s and onward. Similarly, although there are examples of successful practices in HIV prevention and control (such as in Australia), many countries have yet to adopt evidence-based policies.

Theories about the policy-making process, which incorporate recognition of the politics of decision making, start to provide some answers to why evidence is not always taken up. There are, however, other influences that shape public health policy making. Given public health policy-making concerns making a decision about what is beneficial for the society as a whole, there are innumerable factors to be considered: the adequacy and completeness of evidence; the possible benefits and consequences (and their distribution); how to trade off short-term and long-term costs and gains; and how to reconcile potentially conflicting social values, cultural beliefs, and traditions, institutional and political structures, and processes for policy making. Thus, decision making at the population level is more uncertain (Dobrow et al., 2004) and competing demands of stakeholders are ever present. Decision makers may be confronted with both moral and informational uncertainty, as the definition of the problem, the possible solutions, and the nature of evidence that underpins both are contested. Policy making, by its nature, requires making choices that are not value free or reducible to technical inputs (Rodwin, 2001).

Additionally, policy makers may have goals other than clinical effectiveness when producing health policy. Health service policies, which should ultimately improve clinical outcomes, may be made with financial, social, or strategic development goals in mind (Black, 2001). Communities adopt different conceptions of health risk (Beck, 1992), and these notions of risk may be shaped by mass media representation of events. Media can also create political risk by bringing attention to debates or popular concerns (Davies and Marshall, 2000; Marshall et al., 2005). Also, the debate about policy choices may be masked as conflicting perspectives about evidence (Atkins et al., 2005). Politics, ideology, and political economy may thus be more important drivers of policy making, especially when there is scientific and policy uncertainty about the appropriate course of policy action.

Beyond political complexities, there are also practical barriers to evidence-based health policy making. Even with the best intentions, it has not always been possible for researchers and policy makers to connect the results of research with decision making. Researchers and policy makers have been characterized as living in two worlds (Lomas, 2000). There are numerous differences between

Table 4 Two worlds: Different characteristics of researchers and policy makers may prevent connection of research results with decision-making

Characteristic	Researchers	Policy makers
Nature of work	Discrete, planned projects	Continuous, unplanned flow of ever-changing tasks
Incentives	Publications, grants	Re-election, recognition
Time frame for action	Longer	Shorter
Knowledge span	Deep but on narrow issues	Broadly across many issues
Type of evidence used	Empirical data	All forms of information
Basis for decision	Beyond reasonable doubt	On the balance of probabilities
Accountability	Scientific peers and research funding agencies	Politicians and electorate
Constraints	Research funding and research ethics	Political and bureaucratic imperatives

these two groups in terms of imperatives and styles in decision making (Buse et al., 2005; Choi et al., 2005; Brownson et al., 2006) (**Table 4**).

Policy makers are known to complain that they are unable to obtain research evidence when they want or need it, and that what is available often does not address the policy question of concern. These obstacles have previously been highlighted as the critical gaps in need of solution (Gray, 2001). Even when the findings are timely, for policy purposes, policy makers may not know how best to use the information. Weiss (1991) suggests that research outputs may be classified as: (1) data and findings, (2) ideas and criticism, and (3) arguments for action, each being perceived to be useful for different purposes. Research data and findings may be useful for choosing policy options when the nature of the policy problems and possible solutions are clear. Ideas and criticisms may be more useful for policy agenda setting, to obtain attention on policy problems and possible solutions. Arguments for action, however, are likely to require active advocacy by those involved in the policy-making process.

How Can the Evidence Base of Public Health Policies Be Improved (or What Can Researchers Do and What Can Decision Makers Do)?

There are numerous suggestions about how to reduce the gap between researchers and policy makers. These can generally fall into the categories of: (1) content, what should be researched and how; (2) what mechanisms should be put in place; and (3) capacity building and culture change.

In relation to content, Birch (1996) and Macintyre (2003) have suggested that there is need to move from RCTs to gathering evidence about a range of determinants of health, in other words, research to address social variables and populations. Similarly, the National Institutes of Health (NIH) has recognized the need for more interventional research within the social context, utilizing interdisciplinary research teams (NIH, 2006).

Green (2006) advocates more systems thinking and modeling as a way of producing practice-based evidence that will produce more useful evidence for policy making, while Sheldon (2005) and Anderson et al. (2005) promote greater use of systematic evidence and development of quantitative and qualitative synthesis methods. The need for more evaluation policy interventions has also been noted (Nutbeam, 2004). Brownson et al. (2006) suggest that policy research should include: (1) understanding the determinants of policy making and (2) assessing impact of policy implementation, with case studies being a useful methodology.

The mechanisms that have been mooted as useful for improving the links between researchers and policy makers are numerous. The development of a strategic, priority-driven research program has been suggested to be one method for ensuring research will be more overtly directed toward informing policy (and practice) (Nutbeam, 2004). The National Institute for Occupational Safety and Health (NIOSH) involved a broad constituency of users in defining the research agenda (NORA, 1996). Lomas (2000) has promoted knowledge transfer by the use of knowledge brokers who have a role in linking policy makers and researchers through translating questions and findings to one another.

Oldenburg (2000) suggests, however, that effective dissemination involves more than linkage and exchange, and points to the need to invest in factors that support dissemination (such as organizational resources, infrastructure, etc.). Hanney et al. (2002) also argue that a range of strategies are required for research translation, including long-term liaison, knowledge brokers, evidence champions, change agendas, diffusion networks, communication training, and so on. The particular approaches need to suit the stage of policy development, as well as the types of evidence required or in use. The importance of systematic collation and dissemination of international evidence of effectiveness has been recognized in Sweden, the Netherlands, and the UK (Macintyre, 2003) and independent institutions may be in the strongest position to offer trustworthy synthesis of research data as the basis for informing policy debates (Ham et al., 1995).

More fundamentally, changes are needed in researchers' attitudes, funders' understanding, and the way research is conducted (Black, 2001). Capacity building has been recognized as the basis for culture change. Some (Brownson et al., 2006) have suggested that researchers become more involved in the policy process, through development of short policy summaries, presenting data in more understandable forms, and providing testimony at public hearings. They further recommend that public health training programs should ensure communication skills, including working with the media, are imparted on students. Others (Kavanagh et al., 2003) have suggested increasing policy makers' skills for critical appraisal of research and its methodology as one strategy. Ross et al. (2003), however, suggest interactions between researchers and decision makers need to occur within and outside the research process, and decision makers can become involved as formal supporters, responsive audience, and integral partner, depending on the context.

Deliberative processes that bring together different stakeholders to consider context-free and context-sensitive evidence have also been proposed (CHSRF, 2006). Within such a participatory forum, scientific and decision-maker communities can come together to examine different types of evidence, to make values explicit and to promote consensus where possible. Deliberative processes would bring together scientific evidence on effectiveness, scientific evidence on context features, and colloquial evidence (Lomas et al., 2005). Rather than being a policy consultation process, a deliberative process would foster an integration of technical analysis with stakeholder (and lay) views.

The practical steps most commonly advocated for reducing the gap between research and policy can be summarized as in **Table 5** (Lin, 2003b; Buse et al., 2005).

These practical approaches are useful starting points, but do not substitute for the need for institutional cultural change and for having a good information infrastructure that can allow for ongoing monitoring of policy impact, particularly on the health of populations (Lin, 2003b). Many foundations and organizations have taken on board the need for building the capacity within and between organizations, researchers, and policy makers, so as to develop knowledge management infrastructures to enable knowledge transfer, sharing, or translation to take place. In addition, collaborations aiming to make information more accessible to academics, policy makers, and practitioners, and thus play a part in addressing at least some of the obstacles or gaps preventing widespread evidence-based public health policy and practice are increasing. Since the establishment of the Cochrane Collaboration, other collaborative institutions have been created with the aim of producing high-quality systematic reviews of research in the health (and other) fields. Notably, the Campbell Collaboration has been set up as a parallel organization to Cochrane for reviewing interventions in social policy, education, and criminology. Additionally, entities such as the European Observatory on Health Systems and Policies offer a template for systematic tracking of health system development and change.

Further, systematic partnerships are needed not only between researchers and policy makers, but should also involve research funding bodies and civil society organizations, including professional associations, that are part of the policy-making and policy implementation processes. Capacity-building efforts will be needed not only at individual and organizational levels, but across the network of players. Such capacity-building efforts need to build on existing capacities, link local knowledge with more global research evidence, respect the diverse value systems,

Table 5 Practical steps for improving knowledge transfer between researchers and policy makers: Reducing the gap

Steps to be taken by researchers	Steps to be taken by policy makers
Communicate research findings simply through newsletters, summaries, etc.	Set up advisory mechanisms to help identify research priorities
Hold briefings, seminars, and workshops for policy makers	Built evaluation research into programs and budgets and publish findings
Discuss policy implications or include policy recommendations in research	Ensure research funding bodies develop program of strategic, priority-driven research
Target opinion leaders for research disseminations	Develop a culture of learning organization within government departments, including regular seminar programs and sabbaticals for policy analysts
Involve policy makers in all stages of the research process	Develop in-house research capacity, including commissioning of policy research
Conduct more policy-relevant research, including more action research, evaluation research, and systems research	Establish policy research institutions that have ongoing involvement in policy monitoring and analysis
Offer training to policy makers on critical appraisal and commissioning of systematic reviews	Provide training for researchers on, and involve them in, policy development processes

Adapted from Lin V (2003b) Improving the research and policy partnership: An agenda for research transfer and governance. In: *Evidence-Based Health Policy: Problems and Possibilities*, pp. 285–297. Melbourne: Oxford University Press; and Buse K, Mays N, and Walt G (2005) *Making Health Policy* Maidenhead: Open University Press.

challenge mindsets and power differentials, establish positive incentives, and find ways for diverse players to stay engaged in the longer term (Blagescu and Young, 2006).

Knowledge transfer may also require more explicit recognition that a range of individuals are likely to play different roles in the process (Thompson *et al.*, 2006), i.e., opinion leaders exert informal social influence within a specialty area on an on-going basis and community leaders similarly influence civil society understanding about issues. Linking agents (or knowledge brokers) may formally bridge gaps on specific issues or in specific organizational contexts, change agents (or champions), and may promote and drive behavioral and organizational change across groups and issues. As Kerner (2006) suggests, translating research into policy would require a common language and common understanding about the meaning of knowledge translation and the nature of evidence. This effort may well need to be underpinned by more research on how best to disseminate and implement research, as well as dissemination and implementation of research results.

For developing countries, donor organizations and international institutions will have a particular role to play in supporting capacity development. The World Bank Institute, the capacity development branch of the World Bank, is one such example. The aim of the Institute is to not only reach policy makers, researchers, and practitioners across the globe, but to also to share knowledge with parliamentarians, journalists, teachers, youth, and civil society leaders. The World Health Organization also has a similar agenda of removing barriers to research use (WHO, 2005). Civil society organizations and educational institutions may be particularly important in reaching key segments of society, as well as converting local knowledge from anecdote to evidence.

Conclusion

In public health policy, the key question is not just what works, but what works for whom, in what circumstances, and in what ways? Research and evaluation that help answer these questions can assist with the development of appropriately considered policies, thus supporting the creation of a more level playing field in the political marketplace (Marmor and Christianson, 1982), thus allowing for a more balanced set of voices to be heard in the political process of policy making.

The differences between the two worlds of researchers and policy makers are often cited as providing obstacles preventing research from being taken up into policy making. In response to this problem, infrastructure to promote knowledge transfer and capacity building to bridge the gap between these two communities is increasingly being put into place within and between institutions. However, while the two-worlds concept is useful for thinking about the challenges faced in making policy evidence-based, it may be insufficient for incorporating all of the stakeholders and actors in the policy process, especially if the research being funded and conducted is not addressing questions that are central to the concerns of policy players.

Health concerns all of civil society, and so social, economic, cultural, political, and ethical considerations do influence agenda setting, policy formation, and implementation to varying degrees. Therefore, seeking an evidence base for public health policy may mean taking into account many different forms of evidence, in addition to evidence of efficacy and effectiveness. The consideration of local, colloquial, and contextual evidence is increasingly recognized by some within the movement of evidence-based policy for its influence upon all aspects of policy formation and implementation.

In taking such evidence into account, linear models of research utilization for the making of public health policy are too simplistic, because they disregard the many contextual factors influencing decision making, particularly the political process. Research evidence may be more usefully understood as framing issues rather than providing the central picture. The research itself may be better conceptualized as influencing through ideas more so than through data. The language of evidence-informed policy and practice, then, is increasingly being recognized as appropriate for health policy making. Research can improve the evidential basis for public health policies, but this requires that more stakeholders – in civil society, in government, and in the business sector – are both skilled in appraising research as well as being an integral part of the research agenda setting process. More policy evaluation studies and health system observatories may also be useful for both informational and capacity-building purposes.

Acknowledgments

Rachel Canaway, La Trobe University – School of Public Health, for research and editorial comment.

See also: Planning, for Public Health Policy.

Citations

Anderson LM, Brownson RC, Fullilove MT, *et al.* (2005) Evidence-based public health policy and practice: Promises and limits. *American Journal of Preventive Medicine* 28: 226–230.

Atkins D, Siegel J, and Slutsky J (2005) Making policy when the evidence is in dispute. *Health Affairs* 24: 102.

Beck U (1992) *Risk Society Towards a New Modernity.* London: Sage Publications.

Birch S (1996) Equity and health outcomes. In: *Health Outcomes – Integrating Health Outcomes Measurement in Routine Health Care.*

Conference Proceedings. Canberra, Australia: Australian Institute of Health and Welfare.

Black N (2001) Evidence based policy: proceed with care. *British Medical Journal* 323: 275–279.

Blagescu M and Young J (2006) *Capacity development for policy advocacy: Current thinking and approaches among agencies supporting Civil Society Organisations - Working paper 260*, London: Overseas Development Institute.

Bowen S and Zwi AB (2005) Pathways to ''Evidence-Informed'' Policy and Practice: A Framework for Action. *PLoS Medicine* 2: e166.

Bridgman P and Davis G (2004) *The Australian Policy Handbook,* 3rd edn. Crows Nest, NSW: Allen and Unwin.

Brownson RC, Gurney JG, and Land GH (1999) Evidence-based decision making in public health. *Journal of Public Health Management and Practice* 5: 86–97.

Brownson RC, Royer C, Ewing R, and McBride TD (2006) Researchers and policymakers: Travelers in parallel universes. *American Journal of Preventive Medicine* 30: 164–172.

Buse K, Mays N, and Walt G (2005) *Making Health Policy.* Maidenhead, UK: Open University Press.

Choi BCK, Pang T, Lin V, et al. (2005) Can scientists and policy makers work together? *Journal of Epidemiology and Community Health* 59: 632–637.

CHSRF (2006) *Weighing up the Evidence: Making Evidence-Informed Guidance Accurate, Achievable, and Acceptable.* Ottawa, Canada: Canadian Health Services Research Foundation.

Cohen M, March J, and Olsen J (1972) A garbage can model of organizational choice. *Administrative Science Quarterly* 17: 1–25.

Cookson R (2005) Evidence-based policy making in health care: What it is and what it isn't. *Journal of Health Services Research and Policy* 10: 118.

Davies HTO and Marshall MN (2000) UK and US health-care systems: Divided by more than a common language. *The Lancet* 355: 336.

Davies HTO, Nutley SM, and Smith PC (2000) *What Works? Evidence-Based Policy and Practice in Public Service.* Bristol, UK: The Policy Press.

Dawes M, Summerskill W, Glasziou P, et al. (2005) Sicily statement on evidence-based practice. *BMC Medical Education* 5: 1–7.

Dery D (1984) *Problem Definition in Policy Analysis.* Lawrence, KS: University Press of Kansas.

Dobrow MJ, Goel V, and Upshur REG (2004) Evidence-based health policy: Context and utilization. *Social Science and Medicine* 58: 207–217.

Foucault M (2001) Governmentality. In: Faubion JD (ed.) *Power: Essential Works of Foucault, 1954–1984,* vol. 3, pp. 201–222. London: Penguin.

Gelijns AC, Brown LD, Magnell C, Ronchi E, and Moskowitz AJ (2005) Evidence, politics, and technological change. *Health Affairs* 24: 29–40.

Gray JAM (2001) *Evidence-Based Healthcare: How to Make Health Policy and Management Decisions,* 2nd edn. Edinburgh: Churchill Livingstone.

Gray JAM (2005) Evidence-based and value-based healthcare. *Evidence-Based Healthcare and Public Health* 9: 317–318.

Green LW (2006) Public health asks of systems science: To advance our evidence-based practice, can you help us get more practice-based evidence? *American Journal of Public Health* 96: 406–409.

Ham C, Hunter DJ, and Robinson R (1995) Evidence based policymaking: Research must inform health policy as well as medical care. *British Medical Journal* 310: 71–72.

Hanney SR, Gonzalez-Block MA, Buxton MJ, and Kogan M (2002) *The Utilisation of Health Research in Policy-Making: Concepts, Examples, and Methods of Assessment. A Report to the Research Policy and Co-operation Department World Health Organization Geneva.* Uxbridge: Health Economics Research Group Brunel University.

Kavanagh A, Daly J, and Jolley D (2002) Research methods, evidence and public health. *Australia and New Zealand Journal of Public Health* 26: 337–342.

Kavanagh A, Daly J, Melder A, and Jolley D (2003) 'Mind the gap': Assessing the quality of evidence for public health problems. In: Lin V and Gibson B (eds.) *Evidence-Based Health Policy: Problems and Possibilities,* pp. 70–79. Melbourne, Australia: Oxford University Press.

Kerner JF (2006) Knowledge translation versus knowledge integration: A ''funder's'' perspective. *The Journal of Continuing Education in the Health Professions* 26: 72–80.

Kingdon J (1984) *Agendas, Alternatives and Public Policies.* Boston, MA: Little Brown.

Kohatsu ND, Robinson JG, and Torner JC (2004) Evidence-based public health: An evolving concept. *American Journal of Preventive Medicine* 27: 417–421.

Lavis JN (2002) Ideas at the margin or marginalized ideas? Nonmedical determinants of health in Canada. *Health Affairs* 21: 107.

Lin V (2003a) Competing rationalities: Evidence-based health policy? In: Lin V and Gibson B (eds.) *Evidence-Based Health Policy: Problems and Possibilities,* pp. 3–17. Melbourne, Australia: Oxford University Press.

Lin V (2003b) Improving the research and policy partnership: An agenda for research transfer and governance. In: Lin V and Gibson B (eds.) *Evidence-Based Health Policy: Problems and Possibilities,* pp. 285–297. Melbourne, Australia: Oxford University Press.

Lin V and Fawkes S (2005) Achieving effectiveness in health promotion programs: Evidence, infrastructure and action. In: Browning C and Thomas S (eds.) *Behavioural Change: An Evidence-Based Handbook for Social and Public Health,* pp. 17–44. Edinburgh: Churchill-Livingston.

Lomas J (2000) Connecting research and policy. *Isuma: Canadian Journal of Policy Research* 1: 140–144.

Lomas J, Culyer T, McCutcheon C, McAuley L, and Law S (2005) *Conceptualizing and Combing Evidence for Health System Guidance.* Ottawa, Canada: Canadian Health Services Research Foundation.

Macintyre S (2003) Evidence based policy making: Impact on health inequalities still needs to be assessed. *British Medical Journal* 326: 5–6.

Marmor TR and Christianson JB (1982) *Health Care Policy: A Political Economy Approach.* Beverley Hills, CA: Sage.

Marshall MN, Romano PS, and Davies HTO (2005) How do we maximize the impact of the public reporting of quality of care? *International Journal for Quality in Health Care* 16: i57.

Millward LM, Kelly MP, and Nutbeam D (2003) *Public Health Intervention Research: The Evidence.* London: Health Development Agency.

National Institutes of Health (2006) *NIH Roadmap for Medical Research – Initiatives.* National Institutes of Health. http://nihroadmap.nih.gov/initiatives.asp (accessed September 2007).

NORA (1996) *National Occupational Research Agenda (NORA).* National Institute for Occupational Safety and Health (NIOSH). www.cdc.gov/niosh/nora (accessed September 2007).

Nutbeam D (2004) Getting evidence into policy and practice to address health inequalities. *Health Promotion International* 19: 137–140.

Nutley S and Webb J (2000) Evidence and the policy process. In: Davies HTO, Nutley SM and Smith PC (eds.) *What Works? Evidence-Based Policy and Practice in Public Services.* Bristol, UK: The Policy Press.

Oldenburg B, McGuffog ID, and Turrell G (2000) Socioeconomic determinants of health in Australia: Policy responses and intervention options. *Medical Journal of Australia* 172: 489–492.

Pawson R (2002) Evidence-based policy: In search of a method. *Evaluation* 8: 157–181.

Popay J (2006) *Moving Beyond Effectiveness in Evidence Synthesis: Methodological Issues in the Synthesis of Diverse Sources of Evidence.* London: National Institute for Health and Clinical Excellence.

Potter M, Quill B, Aglipay G, et al. (2006) Demonstrating excellence in practice-based research for public health. *Public Health Report* 121: 1–16.

Rix M and Matete S (2005) Is there ever enough evidence? The benefits and limits of evidence-based public health policy: the case of the

Victorian Children's Health and Wellbeing Project. Paper presented at the Australian Social Policy Conference, University of New South Wales, 20–22 July 2005.
Rodwin MA (2001) The politics of evidence-based medicine. *Journal of Health Politics Policy and Law* 26: 439–446.
Ross S, Lavis J, Rodriguez C, Woodside J, and Denis J-L (2003) Partnership experiences: Involving decision-makers in the research process. *Journal of Health Services Research and Policy* 8: S26.
Sabatier PA and Jenkins-Smith H (1993) *Policy Change and Learning: An Advocacy Coalition Approach.* Boulder, CO: Westview Press.
Sackett DL, Rosenberg WMC, Gray JAM, Haynes RB, and Richardson WS (1996) Evidence based medicine: what it is and what it isn't. *British Medical Journal* 312: 71–72.
Sheldon TA (2005) Making evidence synthesis more useful for management and policy-making. *Journal of Health Services Research and Policy* 10: S1.
Short S (1997) Elective affinities: Research and health policy development. In: Gardner H (ed.) *Health Policy in Australia.* Melbourne, Australia: Oxford University Press.
Terris M (1980) Epidemiology as a guide to health policy. *Annual Review of Public Health* 1: 323–344.
Thompson GN, Estabrooks CA, and Degner LF (2006) Clarifying the concepts in knowledge transfer: A literature review. *Journal of Advanced Nursing* 53: 691–701.
United Kingdom Cabinet Office (1999a) *Modernising Government White Paper.* London: Cabinet Office Government of the United Kingdom.
United Kingdom Cabinet Office (1999b) *Professional Policy Making for the Twenty First Century. Report by the Strategic Policy Making Team.* London: Cabinet Office Government of the United Kingdom.
Weiss C (1979) The many meanings of research utilization. *Public Administration Review* 39: 426–431.
Weiss C (1991) Policy research: Data, ideas or arguments? In: Wagner P, Weiss C, Wittrock B and Woman H (eds.) *Social Sciences and Modern States*, pp. 307–332. Cambridge, UK: Cambridge University Press.
WHO (2005) *Bridging the "Know-Do" Gap: Meeting on Knowledge Translation in Global Health.* Geneva, Switzerland: World Health Organization.

Further Reading

Lin V and Gibson B (eds.) (2003) *Evidence-Based Health Policy: Problems and Possibilitie.* Melbourne, Australia: Oxford University Press.

Relevant Websites

http://www.chsrf.ca – Canadian Health Services Research Foundation (CHSRF).
http://www.campbellcollaboration.org – The Campbell Collaboration.
http://www.cochrane.org – The Cochrane Collaboration.
http://www.euro.who.int/observatory – European Observatory on Health Care Systems and Policies.
EPPIWeb/EPPIWeb/home.aspx or EPPIWeb/ – Evidence for Policy and Practice Information and Coordinating Centre (EPPI-Centre).
http://www.joannabriggs.edu.au – The Joanna Briggs Institute.
http://www.nice.org.uk – National Institute for Clinical Excellence (NICE).
http://www.policyhub.gov.uk – United Kingdom Cabinet Office Policy Hub.
http://www.worldbank.org/wbi/home.html – The World Bank Institute.
http://www.who.int/kms/en – World Health Organization (WHO): Knowledge management and health.

Planning, for Public Health Policy

A T Green and T N Mirzoev, University of Leeds, Leeds, UK

© 2008 Elsevier Inc. All rights reserved.

Health Planning – What Is It?

Definition of Health Planning, Overall Purpose of Planning, Relationship to Policy Making

Health planning can be defined as: "a systematic approach to attaining explicit objectives for the future through the efficient and appropriate use of resources, available now and in the future" (Green, 2007: 3).

Many definitions of planning focus on technical aspects such as setting goals, outlining broad strategies and developing detailed activities. Health planning, however, also involves the art of maneuvering between different actors and processes in the context of the health system to achieve desired objectives. It is thus also a political process and one that involves real choices between alternatives, each with different technical and political advantages and disadvantages. The need for planning arises from the shortfall between the available resources and the resources needed to address the perceived health needs that face health systems. This highlights the importance of prioritization as a key feature of health planning.

Health planning can be perceived as a continuation of health policy-making, i.e., translation of policy outputs (statements, documents) into implementation strategies and plans. This 'operationalization' of policy outputs can occur at different levels of a country's health system (e.g., national, regional) and result in different types of plans (e.g., strategic plan, rolling operational plan). Health planning and health policy making are both often described as cycles with clearly defined stages and continuous nature of the process.

A distinction needs to be made between *health planning* and *health-care planning*. The former recognizes the wider determinants of health and the need for multisectoral initiatives while the latter focuses on health services. This article assumes the first, broader scope.

Planning can be interpreted as an attempt to address the following questions:

1. Where are we now?
2. Where do we want to be?
3. How are we going to get there?

Different types of planning focus on different aspects of these questions. For example, strategic planning, which is often seen as an integral part of health policy making, is concerned with defining the priority direction for the development of a sector or a program (the second question). In contrast with this, operational planning is more concerned with the technicalities of the process, as in the third question.

The purpose of planning should not be seen as merely the *production* of plans, but also their *implementation*. As such it includes monitoring and evaluation, which lead to the next cycle of the planning process. Planning is therefore closely linked with both policy making and management. Health planning is also concerned with negotiating priorities and strategies between key actors, which reinforces its links with health policy making.

Historical Roots

Although planning is sometimes described as having emerged as a discipline in industrialized countries after World War II (Rodwin, 1984), it can be argued to have existed earlier. For example, John Snow is often regarded as the father of modern epidemiology, and there are certainly elements of health planning in his work; the Soviet Union introduced 5-year national development plans in 1928 and India has developed national development plans since 1951. Planning is a separate discipline in virtually every sector including health. Furthermore, planning is embedded into almost every aspect of the health system ranging from planning of an individual patient's treatment course to planning sector development for the next decade.

Health Planning – The Main Features

While the rationale for planning (the need to make choices about the use of scarce resources) is common to planning in all sectors, there are some distinctive features to health planning. Health is a very labor-intensive sector with the time needed to train a health professional often being several years. As such long-term human resource planning is critical for the health sector.

A second feature of health planning is the complex power relations between the various actors involved in or influencing decision-making processes. This includes both external (donors, international agencies) and internal (health ministry, professional associations, civil society) stakeholders. Health planning, because of close links with health policy making, is seen as both a technical and a political process with different groups of stakeholders bringing different agendas into the process. Mechanisms of engagement and the degree of influence of various actors may vary (for instance, some may impose conditionality, whereas others may use advocacy as the main instrument of influence). Complex interrelationships between different groups of stakeholders can have an impact on the approaches to, and success of, health planning.

A third characteristic of health planning is the tension between the clinical perspective (focus on individuals) versus the public health perspective (focus on populations). Planning within the health system needs to find an accommodation between both perspectives.

Values in Planning

The technical basis of planning suggests the need for rationality of approach, efficiency, and the use of evidence to support decisions. One important issue in health planning relates to objectivity. While the use of evidence in the planning process is essential, it is also important to recognize both that information or evidence may not be available or reliable and that selection and interpretation of information can also reflect particular values and judgments. Indeed all parts of the planning process involve values. Key ones are those related to equity, gender, human rights, solidarity, and wider choice to patients and communities. Different stakeholders will, of course, have different ideological perspectives and values.

Figure 1 provides a conceptual framework for the planning system showing the relationships of the processes, actors, values, and the wider context.

Each factor resulting from the above elements of the conceptual framework affects the broad approach to planning, use of evidence in the planning processes, as well as the other context-specific characteristics of health planning such as the choice of priorities.

Health planning occurs at different organizational levels of the health system. Priorities and values may differ at the national level from those at the local level.

Links Between Planning and Other Decision-Making Processes

For planning to function effectively, it needs to be embedded in all the decision-making processes within the health sector. Most planning failures can be traced to a lack of consistency between these different systems. This is exemplified in **Table 1** with illustrative planning questions across the main components of the health system.

Questions for planning vary, depending on the level of the health system. For example, national-level policy makers may be more concerned with the priority areas

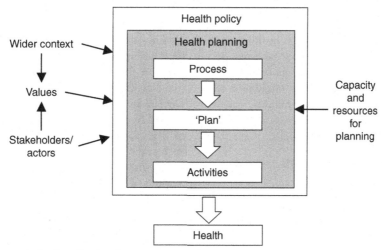

Figure 1 Conceptual framework of health planning.

Table 1 Planning questions across the main components of the health system

Health system component	Illustrative planning questions
Health policy making	• What are the current priority areas for the national health development policy? • Are these likely to change in the next 10 years? • Who should be involved in policy formulation? • How can the use of evidence in health policies be enhanced to promote equity?
Human resources	• How many nurses and doctors do we need now and in the future? • What should their qualification be now and in the future? • What are the ways of ensuring an optimal quantity and quality?
Health financing	• What resources do we need to cover the population's health needs now and in the future? • What is the best way to generate these resources? • What is the best option to ensure value for money in the health sector?
Service delivery	• What approach to service delivery is the most effective and efficient within the given context? • How may this approach change in the future? • What is the best way to ensure the quality of services and care? • What should be the balance between equity and efficiency in providing health services?
Institutional arrangements	• What should be the public–private relationships to ensure generation of adequate resources and availability of affordable high-quality care? • What type of decentralization is the most appropriate to the given context to ensure proper response to the health needs? • What is the best way of assessing performance of health facilities?
Health management information system	• What information do we need for making informed decisions at each level of the health system? • How often should this information be collected? • At what level should the data be processed and analyzed?
Responding to people's expectations	• What is the best way to involve communities in determining their health needs? • What is the best way to conduct health education in the given context?
Acting on the wider determinants of health	• How can other sectors be encouraged to increase health-promotional activities and minimize health-damaging activities?

for a country's overall health policy and the availability of resources including professional staff, while the primary planning issue for local decision makers would be how to ensure an adequate response to the policy direction in terms of service provision.

The need for planning and the type of planning decisions at each level of the health system also depend on the degree of autonomy and wider decision-making practices in society. For example, if budgeting is seen as a bottom-up process the role of the national level will be to respond to locally identified needs, while if the health system is highly centralized and hierarchical, the local level is likely to follow nationally set directives.

Who Should Plan

Health planning should be a shared task at all levels of the health system. Planning is, however, often seen as the responsibility of a separate administrative unit. But planning is wider than this and requires constant interaction between decision makers, managers, and professionals at all levels. This suggests the need for input into planning by decision makers at each health system level with the planning unit performing advisory and facilitatory functions and guiding decisions from a technical perspective. The ultimate decisions would be made by relevant stakeholders such as community leaders, patients, and health professionals.

The Context of Health Planning

Health planning occurs within the political and socioeconomic context involving complex links between the wider societal factors and health planning processes. Key contextual factors include:

- stage of development of a particular country (for example, countries in transition);
- power of different groups directly or indirectly involved in the decision-making process;
- historical decision-making processes;
- resource framework;
- available planning expertise and skills;
- institutional arrangements for implementing plans.

The context in which planning takes place is ever-changing. In particular, the health pattern is changing due to a complex set of factors including demographic and epidemiological transition and the emergence of new diseases such as HIV/AIDS or avian flu; public sector (including health) systems may be reformed; costs are rising and the expectations of users are growing. These and other important factors set the complex contextual environment for health planning.

Planning has moved away from "...intuitive, spontaneous, and subjective projection of activity based on past experience to a much more deliberate, systematic and objective process of mobilizing information and organizing resources" (Reinke, 1988: 3).

Changing Environment

Objectives for health planning may change as health systems develop. One can observe emphasis on different aspects of health and health system at different times. For example, in the eighteenth and nineteenth centuries, efforts were directed mainly toward responding to epidemics and focusing on wider determinants of health, building health systems, and developing health (social) insurance (Hyman, 1982); until the mid-1960s, planning largely focused on managing growth of the health sector; in the 1970s and 1980s, planning efforts were concentrated on improving access to health services and the 1990s were characterized by health sector reforms. New issues for national health planning include integration of global vertical health programs with national health systems and a return to wider social determinants of health.

Since the late 1970s, health planning has been increasingly influenced by international actors and their priorities and policies. One of the first international health planning efforts was the set of elements of the Alma Ata Declaration (Primary Health Care strengthening, Health For All by the Year 2000), which prompted development of PHC in many contexts. More recently, global targets such as the 3-by-5 initiative (treating three million people living with HIV/AIDS by 2005), which was launched by WHO and UNAIDS in 2003, and the adoption of Millennium Development Goals at the UN General Assembly in 2000 have shaped international health; this is also reflected in the increasing number of international agencies and in particular Global Public Private Partnerships such as the GAVI Alliance and the Global Fund to Fight AIDS, TB and Malaria.

Planning for Public–Private Mix and Regulatory Role of the Government/Public Sector

Marketization of the health system was widely advocated in the 1990s and this policy encouraged a greater role for the private sector. The resultant complexity in the public–private mix suggests the need for changes in the approaches from what had often been a primary focus on public sector health services. It suggests the need to develop new planning tools suitable for inducing appropriate change in the private sector. While public-sector planning relies heavily on managerial directives and controls, planning for the private sector requires use of legislative and regulatory tools, advocacy, and the use of incentives.

Planning for Decentralization

Decentralization is another example of a changing context. This may be either part of a wider governance policy or health-sector-specific, and indeed may be part of health plans themselves.

The approach to planning will depend on the type and degree of decentralization of the health sector. For example, devolution (devolution is the most comprehensive form of decentralization, which is different from deconcentration where vertical lines of management control are retained), is likely to result in wider participation of local levels and hence bottom-up planning, and greater opportunities for multisectoral action.

An important aspect of decentralization is the process and criteria whereby central funds are allocated to lower levels. Resource allocation formulae based on needs are being increasingly introduced to replace historical incremental systems of allocation.

Planning Within Emergency and Transitional Countries

Within rapidly changing environments such as emergencies, planning is likely to concentrate on short-term objectives. One example of short-term planning objectives from a public health perspective is provision of safe drinking water to prevent water-borne infections in the wake of a humanitarian disaster.

Planning within transitional countries where the situation changes faster than in more stable contexts may be best done on a rolling or incremental basis.

Technical Issues in Health Planning

In broad terms, approaches to planning can be described as being on a continuum with two extremes: Top-down and bottom-up. The top-down approach implies that the planning process occurs exclusively at the central level with only final decisions (plans) communicated to the local levels. The bottom-up approach encompasses the idea of local levels being closely involved in the planning process through assessment of health needs, identification of priorities, and participation in other planning decisions. Top-down planning is normally found in centralized systems with strong command and control mechanisms with bottom-up planning in genuinely decentralized contexts. The latter provides an opportunity for wider participation and empowerment of stakeholders in decision-making processes including planning, which stems from contemporary disillusionment with top-down processes of command and control. Each approach has its strengths and weaknesses but nowadays there is a preference at the international level for bottom-up health planning, which is partly the result of disillusionment with the effectiveness of top-down processes.

From the perspective of the level of the health system, health planning can occur at country, sector, program, or project levels. Health planning can also be described as strategic or operational. Strategic planning is an integral part of health policy, is normally broad, long-term, and associated with central levels of the health system, while operational planning is short term, more detailed and particularly relevant to the local levels of health system.

Approaches to health planning also relate to the wider decision-making styles and can be divided into three broad categories:

- status quo models, i.e., reproducing previous plans;
- reactive planning, i.e., plan only if it is regarded as necessary – this may include problem-solving approaches;
- rational proactive planning.

Characteristics of these approaches are described in **Table 2**. There will inevitably be intermediate approaches which contain elements from more than one approach. An example of this is incremental planning, which can be described as small adjustments to the status quo in the light of current political circumstances (Buse *et al.*, 2005).

Forecasting can be an important part of health planning. From the health planning perspective, forecasting can be seen as a process of projecting any determinants of health planning such as future health service delivery needs for a particular population. Examples of forecasting can be seen in the models that attempt to predict future health professional requirements to respond to the health needs arising from a projected population growth and/or shifts in disease patterns. It is important to ensure that such forecasting takes account of the particular context of a health system and does not apply uncritically international blueprints.

It can, however, be difficult to differentiate between *evidence-based projections/modeling*, which may be part of rational planning, and *blueprinting*, which shares some characteristics with status quo planning. In contrast with evidence-based projections, an implicit assumption within blueprinting is that the same models (health plans) can be replicated in different contexts. In practice, however, the ever-changing environment provides just one example of the need for contextualization in health planning.

We consider rational planning, which takes account of political influences as optimal, and will focus here on the processes related to this. However, any approach inevitably has downsides and the rational approach is no exception. Some downsides include the significant human resource capacity required, the need for reliable information (evidence), and the ability of key actors to believe in results of rational approaches. It is important also to recognize that in practice the distinction between different approaches is blurred.

Types of Planning

There is no general consensus on the terms for types of health planning. Different perspectives are used to classify different types of health planning. For example, some classifications follow the lines of comprehensive-program-project (Taylor and Reinke, 1988) where comprehensive stands for broad strategic planning and the next steps focus on operational planning. Another perspective distinguishes types of health planning across main levels of planning, e.g., national, regional, and district (Green, 2007).

Health planning is a chain of interrelated processes involving different levels of planning (country, sector, program, project). Within this, the logic of one process being translated into another is evident. This is exemplified in **Table 3**.

Table 2 Characteristics of main approaches to health planning

Criteria	Approach		
	Status quo	Reactive	Rational
Wider context of public sector	Likely centralized system with fixed budgetary framework	Countries in emergencies and transition	Likely decentralized with flexible expenditure framework
Major guiding principles	Often input-based, rarely geographical	Problem and resource-driven	Population- and health needs-based
Use of information (evidence)	Unlikely	Limited to problem-related	Likely at all stages
Consistency between different levels of planning (e.g., strategic, operational)	Only if stable health situation context and resource framework	Unlikely since most planning efforts focused on short-term solutions without wider framework	Most likely
Responsiveness to the health needs	Unlikely, especially with changing health status	Only immediate health needs are responded to with focus being on health project	Most likely with planning focusing around health rather than health projects
Response to wider values such as equity	Only if stable health and socioeconomic context	Unlikely as these are difficult to consider in the short term	Most likely
Flexibility to adapt to the changing context (resource framework, people's expectations, etc.)	Unlikely	Likely in the short term	Likely in the long term
Account of dynamics of resource framework	Unlikely, especially in the changing context	Likely in the short term	Likely in the long term
Human resource capacity (skills) needs	Technical programing and budgeting skills	Needs assessment; technical programing and budgeting	Strategic approach; needs assessment; technical programing and budgeting
Degree of involvement of key stakeholders	Limited to primary decision makers	Expanded to include civil society	Likely to be widest involvement
Transparency and accountability	Often blurred and accountability is unclear	Yes, if a long-term approach is deployed but difficult to monitor/supervise in the short term	Likely

Table 3 Levels and types of planning

PSRPs	Poverty Reduction Strategy Papers (PSRPs) (see World Bank and IMF websites) are normally developed at a country level and represent the broadest type of planning that focuses on the overall public sector. PRSPs are intersectoral initiatives and comprise objectives for all public sectors such as health, economics, agriculture, education, housing, and others. As such, health, although part of the wider societal objective, is not an explicit objective of the PRSP. The strategy, being at a country level, is normally complemented by government's Medium-Term Expenditure Framework – state resource commitments for the next 5–10 years along identified priorities
SWAps	Sector-Wide Approach (SWAp) is an example of sector-specific planning (see the STI and KIT websites). The core of a health SWAp is in shared health development policy with agreed broad health development objectives. Other key elements of a SWAp include the leading role of national government in dialogue with donors, an appropriate expenditure framework, agreed operational procedures and an agreed model for monitoring and evaluation. SWAp is a process that attempts to coordinate efforts to achieve a shared health policy
Policy/strategy	The health policy or strategy is the next level of health planning. The terms health policy and strategy are often used interchangeably. However, the strategy should be seen as a means of achieving the policy. In practice, health ministries often produce a health policy document, which comprises both broad policy direction and more detailed strategic approaches to achieving country health goals. Examples of health policies and strategies from UK DOH can be found here http://www.dh.gov.uk/PolicyAndGuidances/en
Program/project/ operational planning	Program and project planning incorporate the next level of detail (operational aspects) of health planning. Programs (example of TB program is here http://www.emro.who.int/stb/egypt/AboutNTP.htm) are normally broader than projects (an example of a women's health project is here http:/www.health.org/about/index.html) and represent vertical initiatives such as MCH or HIV/AIDS with specific objectives and detailed implementation plans. As health is a cross-sectoral issue, health programs should include actions from other sectors, which is not always the practice. Projects are time-limited specific initiatives within a specific field
Logframe	A logframe, or Logical Framework, approach is a tool often used by donors as a way of mapping out the hierarchy of a health program or project in a concise way. The distinctive feature of this type of planning is the possibility of illustrating the consistency and continuity of different levels of objectives, namely outcomes, outputs, and activities

Another feature of different types and levels of planning is the time-frame. The higher the level of planning the longer the timeframe for achieving objectives. For example, Poverty Reduction Strategy Papers and Sector-Wide Approaches may be processes for 5+ years, while operational planning is usually done on an annual/semi-annual/quarterly basis.

The Rolling Plan (**Figure 2**) is another type of plan that emphasizes the continuous nature of health planning at the operational level.

One theme from the above is the necessity of a clear link between strategic and operational aspects of health planning. We suggest that this is two-way: Operational planning should develop implementation aspects of wider strategy and strategic planning and is an opportunity to scale up positive experience from implementation of operational plans. This is particularly true in the case of pilot initiatives, where innovative ideas are tested.

New techniques for health planning are being continuously developed, including at the international level. Marginal budgeting for bottlenecks (MBB) is an example of a new method developed by UNICEF, WHO, and the World Bank, which attempts to identify bottlenecks (factors negatively affecting implementation) and estimate the marginal cost of eliminating these. As a result of the close relationship between strategic and operational levels of health planning, MBB is seen to be a useful tool to help countries develop their Medium-Term Expenditure Frameworks and align efforts toward more effective and efficient utilization of available resources. MBBs normally comprise three components: Identification of barriers (bottlenecks), costing, and assessment of possible impact (Knippenberg et al., undated).

Stages of the Planning Process

Planning processes can be illustrated in the form of a spiral. Green's planning spiral (**Figure 3**) is a classical example of approaching planning from a rational–comprehensive perspective and illustrating it as a continuous process.

Green's model includes six stages (situational analysis, priority setting, option appraisal, programing, implementation and monitoring, and evaluation). Within the public health context, these broadly correspond to the following five stages of making a decision on the best public health intervention (Walley et al., 2004):

1. assessing health needs (which corresponds to situational analysis stage in the Green's planning spiral);
2. reviewing health services and programs (situational analysis and priority-setting stage);
3. choosing the best interventions (option appraisal stage);
4. listing the activities and drafting an action plan (programing stage);
5. implementing and monitoring (implementation and monitoring and evaluation stages).

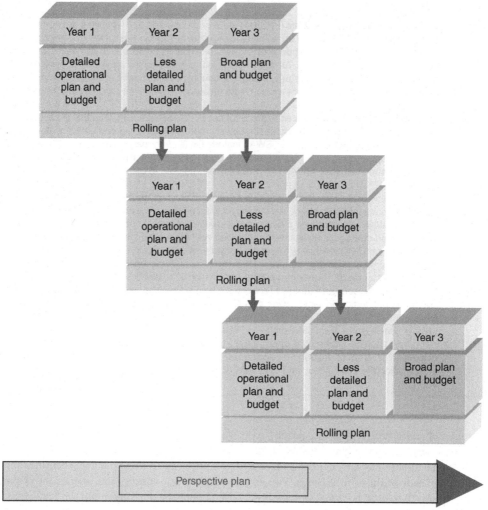

Figure 2 Three-year rolling plan and long-term perspective plan. From Green A (2007) *An Introduction to Health Planning for Developing Health Systems*, p. 292, 3rd edn. London: Oxford University Press, by permission of Oxford University Press.

The process of health planning usually involves iteration (as exemplified by the spiral) and should not be seen as linear.

Situational Analysis

A situational analysis answers the question: Where are we now? The end result of the situational analysis is a map of the health sector that includes a number of elements:

- the demographic, social, political, economic, and institutional context of the health system;
- the health needs and the key factors affecting those health needs;
- the current services provided, their type, ownership, and level of activity and general performance;
- the resources available to the health sector both in terms of finance and real resources;
- identification of key stakeholders and actors related to this issue.

The situational analysis should also look at distributional issues particularly in terms of equity and should estimate the future situation in terms of health needs and resources.

Priority Setting

As indicated earlier, planning is associated with resource constraints. Not all health needs can be met and society must prioritize which interventions are essential for the achievement of desired objectives and which can either be postponed or skipped. Prioritization occurs at different levels and there is no technical standard as to the criteria for assessing and comparing health needs and who should set priorities. The guiding principles may include values (equity, gender, rights) as well as organizational motivation to improve performance such as efficiency. Wider participation of key actors (community, health professionals, policy makers) can improve responsiveness to the *actual* health needs rather than the needs *perceived* by

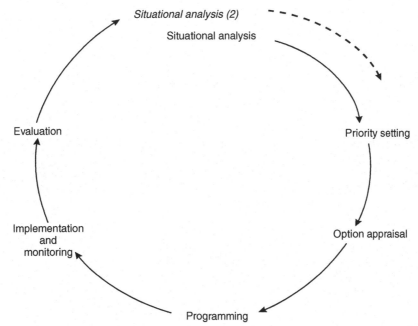

Figure 3 The planning spiral. From Green A (2007) *An Introduction to Health Planning for Developing Health Systems*, 3rd edn. p. 36, London: Oxford University Press, by permission of Oxford University Press.

decision makers. Economic appraisal techniques such as cost per disability-adjusted life year (a health measure introduced by the World Bank in the World Development Report 1993 and increasingly used in health planning afterward) may be used to set priorities based on a criterion of maximum health impact for given resources, but this can be criticized as being a narrow interpretation of goals and incorporating various contestable implicit values. For example, DALYs were recently criticized for taking into account only age, sex, disability period, and time with no consideration of the socioeconomic circumstances and thus focusing more on efficiency at the expense of equity (Anand and Hanson, 1998). Stakeholder analysis, Delphi techniques, multivariable decision-making matrices, and others are also important in prioritization and give greater emphasis to the political nature of planning.

The end result of priority setting stage should be a set of objectives. As shown in **Figure 4**, these are normally across the hierarchy Goal/Aim → Objectives → Targets/Milestones, which often corresponds to the LogFrame approach. The abbreviation SMART is often used as a checklist to appraise objectives against five criteria (specific, measurable, attainable, relevant, and timebound).

Option Appraisal

At this stage, different alternatives for achieving the same objectives are assessed. The criteria for decisions should include underpinning values within the health system such as equity, but are often inappropriately driven only by performance-based judgments such as efficiency and technical and financial feasibility through techniques such as economic appraisal. It is helpful to deploy a holistic approach and include as many relevant criteria for assessing different options as possible to be able to form a comprehensive understanding of hidden issues such as cultural acceptability, sustainability of results in the long term, likely effects on health needs, and/or people's expectations. One of the key criteria that should be considered is feasibility, including acceptability to key stakeholders. The use of stakeholder analysis at this stage is often important.

Techniques for option appraisal are similar to the ones used for priority setting and can be important in technology assessment including the development of Essential Service Packages. Examples of this can be found in the UK National Institute for Health and Clinical Excellence and WHO CHOICE initiative.

Programming

This is the stage when the plan – the tangible output of the health planning process – is produced. The degree of detail within the plan depends on the level at which the document is produced. For example, a 10-year national health plan will have a relatively broad policy direction with fewer details on organizational requirements. In contrast, annual operational plans would outline the budget details, staff needs, supply system, and a detailed description of means of monitoring progress. The plan usually comprises sections, which mirror the stages of planning: background or situational analysis, rationale or priority setting, justification or option appraisal, workplan

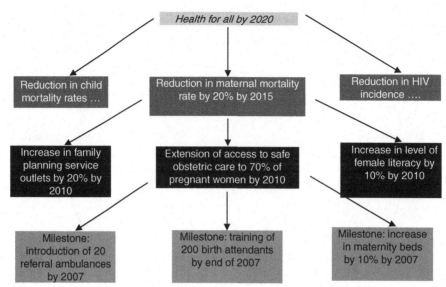

Figure 4 Example of the hierarchy of objectives. From Green A (2007) *An Introduction to Health Planning for Developing Health Systems*, 3rd edn. p. 202, London: Oxford University Press, by permission of Oxford University Press.

with identification of resources needed or programing, and monitoring and evaluation.

LogFrames have often been used as a tool to map out the health project in a concise format. Gantt charts present activities over a period of time. A number of programing tools are readily available, such as Microsoft Project. Costing and budgeting, integral components of programing, are often undertaken using spreadsheet templates designed for a particular program (see examples of WHO tools: the Cost It software tool and the mother-baby package costing spreadsheet).

The end product of this stage is a plan. It is, however, important to remember that the plan is not the end of the planning process but represents an intermediate output.

Implementation and monitoring

Appropriate implementation is critical to the success of planning. Monitoring is the process by which progress is assessed. In many cases, implementation is the responsibility of implementing agencies, whereas the plan itself may be produced by planners alone. Where this is the case, difficulties may arise, including a lack of a comprehensive understanding of the objectives and means of achieving them and inadequate measures to monitor progress. Monitoring can often be based on existing support systems such as health management information systems (HMIS) or, less desirably, may require the establishment of a vertical system to collect, process, and analyze the data or even *ad hoc* surveys. Monitoring should be seen as a tool to support implementation and to help identify problems and adjust actions during implementation rather than as a 'tick box' exercise. The indicators and methods for monitoring should reflect the way of achieving the objectives and should lead to the next stage: evaluation.

Techniques used for programing such as Gantt charts are important for implementation and monitoring. The end product of this stage of planning is the record of implementation of a particular initiative and an assessment of progress during implementation.

Evaluation

Evaluation is the process of assessing whether the objectives set have been achieved and the causes for any deviation from this. It may be formative where it takes place during the implementation phase (allowing the opportunity to learn and adjust, and as such is closely related to monitoring) or summative. Summative evaluations are conducted at the end of a plan or project period. Evaluation often involves a combination of managers involved in the activity to gain access to in-depth understanding and facilitate learning, and outside experts to encourage objectivity. Information gained from an evaluation feeds into the next round of planning and the situational analysis.

The end result of this stage of the evaluation is a report on the implemented set of outputs, outcomes, and impact against its objectives.

Planning for Specific Inputs

The above has described the overarching approach to strategic and operational planning. Another aspect of the process relates to planning for specific inputs, which are briefly considered below.

Human resource planning

As health-care provision is extremely labor-intensive, it is essential that attention be paid to ensuring the right numbers of staff are trained, employed, and retained. Human resource planning is the subdiscipline that deals with this. Inadequate attention has been paid to human resource planning in recent years with the result that many health systems have a mismatch between their service plans and the staffing available. This has been further aggravated recently by international migration. It is essential that health systems analyze the needs for staff and develop appropriate policies acting on both the demand for and supply of staff that align with service plans.

Infrastructure planning

Planning for new buildings and equipment has often been seen as a key part of planning (indeed often, inappropriately, given more priority than service planning). There are particular skills required in this aspect of planning in terms of ensuring that building designs meet user requirements and that the recurrent cost implications of new projects are fully recognized.

Financial planning

We have already referred to the chain of financial allocations that occur and it is essential that planners align their plans with this process. Unfortunately, there is often an organizational mismatch between planning and financial planning, with different authorities for each. Financial planning is an integral element of health planning and is concerned with matching the resources to the existing plan. It is closely related to, but different from budgeting, in that it is concerned with broad matching of available funds with plans rather than specific budgets. Examples of financial planning at a wider public sector level include Medium-Term Expenditure Framework (MTEF) and Public Investment Programme (PIP).

Capacity Required for Health Planning

Planning is not the sole responsibility of health planners. It should be seen as an integral element in the work of everyone who works within the health system, facilitated by specialists. However, the level and type of planning determines its characteristics, and this in turn affects the specialist capacity required.

Capacity for health planning does not only comprise a group of individuals with specific skills and experience. Besides technical skills in traditional disciplines such as epidemiology and economics, adequate planning capacity normally requires skills in other areas such as political analysis and advocacy. Planning also needs to draw on other processes within the health system such as the Health Management Information System.

Actors Involved in Health Planning

Planning occurs at all levels of the health system, with different actors involved in developing pieces of a common jigsaw.

Local-level planners usually develop operational details of the broad nationally determined policy or strategy. However, at a single level, there are inevitably different categories of actors involved in planning. For example, at the national level the health ministry should work closely with the education ministry on medical education issues; within the health system at the district level, the district hospital manager should work in close conjunction with the district primary health-care manager on operational issues, but their actions are also expected to be concerted with other local health-related issues such as transport or employment. Civil society, being often outside of the formal public sector entities, represents another group of actors that can be involved in the health planning.

Mechanisms for engagement

A participatory approach involving key stakeholders is likely to improve the use of evidence, objectivity, and integration of planning efforts and to result in wider ownership of the planning product and prospects for implementation This suggests two issues related to stakeholder engagement in the planning process.

First, how can one ensure adequate participation of decision makers in the planning process? Planning processes need to be set up that fully involve key decision makers as part of their routine activity, which is seen as a key responsibility with appropriate incentives to reward time spent in considering the future as well as the immediate management issues.

Second, some groups of stakeholders such as civil society may not be easy to involve. Even those ostensibly involved in the planning process may not have the opportunity to express their views. There are various techniques for participation and empowerment of communities in the planning process (Rifkin and Pridmore, 2001). Direct involvement of representatives from these groups in the planning process via planning boards and workshops with appropriate training and support may help to empower such groups and to consider their views in the planning process.

Challenges in Planning

Earlier sections raised various challenges facing health planning, in particular:

- developing a balance between national and decentralized planning;
- responding to increasing international influences;

- achieving an appropriate balance between technical and political characteristics of health planning;
- forecasting – the balance between projections and blueprinting;
- scaling up positive experiences;
- harnessing new approaches to planning.

Development of Balance Between National and Decentralized Planning

A balance is needed between national and local level planning, and the systems at each level need to be developed appropriately and consistent with each other. Many countries, such as former Soviet states, still deploy top-down approaches as a means of communicating policy decisions and ensuring consistency of local planning initiatives with nationally determined agenda. However, top-down processes of command and control are increasingly seen as ineffective approaches, with health planning decisions often failing to recognize the local health needs or failing to be implemented. Deliberate strategies to develop local planning capacity and to shift national-level roles to reflect the changing approach to planning.

Responding to increasing international influences

As health systems become more closely affected by the international context through the globalization of health, and new financial instruments such as Global Public Private Partnerships, national planners need to be able to respond to resultant pressures and complexity (Buse and Harmer, 2007). For example, the changing complexity of the aid architecture has led to approaches to donor support such as SWAps.

Managing the tension between planning techniques and the politics of planning

Planning uses, as we have seen, various techniques. Planning involves making difficult choices about use of resources that will almost inevitably result in some groups becoming 'losers'. As such, it is inevitably a political process and health planners need to be aware of this and develop ways of managing this tension. Many techniques (such as cost-effectiveness and the use of DALYs as outcome measures) appear to be technical and as such politically neutral, and yet implicit within them are value judgments. There is a need to achieve a balance between political, value-driven outputs and technically justified planning decisions.

Forecasting – finding the right balance between modeling and blueprinting

Modern technology is increasingly likely to allow the possibility of developing models for projections in areas such as epidemiological trends, human resources, and resource requirements for health care. However, such models need to be context-specific and driven by the local situation.

Scaling up for MDGs

Global influences such as Millennium Development Goals, WHO's 3-by-5 HIV/AIDS initiative, UNAIDS 'road towards universal access' to HIV prevention and AIDS treatment care and support by 2010 and others call for scaling up different interventions in many countries in order to achieve international targets. This puts significant pressure on health planning systems at different levels (subnational, national/country, region) to align health resources for the achievement of objectives both at the program level and at the wider health system level.

This poses an important and difficult planning question: What interventions will work on a larger scale as effectively as they were piloted? Many small-scale initiatives at the subnational level may not be appropriate to the whole country. On the other hand, issues such as social insurance may only be applicable at the larger scale.

Developing and harnessing new approaches to health planning

Health planning needs to evolve constantly and is developing for new techniques. There are significant potential opportunities becoming available through technology to collect and analyze data in ways that have the potential to enhance planning decisions. Geographical mapping and the linkage of local information to IT-based HMIS systems such as the application of geographical information systems for epidemiological surveillance (WHO, 1999) or establishment of a seasonal climate forecasting system for operational use by different sectors, including planning the health services (Thomson et al., 2000) provide exciting possibilities for understanding health needs and exploring options to respond to these.

Key Summary

Health planning is a complex process with at least three distinctive features (health being a labor-intensive sector, complex relationships between different actors, and the balance between clinical and public health perspectives). Planning is the product of values, techniques, and power relationships between different groups. Health planning is a continuous process and the production of a plan should not be seen as the end product of this process.

Approaches to planning will vary depending on the wider societal principles of decision making. There are various stages within the health planning cycle, with inevitable iterations. Presently, health planning faces a number of challenges and ultimately is an art of maneuvering within existing circumstances to achieve the desired objectives.

See also: Demand and Supply of Human Resources for Health; Global Health Initiatives and Public Health Policy; Health Policy: Overview; Resource Allocation: International Perspectives on Resource Allocation; The State in Public Health, The Role of.

Citations

Anand S and Hanson K (1998) DALYs: efficiency versus equity. *World Development* 26(2): 307–310.
Buse K, Mays N, and Walt G (2005) *Making Health Policy.* Maidenhead, UK: Open University Press.
Buse K and Harmer AM (2007) Seven habits of highly effective global public-private health partnerships: Practice and potential. *Social Science and Medicine* 64(2): 259–271.
Green A (2007) *An Introduction to Health Planning for Developing Health Systems,* 3rd edn. London: Oxford University Press.
Hyman H (1982) History. In: Hyman H (ed.) *Health Planning: A Systematic Approach,* pp. 1–24. Rockville MD: Aspen Systems Corporation.
Reinke W (1988) *Health Planning for Effective Management.* New York: Oxford University Press.
Rifkin S and Pridmore P (2001) *Partners in Planning – Information, Participation and Empowerment.* London: MacMillan Education.
Rodwin V (1984) *The Health Planning Predicament.* Berkeley, CA: University of California Press.
Soucat A, Vanerberghe UW, Diop F, Nguyen S, and Knippenberg R (2002) Marginal budgeting for bottlenecks: a new costing and resource allocation practice to buy health results: using health sector's budget expansion to progress towards the Millennium Development Goals in Sub-Saharan Africa. Washington, DC: The World Bank.
Taylor C and Reinke W (1988) The process, structure and functions of planning. In: Reinke W (ed.) *Health Planning for Effective Management,* pp. 5–20. Oxford, UK: Oxford University Press.
Thomson MC, Palmer T, Morse AP, Cresswell M, and Connor SJ (2000) Forecasting disease risk with seasonal climate predictions. *The Lancet* 355(9214): 1559–1560.
Walley J, Wright J, and Hubley J (2004) *Public Health an Action: Guide to Improving Health in Developing Countries.* New York: Oxford University Press.
WHO (1999) Geographic Information Systems (GIS): Mapping for epidemiological surveillance. *Weekly Epidemiological Record* 74(34): 281–285.

Further Reading

Easterly W (2006) *The White Man's Burden: Why the West's Efforts to Aid the Rest Have Done So Much Ill and So Little Good.* London: Penguin Press.
Green A and Collins C (2006) Management and planning for public health. In: Merson MH, Black RE, and Mills AJ (eds.) *International Public Health,* 2nd edn., pp. 553–599. Jones and Bartlett.

The State in Public Health, Role of

A Alvarez-Rosete, Health Policy Researcher, London, UK

© 2008 Elsevier Inc. All rights reserved.

This article explains the roles of state and its executive branch, the government, in public health policy. In contemporary complex societies, the state holds the political authority over the population of a given territory, and its diverse roles and functions (including policymaking) are executed by the government. This entry describes how both roles have been evolving since the second half of the twentieth century.

Such evolution can be divided into three broad stages: the 1950s and 1960s; the 1970s and 1980s; and the 1990s to the present. Simultaneously, transformations have occurred in the following three dimensions. First, the responsibility of the state for ensuring public health has evolved. This has been accompanied by debate about the nature of the state's responsibility in providing for public health. Second, the way in which governments have intervened in public health has also changed. Governments have now at their disposal new tools for influencing the lifestyles of citizens and organizations and for gathering information for promoting public health. Third, the process of making public health policies and the number and identity of actors and the arenas for policymaking have evolved. In this more complex scenario, governments are developing new approaches to the governance of public health and adopting new strategies for improving public health policymaking.

The Evolution of the State's Responsibility over Public Health

Despite the intensification of state involvement in promoting public health in these last decades, public authorities since ancient civilizations such as the Incas, the Etruscans, and the Romans have been concerned with public health. In the Italian city-states of the middle ages, public infrastructures for providing safe water and sanitation (such as cisterns and sewers), cleaning streets, and fighting diseases and epidemics were developed and managed by public boards of health (Beaglehole and Bonita, 2004).

Gradually since the Middle Ages, first in Western Europe, states have become the preferred institutional configuration to collectively organize political societies. The nation-state replaced other political entities such as tribes, feudal societies, or city-states, monopolizing the legitimate use of physical force over a group of people, who shared a common identity as a nation, within a given territory. The state organizes through a number of institutions, including legislative assemblies, the executive or government, the judiciary, the civil bureaucracy, the police, and the armed forces.

The origins of the idea of state responsibility for the health and well-being of citizens can be traced back to the eighteenth century, but the idea was not translated into legislation and other central government interventions until the nineteenth century. The consequences of the industrial revolution forced states to intervene and regulate the working conditions in factories. This, however, was not without debate on whether the state had the right and duty to intervene in order to correct the shortcomings of capitalist development. In Britain, the first national health law was the British Public Health Act of 1848 (Beaglehole and Bonita, 2004) and a general board of health was set up. Public health actions were still, however, fragmented and usually undertaken by local authorities and religious organizations.

In the interwar years of the twentieth century, more comprehensive systems of health and health care developed across the world. Totalitarian regimes, such as the communists in the Soviet Union between the 1920s and the 1950s, or the Nazis in Germany in the 1930s, were very active in promoting public health, implementing programs such as promoting exercise among the population (especially among children and young people), combating smoking, and preventing infectious diseases.

The epitome of the state assuming responsibility for the welfare of the population was the establishment of national health systems following the end of the Second World War. These systems were funded by taxation and free at the point of use and were accompanied by comprehensive education, social care, and unemployment programs. William Beverage's report *Social Insurance and Allied Services* in the United Kingdom (UK), published in 1942, is usually cited as the first systematization of such reform programs which came to be known as the welfare state. The British National Health Service (NHS) was subsequently created in 1948. However, the welfare state prioritized health care over public health. The welfare state marked the triumph of the 'clinical care model,' which emphasizes health care provided to individuals by specialized physicians in hospitals.

Following independence in the 1950s and 1960s, a number of newly independent former colonies in the developing world adopted socialist and Marxist ideologies. These ideologies advocated total state control over the economy through the use of public enterprises and huge bureaucracies. Soviet and Chinese socialism provided examples for many other countries. The state took full responsibility for public health and health care, even if this was limited in its delivery in practice.

In 1970s and 1980s, in the midst of a profound international economic crisis, the welfare state and, more widely, the idea of state responsibility for people's welfare, was challenged. In the First World, a series of welfare reforms aimed to limit the exponential growth of the welfare state were introduced. For many, these reforms represented a 'retrenchment' (affecting less important areas of the welfare state such as employment policies or social care, not core services such as health and education), rather than a full 'dismantling' of the welfare state. In communist countries, the financial crisis also led to the cutting of public health and other welfare programs, with a resulting dramatic worsening of the health of the population as reflected in different health indicators.

The economic crisis fuelled criticisms of the role of the state by a resurgent neoliberal ideology in the form of two connected arguments. The first argument challenged the notion that the government should be principally responsible for public service financing and provision and emphasized instead the role and duty of individuals to provide for themselves rather than to rely on the state. Governments, it was argued, should intervene less in social and economic affairs. For the neoliberal ideology, public health interventions are regarded as 'nanny statist,' and as 'unnecessary intrusions into people's lives' (Jochelson, 2006).

The second argument was that even if one accepted that government had a role to play, governments increasingly appeared to lack the capacity to intervene effectively and to deal with increasingly complex public matters. In the 1970s, the thesis of the 'ungovernable state' (also referred to as 'overload') grew from both neoliberal and neo-Marxist positions. For the overload thesis, the continuous growth of the state since the 1940s, increasing public expectations of what the state could deliver, and the demands of pressure groups had led to a situation of 'ungovernability' and financial crisis (Richards and Smith, 2002). Added to these domestic pressures, globalization and supranational integration (e.g., the European Union (EU)) challenged the way national states performed traditional functions. For example, as decision-making power was being increasingly transferred to the EU, many policies were not decided at the national level, although it was the responsibility of the member states to fully implement them.

Public health was affected by these wider changes. Overall, the economic and public sector reforms introduced during the 1970s and 1980s had a negative impact on public health by increasing poverty and inequality rates. Public sector reforms tended to target those policy areas, such as public health and social care, which were not supported by strong public constituencies and therefore were unlikely to have big political costs for the politicians responsible for the reforms.

Since the 1990s, a more pronounced role for the state in public health has again been advocated. Governments had articulated their commitment to public health in the 1978 Alma-Ata Declaration. The need for government action on public health was put forward by the worldwide People's Health Movement in their 2000 People's Charter for Health and the 2004 Mumbai Declaration. As a relative measure of the salience of public health and the responsibility of the state for promoting it, public spending on public health and disease prevention has been increasing over the last two decades in many countries (Allin et al., 2004).

In contemporary political thinking, those claiming that the state has (at least some) responsibility for promoting and protecting public health have suggested several images of the government as 'catalyst,' 'enabler,' 'steward,' and so forth. The 'catalyst' and 'enabler' categories are based on the idea that the role of the state is to help people to help themselves, that is, to enable individuals to make their own choices about their lifestyles rather than for the state to impose forms of behavior.

However, for others, the categorizations of the state as 'enabler' or 'persuader' still place too much emphasis on individual responsibility for public health. 'Stewardship' has been suggested as a better term to justify the state's intervention in public health (Saltman and Ferroussier-Davis, 2000; Jochelson, 2006). 'Stewardship implies government has a responsibility for protecting national health, and to serving in the public interest and for the public good' (Jochelson, 2006: 1153). This renewed emphasis on the responsibility of the state does not, however, imply a traditional role for citizens as passive recipients of public services. In this new narrative, individuals have responsibility to play an active role in relation to public health. Stewardship does not necessarily imply that the state should be the provider of public health, but that the state should be responsible for ensuring that public interventions are funded, delivered, and effective.

All these images recognize that public health is a 'public good' (Bobak et al., 2004; Buse et al., 2005). Public goods benefit the entire population whether or not each individual has actively sought them, has explicitly paid a price for the cost of them, or even agrees with them being provided. For example, someone may be opposed to policies which ban smoking in public places, but he or she receives the benefit of cleaner air if such policies are implemented. In that sense, just as transport infrastructures, defense policy, and other public goods are nonexcludable, so is public health – 'if provided to one, it is available to all' (Hughes, 2003: 78; Buse et al., 2005). Even if the market could provide public health interventions, they are socially desirable so there are benefits to the whole society by some government involvement. For example, vaccination brings benefits for the entire population, despite the fact that it could be made available only to those who can afford to pay (Hughes, 2003: 78).

Government and Its Tools for Promoting Public Health

The government is the state institution operating at the national level which embodies the formal authority of the state. In any political regime (i.e., democratic, authoritarian, totalitarian), in any state configuration (i.e., unitary, federal, parliamentary monarchy, presidential, etc.), at the federal/national level, there is a government which substantiates the formal exercise of power. Although there can be a legislative branch formed by two bodies (e.g., two houses, a senate and a congress), there can only be one national government. In non-democratic regimes, the power of government is even more pronounced.

The core functions of government are to make and implement policy. To carry out these functions, the government employs the resources of the state – principally, the civil service.

Governments have at their disposal various forms of organizations to develop and implement policy and to deliver services. These instruments include public corporations, private sector contractors, and public-private partnerships (Hood, 2006). In public health policy, these tools have evolved in response to the changing policy environment and the dominant ideology prevailing at any one time.

Another way of understanding the instruments available to government is by classifying them according to the objectives they seek. Thus, they can be broadly classified as tools for gathering information and tools for modifying the behavior of citizens and organizations (Hood, 2006). These instruments have been changing as a result of information-age technology, especially detecting tools for gathering information, to the extent that governments have now at their disposal new tools to obtain useful information for promoting public health, including the use of indicators, systematic screening of populations, cross-national data, surveys, and so forth.

In the 1950s, the paradigm for administering the state was the 'bureaucratic' model, which has been described by Max Weber as bearing the characteristics of centralization, formality, and hierarchy, supported by a politically neutral civil service. In the postwar bureaucratic state, public policies were formulated within central government and developed by the civil service. Ministries and departments were responsible for policy areas such as education, defense, foreign policy, and health, and 'joined-up,' cross-departmental work was rare.

Public health policy was placed under the remit of the ministries of health, which were established across the world in the 1950s (with the exception of some pioneering examples which came earlier (e.g., UK in 1919 or Costa Rica in 1927). State bureaucracies were responsible for the direct provision of health and health-care services. Responsibility for many public health programs was transferred to public corporations at the national or local level.

Banning alcohol consumption, taxing smoking, or subsidizing sanitation programs were typical behavior-modifying tools employed by governments to promote public health. Tools for identifying population health needs or risks, however, were little developed.

Such a strong role for central executives and central bureaucracies in the financing and provision of services also characterized public administration in the colonies and, following independence, in the new countries (Hughes, 2003), and was even more marked in totalitarian and authoritarian regimes. In Botswana, for example, after independence in 1966, the government implemented a program of groundwater drilling and water network construction and provided incentives to rural households to build latrines by subsidizing them (Oxfam, 2006).

Under the influence of the neoliberal ideology, during the 1970s and 1980s, countries across the world embarked upon ambitious reforms of their public sector and the administrative structures of the state. Despite their differences, these reforms, which have been labeled as 'new public management' (NPM), reflected the neoliberal principles of a minimal state, a preference for market-based solutions rather than direct public sector provision, and the belief that the capacity of governments to intervene effectively is very limited. NPM advocated a new role for governments: 'to steer rather than row' and to oversee market competition.

For NPM advocates (among which the World Bank and the International Monetary Fund stood out), enabling private providers to compete in a marketplace was a more efficient way of providing services than direct public provision. The introduction of market mechanisms became a fashionable solution in the 1980s across the world. Many developed and developing countries such as the UK, New Zealand, South Africa, Chile, Thailand, and India adopted the NPM principles, undertaking major privatization reforms of their public sectors (Hughes, 2003).

As a result, NPM reforms across the world led to the cutting of public health programs, as happened with federal funding for public health in the United States and the decision by the UK Conservative Government to reduce the funding for the Health Education Authority for England (Beaglehole and Bonita, 2004). Many countries also introduced separate agencies to promote public health, thus leading to institutional fragmentation (Beaglehole and Bonita, 2004). Despite these reforms, many countries put in place national public health policies and strategies to promote collaborative work, especially between national and local governments and agencies, but institutional barriers made this aim very difficult to achieve.

As quality, equity, competition, and efficiency need to be guaranteed in the public sector, the state had to regulate the behavior of providers and the performance of markets. The most common regulatory mechanism has been establishing independent bodies at arm's length from government – known as 'quangos,' nondepartmental public bodies, independent agencies, and so forth.

The NPM advocated practices such as the use of goals and targets for measuring performance and monitoring progress of public services. In 1980, the United States established quantifiable objectives to improve the health of the nation, reduce health risks, and improve services and protection (Allin et al., 2004). In 1985, the World Health Organization (WHO) introduced regional targets, called the Health for All programe (Allin et al., 2004; Beaglehole and Bonita, 2004). Despite the fact that these targets reflected the narrow purpose of achieving improved efficiency and efficacy, they dramatically improved the detecting tools for governments and paved the way for better monitoring and evaluation.

Today, governments make use of many forms of organizations to provide services. Together with direct provision by public corporations and contracting out to private sector providers, public-private partnerships are being deployed in public health to promote, for example, anti-smoking initiatives, road safety, and alcohol misuse education campaigns or to undertake community renewal interventions. Partners typically include private sector or voluntary not-for-profit organizations, independent public agencies, governmental bodies such as ministerial departments, local authorities, universities, schools, and civil society groups, for example.

From the point of view of the tools used either to modify lifestyles or to gather information, both traditional and new policy instruments are being used. Traditional policy instruments for modifying behavior such as taxation, regulation, and government-led campaigns continue to prove effective. Taxation of alcohol or tobacco leads to a reduction in consumption and, therefore, to positive effects on health outcomes and, particularly in the case of alcohol, to better public safety (e.g., fewer motor vehicle fatalities, fewer homicides, less domestic violence and child abuse) (Jochelson, 2006). Examples of effective regulation to restrict the consumption of alcohol and tobacco include tougher licensing laws for pubs' opening hours or the banning of smoking in public places and of tobacco advertising (Jochelson, 2006). The 'total sanitation campaign' in India (Oxfam, 2006) and the 'free school meals' campaign in Sri Lanka (Oxfam, 2006) are examples of public health campaigns directly led by government which have met with variable success.

At the same time, governments throughout the world are exploring the use of new tools for influencing the lifestyles of citizens and organizations. Such tools include voluntary codes of conduct, financial incentives, benchmarking, performance league tables, the coproduction of policies and initiatives, and so on. For example, in Spain, voluntary codes of conduct have been adopted by the food industry, which has agreed to refrain from the aggressive advertising of 'fast food' to children, reduce fat and sugar levels through the food manufacturing process, and improve the information provided on food packaging.

As a result of information-age technology, governments can use new tools through which to gather useful information for promoting public health, including the use of indicators, systematic screening of populations, cross-national data, surveys, etc. The WHO provides a great deal of epidemiological and statistical information which is freely available online, including systems for managing information about disease outbreaks. With the support of the WHO and other international organizations such as the Organization for Economic Co-operation and Development (OECD) and the EU, countries are making efforts to standardize public health information data collection.

The Process of Making Public Health Policy

The process of making public health policies since the 1950s has been evolving as well. The actors participating in the policy process, the venues or arenas where policies are formulated and implemented, and the way ideas enter the process and influence actors are now different from those of the mid-twentieth century (Richards and Smith, 2002; Buse et al., 2005). Today, governments do not seem to have the same level of autonomy and capacity to shape the policymaking process that they once enjoyed.

In the 1950s and 1960s, the process of formulating public health usually took place at the national government level and was led by politicians and senior civil servants within central executives and central bureaucracies. The civil service held the monopoly for policy advice to politicians and decision makers, thereby limiting the pluralism of ideas and policy solutions. At that time, only the medical profession, usually organized through formal corporatist bodies (such as medical councils or colleges), and powerful economic interests (such as the tobacco, food, and pharmaceutical industries) enjoyed any significant degree of leverage over the policymaking process.

Political parties, although crucially important in mobilizing people and channeling the selection and recruitment of political leaders and cadres, have always had a secondary role in formulating public policy (Buse et al., 2005). Parties do generate alternatives while in opposition or in the running up to an election, but once in office, it is the government which takes the lead in formulating and implementing policy.

The executive and the legislative branches were the arenas for public health policymaking. In unitary states, where hierarchical subordination exists between national central governments and lower units of government at the regional or local levels, public health laws were passed by the national executives and legislative branches and the lower levels of government were in charge of implementing them. In federal systems, where political power is shared by federal and subnational governments and legislatures, the latter have always had a major responsibility for formulating and implementing public health policies (Buse et al., 2005).

Policy implementation, despite requiring participation from local authorities and 'street-level bureaucrats' (i.e., implementers), was understood as a top-down process directed by central government. Implementation failure would simply be seen as a problem of compliance by the lower administrative levels.

During the 1970s and 1980s, the emergence of a strong international public health movement allowed new actors to enter the public health policy process at both the international and national levels (Reich, 2002). International organizations such as the World Bank competed with the WHO to promote international health. Especially in developing countries, international donors and individual experts have been advising governments on public health. As NPM reforms were rolled out, the newly created executive agencies, local and national bodies, and independent providers of public services became new actors in formulating, but especially implementing, public health policies.

In the early twenty-first century, due to NPM reforms and to wider socioeconomic and political trends (globalization, processes of regional economic integration, etc.), the public health policy process is even more complex than ever. The trend of new actors entering the process has intensified. For example, in the health sector, the number of patient associations and health consumer groups has been growing in countries across the world, although their leverage over the policy process is still a matter of discussion.

The media is a powerful actor, capable of shaping the public agenda. For example, in 2002–03, the media coverage in the UK of the potential risk of autism associated with receiving the combined measles, mumps, and rubella (MMR) vaccination exemplifies how influential the media can be in bringing an issue to the forefront (Buse et al., 2005). Although in this particular example the government managed to resist the pressure to change its childhood immunization policy, on many occasions, high political costs incline governments to follow the flow of public opinion.

Not only have new participants now entered the policymaking process to develop public health policy, but the way old and new actors interact has been changing as well. Formal and informal contacts and relationships between state and nonstate actors, either from inside or outside government, take the form of 'networks.' The concept of policy networks reflect the existence of groups of people (politicians, civil servants, academics, interest groups, etc.) with common interests in the policy area to which the network is dedicated, who share common values over policy problems and solutions and who are keen to exchange resources (information, authority, legitimacy, nodality, etc.) to pursue common goals. For many scholars, policy networks are the quintessence of contemporary government.

Processes of regional economic integration and intergovernmental organizations across the world have brought about new arenas for policymaking (Reich, 2002). The EU has been developing a strong interest in public health. Treaties, such as the Maastricht Treaty of 1992 or the 1999 Treaty of Amsterdam envisage an important role for the European Community in contributing to the attainment of a high level of health protection for its citizens, therefore providing the EU with new competencies in public health. The Commonwealth, an association of 53 independent states, promotes cooperation between members on public health issues such as combating HIV/AIDS or promoting maternity and child health.

Another change to the venue of policymaking is a growing trend in countries across the world to devolve power to lower levels of government (Reich, 2002). Devolved administrations have been assuming more functions and roles to develop public health policy. Devolution in Scotland, for example, opened up a window of opportunity to develop more radical smoking control policies than in the rest of the UK. Groups advocating the banning of smoking in public places were able to influence policy through the Scottish Parliamentary procedures after devolution, whereas they had been unsuccessful in attempts to exert the same leverage at the UK policy process level (Cairney, 2007).

As a result of the increasing number of actors and arenas for policymaking and the effect of the information-age technology, ideas and policy solutions now flow more freely. Consequently the transfer of public health ideas and solutions across the world is more intense than ever before.

The multiplication of actors and arenas for policymaking also affects the process of implementing public health policies. Most of the time, policies are not implemented as originally intended by decision-makers, because many actors at the front line have some discretion to introduce changes, or various institutional factors impede or put obstacles in their path. This transformation of the policy process has been affecting both nondemocratic and democratic political regimes across the world. In democratic states, political power is exercised by the people, usually through systems of representation which require free elections. This implies that, at least formally, different economic, social, and political groups and individuals have the possibility to influence the policy process. In nondemocratic regimes, political power is concentrated upon a single individual or a group (such as a single political party or the military). The policy process is monopolized by a very limited number of actors, predominantly from within the regime. Intense popular mobilization makes it easy for a country to launch and implement public health programs successfully, as illustrated by the case of the quarantine policy for people with HIV infection, implemented by the Cuban communist regime between 1986 and 1993, which involved mass testing and the isolation of the infected in sanatoriums. Despite the fact that nondemocratic regimes have more capacity and autonomy to steer the policy process, globalization and wider socioeconomic and political trends shape their health policy agendas as well. Cuba's health achievements with respect to nutrition and child survival, for example, are currently under threat from several causes, including the United States trade embargo, the collapse of the Soviet Union, and the effect of natural disasters (Beaglehole and Bonita, 2004). Other nondemocratic regimes have been forced to take on board demands for radical reforms imposed by external actors such as the World Bank and the International Monetary Fund.

How Can Governments Tackle Public Health Issues Today?

At the beginning of the twenty-first century, as a result of wider economic, political, social, technological, and cultural changes, public health problems appear to be now more difficult to tackle than before. The public policy literature coined the term 'wicked problems' to refer to complex, contested issues of interest to multiple policy actors which therefore require addressing them from different policy domains and deploying a multi-agency strategy (Blackman *et al.*, 2006).

Public health issues are usually 'contested' issues. Their nature is subject to competing definitions, in other words, they are 'political' issues in their very nature. For example, policies to ban smoking in public places usually encounter the fierce opposition of the hospitality sector and the tobacco industry, which claim that such measures would affect their business negatively.

The term 'wicked issues' is also useful to understand how public health policy usually deals with cross-cutting issues, which transcend a single policy domain and fall under the responsibility of different authorities and state structures. For example, social, economic, and cultural factors constitute the major determinants of (ill) health, and this implies that 'the policy response to improve health needs to be interdisciplinary and multisectoral' (Bobak et al., 2004: 135). Also, global public health problems transcend state borders. In consequence, public health interventions require interagency collaboration and complex coordination between local, regional, national, and supranational levels of government.

Given the complexity of current public health issues, the pressures modern governments have to face 'from above, from within, from below' (Reich, 2002) as reflected in the increasingly complex policymaking process, and given that public health policy is inherently a political process, governments around the world have been trying new approaches to public health policymaking.

The Public Governance paradigm, it is argued, can provide a more fruitful approach for tackling wicked health issues than the traditional administration approach or new public management (NPM). For Bovaird and Löffler (2003), the public governance paradigm incorporates the NPM concerns for measuring results in terms of outputs and achieving efficiency and value for money, but stresses the distinctive nature of the public sector and the centrality of political processes. In the public sector, it is not all about how good policies are (in terms of efficiency, value for money, technical viability, outputs, etc.) but also how policies have been made. The processes by which different stakeholders interact are also seen to have a major importance in themselves. Ensuring that the public policy process is inclusive and democratic, that decision makers are accountable, and that equity and fairness informs policymaking as much as efficiency and value for money are key issues for public governance theorists.

International organizations have been attracted by the governance agenda. The 1999 Manila Declaration on Governance defined 'good governance' as a 'system that is transparent, accountable, just, fair, democratic, participatory and responsive to people's needs.' The EU White Paper on governance proposed the following five principles of good governance: 'openness, participation, accountability, effectiveness, and coherence.' The UK Labour Government's program for modernizing government incorporates many of the public governance concerns. The 1999 Cabinet Office White Paper, *Modernising Government*, and the subsequent documents and initiatives that followed, in particular the 1999 Cabinet Office report *Professional Policy Making for the Twenty-first Century*, suggested a model of 'modern' policymaking based upon nine 'core competencies': forward looking; outward looking; innovative, and creative; evidence-based; inclusive; joined up; uses evaluation; employs reviews; learns lessons (see http://www.policyhub.gov.uk).

As a result, there is now a growing concern among governments with using good evidence, developing cross-cutting work among stakeholder organizations, opening up mechanisms for public participation, avoiding implementation failures, and using evaluations in policymaking.

Evidence-Based

When making public policy, especially when facing complicated problems, policymakers need to review the evidence of what works and how it works best. This includes an assessment of what impact different proposals will have on various situations. Research also helps identify and clarify the policy problems which require action.

Research should be conducted throughout the entire policy process, not only during the policy formulation and design stage, at which policymakers define what problems require action and search for how to solve them. Pilots are useful tools for testing whether a policy will work as planned. Process evaluations, conducted while the policy is being implemented, can help to quickly identify unforeseen obstacles and recommend immediate action.

To tackle wicked public health issues, it is especially important to improve the quality of health data. Health reporting is a crucial tool for identifying population needs and risks (Allin et al., 2004). The WHO has been promoting consistent approaches to collecting and analyzing noncommunicable disease risk factors to enable countries to set up compatible surveillance systems (WHO, 2002).

Although many governmental departments conduct research in-house, most of the time evidence comes from a variety of sources, ranging from different public organizations and private stakeholders to national and international groups. Researchers and policymakers need to evaluate the quality of the evidence they gather. This requires developing the analytical capacity of governments. To achieve this, governments have been setting up analytical units across departments and sharing information among local, national, and international organizations.

Cross-Cutting Work

Public health policy requires cross-sectoral interventions in areas such as housing, transport, education, and, of course, health care. To address this, governments are creating horizontal structures such as task forces, cross-departmental bodies, and central–local partnerships to overcome institutional obstacles in order to better tackle cross-cutting issues.

In the UK, the Cabinet Office Social Exclusion Task Force, previously the Social Exclusion Unit, coordinates policy against social exclusion. Recognizing that health is often linked to other forms of exclusion, much of the task force work on critical health issues such as teenage pregnancy and health inequalities has sought to promote multi-agency, cross-departmental work.

The Public Health Agency of Canada has the same remit of providing leadership and promoting collaboration with provinces and territories on public health. The agency coordinates the efforts of federal and provincial governments, academia, and nongovernmental organizations to prevent chronic diseases; identify, prevent, and reduce public health risks; and respond to health crises.

At the same time, national governments also need to coordinate efforts with local authorities and other governments at the international level. Sweden provides a good example of how to promote synergies between the national and local levels of government in public health (Beaglehole and Bonita, 2004). Another example of good practice is the Australian National Public Health Partnership, set up in 1996 to coordinate public health initiatives between all levels of government in Australia (Allin et al., 2004). For Beaglehole and Bonita, 'an ideal approach would combine strong and progressive national guidelines, appropriate legislation and inter-sectoral support, with local initiatives and responsibilities' (Beaglehole and Bonita, 2004: 215–216).

Inclusive Policymaking

Citizens are no longer passive users of public services. They are increasingly aware of their rights to express their own views and needs, participate in the design of services, choose services according to their interests, and demand accountability over the quality of services. Policies should be developed in consultation with stakeholders who have a particular interest in them.

Democratic governance, especially at the local level, is crucial for health development. Best practice relevant for public health policy can be found in Uganda and in the Indian state of Kerala. The Ugandan Participatory Poverty Assessment Project brought together government and civil society groups in developing a comprehensive health plan (Oxfam, 2006). The 1996–2001 Kerala People's Campaign for Decentralized Planning encouraged local democratic participation in producing projects according to the health needs of the people (Elamon et al., 2004).

Implementation

Good policy design has to consider whether the policy is workable, sufficient resources are at the disposal of implementers, and the timing is right, as well as how the success or failure of the policy is going to be measured. Consulting those with responsibility for implementing the policy during its design and development increases the chances of getting the policy content right and, therefore, making the policy successful.

Evaluation

Policymakers are increasingly acknowledging the usefulness of conducting evaluations of past public health interventions to inform policymaking. Traditionally, evaluation was considered to be the last and least important stage of the policy process to the extent that it was not considered part of it at all. Evaluation, however, is a key element, comprising early assessments, pilots, informal 'feedback loops,' and formal and systematic reviews of past or ongoing policies. This implies that provisions for evaluation need to be included at early stages of the policy process, ideally during policy formulation and design.

Australia provides an example of good practice of the use of economic evaluations of public health interventions, although, according to Allin et al. (2004), their outcomes are not systematically used for decision making.

Conclusion

Since the 1950s, both the responsibility of the state over public health and the way government has intervened in public health have been changing, and the policymaking process has become increasingly complex. Presently, most states retain an important role in promoting public health. The foreseeable future is that, facing continuous pressures 'from above, from within, from below,' the state and its executive branch will need to continue searching for tools for governing public health effectively and to develop new approaches for improving public health policymaking.

See also: Agenda Setting in Public Health Policy; Alma Ata and Primary Health Care: An Evolving Story; Evidence-Based Public Health Policy; Global Health Initiatives and Public Health Policy; Interest Groups and Civil Society, in Public Health Policy; People's Health Movement; Planning, for Public Health Policy.

Citations

Allin S, McKee M, and Holland W (2004) *Making Decisions on Public Health: A Review of Eight Countries.* London: European Observatory on Health Systems and Policies.

Beaglehole R and Bonita R (2004) *Public Health at the Crossroads. Achievements and Prospects,* 2nd edn. Cambridge, UK: Cambridge University Press.

Blackman T, Greene A, Hunter DJ, et al. (2006) Performance assessment and wicked problems: The case of health inequalities. *Public Policy and Administration* 21(2): 66–80.

Bobak M, McCarthy M, Perlman F, and Marmot M (2004) Modernizing public health. In: Figueras J, McKee M, Cain J and Lessof S (eds.) *Health Systems in Transition: Learning from Experience,* pp. 135–142. London: World Health Organization, European Observatory on Health Systems and Policies.

Bovaird T and Löffler E (2003) Understanding public management and governance. In: Bovaird T and Löffler E (eds.) *Public Management and Governance,* pp. 3–12. London: Routledge.

Buse K, Mays N, and Walt G (2005) *Making Health Policy.* Maidenhead, UK: Open University Press.

Cairney P (2007) Using devolution to set the agenda? Venue shift and the smoking ban in Scotland. *British Journal of Politics and International Relations* 9(1): 73–89.

Elamon J, Franke RW, and Ekbal B (2004) Decentralization of health services: The Kerala People's Campaign. *International Journal of Health Services* 34(4): 681–708.

Hood C (2006) The tools of government in the information age. In: Moran M, Rein M and Goodin RE (eds.) *The Oxford Handbook of Public Policy*, pp. 469–481. Oxford, UK: Oxford University Press.

Hughes OE (2003) *Public Management and Administration. An Introduction.* Basingstoke, UK: Palgrave.

Jochelson K (2006) Nanny or steward? The role of government in public health. *Public Health* 120: 1149–1155.

Oxfam International, Wateraid (2006) *In the Public Interest. Health, Education and Water and Sanitation for All.* Oxford, UK: Oxfam International.

Reich MR (2002) Reshaping the state from above, from within, from below: Implications for public health. *Social Science and Medicine* 54: 1669–1675.

Richards D and Smith MJ (2002) *Governance and Public Policy in the UK.* Oxford, UK: Oxford University Press.

Saltman RB and Ferroussier-Davis O (2000) The concept of stewardship in health policy. *Bulletin of the World Health Organization* 78(6): 732–739.

World Health, Organization (2002) *The World Health Report 2002: Reducing Risks, Promoting Healthy Life.* http://www.who.int/whr/2002/en/ (accessed August 2007).

Further Reading

McKee M and Pomerleau J (2005) The emergence of public health and the centrality of values. In: Pomerleau J and McKee M (eds.) *Issues in Public Health*, pp. 7–23. Maidenhead, UK: Open University Press.

Alma-Ata and Primary Health Care: An Evolving Story

J H Bryant, Johns Hopkins School of Public Health, Baltimore, MD, USA
J B Richmond, Harvard Medical School, Boston, MA, USA

© 2008 Elsevier Inc. All rights reserved.

Overview

The story of how Alma-Ata and Primary Health Care gained the attention of the world's health leadership must be seen as one of the most intriguing in the history of health and development. The postcolonial years in the developing world saw health care that was largely hospital-based and curative in its orientation, which meant, of course, that most people who needed health care had little or no access to it. The shift to community-oriented care with outreach beyond hospitals to health centers and even to households called for dramatic changes in all aspects of the health sector.

It was during those years that WHO was shifting its concerns from issues such as malaria eradication (which could not be accomplished) to the development of basic health services. In the cluster of years prior to Alma-Ata, 1978, WHO went through an exploratory process, partnering with interested organizations, conceptualizing various aspects of health care, culminating in the notion of primary health care, which was refined for and fully accepted at the Alma-Ata Conference.

This was the era of Halfdan Mahler, who became director general of WHO during these years and provided charismatic leadership that led to the planning for and remarkable outcomes of Alma-Ata. The WHO staff was initially mixed in its perceptions of this process, but then turned in the direction of strong support of what turned out to be one of the signal events in the history of the organization.

The Conference in Alma-Ata was a splendid event, well planned, widely attended, and focused on problems of major importance, with the policy-related product of Primary Health Care and Health for All by 2000. It was seeking ways to translate the emerging knowledge base into health care for people all over the world.

Following Alma-Ata, a major interest, reaching to present times, has been to follow implementation of the concepts, policies, and actions integral to primary health care in various parts of the world, and also to note conflicting concepts, policies, and processes. Here follows a listing of major relevant events, preceding and following Alma-Ata, up to the present, including relevant documentation (the time period that is the focus of each of the referenced materials will be noted, followed by the reference):

- The Christian Medical Commission and WHO's PHC Approach (late 1960s and 1970s), (Litsios, 2004);
- Alma-Ata Revisited (1970s to present), (Tejada, 2003);
- Alma-Ata 1978 – Primary Health Care; Declaration of Alma-Ata (Alma-Ata, 1978);
- Selective Primary Health Care, 1979 (1978 to present), (Cueto, 2004);
- The Ottawa Charter – 1st International Conference on Health Promotion (WHO/HPR/HEP, 1986);
- From Alma Ata to the Year 2000 – Reflections at the Midpoint, Riga, USSR, 1988 (World Health Organization 1988);
- Alma-Ata and After (1978 – present), (Venediktov, 1998);
- Primary Health Care – 21 Almaty, Kazakhstan, 1998 (WHO, 2000);
  1. Foreword, G. Brundtland
  2. Conclusions, D. Sanders

- Global Review of Primary Health Care, Madrid, 2003, Emerging Messages;
- Renewing PHC in the Americas, 2005 (PAHO, 2007);
- Commission on Macroeconomics and Health;
- Millennium Development Goals, and Millennium Project;
- The Commission on Social Determinants of Health;
- Primary Health Care and the new Director General of WHO, Dr. Margaret Chan;
- Addendum to Alma-Ata and Primary Health Care. An Evolving Story Buenos Aires 30/15 International Conference, August 2007 From Alma-Ata to the Millennium Declaration: *Towards Equity-Based Comprehensive Health Care;*
- Building from Common Foundations. The World Health Organization and Faith-Based Organizations in Primary Health Care (World Health Organization 2008).
- Unequivocal regional support for Margaret Chan's commitment to primary health care. (*Lancet*, Correspondence, June 19, 2008).

Historical Reflections On Factors Leading to and Following Alma-Ata 1978

The Christian Medical Commission and WHO's PHC Approach (late 1960s and 1970s)

The 1968–1975 period saw dramatic changes in the priorities that governed the work program of WHO. For more than a decade, the global malaria eradication campaign had been WHO's leading program. Initiated in the mid-1950s, it was a strictly vertical program based on the insecticidal power of DDT. As it became evident that malaria eradication would not be achieved, greater priority was given to the development of basic health services. Over the ensuing years, various steps were taken to focus attention on the importance of health services and how they might be pursued (Litsios, 2004).

The primary health care approach was introduced to the Executive Board of WHO in 1975. It is useful to review the changes that took place in the preceding years that made it possible for such a radical approach to health services to emerge when it did. Here, we will review the parallel approaches being taken by WHO and by the Christian Medical Commission (CMC) of the World Council of Churches and how they came into useful association.

Dr. Halfdan T. Mahler became assistant director general of WHO in September, 1970, and Director General in 1973. Working with Dr. Ken Newell, a new division, Strengthening of Health Services, was created in 1972 with Newell as director.

In May, 1973, the 26th World Health Assembly adopted resolution WHA26.35, titled 'Organizational Study of Methods of Promoting the Development of Basic Health Services.' Among other things, this resolution confirmed the high priority to be given to the development of health services that were both accessible and acceptable to the total population, suited to its needs, to the socioeconomic conditions of the country, and at the level of health technology considered necessary to meet the problems of that country at a given time.

The search for new approaches led to two important WHO publications in 1975:

- *Alternative Approaches to Meeting Basic Health Needs of Populations in Developing Countries*, edited by V. Djukanovic and E.P. Mach, (Djukanovic and Mach, 1975)
- *Health by the People*, edited by K. Newell (Newall, 1975).

These were products of Newell's Division of Strengthening Health Services.

Establishment and Early Work Program of the Christian Medical Commission

The Christian Medical Commission (CMC) was established in 1968 as a semiautonomous body to assist the World Council of Churches (WCC) in its evaluation and assistance with church-related medical programs in the developing world. Of particular concern to the WCC was the fact that many of the more than 1200 hospitals that were run by affiliated associations were rapidly becoming obsolete, with operating costs increasing dramatically. What was needed were some criteria for evaluating these programs that would help reorient the direction for their future development.

Key contributions to the formulation of the mandate of the commission came from the Rockefeller Foundation and its extensive study of 'Health and the Developing World' (Bryant, 1969). This book was, 'one of the most definitive resources for all engaged in health care in the lesser developed countries' (McGilvray, 1981). Its author, John Bryant, became the first chairman of the Christian Medical Commission.

The CMC was composed of 25 members from diverse countries and levels of health development that met annually and was served by an executive staff of a director and three others. Its purpose was to engage in surveys, data collection, and research into the most appropriate ways of delivering health services that could be relevant to local needs and the mission and resources of the Church.

The first director of the CMC, James C. McGilvray, found the contribution of Dr. Robert A. Lambourne to be most significant, reporting a disturbing picture of the manner in which modern care was at odds with the quest for health and wholeness (McGilvray, 1981). Hospitals became a factory for repair of things rather than a hospice for the care of souls. The growth of medical specialization tended to break down the patient into pathological parts so that he is regarded or treated less and less as a whole patient.

Lambourne's concept of health and wholeness had strong implications for the congregation. It is only when the Christian community serves the sick person in its midst that it becomes itself healed and whole, suggesting a moral basis for individuals and communities to be involved in any consideration of how resources are to be used to promote their health.

The theological basis for health and healing became important points of discussion during the CMC's first meetings. These took the form of a dialogue between John Bryant, the commission's first chairman and a professor of public health, and David E. Jenkins, a commission member and a theologian. Even though there were differences of opinion between them, both were committed to a distribution of resources that improved the lots of those worst off (Bryant and Jenkins, 1971; Bryant, 1977).

CMC staff and members of the commission searched for community-based experiences around the world that would shed light on how best to develop programs that were comprehensive, part of a network of services ranging from the home to specialized institutions, and would incorporate human resources ranging from church members to specialist professionals, including auxiliary and midlevel health workers.

Three community-based experiences presented to the CMC between 1971 and 1973 proved to be critical in WHO's conceptualization of primary health care:

- Central Java, Dr. and Mrs. (Dr.) Gunawan Nugroho
- Jamkhed, India, Drs. Raj and Mabelle Arole
- Chimaltenango, Guatemala, Dr. Carroll Behrhorst.

These programs were strongly community-based, reaching out to those in greatest need, in continuous partnership with the community, and committed to community empowerment. They reached beyond health programs to other sectors – agricultural productivity, shelters, education, water, and sanitation – that were seen as important to community well-being and often directly supportive of health.

These programs and others similar to them were given wide publicity by the CMC through its publication *Contact* (Christian Medical Commission, 1979). These discoveries were not only exciting in themselves but they were illustrative of the growing awareness that health-care systems must respond to the basic needs of people for social justice.

WHO and CMC Join Forces

By the summer of 1973, the CMC had brought to the world's attention many projects that offered innovative ways to improve the health of populations in developing countries. The first official meeting of WHO and the CMC took place in 1974. A joint working group was established, with Dame Nita Barrow and Dr. Ken Newell designated as representatives from CMC and WHO respectively.

Primary Health Care: WHO's New Approach to Health Development

The World Health Assembly in 1974 called on WHO to report to the 55th Executive Board in January 1975 on steps undertaken by WHO to assist governments toward their major health objectives, with priority being given to the rapid and effective development of the health delivery system. This was at the time the smallpox campaign was concluding. It provided Mahler and Newall with the opportunity to introduce primary health care in a comprehensive manner, drawing on the work of the previous 2 years.

The paper presented to the board argued that the resources available to the community needed to be brought into harmony with the resources available to the health services. For this to happen, a radical departure from the conventional health services approach is required, one that builds new services out of a series of peripheral structures that are designed for the context they are to serve, including the reorientation of existing health services so as to establish a unified approach to primary health care.

Conclusion

How dramatic a change primary health care was for WHO can be seen in the contrast between it and the ideas and approaches being promoted several years earlier concerning how best to develop national health systems. Instead of the top-down perspective of health planning and systems analysis, priority was now being given to the bottom-up approaches of community involvement and development, but without losing sight of the importance of planning and informed decision making.

It needs to be appreciated that real courage was required for Mahler to challenge the organization to rethink its approach to health services development or for Newell to respond to that challenge in the way he did.

In January 1975, Newell formally created the Primary Health Care program area, whose members included those who had drafted the report to the executive board. While there was mixed reaction within WHO to this new priority, a wide range of nongovernmental organizations (NGOs) joined forces in what soon became the NGO Committee on Primary Health Care, which worked in close support of WHO's PHC group. This group of organizations prepared for the International Conference on Primary Health Care held at Alma-Ata in September 1978 in an independent manner, thus helping to keep WHO on track. The CMC continued its constructive relationship with WHO, learning as it was contributing (CONTACT, Christian Medical Commission, 1979).

Alma-Ata Revisited, Reflections of Dr. David Tejada (1970s to present)

By the end of the 3-day event, nearly all of the world's countries had signed on to an ambitious commitment. The meeting itself, the final Declaration of Alma-Ata and its Recommendations, mobilized countries worldwide to embark on a process of slow but steady progress toward the social and political goal of Health for All. Since then, Alma-Ata and Primary Health Care have become inseparable terms (Tejada, 2003).

Looking back, the 1970s saw the cresting of the scientific and technological revolution that began with the end of World War II, a revolution that produced, among other major changes, what is today known as globalization. But there was also recognition of growing inequality among the vast sectors of the world's population. This recognition provided the impetus during the 28th and 29th World Health Assemblies in 1975–76 for the commitment to Health for All in the Year 2000.

For Mahler and others, 'Health for All' was a social and political goal, but above all a battle cry to incite people to action. Its meaning, however, has been misunderstood, and confused with a simple concept of programming that is technical rather than social and more bureaucratic then political.

When Mahler proposed Health for All in 1975, he made it clear that he was referring to the need to provide a level of health that would enable all people without exception to live socially and economically productive lives. The reference to the year 2000 meant, as of that date, all the world's countries would have developed the appropriate political strategies and be carrying out concrete measures toward achieving this social goal, albeit within different time frames.

Perhaps because of what might be called professional deformation, it was not really understood that health is a social phenomenon whose determinants cannot be neatly separated from other social and economic determinants. Nor can it be assigned solely to one bureaucratic-administrative sector of the state. Nor was it understood sufficiently – though it was spelled out clearly – that health is, above all, a complex social and political process that requires political decision making not only at the sectorial level but also by the state, so that these decisions are binding upon all sectors without exception.

There is a fundamental difference between integral health care for everyone and by everyone – care that is multisectoral and multidisciplinary, health-promoting and preventive, participatory and decentralized – and low-cost (and lower-quality) curative treatment that is aimed at the poorest and most marginalized segments of the population and, what is worse, provided through programs that are parallel to the rest of the health-care system without the direct, effective participation of the population.

It was at the 28th World Health Assembly in 1975 that the urgent need for new approaches to health care for everyone and by everyone was finally recognized. This is how the notion of primary health care emerged, and it was a victory for the developing world. No one thought about an international conference on the subject, and during the 28th assembly, the prevailing wisdom was that new experiences were needed in this area.

A Soviet Proposal

In January 1976, at the meeting of WHO's Executive Board, Dmitri Venediktov, the powerful Soviet vice-minister for international affairs in the Ministry of Health, proposed a major international conference on primary health care and offered $2 million as an extraordinary contribution by the Soviet Union.

The idea was formally accepted 4 months later at the World Health Assembly, and the conference was scheduled for 1978, to be held in Alma-Ata, Kazakhstan, USSR. Dr. Tejada was designated by the director-general as the general coordinator in charge of the technical, logistical and political aspects. Importantly, the conference was co-hosted and jointly organized with UNICEF, as the product of several years of interaction.

A New Era

The conditions that led to the social and political goal of Health for All and to the strategy of primary health care still exist and are, indeed, even more pronounced. However, there remain gaping inequities and social injustice that leave large segments of populations without integral health care. Poverty is on the rise, and the few resources that societies have for education and health are invested and spent in misguided and unfair ways. The confusion between health and curative medical treatment that is focused on a few diseases inexplicably still prevails. Health systems have not been decentralized effectively, and both citizen participation and social control in health remain distorted concepts.

In today's globalized, unipolar world, where national sovereignty is increasingly threatened, one of the few ways in which countries can still control their own destiny is through the development of genuine decentralized and participatory democracies. Nowadays it is essential to transfer, or rather, to return political power for social decision making to its point of origin, that is, the citizenry.

Integral health care for all and by all – perhaps the best way to phrase Alma-Ata's call for genuine primary health care – is a necessity not only for health but also for the future of countries that aspire to remain sovereign nations in an increasingly unjust world.

There have been major global changes and many important new experiences in the world during the 25 years since the first International Conference on Primary Health Care. Perhaps it is time to convene an Alma-Ata II, to set forth again, without distortions, the original concept that led to the conference in 1978.

Alma-Ata 1978 – Primary Health Care Report of the International Conference on Primary Health Care, Alma-Ata, 6–12 September 1978

Declaration of Alma-Ata

The International Conference on Primary Health Care, meeting in Alma-Ata this twelfth day of September in the year Nineteen hundred and seventy-eight (World Health Organization, 1978), expressing the need for urgent action by all governments, all health and development workers, and the world community to protect and promote the health of all the people of the world, hereby makes the following Declaration:

I

The Conference strongly reaffirms that health, which is a state of complete physical, mental, and social well-being, and not merely the absence of disease or infirmity, is a fundamental human right and that the attainment of the highest possible level of health is a most important worldwide social goal whose realization requires the action of many other social and economic sectors in addition to the health sector.

II

The existing inequality in the health status of people particularly between developed and developing countries as well as within countries is politically, socially, and economically unacceptable and is, therefore, of common concern to all countries.

III

Economic and social development, based on a New International Economic Order, is of basic importance to the fullest attainment of health for all and to the reduction of the gap between the health status of the developing and developed countries. The promotion and protection of the health of the people is essential to sustained economic and social development and contributes to a better quality of life and to world peace.

IV

The people have the right and duty to participate individually and collectively in the planning and implementation of their health care.

V

Governments have a responsibility for the health of their people which can be fulfilled only by the provision of adequate health and social measures. A main social target of governments, international organizations, and the whole world community in the coming decades should be the attainment by all peoples of the world by the year 2000 of a level of health that will permit them to lead a socially and economically productive life. Primary health care is the key to attaining this target as part of development in the spirit of social justice.

VI

Primary health care is essential health care based on practical, scientifically sound, and socially acceptable methods and technology made universally accessible to individuals and families in the community through their full participation and at a cost that the community and country can afford to maintain at every stage of their development in the spirit of self-reliance and self-determination. It forms an integral part both of the country's health system, of which it is the central function and main focus, and of the overall social and economic development of the community. It is the first level of contact of individuals, the family and community with the national health system bringing health care as close as possible to where the people live and work, and constitutes the first element of a continuing health care process.

VII

Primary health care:

1. reflects and evolves from the economic conditions and sociocultural and political characteristics of the country and its communities and is based on the applications of the relevant results of social, biomedical, and health services research and public health experience;
2. addresses the main health problems in the community, providing promotive, preventive, curative, and rehabilitative services accordingly;
3. includes at least education concerning prevailing health problems and the methods of preventing and controlling them; promotion of food supply and proper nutrition; an adequate supply of safe water and basic sanitation; maternal and child health care, including family planning and immunization against the major infectious diseases; prevention and control of locally endemic diseases; appropriate treatment of common diseases and injuries; and provision of essential drugs;

4. involves, in addition to the health sector, all related sectors and aspects of national and community development, in particular agriculture, animal husbandry, food, industry, education, housing, public works, communications, and other sectors, and demands the coordinated efforts of all those sectors;
5. requires and promotes maximum community and individual self-reliance and participation in the planning, organization, operation and control of primary health care, making the fullest use of local, national, and other available resources; and to this end develops through appropriate education the ability of communities to participate;
6. should be sustained and integrated, functional and mutually supportive referral systems, leading to the progressive improvement of comprehensive health care for all, and giving priority to those most in need;
7. relies, at local and referral levels, on health workers, including physicians, nurses, midwives, auxiliaries, and community workers as applicable, as well as traditional practitioners as needed, suitably trained socially and technically to work as a health team and to respond to the expressed health needs of the community.

VIII

All governments should formulate national policies, strategies, and plans of action to launch and sustain primary health care as part of a comprehensive national health system and in coordination with other sectors. To this end, it will be necessary to exercise political will, to mobilize the country's resources and to use available external resources rationally.

IX

All countries should cooperate in a spirit of partnership and service to ensure primary health care for all people since the attainment of health by people in any one country directly concerns and benefits every other country. In this context, the joint WHO/UNICEF report on primary health care constitutes a solid basis for the further development and operation of primary health care throughout the world.

X

An acceptable level of health for all people of the world by the year 2000 can be attained through a fuller and better use of the world's resources, a considerable part of which is now spent on armaments and military conflicts. A genuine policy of independence, peace, détente, and disarmament could and should release additional resources that could be devoted to peaceful aims and in particular to the acceleration of social and economic development of which primary health care, as an essential part, should be allotted its proper share.

Primary Health Care

Primary Health Care is essential health care made universally accessible to individuals and families in the community by means acceptable to them, through their full participation and at a cost that the community and country can afford. It forms an integral part both of the country's health system of which it is the nucleus and of the overall social and economic development of the community.

Primary health care addresses the main health problems in the community, providing promotive, preventive, curative, and rehabilitative services accordingly. Since these services reflect and evolve from the economic conditions and social values of the country and its communities, they will vary by country and community, but will include at least promotion of proper nutrition and adequate supply of safe water; basic sanitation; maternal and child care, including family planning; immunization against the major infectious diseases; prevention and control of locally endemic diseases; education concerning prevailing health problems and methods of preventing and controlling them; and appropriate treatment for common diseases and injuries.

In order to make primary health care universally accessible in the community as quickly as possible, maximum community and individual self-reliance for health development is essential. To attain such self-reliance requires full community participation in the planning, organization, and management of Primary Health Care. Such participation is best mobilized through appropriate education that enables communities to deal with their real health problems in the most suitable ways. They will thus be in a better position to make rational decisions concerning primary health care and to make sure that the right kind of support is provided by the other levels of the national health system. These other levels have to be organized and strengthened so as to support primary health care with technical knowledge, training, guidance and supervision, logistic support, supplies, information, financing, and referral facilities, including institutions to which unsolved problems and individual patients can be referred.

Primary health care is likely to be most effective if it employs means that are understood and accepted by the community and applied by community health workers at a cost the community and the country can afford. These community health workers, including traditional practitioners where applicable, will function best if they reside in the community they serve and are properly trained socially and technically to respond to its expressed health needs.

Since primary health care is an integral part both of the country's health system and of overall economic and social development, without which it is bound to fail, it has to be coordinated on a national basis with other levels of the health system, as well as with the other sectors that contribute to a country's total development strategy.

Selective Primary Health Care (1978 to Present)

The Alma-Ata Declaration was criticized for being too broad and idealistic, with an unrealistic timetable. A common criticism was that the slogan Health for All by 2000 was not feasible. Concerned about the identification of the most cost-effective strategies, in 1979 the Rockefeller Foundation sponsored a small conference entitled Health and Population in Development at its Bellagio Conference Center in Italy. The goal of the meeting was to examine the status and interrelations of health and population programs as the organizers felt there were 'disturbing signs of declining interest in population issues.'

The conference was based on a published paper by Julia Walsh and Kenneth Warren entitled: 'Selective Primary Health Care, an Interim Strategy for Disease Control in Developing Countries' (Walsh and Warren, 1979). The paper sought specific causes of death, paying special attention to the most common diseases of infants in developing countries such as diarrhea and diseases produced by lack of immunizations. In the paper, and at the meeting, selective primary health care was introduced as the name of a new perspective. The term meant a package of low-cost, technical interventions to tackle the main disease problems of poor countries.

The interventions were known as GOBI, meaning growth monitoring, oral rehydration techniques, breast feeding, and immunizations. These four interventions appeared easy to monitor and evaluate. Moreover, they were measurable and had clear targets. Funding appeared easier to obtain because indicators of success and reporting could be produced more rapidly. Later, some agencies added FFF (food supplementation, female literacy, family planning) to the acronym GOBI, creating GOBI-FFF.

One participant of the Bellagio meeting who was strongly influenced by the new proposal was James Grant of UNICEF. A Harvard-trained economist and lawyer, Grant was appointed executive director of UNICEF in January 1980 and served until January 1995. Under his dynamic leadership, UNICEF began to back away from a holistic approach to primary health care. Like Mahler, he was a charismatic leader who had an easy way with both heads of state and common people. A few years later, Grant organized a children's revolution and explained the four inexpensive interventions contained in GOBI (Cueto, 2004).

A debate between the two versions of primary health care was inevitable.

The Debate

The supporters of comprehensive primary health care accused selective primary health care of being a narrow, technocentric approach that diverted attention away from basic health and socioeconomic development, did not address the social causes of disease, and resembled vertical programs. The debate between these two perspectives evolved around three questions: What was the meaning of primary health care? How was primary health care to be financed? How was it to be implemented?

The passage of time has not resolved these differences. They have persisted, with positions reshaped by evolving local, national, and global contexts. The history of primary health care and selective primary health care analyzed in this paper illustrate two diverse assumptions in international health in the twentieth century. First, there was a recognition that diseases in less-developed countries were socially and economically sustained and needed a political response. Second, there was an assumption that the main diseases in poor countries were a natural reality that needed adequate technological solutions. These two ideas were taken – even before primary heath care – as representing a dilemma, and one path or the other had to be chosen.

A lesson of this story is that the divorce between goals and techniques and the lack of articulation between different aspects of health work need to be addressed. A holistic approach, idealism, technical expertise, and finance should – must – go together. There are still problems of territoriality, lack of flexibility, and fragmentation in international agencies and in health programs in developing countries. Primary and vertical programs coexist. One way to enhance the integration of sound technical interventions, socioeconomic development programs, and the training of human resources for health is the study of history.

Ottawa Charter

The first International Conference on Health Promotion, meeting in Ottawa this 21st day of November 1986, hereby presents this CHARTER for action to achieve Health for All by the year 2000 and beyond.

This conference was primarily a response to growing expectations for a new public health movement around the world. Discussions focused on the needs in industrialized countries, but took into account similar concerns in all other regions. It built on the progress made through the Declaration on Primary Health Care at Alma-Ata, the World Health Organization's Targets for Health for All document, and the recent debate at the World Health Assembly on intersectoral action for health.

Health Promotion

Health promotion is the process of enabling people to increase control over, and to improve, their health. To reach a state of complete physical, mental, and social well-being, an individual or group must be able to identify and to realize aspirations, to satisfy needs, and to change or cope with the environment. Health is, therefore, seen as a resource for everyday life, not the objective of living. Health is a positive concept emphasizing social and personal resources, as well as physical capacities. Therefore, health promotion is not just the responsibility of the health sector, it goes beyond healthy life-styles to well-being.

Commitment to Health Promotion

The participants in this Conference pledge:

- to move into the arena of health public policy and to advocate a clear political commitment to health and equity in all sectors;
- to counteract the pressures toward harmful products, resource depletion, unhealthy living conditions and environments, and bad nutrition, and to focus attention on public health issues such as pollution, occupational hazards, housing, and settlements;
- to respond to the health gap within and between societies and to tackle the inequities in health produced by the rules and practices of these societies;
- to acknowledge people as the main health resource, to support and enable them to keep themselves, their families, and friends healthy through financial and other means, and to accept the community as the essential voice in matters of its health, living conditions, and well-being;
- to reorient health services and their resources toward the promotion of health and to share power with other sectors, other disciplines, and, most importantly, with people themselves;
- to recognize health and its maintenance as a major social investment and challenge; and to address the overall ecological issue of our ways of living.

The Conference urges all concerned to join them in their commitment to a strong public health alliance.

Call for International Action

The Conference calls on the World Health Organization and other international organizations to advocate the promotion of health in all appropriate forums and to support countries in setting up strategies and programmes for health promotion.

The Conference is firmly convinced that if people in all walks of life, nongovernmental and voluntary organizations, governments, the World Health Organization, and all other bodies concerned join forces in introducing strategies for health promotion, in line with the moral and social values that form the basis of this charter, Health For All by the year 2000 will become a reality.

Reflections on the Ottawa Charter

It is notable that the Ottawa Charter was followed by an international insistence on the further development of health promotion as a conceptual and policy centerpiece of international health. This led, in turn, to establishing in WHO the Department of Chronic Diseases and Health Promotion. A dramatic indication of its evolving strength was the establishment in 2005 of the Bangkok Charter for Health Promotion, with strong international support (WHO/HPR/HEP, 1986).

From Alma-Ata to the Year 2000, Reflections at the Midpoint, Riga, Latvia

The first of several meetings celebrating the anniversaries of Alma-Ata took place in Riga, Latvia Republic, USSR, 1988 (World Health Organization, 1988). The meeting reflected the intense interest of multiple parties in the consequences of the Alma-Ata conference and what had happened to the key concepts of Health for All and primary health care. Following are comments by John Bryant, who was on the U.S. Delegation to Alma-Ata, and helped to plan and organize the Riga meeting, and Halfdan Mahler, then Director General of WHO.

- Bryant. In reviewing the successes and failures since Alma-Ata, we have concluded that there is no doubt that health for all and primary health care have served the world well. At the same time, despite substantial gains in most countries, there has been a slowness and even stagnation in many countries. If you look from now, in 1988, at projections for the year 2000, you will find a large number of African and South Asian countries where infant, young child, and maternal mortality rates will still be at levels that the world must consider completely unacceptable.

  This was a turning point at Riga: The recognition that what is being done is not enough. As WHO turns the corner of the first decade after Alma-Ata, it needs to ready itself for new sets of problems. Tomorrow will not be yesterday, and yesterday's answers, though they brought glory, will not serve tomorrow. So there was a call for new forms of analysis, new partnerships, new mechanisms of action, and new resources.

  Reflecting on the debate at Riga, the result was Alma-Ata reaffirmed at Riga – a statement of renewed and strengthened commitment to health for all by the year 2000 and beyond. But this was not simply a self-congratulatory exercise. There was an acknowledgement of the important shortfalls, that serious problems remained almost untouched by the Health for All effort, and new problems are emerging that are already defying solutions. An example would be the emergence of the HIV/AIDS pandemic. To address this range of persisting and emerging problems, the meeting at Riga suggested a number of actions to be taken, including empowering people, strengthening district health systems based on primary health care; overcoming problems that continue to resist solution, and finally a special priority initiative in support of the least developed countries.

The last point, about the least developed countries, is based on the fact that, while most countries have benefited from the Health for All movement, a tragic residuum remains. These nations are not the causes of the problems of severe underdevelopment, they are the victims of it. They have been marginalized by it and, to a large extent, abandoned to it. The resources and processes involved in international development have failed these people, and Health for All to date has failed them as well. And so a special initiative is proposed, which should be strongly intersectoral in nature as well as long term. Finally, we believe that WHO should monitor the rate of progress, which should serve as an indicator of the resolve of WHO and the Member States to deal with this most fundamental of challenges, namely the needs of countries which, without effective help, will likely slip further down the spiral of development failure.

The comments of Dr. Halfdan Mahler are of special interest, both because of his commitment to the underlying values and principles of Health for All and primary health care, and because this was one of the last events in his professional life as Director General of WHO.

- Mahler. There is one last point, which is very close to my heart, especially as I leave WHO. We must have an obsession, a moral obsession, about the least developed of the developing countries. They are missing out totally, as Jack Bryant said, in the development process. It is development gone wrong. They are marginalized in the cynical economic climate of the contemporary world. With the kind of platform we are talking about, with UNICEF and WHO together with UNFPA and other multilateral agencies, we can look at how we can address the problems of their predicament at this time in history. They must be brought on board in a real and true sense before the year 2000. It is indispensable, not so that they survive in misery, but that they survive so their children can realize their physical, social and spiritual potential.

If we could make a real entry point into the development dilemma of these countries through health for all and primary health care, I think we could also challenge the other partners in development, and somehow shame them into saying that this cannot possibly go on if we have the minimum of morality on spaceship earth.

Alma-Ata and After – Dmitry Venediktov (1978 to present)

Of particular interest are the reflections of Dmitry Venediktov relating to the Alma-Ata Conference (Venediktov, 1998). He played a key role in representing the Russian government in negotiating with WHO in favor of an international conference on health system development and also for having the conference in a Russian city, which turned out to be Alma-Ata. He was serving at that time on the Executive Board of WHO and was one of the most influential persons in concepts, events, and decisions leading to Alma-Ata.

We have known Venediktov for many years, beginning during the latter years of planning for Alma-Ata, and served with him on the Executive Board of WHO for a number of years. We have also seen him on occasion in more recent years. He contributed an exceedingly interesting article to the World Health Forum in 1998 in which he reflects on various issues relating to Alma-Ata (Venediktov, 1998). At the end of the article, which analyzes a variety of issues relating to the conference, he offers three lessons from Alma-Ata.

First, it marked the beginning of a new international understanding of the real dimensions of health-care needs, especially in developing countries, and of the enormous social and economic problems involved. It made it clear that meeting these needs was one of the foremost responsibilities of any government.

Second, it brought to a close the era in which technical assistance and efforts at disease eradication could be thought of as a sufficient activity for WHO. By showing that it was both necessary and possible to redesign health systems on the basis of primary health care, it pointed the way toward national self-reliance in health.

Third, it opened up new prospects for international cooperation in health. Long before the current talk of globalization, it demonstrated not only the advantages but the necessity of sharing information and strategies for promoting health and preventing and controlling disease.

The conviction that health is a human right and that governments must uphold that right for present and future generations is the most important message that comes to us from Alma-Ata as we approach the year 2000.

Primary Health Care – Everybody's Business, 20 Years after Alma-Ata, Meeting in Almaty, Kazakhstan 1978

Primary Health Care 21, Gro Brundtland, Director General, WHO

The Alma-Ata Declaration of 1978 emerged from the International Conference on primary health care as a major milestone of this century in the field of Public Health. Motivated by gross inequality in health status within and between countries and arguing that health is essential to social and economic development, the declaration identifies primary health care as the key to the attainment of Health for All by the people of a level of health that will permit them to lead a socially and economically productive life. It advocates the essential elements and intersectoral nature of primary health care (World Health Organization, 2000).

As we move into the next millennium, we have new challenges, new opportunities, and unfinished agendas. Accessibility to essential care remains a challenge. Most affected is the growing number of poor and economically dependent, such as the aged who are unable to afford basic health care. Intersectoral action for health, at all levels of society, and particularly in communities where people live and work, has become a critical element of any approach to public health that aims to improve the health outcomes and help people maintain and improve their health. While the delivery of essential health care and cost-effective interventions is critical, the social relevance of health systems plays an equally if not more important role in sustaining acceptable and affordable health services. Ultimately, it is the individual, the family and the community who make the most important decisions about their health. The degree to which they are able to respond to the health challenges they encounter contributes to their ability to maintain their health and to the effectiveness of the health and social services available to them. These are key aspects of primary health care, which remain relevant and need to be an integral part of any effort to strengthen national health systems.

In today's context, I am emphasizing the need for a new universalism that includes a commitment to primary health care to maximize the efficiency and equity gains and create a win/win situation in poorer countries with larger burden of disease. Practical steps toward universal coverage need to be taken. There is no single blueprint available for replication in all countries. We are living a world of increased democratization with expanding free market forces, which affect all sectors. Within that context, we must find ways of using these forces to incorporate the values and principles of primary health care together with partners in the private sector and civil society.

Primary health care remains a key strategy in implementing the policy of HFA. We will continue to work with our partners in UNICEF as well as new partners including the World Bank, United Nations Development Programme (UNDP) and the United Nations Population Fund (UNFPA) in ensuring that the primary health care movement continues and builds on the lessons learned and the gains achieved and the leadership and commitment of the many who have tirelessly worked to make primary health care a reality.

Primary Health Care 21, Dr. David Sanders, University of Western Cape

Conclusions

While there have been significant achievements, it is clear that progress toward Health for All has been uneven. Gains made are at risk from a complex and accelerating process of globalization and economic policies that have a negative impact on the livelihoods and health of an increasing percentage of the world's population and the large majority in developing countries. Although the global primary health care initiative has been successful in disseminating a number of effective technologies and programs that have substantially reduced the impact of certain (mostly infectious) diseases, its intersectoral focus and social mobilizing roles – which are the keys to its sustainability – have been neglected, both in discourse but also in implementation.

Governments enthusiastically promoting partnerships between sectors, agencies, and communities to develop intersectoral policies that address the determinants of inequities and ill health can halt, and reverse, this trend. The policy development process needs to be inclusive, transparent, and supported by legislative and financial commitment.

WHO has the opportunity to lead in the development of a strategy for primary health care by working in collaboration with Member States and national and international health agencies and professional organizations. The strategy should capture the diversity of needs and capacities and aim to establish linkages between primary care services, disease prevention, and health promotion at local levels.

A defined research agenda, and lessons about what is being learned about the impact of different primary health care models and effective approaches to disseminating best practice, will underpin all these activities.

In promoting the above move from policy to action, WHO has to play a much bolder role in advocating for equity and legislation to facilitate its achievement; pointing out the dangers to health of globalization and liberalization; stressing the importance of partnerships between the health sector and other sectors; integrating its own internal structures and activities to ensure that comprehensive primary health care programs are developed; entering into partnerships with and influencing other multilateral and bilateral agencies and donors as well as nongovernmental organizations and professional bodies toward a common vision of primary health care; and arguing for major investment in health, especially in human resource development, without which Health for All will remain a mere statement of intent.

Global Review of Primary Health Care: Emerging Messages

The Global Report by WHO in 2003 is based on a review of primary health care derived from the six regions of WHO (World Health Organization, 2003a).

Primary Health Care in a Changing World. What's New?

- Since Alma-Ata there have been dramatic changes in the pattern of disease, in demographic profiles, and in the socioeconomic environment, which present new challenges to primary health care.
- There have been significant changes in how governments are interpreting their roles and this has implications for both policy development and globally driven health programs.
- The policy environment now includes the widespread presence of nongovernmental organizations (NGOs) as major stakeholders in health and health care.
- The delivery of a wide range of WHO's own strategies is dependent on there being appropriate primary health care capacity at a local level.
- Both the recommendations of the Commission on Macro-economics and Health and the Millennium Development Goals (MDGs) set out a future agenda that would see major new investments in health systems. It will be vitally important for WHO to offer guidance on the most effective health solutions, including a contribution that can be expected from primary health care close-to-client services.
- It is unrealistic to expect the achievement of the MDGs without an organized primary health care.

Primary Health Care and Evidence

Many countries have included PHC as a policy cornerstone in their health system reforms. As part of these reforms, many have carried out reviews of the available and relevant evidence. An earlier review of international literature noted that the paucity of rigorous evaluation research in such a broad policy area as primary health care delivery is striking. Whatever policies are contemplated for the reform of primary health care systems around the world, their implementation should be considered in the context of a strong policy-informing research agenda.

Responding to the Typology for Development

There are three scenarios that could be the basis for identifying development needs and taking forward PHC policies and models in the twenty-first century.

Scenario 1

The first scenario involves completing implementation. The challenge to key stakeholders is to understand why implementation is failing and plan remedial action to secure the benefits of primary health care for their populations. For example:

- Lack of political commitment, leadership, and insufficient policy continuity.
- Initial objectives were unrealistic.
- Local primary health care services were seen as inappropriate.
- Lack of integration between primary health care and other parts of the health system.
- Primary health care staff have the wrong skills and are not motivated.
- An effective intersectoral approach has not been developed.
- PHC policies and models are not sustainable.
- Community involvement is not working.

Scenario 2

The second scenario involves strengthening PHC to meet new challenges.

- To be successful community participation must become part of a community's common experience and not just imposed from the outside.
- Strengthening the primary health care model at the local level.
  1. Making the primary health care model problem-oriented;
  2. Reinforcing community involvement;
  3. Reinforcing intersectoral collaboration;
  4. Strengthen integration of primary health care with other health care organizations;
  5. Building leadership capacity in change management within the local primary health care team.
- Policy alignment at a national level. The impact of central policies which promote PHC will be less if:
  1. intersectoral collaboration is not reinforced at government level;
  2. tensions between vertical programs for health improvement and PHC are not addressed;
  3. the drive for integration of PHC with other parts of the health care system is undermined.

Scenario 3

The third scenario involves locating primary health care in a new paradigm, such as integrating health goals in the larger and transcendent goals of social justice, human rights, and equity. For example:

- Promote wider social change in areas such as gender, children's rights, education, employment.
- Changes in leadership to reflect concern for social justice, human rights, and equity.
- Change education of primary health care practitioners to reinforce a values system concerned with social justice, human rights, and equity.
- Focus primary health care attention on those who suffer most from inequality and social injustice.

Renewing Primary Health Care in the Americas

The Pan American Health Organization is in a global leadership role in reviewing problems and current inadequacies in primary health care and in proposing corrective patterns that are strongly responsive to global challenges.

Director's Letter

> Nothing great in the world has ever been accomplished without passion. Hebbel, 1818–1863

In 2003, motivated by the 25th Anniversary of Alma-Ata Conference and at the behest of its member countries, the Pan-American Health Organization decided to re-examine the values and principles that a few decades ago inspired the Alma-Ata Declaration in order to develop its future strategic and programmatic orientations in primary health care. The resulting strategy, presented in this article, provides a vision and renewed sense of purpose for health systems development: That of the Primary Health Care-Based Health System. This position paper reviews the legacy of Alma-Ata in the Americas, articulates components of a new strategy for primary health care renewal, and lays out steps that need to be taken in order to achieve this ambitious vision.

The process of developing the position paper has helped to invigorate debate about the meaning of health systems and their relationship to other determinants of population health and its equitable distribution in societies. Initial discussions about PHC renewal moved quickly from technical talk about health services to reflection about social values as fundamental determinants of health and health systems. Country consultations and meetings revealed a desire to assure that technical discussions about health policies continue to reflect the real meanings such policies have on the lives of citizens within the region.

The vision of a primary health care-based health system is well within the spirit of Alma-Ata, while acknowledging new developments such as the Ottawa Charter for health promotion, the Millennium Declaration, and the Commission on the Social Determinants of Health.

This document presents the work of numerous individuals and organizations and thus the extent and ambition of its vision reflects the diversity of its architects. The position paper focuses on the core values, principles, and elements likely to be present in a reinvigorated primary health care approach, rather than describing an all-encompassing mold into which all countries are expected to fit. Each country will need to find its own way to craft a sustainable strategy for basing their health system more firmly on the primary health care approach.

The road to achieving this vision is not expected to be a simple one, but few things of value come without dedication. Challenges include the need to invest in integrated networks of health and social services that have in many areas been inadequately staffed, equipped, or supported and inequitably distributed. This overhaul needs to take place within the context of shrinking budgets, which will require more rational and more equitable resource utilization, especially if they want to reach those with greater needs. The best available evidence supports the contention that a strong primary health care orientation is among the most equitable and efficient ways to organize a health system, although we must continue to strengthen the evidence base on innovations in primary health care and learn how to maximize and sustain their impact over time.

The position paper 'Renewing Primary Health Care in the Americas' is intended to be a reference for all countries moving forward to strengthen their health care systems, bringing health care to people living in urban and rural areas, regardless of their gender, age, ethnicity, social status, or religion. We invite you to read this document conveying the view and feelings of a great diversity of individuals living and working in the Americas as well as many experts from around the world and look forward to continuing this ongoing dialogue as we embark together on this ambitious endeavor.

Mirta Roses Periago

Director, PAHO

Executive Summary, February 2007

For more than a quarter of a century primary health care has been recognized as one of the key components of an effective health system. Experiences in more developed and less developed countries alike have demonstrated that primary health care can be adapted and interpreted to suit a wide variety of political, social, and cultural contexts. A comprehensive review of primary health care – both in theory and practice – and a critical look at how this concept can be renewed to better reflect the current health and development needs of people around the world, is now in order. This document – written to fulfill a mandate established in 2003 by a resolution of the Pan American Health Organization (PAHO) – states the position of PAHO on the proposed renewal of PHC. The goal of this paper is to generate ideas and recommendations to enable such a renewal, and to help strengthen and reinvigorate primary health care into a concept that can lead the development of health systems for the coming quarter century and beyond.

There are several reasons for adopting a renewed approach to primary health care, including: The rise of new epidemiologic challenges that primary health care must evolve to address; the need to correct weaknesses and inconsistencies present in some of the widely divergent approaches to primary health care; the development of new tools and knowledge of best practices that primary health care can capitalize on to be more effective; and a growing recognition that primary health care is an approach to strengthen society's ability to reduce inequities in health. In addition, a renewed approach to primary health care is viewed as an essential condition for meeting the commitments of internationally agreed-upon development goals, including those contained in the United Nations Millennium Declaration, addressing the social determinants of health, and achieving the highest attainable level of health by everyone.

By examining concepts and components of primary health care and the evidence of its impact, this document builds upon the legacy of Alma-Ata and the primary health care movement, distills lessons learned from primary health care and health reform experiences, and proposes a set of key values, principles, and elements essential for building health systems based on primary health care. It postulates that such systems will be necessary to tackle the unfinished health agenda in the Americas, as well as to consolidate and maintain progress made and rise to the new health and development challenges and commitments of the twenty-first century.

The ultimate goal of the renewal of primary health care is to obtain sustainable health gains for all. The proposal presented here is meant to be visionary; the realization of this document's recommendations, and the realization of primary health care's potential, will be limited only by our commitment and imagination.

The main messages include:

- Throughout the extensive consultation process that formed the basis for this paper, it was found that primary health care represents, even today, a source of inspiration and hope, not only for most health personnel, but for the community at large.
- Due to new challenges, knowledge, and contexts, there is a need to renew and reinvigorate primary health care in the region so that it can realize its potential to meet today's health challenges and those of the next quarter-century.
- Renewal of primary health care entails recognizing and facilitating the role of primary health care as an approach to promote more equitable health and human development.
- Primary health care renewal will need to pay increased attention to structural and operational needs such as access, financial fairness, adequacy and sustainability of resources, political commitment, and the development of systems that assure high-quality care.
- Successful primary health care experiences have demonstrated that system-wide approaches are needed, so a renewed approach to primary health care must make a stronger case for a reasoned and evidence-based approach to achieving universal, integrated, and comprehensive care.
- The proposed mechanism for primary health care renewal is the transformation of health systems so that they incorporate primary health care as their basis.
- A primary health care-based health system entails an overarching approach to the organization and operation of health systems that makes the right to the highest attainable level of health its main goal while maximizing equity and solidarity. Such a system is guided by the primary health care principles of responsiveness to people's health needs, quality orientation, government accountability, social justice, sustainability, participation, and intersectoriality.
- A primary health care-based health system is composed of a core set of functional and structural elements that guarantee universal coverage and access to services that are acceptable to the population and that are equity-enhancing. It provides comprehensive, integrated, and appropriate care over time, emphasizes prevention and promotion, and assures first-contact care. Families and communities are its basis for planning and action.
- A primary health care-based health system requires a sound legal, institutional, and organizational foundation as well as adequate and sustainable human, financial, and technological resources. It employs optimal organization and management practices at all levels to achieve quality, efficiency, and effectiveness and develops active mechanisms to maximize individual and collective participation in health. A primary health care-based health system develops intersectorial actions to address other determinants of health and equity.
- International evidence suggests that health systems based on a strong primary health care orientation have better and more equitable health outcomes, are more efficient, have lower health care costs, and can achieve higher user satisfaction than those whose health systems have only a weak primary health care orientation.

- The reorientation of health systems toward primary health care requires a greater emphasis on health promotion and prevention. This is achieved by assigning appropriate functions to each level of government, integrating public and personal health services, focusing on families and communities, using accurate data in planning and decision making, and creating an institutional framework with incentives to improve the quality of services.
- Full realization of primary health care requires additional focus on the role of human resources, development of strategies for managing change, and aligning international cooperation with the primary health care approach.
- The next step to renewing primary health care is to constitute an international coalition of interested parties. The tasks of this coalition will be to frame primary health care renewal as a priority, develop the concept of primary health care-based health systems so that it represents a feasible and politically appealing policy option, and finds ways to capitalize on the current window of opportunity provided by the recent 25th anniversary of Alma-Ata, the international consensus on the importance of attaining the Millennium Development Goals (MDGs), and the current international focus on the need for strengthening health systems.

Building Primary Health Care-Based Health Systems

The conceptual framework presented here is meant to serve as a foundation for organizing and understanding components of a primary health care-based health system; it is not meant to define, exhaustively, all of the necessary elements that constitute or define a health system. Due to the great variation in national economic resources, political circumstances, administrative capacities, and historical development of the health sector, each country will need to design their own strategy for primary health care renewal. It is hoped that the values, principles, and elements described below will aid in that process.

A. Values
- Right to the highest attainable level of health
- Equity
- Solidarity.

B. Principles
- Responsiveness to people's health needs
- Quality-oriented
- Government accountability
- Social justice
- Sustainability
- Participation
- Intersectoriality.

C. Elements
- Universal coverage and access
- First contact
- Comprehensive, integrated, and continuing care
- Family- and community-based
- Emphasis on promotion and prevention
- Appropriate care
- Active participation mechanisms
- Sound policy, legal, and institutional framework
- Pro-equity policies and programs
- Optimal organization and management
- Appropriate human resources
- Adequate and sustainable resources
- Intersectorial actions.

The Commission on Macroeconomics and Health

The Commission was launched by Gro Brundtland, Director General of WHO, in the year 2000, with Jeffrey Sachs as its director, with the mandate of examining the interactions of health and economic development. The Commission argued that by taking essential interventions to scale and making them available worldwide, eight million lives could be saved each year by 2010. To achieve these huge gains in health and economic development, the Commission called for a major increase in the resources allocated to the health sector of the next few years. Then, on a very practical note, the Commission recommends that the most effective interventions can be delivered through health centers and similar facilities and through outreach, which they collectively describe as close-to-the-client (CTC) systems. This can be seen as an important endorsement of PHC principles and practice (CMH, 2000).

The Millennium Development Goals Coupled with the Millennium Project

The MDGs were the product, in the year 2000, of 189 countries signing the UN Millennium Declaration. This historic call to action – at the dawn of the new century – set forth an ambitious agenda for improving the lives of the world's poorest citizens by 2015, through a joint effort of both developed and developing countries. The key goals were then expanded, refined and operationalized as the MDGs, including concrete targets and a specific timetable, with accountability at all levels: international, regional and country, as well as municipal and community (Sachs, 2005).

Given the ambitious range and the global complexities of the MDGs, it became apparent that further refinement of strategies would be required, thus the establishment of the UN Millennium Project in 2002 under the leadership of Jeffrey Sachs. Thirteen task forces were formed to address the goals and targets, and their work culminated in a final report in 2005: *Investing in Development – A Practical Plan to Achieve the MDGs*.

This must be seen as a remarkable process encompassing threats to the health and well-being of humanity, and the need to extend responsive actions not only to diverse national settings, but onward to community levels. This is well stated by Jeff Sachs.

> Our Project has been a microcosm of a larger truth: achieving the MDG will require a global partnership suitable for an interconnected world. Another special aspect of the Project is the rare and powerful opportunity to help give voice to the hopes, aspirations, and vital needs of the world's poor and most voiceless people. We have met countless heroes and heroines of development in the three years of our work – in the villages and slums of Africa, Asia, Latin America and other parts of the developing world (Sachs, 2005).

Not surprisingly, multiple flaws in the nature of responses and coverage relating to populations in need have been identified in the MDGs, and the insights of the Millennium Project have covered many of them. Indeed, it is impressive to see the realities specified by the task forces of the project.

Overall, there is no doubting the implications of these global developments for PHC. They provide a new platform for PHC policy and program development, with profound potential for constructive change.

The Commission on Social Determinants of Health

Established by the Director General of WHO in 2005, the Commission on Social Determinants of Health (CSDH) is a strategic mechanism to promote a global health agenda to improve equity in health and health through action on the social determinants of health at global, regional, and country levels.

The CSDH states that today, an unprecedented opportunity exists to improve health in some of the world's poorest and most vulnerable communities by tackling the root causes of disease and health inequalities. The most powerful of these causes are the social conditions in which people live and work.

In assessing the general field of health and development, the founders of the Commission have reflected on the policies and processes that have been supportive of social factors in health and those that have been conflictual. It is interesting to include PHC in those considerations as it is closely related to social determinants of health.

One factor of importance has been intersectoral action, which was central to the model of comprehensive primary health care proposed to drive the Health for All agenda following the 1978 conference at Alma-Ata, USSR.

One of the conflictual approaches was that of selective primary health care, introduced in 1979, which focused on a small number of cost-effective interventions and downplayed the social dimensions of health.

Like other aspects of comprehensive primary health care, action on social determinants was weakened by the neoliberal economic and political consensus that was dominant in the 1980s and beyond, with its focus on privatization, deregulation, shrinking states, and freeing markets. A key postulate of the neoliberal economic orthodoxy of the 1980s and 1990s was that, since economic growth was the key to rapid development and ultimately to a better life for all, countries should rapidly and rigorously implement policies to stimulate growth, with little concern for the social consequences in the near term.

Another major factor related to neoliberal doctrines was the structural adjustment programs (SAPs) imposed on a large number of countries as a condition for debt restructuring, access to new development loans and other forms of international support. The SAPs were implemented in many countries of Africa, Asia, and Latin America under the guidance of the International Financial Institutions (IFIs). A central principle of SAPs was sharp reduction in government expenditures, in many cases meaning drastic cuts in social sector budgets. These cuts affect areas of key importance as determinants of health, including education, nutrition programs, water and sanitation, transport, housing, and various forms of social protection and safety nets, in addition to direct spending in the health sector. In addition, many SAPs demanded large and abrupt cuts in public sector payrolls. The negative impacts on primary health care as well as social determinants of health were striking (World Health Organization, 2005).

In contrast, the Millennium Development Goals (MDGs) shape the current global development agenda in strongly positive ways. The MDGs recognize the interdependence of health and social conditions and present an opportunity to promote health policies that tackle the social roots of unfair and avoidable human suffering.

It is interesting, indeed, to see that although several global processes or policies, like neoliberal perspectives and structural adjustment programs, have had distinctly negative impacts on the social side of health development where primary health care resides in the development process, other actions, such as the Commission on Macroeconomics and Health, the MDGs, and the Commission on Social Determinants of Health, are being envisaged and implemented that are strongly supportive of the social and economic base for health development for poor populations. How timely it is to recall Mahler's comments in his address to the 1978 World Health Assembly: 'Health and economic development are indivisible; cutting back on health programs retards economic development.'

Primary Health Care and the New Director General of WHO, Dr. Margaret Chan

It has been dramatic, indeed, to hear the remarks of the new Director General of WHO, Dr. Margaret Chan, regarding her perspectives on health and health care. Here are excerpts of her presentation to the World Health Assembly, November, 2006. (The sequence of these remarks has been modified from the presentation)

> So let me be clear about the results that matter most. Reducing burden of disease is important. Improving the strength of health systems is important. Reducing the threat of risk factors for disease is important.
>
> These are all vital. But what matters to me is people. And two specific groups of people in particular. I want us to be judged by the impact we have on the health of the people of Africa, and the health of women.
>
> Health systems are the tap root for better health. When we talk about capacity, we absolutely must talk about the importance of primary health care. It is the cornerstone of building the capacity of health systems. I plan to promote primary health care as a strategy for strengthening health systems. The reason is simple: It works. This is the only way to ensure fair, affordable, and sustainable access to essential care across a population. We have the evidence. I have experienced this personally. During my tenure in Hong Kong, I introduced primary health care from the diaper to the grave.

There have been numerous enthusiastic responses to her call for special attention to primary health care. She has sought advice from Halfdan Mahler and others with close familiarity with the Alma-Ata story and its contemporary challenges. There will be a Conference on Primary Health Care in Buenos Aires, Argentina, August 13–18, 2007, sponsored by PAHO, with the title 'Rights, Facts, and Realities, strengthening PHC and health systems to achieve the MDGs'. This conference is seen as setting the stage for another conference to be held in 2008 to celebrate the 30th Anniversary of Alma Ata and the 60th Anniversary of the founding of WHO, including the possibility of organizing an Alma-Ata II!

Addendum to Alma-Ata and Primary Health Care: An Evolving Story. Buenos Aires 30/15 International Conference, August 2007 From Alma-Ata to the Millennium Declaration: *Towards Equity-Based Comprehensive Health Care*

Background

The interest in and commitment to primary health care, which found its origin at the WHO/UNICEF International Conference on Primary Health Care at Alma-Ata in 1978, has been increasing globally. Important support has come from Dr. Margaret Chan, the new Director General of WHO, who has called for a global rejuvenation of primary health care. Virtually all of the six regions of WHO have been taking supportive steps. The support of the Pan American Health Organization has been particularly strong, as illustrated by the publication in 2005 of its position paper on *Renewing Primary Health Care in the Americas*.

These factors coalesced into the convening of the International Conference – From Alma Ata to the Millennium Declaration, Buenos Aires 30/15. The title of the conference is revealing – 30 years since Alma Ata, and now near the mid-point in the countdown to 2015, the year given so much significance and promise by the Millennium Declaration and its goals.

The conference brought together a wide range of persons who have had major impacts on global health policies with special interest in Primary Health Care. The following presentations are illustrative of the broad international support given to the Buenos Aires Conference:

- Gines Gonzalez Garcia, Minister of Health of Argentina: *Prologue*;
- Halfdan T. Mahler, Director General, WHO, at the time of the International Conference, Alma Ata in 1978: *Leadership and Equity in Health*;
- Michael Marmot, Chairman, Commission on Social Determinants of Health, WHO: *Social Determinants of Health. Global Context and Challenges*;
- Ravi Narayan, Coordinator of the Peoples Health Movement: *Health for All – A Supreme Challenge*;
- Margaret Chan, Director General, WHO: *Contribution of Primary Health Care to the Millennium Development Goals*;
- Mirta Roses Periago, Director, PAHO: *Closing Statement*.

The Conference Report concludes with the Buenos Aires Declaration: *Towards a Health Strategy for Equity-Based Primary Health Care*, which deserves special attention, as it expresses the concern of the participants for equity-based comprehensive care, accessible to all including those who are most disadvantaged.

Prologue

Gines Gonzalez Garcia, Minister of Health of Argentina

The main challenges for world health systems are the access to quality services for all, a more humanized care at health centers, and an equity-based distribution of resources and sanitary results.

These were the conclusions of the Buenos Aires 30/15 International Conference, held in August, 2007, which gathered specialists and representatives from over 60 countries and was attended by more than 3000 people.

The two major breakthroughs in the interests of the right to health for our people have been the Universal Declaration of Human Rights (1948) and the Alma-Ata Conference (1978). The 30-year period between both milestones outlined the most important paradigm in public health policies: primary health care.

In a few months, another 30 years will have passed. The objective of the Conference held in Buenos Aires was to relaunch primary health care as essential approach to tackle new and old health problems.

During Buenos Aires 30/15, we all realized that the primary health care strategy is still producing very good results in the countries of the region. But there is still a lot to be done. This is why we must deepen the reforms, turning this strategy into the core of the whole system. Our main struggle is not against biological agents, but against society and behavior models that bring disease and death to millions of people.

Recent experience in the region has shown that the sanitary reforms that focused on primary health care produced excellent results, and Argentina is a good example. This forces us to deepen the ongoing transformations. If we can adequately implement the ideas set out in Buenos Aires 30/15, we will be closer to the scenario where everyone has the opportunity to live a long and healthy life.

Leadership and Equity in Health

Halfdan Mahler, Former Director General of WHO

I am morally and intellectually convinced that the Health for All approach and the primary health care strategy provide significant initial strengths and have added impetus to health development in the whole world.

I see amazing inequity patterns in health indicators throughout our whole miserable world. I am not talking about the first, second, or third world. I am talking about one single world, the only one that we have to share and take care of. Therefore, I will continue supporting everything that contributes to providing health levels to allow all the people in this one world to have a productive and both socially and economically satisfactory life.

What hundreds of millions of people around the underprivileged world need and want is the same as everyone in any part of the world needs and wants: The well-being of their loved ones and a better future for their children, the eradication of the increasing injustice, and the beginning of hope.

Equity, understood as assurance of satisfaction of basic needs in terms of health as well as social and economic needs, especially in connection with vulnerable groups, such as the poor, children, women, the elderly, and the handicapped, is for me the fundamental objective of every development.

Actually, I consider equity as a moral imperative that involves all social and economic activities.

This morally binding commitment of Health for All was the basis of the primary health care strategy, which implied a commitment not only to the reorientation of traditional health care systems – which should be called medical palliative systems – but also to a change where people have their own control over their health and well-being, up to the point when they actually lead to deep social reforms in the health care field. This implies a process of permanent empowering, by means of which people acquire a skill and the desire to become a social agent of their own health and well-being.

This is why I actually believe that the fundamental values of social justice and equity are the essence of the Health for All approach and the primary health care strategy. And this approach and strategy can actually become true and constitute a powerful force and conduction line to achieve equity and social justice. Health might not be all, but without health there will be very little well-being.

Social Determinants of Health Global Context and Challenges

Michael Marmot, Chairman, Commission on Social Determinants of Health, WHO

It's a pleasure to be here in this most important conference.

I have one clear point: When we rediscover the importance of primary health care, we should also rediscover the importance of the social determinants of health. They are not the same. I think that saying that social determinants of health are simply a part of primary health care is liable to cause confusion. They need each other. There should be a partnership between social determinants of health and the redevelopment of primary health care.

A central task of the Commission on Social Determinants of Health is to gather and synthesize evidence in such a way that it can lay the basis for action. The problem with which the Commission is concerned is health inequalities between and within countries.

There are substantial health differences within countries. For example, in the 25-year follow-up of the first Whitehall Studies of British Civil Servants, we showed that for men classified according to grade of employment in the civil service, the higher the position in the hierarchy, the lower the mortality. The importance of this Whitehall study is that it shows that we are not dealing only with absolute deprivation. Even people at the bottom of the British Civil Service are not poor. Twenty percent of the national population of Argentina lives on $2 a day or less.

No one in the British Civil Service lives on $2 a day or less – they are not poor in the sense of absolute deprivation. Yet there is a remarkable social gradient in health, running from the top to the bottom of the society. In the United States, we see a 17-year gap in life expectancy between poor Blacks in downtown, Washington, DC, and richer Whites of nearby Montgomery County, Maryland.

The Commission is action-oriented. High-quality academic work is an important foundation of our deliberations but we want to see academic work translated into action. We want to create a global movement that places fair health, health equity, at the head and heart of social policy. Coming to Argentina, I felt the need to read your most famous author, Jorge Luis Borges, who said "My humanity is in feeling we are all voices of the same poverty." That, colleagues, is what the Commission is trying to deal with.

The People's Health for All Movement

Ravi Narayan, Coordinator, People's Health Movement Global Secretariat

How can we go beyond the market forces that operate all over the world and prevent health from being only for those who can afford it? I represent the people who are being left out of our current health programs. On their behalf, I would like to say that the first step any of you as decision makers and political scientists must take is to listen to the people. What are people saying?

Today, I would like to show you the evidence, the proof people gave us and the way we interpreted it. People come to see us with a cough and we give them cough syrup. But if we sit down and listen to their life stories, they tell us stories of poverty, injustice, discomfort, exploitation. Is the cough syrup enough?

In the lives of ordinary people, then, to summarize what people are saying, there are social, political, economic factors that impact our lives, our access to health care, our access to all types of public policies, and unless we address these determinants health for all cannot be a reality.

Finally, I would like to emphasize, together with all of you and all of the people of the world, that health for all needs a new paradigm. We have to confront WHO and the World Bank and other international health players to ensure that their policies have the needs of the people at the center, and not the market economy: that the Millennium Development Goals (MDGs) become more sustainable. We have to make sure that the MDGs are not only eight stand-alone vertical programs, but that there must be a more integrated and holistic approach. We cannot have MDG 3, empowering women, and MDG 5, that of children, being tackled separately. We have to move from top-down, vertical globalization to a people-led globalization involving everybody from the bottom up.

We are glad that PAHO has quoted our people's health charter and emphasized that for a good PHC service in the new millennium we should "encourage community participation, prepare accountable health programs, provide appropriate services for all, and we have to make sure that services become accessible regardless of people's ability to pay."

Contribution of Primary Health Care to the Millennium Development Goals

Margaret Chan, Director General of WHO

The topics explored in this conference embrace some of the most pressing issues in public health today. Obviously, if we want better health to work as a poverty reduction strategy, we must reach the poor. And we must do so with appropriate high-quality care.

What role can primary health care play in this quest?

What are our prospects of reaching the health-related MDGs?

More specifically, how can we overcome major barriers, such as weak health systems, inadequate numbers of health-care staff, and the challenge of financing care for impoverished people?

When I took office at the start of this year, I called for a renewed emphasis on primary health care as an approach to strengthening health systems.

The experiences and recommendations coming from this conference are extremely relevant to public health today, both within countries and for the work of WHO.

1. Millennium development goals. We are near the midpoint in the countdown to 2015, the year given so much significance and promise by the Millennium Declaration and its Goals. These goals represent the most ambitious commitment ever made by the international community. Their achievement would make the biggest difference in the lives and future prospects of impoverished populations in the history of humanity.
2. Health for all. Looking back, we are approaching the 30th anniversary of another historical set of commitments: the Declaration of Alma-Ata. That document promoted primary health care as the key to attaining an acceptable level of health for all people in this world. This was the heart of the Health for All movement.

Apart from its passionate call for equity and social justice, Health for All also launched a political struggle on at least three fronts.

- First, it sought to make health part of the political agenda for development, to upgrade the profile of health and increase its prestige.
- Second, it sought to broaden the approach to health, to move away from the narrow medical model of curative care. It acknowledged the power of prevention. And it recognized that health has multiple

determinants, including some in sectors other than health.
- Third, the Declaration of Alma-Ata argued that better health for populations should go hand in hand in a mutually supportive way, with better economic and social productivity.

These, then, were some of the political struggles surrounding a movement launched in the name of social justice and for the good of our common humanity. But the Health for All movement paved the way for even more ambitious goals agreed on at the start of this century.
- First, the goals place health firmly at the center of the development agenda.
- Second, the goals make intersectoral collaboration a prerequisite for success. They attack the root causes of poverty and acknowledge that these causes interact.
- Third, by making better health a poverty reduction strategy, the goals move the health sector from a mere consumer of resources to a producer of economic gains.

3. Present situation. It is by no means certain that we will reach the health-related Millennium Development Goals. We are still not reaching underserved populations with sustainable, equitable, and comprehensive care on an adequate scale. In 2005, the Millennium Project Task Force issued its assessment of the prospects for achieving the goals for child and maternal health. "The health system that should make interventions available, accessible, and utilized is in a crisis. Only a profound shift in how the global health and development community thinks about and addresses health systems can have the impact necessary to meet the Goals." When I think about this dilemma, I reach two conclusions.
- First, in matters of health, I believe our world is out of balance, possibly as never before in history. We have never had such a sophisticated arsenal of technologies for treating disease and prolonging life. Yet, the gaps in health outcomes keep getting wider. Life expectancy can vary by as much as 40 years between rich and poor countries. This is unacceptable.
- My second conclusion relates directly to the topic of this conference. I do not believe we will be able to reach the Millennium Development Goals unless we return to the values, principles, and approaches of primary health care. Decades of experience tell us that primary health care is the best route to universal access, and the best way to ensure sustainable improvements in health outcomes.

Having said this, I want to commend PAHO and its member states for their enduring commitment to primary health care.

I would now like to suggest four principles that can guide us as we explore ways to achieve equity-based comprehensive health care and look at the contribution of primary health care.

- First, we must maintain our commitment, determination, and above all, our sense of urgency. As Dr. Mahler stated almost 30 years ago, our determination must be absolute. We must refuse to retreat.
- Second, we must hold our politicians accountable for the promises they make, whether to their voting constituency or at international summits.
- Third, if we want politicians to make the right priorities and keep them, we must provide solid evidence. Evidence gives health arguments persuasive power at the policy level. As I have said, what gets measured gets done.
- Finally, we must never underestimate the power of human ingenuity. This power goes hand in hand with resolute determination to reach a goal.

As my last remark, I believe that, when we talk about primary health care, we must also acknowledge the great ingenuity of communities. Human nature has certain commonalities that transcend differences of place, race, religion, and culture. Time and time again we see how, when communities are given opportunities they want and programs they can own, they are empowered to achieve the lives they desire. Given a hand up, they can indeed lift themselves out of poverty and improve their health.

This, then, is part of our common humanity, as expressed in the Millennium Declaration. These are our shared traits of compassion, inspiration, aspiration, and great ingenuity. Our common humanity gives us reason to care. It is why we must act with urgency in the face of an emergency. It is also why we have so much to gain, in the name of social justice.

Toward an Equity-Based Comprehensive Health Care

Mirta Roses Periago, Director, Pan American Health Organization

We have arrived at the final moment of this Buenos Aires 30/15 International Conference. It has been a very intense week for the delegations that are present, with many months of preparation and fruitful participation from across the world.

At first glance, Buenos Aires 30/15, and the Declaration that it has produced, are very important symbolically because they come 30 years after the International Conference in Alma-Ata, and at the halfway point of the period set for the fulfillment of the Millennium Development Goals (MDGs).

There is historical continuity between the most important political and doctrinal definition of public health in the world, which established a noble and ambitious goal (Health for All) and put us on the road to achieve it (Primary Health Care), and the most ambitious commitment to combat poverty ever undertaken by the international community, the Millennium Development Goals.

What is the Legacy of Alma-Ata? The social and health policy itinerary from 1978 to 2007 shows us that PHC has had an enormous influence on public policies, on the configuration of health systems, and on the thinking and actions of health workers.

Developments derived from Alma-Ata are consolidated and enriched by contributions from political and moral philosophy and the economy of development (as pointed out in the work of Amartya Sen), which have produced a reconfiguration of frameworks for social policy and governmental action. Along the way there has arisen a new vision of sustainable human development and the relationship between economic development, democracy, and social protection that has led to a new view of social and health policies and the contribution of health systems.

The view from this perspective of the fundamental social determinants of health and human development has assigned health a more important place on the global development agenda and has strengthened the role of health in public policies. Health is not only an input for economic growth, but rather, and principally, an essential component of human development.

Following Sen, this new approach regards health as a basic human capacity, as a fundamental requirement for human beings to be able to carry out their life projects and achieve their maximum life potential, and as an essential human right and a dimension of freedom.

We can say that as long as social and health inequities persist and social exclusion in health continues, the ideal, as well as the principles and values of Alma-Ata will remain in force.

It is on that axiological and ethical legacy, and on the enormous experience of public health workers accumulated over 30 years, that we can and should build a new vision of the role of PHC in health systems in order to make them capable of achieving health for all. This is to say health systems based on PHC.

Reflections and Looking Ahead

At least three generations have met here, inspired by Alma-Ata and under the wise and firm guidance of the founders, and they are now carrying the torch forward as in the Olympics.

From these days of work, three points remain clear for all of us.

- We do not need weak, selective, or incomplete PHC that, as we say, is like a poor man's blanket that when stretched to one side leaves the other side uncovered. We want something that covers us all, not a PHC with basic packages only for the poor, or for rural areas, or for marginal areas.
- We need and we want PHC that has equity, universality, solidarity, and social participation, that reflects a rich encounter of knowledge, that is intersectoral, that makes it possible for us to successfully address the social determinants of health, and that affirms and ensures the right to health care.
- We need and we want the PHC of Alma-Ata firmly rooted in the passion and commitment of 1978 and with the projection and capacity to transform current health systems, because we need them urgently, and because they are indispensable to the viability and sustainability of human society in the twenty-first century, when we will all have to share the same and only planet.

Buenos Aires 30/15 Declaration Towards a Health Strategy for Equity, Based on Primary Health Care August 17th 2007

We, the Ministers of Health and representatives of the Ministries of Health attending the International Conference of Health for Development: Rights, Facts and Realities, have gathered in the City of Buenos Aires on August 16th and 17th, 2007, to analyze the achievements and difficulties in the implementation of the Primary Health Care Strategy and with the object to foster the strengthening of already established consensus and generate new proposals, tending toward the establishment of a strategy of an equity-based comprehensive health care.

Whereas, and taking into account that:

1. We reaffirm that the enjoyment of the highest attainable standard of health is one of the fundamental rights of every human being without distinction as to race, religion, political belief or economic or social condition. This is a key responsibility of the State, together with the participation of the citizens.
2. We acknowledge that the efforts of the public policies and societies must be oriented towards human development. This implies that said efforts require an orientation towards the improvement of quality of life for the people, against poverty and exclusion, ensuring equal opportunities and the development of the capacities of the persons and their communities.
3. Health is an outcome of different and dynamic social, economic, cultural, and environmental determinants. Responsibility for it belongs to everyone. Although it goes far beyond the curative, disease-oriented medical care, health services systems have a key role in bringing sectors together including the community. This

implies a need for policies by the State and the collaboration and commitment from all the sectors: public organizations, private sector, community organizations, international organizations, and each citizen.
4. We acknowledge that health is fundamental to secure the objectives of development agreed to internationally, including those stated in the Millennium Declaration, and that these objectives create an opportunity to integrate health as an essential part of development and therefore, to increase the political commitment and the resources destined to the sector.
5. We affirm that equity, solidarity, and universality should govern health and development systems and policies.
6. The Primary Health Care (PHC) Strategy is based on values and principles that remain relevant and which must guide the structure and operation of the health systems at all levels and for all.
7. Health problems do not respect boundaries between states and jurisdictions. Furthermore, old problems of poverty and exclusion still exist today, and new challenges exist related to the environment, demographic changes, unhealthy lifestyles, and emerging and re-emerging diseases.
8. The Primary Health Care (PHC) Strategy must be capable of dealing with both old health problems as well as the new and emerging ones.
9. Nearly 30 years after the Alma-Ata Declaration the health situation of a great part of humanity is deplorable and large parts of humanity do not enjoy equitable, comprehensive, or even basic health care.
10. Health human resources are generally not trained to respond to socially complex health problems involving prevention, promotion, intersectoral cooperation, client–provider relations, and community participation.
11. We are very far from reaching the goals related to health contained in the Millennium Declaration. We acknowledge that international and national policies, including social and economic policies, have affected our ability to meet the MDGs and develop equitable health systems.
12. It is imperative that we solve these difficulties and develop a new implementation plan for the strategy that brings us nearer not only to reaching the objectives of the Millennium Declaration, but to the full implementation of the values and principles of Primary Health Care.

We accept the following principles:
13. Health is a cause and generating factor of development and growth of a nation. For this reason, we consider health as an investment and not as an expenditure, and also a responsibility of the State and society as a whole.
14. Equitable health care is a key factor for development and can stimulate equitable approaches in other fields. This requires priority and strong public policies which involve all stakeholders.
15. In order to achieve equity-based health care, it is imperative to strive towards universal and comprehensive coverage. In doing so, policies and programs need to be gender-responsive, inclusive, nondiscriminatory, and prioritize vulnerable groups.

Therefore we commit to develop processes that:
16. Take into account the values and principles of primary health care, to guide the policies, structure, and functions of the health systems at all levels for all.
17. Support the leadership and stewardship role of the State and the participation of families, communities and all other stakeholders in guiding planning and where appropriate, in the implementation and support of health programs and services in a comprehensive and intersectoral manner.
18. Determine the set of programs and services necessary to achieve equity-based health care, that the countries can implement according to their national contexts.
19. Assure adequate financing of the programs and services that are considered necessary for each country, ensuring sustainability and working towards universal coverage.
20. Incorporate into the design and implementation of health and development policies, factors such as socioeconomic status, culture, ethnicity, gender, age, and disability.
21. Strive to eliminate inequities in the quality of health services within the countries.
22. Ensure that health systems do not reproduce inequities found in other sectors and engage in intersectoral collaboration to promote social inclusion and poverty reduction public policies.
23. Strengthen relationships between the health authorities and educational institutions to meet the needs of the population by training health workers to use interdisciplinary approaches for new social, environmental and health problems.
24. To involve the health authorities in intersectoral collaboration to help develop public policies of other sectors when they affect health, such as those aimed at improving access to drinking water, safe food, decent work, a healthy environment, and adequate shelter.
25. Include in official publications indicators to measure equity.
26. Strengthen joint cooperation between countries and institutions in managing health issues of local, national, and international concern.
27. Support rapid implementation of the above-mentioned actions, in a framework of equity and

social justice, to achieve the enjoyment of the highest attainable standard of health, which is one of the fundamental rights of every human being without distinction as to race, religion, political belief or economical or social condition.

Building from Common Foundations: The World Health Organization and Faith-Based Organizations in Primary Health Care. WHO 2008

The World Health Organization worked closely with faith-based organizations (FBOs) in preparing for the Alma-Ata Declaration of 1978. The role of the Christian Medical Commission was particularly notable in that process. Together they gained a clearer picture of healthcare in the developing world, and then established the concept of primary health care. This report of WHO focused on FBOs is intended to assist in the process of rejuvenating dialogue and partnership with FBOs in the face of widespread health challenges in communities around the world, not least of which is HIV/AIDS. The revival of the primary health care model within WHO underscores that if this framework is to be promoted as a more sustainable system of health servicing and delivery, then the inclusion of FBOs will add greater potential for breadth and effectiveness.

In 2006, WHO commissioned South Africa-based African Religious Health Assets Programme (ARHAP) to conduct an extensive survey of FBO healthcare delivery in two South African countries. The study concluded that the proportion of faith-based health service provision averages about 40 percent in many sub-Saharan African nations.

Thus, the current scale of FBOs' involvement in health care in sub-Saharan Africa makes a compelling case that religious entities (not only Christian) could become significant players in the new primary health care approach to strengthening health systems globally, especially related to achieving the goal of universal access.

Conclusion: Much can be achieved in renewed interaction and cooperation between WHO and FBOs. This requires a clear long-term commitment to dialogue and mutual learning. The next step should involve forming a road map that interested parties can commit to so they can embark on the next stage of the journey together.

Unequivocal Regional Support for Margaret Chan's Commitment to Primary Health Care. (*Lancet*, Correspondence, June 19, 2008.)

An exceedingly interesting dialogue was prompted by an editorial written by Richard Horton, Editor of *Lancet*, published May 31, 2008, highlighting that Dr. Chan had placed PHC at the center stage at the WHO. Mr. Horton had attended a Technical Briefing on PHC during the May World Health Assembly, which was very well-attended and well-received. While applauding the DG's PHC prioritization, *Mr. Horton questioned whether the WHO's six Regional Directors (RDs), who as he stressed, have influence at country level, would support the DG's PHC agenda.* This sentence caused an immediate reaction among the six RDs. Drafts were exchanged back and forth among the RDs and Dr. Chan. It seems unlikely that *The Lancet* ever anticipated this reaction!

The Lancet issued a press release, June 19, stating *WHO DG's quest to revitalize Alma-Ata gets unqualified and unprecedented support from her lieutenants.* In that press release, Mr. Horton said

"...the alignment and combined advocacy of WHO's global leadership is an unprecedented moment in WHO's history. Revitalizing PHC is the single most important action that countries and donors can do to save lives and avoid disability. WHO is now perfectly poised to lead this new movement for PHC..."

The RDs issued a statement in *The Lancet*, Correspondence, June 19:

"Dr. Chan's commitment to primary health care is in itself an expression of the unequivocal support from the six regional directors and of the unanimity of views among the senior management of the organization with regard to primary health care. Despite the wide variation across and within regions with respect to health challenges and the responses required to address these, there is mutual agreement that primary health care will continue to be central to WHO's strategy to strengthen health system towards the vision of 'Health for All'".

Concluding Comments

The Alma-Ata story is truly inspirational with reference to several issues.

First, to have been at Alma Ata, as the authors of this article were (as members of the U.S. Delegation), to have played a small part in the formulation of the Declaration, was truly one of the great honors of our professional lives.

Second, to have absorbed the major features of Alma-Ata as it happened, and to now be tracking the diverse events and processes that have followed, many of them unpredictable, some with negative impacts, others positive, but still building on the solid base that Alma-Ata provided, is exhilarating.

Third, to have experienced the Buenos Aires Conference, August 2007, entitled: From Alma-Ata to the Millennium Declaration: Towards Equity-Based Comprehensive Health Care, in the presence of Margaret Chan,

Mirta Roses Periago (Director, PAHO) and Halfdan Mahler (Director General, WHO, at the time of Alma-Ata), was so uplifting. It was filled with clear expressions of local, regional, global commitment to primary health care. Of special interest was that such commitment was often expressed in new terms, new values, new concepts, reaching beyond the solid foundation of Alma-Ata. This is not to diminish the importance of the original perspectives, but to show that there is room for expanding the conceptualization and actions of Alma-Ata.

Fourth, at this very moment we are seeing the new initiative of WHO as it seeks constructive interaction with faith-based organizations in global pursuit of primary health care. And to have the new Director General of WHO, Dr. Margaret Chan, herself championing primary health care in this way is an extremely important positive factor.

Fifth, is an intriguing example of the support Margaret Chan is gaining in her call for the revitalization of primary health care. Richard Horton, Editor of *Lancet*, was congratulating WHO on its support for primary health care, but in the process asked if the regional directors of WHO were in full support of that process. Surprised by that question, Dr. Chan and the Regional Directors came forward with strong support, which led Horton to add an editorial in *The Lancet*, in which he stated: WHO DG's quest to revitalize Alma-Ata gets unqualified and unprecedented support from her lieutenants! Further, the alignment and combined advocacy of WHO's global leadership is an unprecedented moment in WHO history.

Sixth, and finally, to look around the world and sense the myriad people who have benefited from the Alma-Ata story, and to know that there will be many more in the future, gives one a sense of encouragement that our world will allow and support such processes. And, we who are involved in those processes are indeed honored.

Citations

Alma-Ata (1978) *Primary Health Care*. Report of the International Conference on Primary Health Care.
Bryant J (1969) *Health and the Developing World*. The Rockefeller Foundation. Ithaca, NY: Cornell University Press.
Bryant JH (1977) Principles of justice as a basis for conceptualizing a health care system. *International Journal of Health Services* 7: 707–719.
Bryant J and Jenkins (1971) Dialogue on Moral Issues and Health Care – Issue No. 4. Geneva, Switzerland: WHO.
Building from Common Foundations: *The World Health Organization and Faith-Based Organizations in Primary Health Care*. WHO 2008.
CONTACT Christian Medical Commission (1979) *Contact, Primary Health Care*. Special Series, No. 1. Geneva, Switzerland: WHO.
Cueto M (2004) The origins of primary health care and selective primary health care. *American Journal of Public Health* 94: 1864–1874.
Djukanovic V and Mach EP (eds.) (1975) *Alternative Approaches to Meeting Basic Health Needs of Populations in Developing Countries*. Geneva, Switzerland: World Health Organization.
Gezairy, Hussain A et al. (Regional Directors, WHO). Unequivocal regional support for Margaret Chan's commitment to primary health care. *Correspondence*, The Lancet, June 19, 2008.
Litsios S (2004) The Christian Medical Commission and the Development of the World Health Organization's Primary Health Care Approach. *American Journal of Public Health* 94: 1884–1893.
Macinko J and Guanais F (2005) *Annotated Bibliography on Primary Health Care*. Washington, DC: Pan American Health Organization.
McGilvray JC (1981) *The Quest for Health and Wholeness*. Tubingen, Germany: German Institute for Medical Mission.
Newall D (ed.) (1975) *Health by the People*. Geneva, Switzerland: World Health Organization.
Sachs JD (2005) *Investing in Development. A Practical Plan to Achieve the Millennium Development Goals. Overview. Millennium Project*. London: Earthscan.
Tajada Rivero D (2003) Alma-Ata Revisited. Perspectives in Health 8. Magazine of PAHO, Regional Office of WHO.
Venediktov D (1998) Alma-Ata and After. *World Health Forum* 19: 79–86.
Walsh J and Warren K (1979) Selective primary health care, an interim strategy for disease control in developing countries. *New England Journal of Medicine* 301: 967–974.
WHO/HPR/HEP (1986) *Ottawa Charter for Health Promotion*. First International Conference on Health Promotion Ottawa, 21 November 1986, WHO/HPR/HEP/95.1. http://www.who.int/hpr/NPH/docs/ottawa_charter_hp.pdf(accessed October 2007).
World Health Organization (1978) Health Care, Alma-Ata, USSR, 6–12 September, 1978. Jointly sponsored by WHO and UNICEF.
World Health Organization (1988) *From Alma-Ata to the Year 2000. Reflections at the Midpoint, Riga, Latvia*. Geneva, Switzerland: World Health Organization.
World Health Organization (2000) *Primary Health Care 21 "Everybody's Business" An International Meeting to Celebrate 20 Years After Alma-Ata, Almaty, Kazakhstan, 27–28 November, 1998* Geneva, Switzerland: World Health Organization.
World Health Organization (2003a) *A Global Review of Primary Health Care: Emerging Messages*. Geneva, Switzerland: World Health Organization.
World Health Organization (2003b) *Primary Health Care and the Millennium Development Goals: Issues for Discussion*. Geneva, Switzerland: World Health Organization.
World Health Organization (2005) *Action on the Social Determinants of Health: Learning from Previous Experiences*. A background paper of the Commission on Social Determinants of Health, March 2005 Geneva, Switzerland: World Health Organization.
World Health Organization (2007) *Renewing Primary Health Care in the Americas*. A Position Paper of the Pan American Health Organization/WHO.

Further Reading

African Religious Health Assets Programme (2006) Appreciating assets: the contribution of religion to universal access in Africa. Report for the World Health Organization. Cape Town: ARHAP.
Bankowski Z and Bryant J (1994) *Poverty, Vulnerability and the Value of Human Life. A Global Agenda for Bioethics*. Geneva, Switzerland: CIOMS.
Bankowski Z, Bryant J, and Gallagher J (1997) *Ethics, Equity and Health for All*. Geneva, Switzerland: CIOMS.
Bryant J, Khan KS, and Hyder A (1997) Ethics, equity and renewal of WHO's health-for-all strategy. *World Health Forum* 18: 107–115; discussion 116–162.
Marmot M (2004) *The Status Syndrome – How Social Standing Affects Our Health and Longevity*. New York: Times Books.
Smith D and Bryant J (1988) Building an infrastructure for primary health care: An overview of vertical and integrated approaches. *Social Science and Medicine* 26: 909–927.
Yach D (1996) Renewal of the health-for-all strategy. *World Health Forum* 17: 321–326; discussion 327–349.

Health Issues of the UN Millennium Development Goals

M Claeson and P Folger, The World Bank, Washington, DC, USA

© 2008 Elsevier Inc. All rights reserved.

The Millennium Development Goals for Health

In the 1990s, the international community recognized the importance of health in development. Development assistance for health rose in spite of overall decline in aid. This period also saw an increased global concern over the debt in the developing world. Debt relief, in response to the unsustainable debt burden of the poorest countries, was explicitly geared to channel freed resources into the health and other social sectors. The 1990s also saw the development of major new global health initiatives and partnerships to control, for example, HIV and AIDS, TB, malaria, and vaccine-preventable childhood infections. These initiatives brought not only new resources – funds, ideas, energy, and mechanisms – but also new challenges to harmonization. Attempts were made to better coordinate and link global goals with local actions in the fight against disease, death, and malnutrition in the developing world.

As the 1990s closed, the international community decided that more was needed to be done to accelerate progress. At the United Nations Millennium Summit in September 2001, heads of 147 states endorsed the Millennium Development Goals (MDGs) to be achieved by 2015, of which nearly half concern health, as shown in **Table 1**. Several goals are indirectly related to health – for example, the goals on education and gender, which are both important to promoting good health and survival among children. The MDGs evolved from earlier International Development Goals, and the baseline date for the new targets was 1990.

The MDGs matter in all countries, for several reasons. Faster progress is important even if targets are missed. Progress in health can be accelerated in all countries through a judicious mix of spending, policy, and institutional reform. The MDGs can facilitate benchmarking and monitoring of results. Communities can hold governments and development partners accountable for achieving these health goals by tracking their progress, or the lack of it. Because the goals focus on a limited set of outcomes, monitoring and evaluating progress toward the MDGs can show what is achievable and where faster progress can be made.

One of the limitations of the MDG target is that they are national averages. Distributional analysis of MDG trends, as discussed in the World Bank report *The Millennium Development Goals for Health: Rising to the Challenges*, reminds us that progress needs to be for everyone, not just the better off (Wagstaff and Claeson, 2004). Focusing attention on the MDGs for different income groups forces countries to consider how the benefits of progress are distributed among the rich and poor within each country – the poor risk being left behind even in countries making progress overall. Progress has been uneven, with the poorer countries lagging behind the rest, and under-5 mortality as trends show, the poor within countries are lagging behind the rest of the population.

The MDG indicators, such as maternal mortality and HIV prevalence rates, are often difficult to measure and not very useful for program managers to measure routinely to inform planning or problem solving. Several more useful proximate indicators, or proxies, have been defined for the purpose of regular monitoring and to assess short-term progress toward the MDGs, as shown in **Table 2**.

The Millennium Development Goals for Health: Current Progress Report

In-depth analysis of the health-related MDGs by Adam Wagstaff (and others) shows a progress in some areas and not much in others (Wagstaff and Claeson, 2004). For the malnutrition target, 77% of the developing world's people lived in a country on track to achieve the goal by 2008 (i.e., in the year 2000 compared with the 1990 baseline),

Table 1 The health-related MDGs, 1990–2015

Goal 1: Eradicating extreme poverty and hunger. Target is to reduce by one-half the proportion of people who suffer from hunger, with progress to be measured in terms of the prevalence of underweight children under 5 years of age. The target implies an average annual rate of reduction of 2.7%

Goal 4: Reducing child mortality. Target is to reduce by two-thirds the under-5 mortality rate, equivalent to an annual rate of reduction of 4.3%

Goal 5: Improving maternal health. Target is to reduce by three-quarters the maternal mortality ratio, equivalent to an annual rate of reduction of 5.4%

Goal 6: Combating HIV/AIDS, malaria, and other diseases. Target is to halt and begin to reverse the spread of these diseases

Goal 7: Ensuring environmental sustainability. Target is to reduce by one-half the proportion of people without sustainable access to safe drinking water

Goal 8: Developing a global partnership for development. Target is to provide access to affordable essential drugs in developing countries

Wagstaff A and Claeson M (2004) *The Millennium Development Goals for Health: Rising to the Challenges.* Washington, DC: The World Bank.

Table 2 Recommended intermediate (proxy) indicators for health and nutrition MDGs, 1990–2015

Millennium development health and nutrition targets	Recommended options: examples of intermediate (proxy) indicators
Target: Reduce by one-half % people who suffer from hunger	• Prevalence of underweight children under 5 • % infants under 6 months who are exclusively breastfed • % children 6–59 months who received 1 dose of vitamin A in the past 6 months
Target: Reduce by two-thirds under-5 mortality rate	• % 1-year-old children immunized against measles • % children with diarrhea in the past 2 weeks who received oral rehydration therapy (ORT) • % children with fast or difficult breathing in the past 2 weeks who received an appropriate antibiotic
Target: Reduce by three-quarters the maternal mortality ratio	• % pregnant women with any antenatal care • % births with skilled birth attendant and/or institutional delivery • Contraceptive prevalence rate
Target: Halt and have begun to reverse the spread of HIV/AIDS	• % persons using a condom at last higher-risk sex • % sexually transmitted infection clients who are appropriately diagnosed and treated • % HIV-positive women receiving antiretroviral treatment during pregnancy
Target: Halt and have begun to reverse the incidence of malaria and other major diseases	• % patients with uncomplicated malaria who received treatment within 24 hours of onset of symptoms • % children/pregnant women sleeping under insecticide-treated nets • % women receiving antenatal care who received at least 2 or 3 intermittent preventive malaria treatments during pregnancy • % registered new smear-positive TB cases in a cohort that were successfully treated • % estimated new smear-positive TB cases that were registered under DOTS approach

For a complete list of recommended core intermediate and optional indicators, see World Bank (2001) Health, nutrition and population development goals: Measuring progress using the poverty reduction strategy framework. *Report of a World Bank Consultation.* Washington, DC: The World Bank.

but in sub-Saharan Africa only 15% of the people lived in an on-track country. Under-5 mortality in the developing world was reduced by an average of only a 2.5% in the 1990s, well short of the 4.3% required to meet the target. Regional differences are pronounced, with sub-Saharan Africa faring worse than other regions. In Africa, trends in reducing under-5 mortality and underweight in children were barely above 0 during the 1990s, and maternal mortality fell on average by just 1.6% a year compared with the annual target rate of 5.4% (Wagstaff and Claeson, 2004).

Evidence on how the poor are faring within countries is mixed. For malnutrition, the poorest 20% of the population within countries appears, on average, to have been experiencing broadly similar rates of reduction to that of the population as a whole. However, for under-5 mortality, the rate has been falling more slowly among the poor, while families who are better off are seeing faster rates of progress.

The Millennium Development Goals for Health: 2008 and Beyond

As a comparison of the child mortality experiences in the 1980s and 1990s demonstrates, past performance is not necessarily a good predictor of future performance. That a country is on track on the basis of its performance during the 1990s does not guarantee that it will maintain the required annual rate of reduction of malnutrition or mortality during the second half of the MDG period up to 2015. Countries that have been off track can get back on if they can combine good policies with expanded funding for programs that address both the direct and the underlying causes of the health-related goals.

The World Bank (2003a) estimates that economic growth will fall somewhat in East Asia and the Pacific from 2000 to 2015, while the positive trend will continue in Europe and Central Asia as well as sub-Saharan Africa, and increase somewhat in Latin America and the Caribbean, the Middle East and North Africa, and South Asia. Primary education completion rates will probably grow faster in the new millennium as a result of the global education initiatives. The gender gaps in secondary education are already narrowing and doing so faster in the new millennium than in the 1990s as a result of the gender MDG (i.e., goal 3, which is to eliminate gender disparity in primary and secondary education by 2005 and in all levels of education no later than 2015). To achieve parity with boys by 2015 in the proportion of the population who are age 15 and have completed secondary education, girls will have to achieve a faster growth in completion rates in the new millennium than in the 1990s in most regions, especially in South Asia and in East Asia and the Pacific. If the water MDG – ensuring that households have access to safe drinking water – is to be reached, access rates will need to grow much faster during 2000 to 2015, especially in sub-Saharan Africa. Gender equality in school and access to clean water will have a positive effect on progress toward the health MDGs (**Figure 1**).

Even with economic growth and faster progress on the nonhealth goals, many regions will still miss many of the health targets. The picture is bleakest for under-5 mortality and for sub-Saharan Africa.

Accelerating Progress – Overcoming the Obstacles to Health Development

A lack of effective interventions is not the primary obstacle to faster progress toward the MDGs, although new technologies could greatly improve progress – for example, malaria or HIV vaccines and effective vaginal microbicides to block the spread of HIV and other sexually transmitted infections. The main obstacle is the low levels of use – especially among the poor – of existing effective interventions. For example, if use of all the proven effective preventive and treatment interventions for childhood illness were to rise from current levels to reach all, the number of under-5 deaths worldwide could fall by as much as 63%, as estimated by the Bellagio Study Group for Child Survival, and published in *The Lancet* series on child survival (Bellagio Study Group, 2003). And, 70% of maternal deaths could be reduced if we could reach 90% coverage of available cost-effective interventions.

Array of Interventions, Programs, and Service Modalities to Reach the MDGs

The available interventions constitute a powerful arsenal for preventing and treating the main causes of malnutrition and death, as shown in **Table 3**. The major diseases and conditions that the MDGs aim to prevent and control, and the best buys in prevention and treatment, are reviewed in the *Disease Control Priorities in the Developing World*. In the case of child mortality, for example, diarrheal diseases, pneumonia, and malaria account for 52% of deaths worldwide. For each of these major causes of childhood mortality, at least one proven effective preventive intervention and at least one proven effective treatment intervention exist, capable of being delivered in a low-income setting. In most cases, several proven effective interventions exist (**Figure 2**). For diarrhea – the second leading cause of child deaths – no fewer than five proven preventive and three proven treatment interventions are available.

Effective Interventions Reaching Too Few People

The slow pace in reaching the health MDGs, causing high rates of malnutrition and death in the developing world has several causes. First, people do not receive the effective interventions that could save their lives or make them well-nourished. In middle- and high-income countries, 90% of children are fully immunized, more than 90% of deliveries are assisted by a medically trained provider (i.e., a doctor, nurse, or trained midwife, excluding traditional birth attendants), and more than 90% of pregnant women have at least one prenatal visit, according to UNICEF (2001). In South Asia, fewer than 50% of pregnant women receive a prenatal checkup, and only 20% of deliveries are assisted by a trained provider. The story is similar for other interventions for other goals. Condom use to prevent transmission of HIV is low in much of

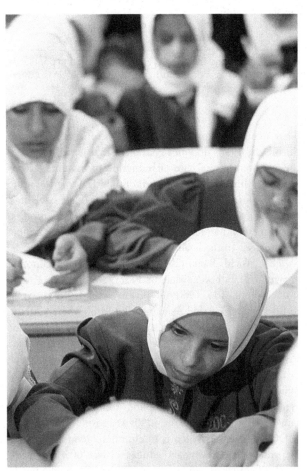

Figure 1 Gender equality in school will have a positive effect on health MDGs. Courtesy of the World Bank.

Table 3 Effective interventions to reduce illness, deaths, and malnutrition

MDG	Preventive interventions	Treatment interventions
Child mortality	Breastfeeding; hand washing; safe disposal of stool; latrine use; safe preparation of weaning foods; use of insecticide-treated bed nets; complementary feeding; immunization; micronutrient supplementation (zinc and vitamin A); prenatal care, including steroids and tetanus toxoid; antimalarial intermittent preventive treatment in pregnancy; newborn temperature management; nevirapine and replacement feeding; antibiotics for premature rupture of membranes; clean delivery	Case management with oral rehydration therapy for diarrhea; antibiotics for dysentery, pneumonia, and sepsis; antimalarials for malaria; newborn resuscitation; breastfeeding; complementary feeding during illness; micronutrient supplementation (zinc and vitamin A)
Maternal mortality	Family planning (lifetime risk); intermittent malaria prophylaxis; use of insecticide-treated bed nets; micronutrient supplementation (iron, folic acid, calcium for those who are deficient)	Antibiotics for preterm rupture of membranes, skilled attendants (especially active management of third stage of labor), basic and emergency obstetric care
Nutrition	Exclusive breastfeeding for 6 months, appropriate complementary child feeding for next 6–24 months, iron and folic acid supplementation for children, improved hygiene and sanitation, improved dietary intake of pregnant and lactating women, micronutrient supplementation for prevention of anemia and vitamin A deficiency for mothers and children, anthelmintic treatment in school-age children	Appropriate feeding of sick child and oral rehydration therapy, control and timely treatment of infectious and parasitic diseases, treatment and monitoring of severely malnourished children, high-dose treatment of clinical signs of vitamin A deficiency
HIV/AIDS	Safe sex, including condom use; unused needles for drug users; treatment of sexually transmitted infections; safe, screened blood supplies; antiretrovirals in pregnancy to prevent maternal-to-child transmission and after occupational exposure	Treatment of opportunistic infections, co-trimoxazole prophylaxis, highly active antiretroviral therapy, palliative care
Tuberculosis	Directly observed treatment of infectious cases to prevent transmission and emergence of drug-resistant strains and treatment of contacts, bacillus Calmette-Guérin immunization	Directly observed treatment to cure, including early identification of tuberculosis symptomatic cases
Malaria	Use of insecticide-treated bed nets, indoor residual spraying (in epidemic-prone areas), intermittent presumptive treatment of pregnant women	Rapid detection and early treatment of uncomplicated cases, treatment of complicated cases (such as cerebral malaria and severe anemia)

Wagstaff A and Claeson M (2004) *The Millennium Development Goals for Health: Rising to the Challenges.* Washington, DC: The World Bank.

sub-Saharan Africa and South Asia, and inexpensive one-time treatment with antiretroviral medicine to prevent transmission from mother to child covers only a small fraction of at-risk pregnant women in most of the developing world. In Asia, where more than 7 million people are living with HIV/AIDS, no country has yet exceeded 5% antiretroviral therapy coverage among those who could benefit from it, and the effective coverage of preventive interventions among vulnerable groups at high risk remains too low to contain epidemics fueled by injecting drug use and unsafe sex.

Just as shortfalls in coverage vary across countries, so do they vary within countries, with the poor and other deprived groups consistently lagging. These groups are less likely to receive full basic immunization coverage, to have their deliveries attended by a trained provider, and to have at least one prenatal care visit to a medically trained provider. On the positive side, the poor are often making fastest progress in coverage, reflecting in part that the better off already have high coverage rates for many interventions.

What Countries Can Do to Accelerate Progress

Development assistance has a stronger effect in countries with strong policies and institutions than in countries with only average-quality policies and institutions – and an insignificant effect in countries in which policies and institutions are weak (Wagstaff and Claeson, 2004). In principle, well-governed countries with good policies and institutions could achieve the health MDGs simply by scaling up their expenditures on existing programs in relation to current allocations. In practice, however, the amount of extra spending required would be difficult to

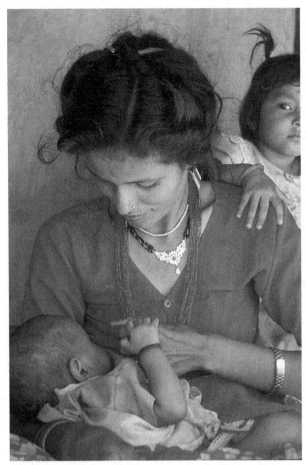

Figure 2 Effective preventive interventions, like exclusive breastfeeding, need to be scaled up among all income groups. Courtesy of the World Bank.

attain on present trends and would even be prohibitively expensive. Poorly governed countries cannot expect to make much progress toward the MDGs simply by scaling up their expenditures on existing programs. They will need to target additional government spending into activities that will have the largest effect on reaching the MDGs – high-impact interventions – and develop good policies and institutions, as discussed in the following section.

Targeting for Millennium Development Goals

Wagstaff and Claeson (2004) recommend that countries include a number of well-targeted efforts, with help from donors, to build stronger policies and institutions such as:

- *Geographic targeting to favor geographic zones that are furthest behind.* Targeting resources to poor regions and provinces may be most effectively implemented through nontraditional mechanisms for priority setting and implementation, such as social investment funds.
- *Changing the allocation of spending across care levels.* Spending on health in developing countries is characterized by a high concentration of spending on secondary and tertiary infrastructure and personnel.
- *Targeting specific programs.* Programs such as those delivering directly observed treatment short course (DOTS) for tuberculosis, or integrated management of childhood illness (IMCI), are good examples of programs that may yield high returns to government spending at the margin. Successful public health programs have several factors in common: technical innovation and stakeholder consensus, strong political leadership, coordination across agencies and management, effective use of information and financial resources, and participation of the beneficiary community.
- *Targeting specific population groups.* Many countries subsidize all government health services for everyone. These blanket subsidy schemes fail to disproportionately benefit the poor – despite the stronger equity case for subsidizing their care and that they tend to bear a disproportionate burden of malnutrition as well as child and maternal mortality. There are many proven ways to target the poor – for example, by delivering essential services in clinics or health posts that poor families are likely to attend or by promoting and delivering services in a way that segments the market and appeals to those in low-income households.
- *Targeting spending to remove bottlenecks.* A planning and budgeting approach is to assess – for a country – the health sector impediments to faster progress, to identify ways of removing them, and to estimate both the costs of removing them and the likely effects of their removal on MDG outcomes, as discussed in the marginal budgeting for bottlenecks approach, by Agnes Soucat and others. Important health systems bottlenecks, such as human resources, drug availability, and health-care management, are essential for achieving the health MDGs.

Improving Policies toward Households

Households are at the center of any efforts to scale up; they not only demand and consume care, but they are also important producers of prevention and care. Low income is a barrier to the use of most health interventions, and economic growth is an important weapon in the war against malnutrition and mortality. Improving poor households' access to services can be done by lowering financial barriers. One part of the affordability equation is price. User charges for MDG interventions are to be discouraged, since many of those interventions involve benefits that spill over to people who do not receive the intervention; high coverage of immunization is a classic example. However, an equity case also can be made for reducing prices facing the poor and near poor, even where no spillovers occur. Subsidies should be targeted to services with spillovers and to the poor.

Providing Information and Enhancing Knowledge

Lack of knowledge is a major factor behind poor health. It results in people not seeking care when needed, despite the absence of price barriers, and it also results in people – especially poor people – wasting limited resources on inappropriate care. Ignorance may also result in people not getting the maximum health gain out of inputs they have available to them and use. Many people do not know that hand washing confers much of the health benefit of piped water, for example. Not surprisingly, piped water has a much greater effect on the prevalence of diarrhea among the children of the better off and better educated, as shown, for instance, in India.

Improving Health Service Delivery

Health providers – in the public and private sectors, as well as in both formal and informal sectors – should deliver interventions of relevance to the MDGs (UN Millennium Project, 2005). The quality of management can make a difference. Better management means a clearer delineation of responsibilities and accountabilities inside organizations and a clear link between performance and reward. Management means getting accountabilities right within an organization. Another way to make a difference is getting accountabilities right between the organization and the public (World Bank, 2003). Governance, the accountability of provider organizations to the public, can also be improved through contracting of services to nongovernment organizations, which has been shown to benefit the poor in resource-constrained settings such as Cambodia and Afghanistan.

Strengthening Core Public Health Functions

Vulnerable populations need to be informed, educated, and protected from risks and damages. Public health laws and regulations need to be established and enforced. Infrastructure needs to be in place to detect early and reduce the impact of emergencies and disasters on health. All this action needs to be implemented through a public health system that is transparent and accountable. Governments in developing countries generally recognize that these public health functions are important, but they often lack the capacity and financial resources to implement them. Indeed, few low-income countries receive support for the core public health functions that should serve as the backbone of any well-functioning and sustained health system, including collection and dissemination of evidence for health policies, prevention and control of diseases, human resource development, and intersectoral action for better health.

Intersectoral Synergies – Actions Beyond the Health Sector

A review of the evidence base for the key determinants of the health and nutrition MDGs identifies significant potential for intersectoral synergies (Wagstaff and Claeson, 2004). Although roads and transport are vital for health services, especially for reducing maternal mortality, it is not just the physical infrastructure that matters. Also important are the availability of transportation and the affordability of its use. Transportation and roads complement health services. A 10-year study in Rajasthan, India, found that better roads and transportation helped women reach referral facilities, but many women still died because no corresponding improvements took place at household and facility levels. Improved hygiene (hand washing) and sanitation (use of latrines and safe disposal of children's stools) (**Figure 3**) are at least as important as drinking water quality in shaping health outcomes, specifically in reducing diarrhea and associated child mortality as shown by Esrey *et al.* (1991). Constructing water supply and sanitation facilities is not enough to improve health outcomes; sustained human behavior change must accompany the infrastructure investment.

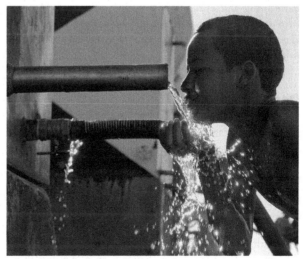

Figure 3 Increased access to water and improved hygiene and sanitation can make significant contributions to the health MDGs. Courtesy of the World Bank.

Development Assistance and the Health Millennium Development Goals

Additional health spending will be required in many countries to accelerate progress toward the health goals. The global estimates of what it would cost to achieve the health MDGs range from an additional US$20–70 billion a year. A World Bank study estimates that the additional official development assistance required to meet the health goals is in the range of US$20–25 billion per year, which is roughly four times the amount of official development assistance spending for health in 2002 (US$6.5 billion) and three times all external financing, including that of foundations and loans from multilateral sources (Wagstaff and Claeson, 2004). Another analysis conducted by the Commission on Macroeconomics and Health (WHO, 2001) estimated that an additional US$40–52 billion annually would be required until 2015 to scale up the coverage for malaria, tuberculosis, HIV/AIDS, childhood mortality, and maternal mortality. Whatever the method of analysis, all global estimates show that reaching the MDGs will require significant additional resources compared with the current levels of funding for health.

Official development assistance tends to account for a larger share of government health spending in poorer countries. Development assistance for health is especially important in sub-Saharan Africa: 12 countries had external funding exceeding 35% of total health expenditures in 2000, and increased development assistance is needed to achieve the MDGs. Development assistance, however, is not without its drawbacks. Consensus on how to improve aid effectiveness is growing among development partners. At the High Level Forum on Health MDGs in Geneva and Abuja, 2004, the agenda included support for countries in developing more MDG-responsive Poverty Reduction Strategy Papers, tracking resource flows, strengthening monitoring and evaluation, and more effectively dealing with the human resources crisis in health (Haines and Cassels, 2004; WHO, 2005; see also under the section titled 'Relevant websites').

Conclusion

All countries can make some progress toward the health MDGs and ensure that the poor do not lag behind. The second half of the period 1990–2015 can go better than the first half. The focus on the MDGs at the start of this decade has contributed to a shift in the attention given by development partners – donors and governments – to health outcomes and to the contributions of multiple sectors to health. However, the attention span is often of short duration and it is always a challenge in global health to keep the momentum going and sustain the commitment to any health goal, be it disease-specific goals or broader development goals such as the MDGs. What could make a significant difference would be for communities and civil society to take greater ownership of the MDGs and use MDG monitoring to keep local, national, and global leadership accountable for the commitment they made to achieve the MDGs for all.

See also: Alma Ata and Primary Health Care: An Evolving Story; People's Health Movement; Health Inequalities; Health Finance, Equity in; Universal Coverage in Developing Countries, Transition to; Patient Empowerment in Health Care.

Citations

The Bellagio Study Group on Child Survival (2003) Knowledge into Action for Child Survival. *Lancet* 326: 323–327.
Disease Control Priorities Project (2006) *The Disease Control Priorities in Developing Countries*, 2nd edn. http://www.dcp2.org (accessed October 2007).
Esrey SA, Potash JB, and Roberts L (1991) Effects of improved water supply and sanitation on ascariasis, diarrhoea, dracunculiasis, hookworm infection, schistosomiasis, and trachoma. *Bulletin of the World Health Organization* 69: 609–621.
Haines A and Cassels A (2004) Can Millennium Development Goals be attained? *British Medical Journal* 329: 394–397.
UNICEF (2001) Progress since the World Summit for Children. *A Statistical Review.* New York: UNICEF.
UN Millennium Project (2005) *Who's Got the Power? Transforming Health Systems for Women and Children. Task Force on Child Health and Maternal Health. The Millennium Development Project.* http://www.unmillenniumproject.org/documents/ChildHealthEBook.pdf.
Wagstaff A and Claeson M (2004) *The Millennium Development Goals for Health: Rising to the Challenges.* Washington, DC: The World Bank.
World Bank (2001) Health, nutrition and population development goals: Measuring progress using the poverty reduction strategy framework. *Report of a World Bank Consultation.* Washington DC: The World Bank.
World Bank (2003) *World Development Report 2004: Making Services Work for Poor People.* Washington, DC: Oxford University Press.
World Bank (2003a) *Global Economic Prospects and the Developing Countries.* Washington, DC: The World Bank.
World Health Organization (2001) *Commission on Macroeconomics and Health: Investing in Health for Economic Development.* Geneva, Switzerland: WHO.
World Health Organization (2005) *Health and the Millennium Development Goals.* Geneva, Switzerland: WHO.

Further Reading

Achieving the Millennium Development Goals for Health: So far, progress is mixed-can we reach our targets? http://www.dcp2.org/file/67/DCCP%20 – %20MDGs.pdf

Relevant Websites

http://www.hlfhealthmdgs.org – High-Level Forum on the Health MDGs.
http://www.undp.org/mdg – United Nations Development Programme, Millennium Development Goals (MDGs).
http://www.un.org/millenniumgoals – The UN Millennium Development Goals.
http://www.developmentgoals.org – The World Bank Group, Millennium Development Goals.
http://www.who.int/mdg/en/ – WHO, Health and the Millennium Development Goals.

Health Inequalities

P Braveman, University of California, San Francisco, CA, USA

© 2008 Elsevier Inc. All rights reserved.

Introduction

A woman in Panama is 80 times as likely to die from childbirth-related causes as a woman in Sweden (WHO, 2004). A baby born in Pakistan is 27 times as likely to die in infancy as a baby born in Singapore. A child born in Chad is 50 times as likely to die before reaching her or his fifth birthday as a child born in Japan (Bellamy, 2004). Such disturbing contrasts reflecting unequal health between countries are probably familiar to the public and to public health professionals in many countries; fewer are aware that substantial differences also exist within countries. In Indonesia, for example, children in the poorest one-fifth of the population are 3.5 times as likely to die before reaching age 5 as children in the wealthiest fifth (Badan Pusat Statistik-Statistics Indonesia and ORC Macro, 2003). In both Bolivia and Egypt, infant mortality is nearly three times as high among babies born to mothers in the poorest fifth of the population as among those born to mothers in the wealthiest fifth of the population (Sardán et al., 2004; El-Zanaty and Way, 2006). In the United States, babies born to mothers of African-American backgrounds are twice as likely to die before reaching their first birthday as babies born to mothers of European-American backgrounds. What do these between- and within-country comparisons have in common? What concepts and values underlie such comparisons and the inequalities they represent? What are the implications for policy and action of making such comparisons? Should societies routinely measure, monitor, and seek to reduce such inequalities and, if so, why those and not other differences? This article explores the concept of health inequalities, the values behind it, and the implications for how we understand, measure, and take action to address those differences.

What Do We Mean by Health Inequalities?

Over the last 25 years, the term 'health inequalities' has become familiar to researchers and many public health and medical practitioners around the world. The term 'health disparities' is more often used in the United States, while globally, many prefer to use 'health inequalities' or 'inequities'; arguments for and against each of these terms are discussed later. Health inequalities are generally understood to refer to differences in health between groups of people who are better or worse off socioeconomically, as reflected by, for example, their occupational standing, levels of income, expenditures, wealth, or education, or by economic characteristics of the places where they live; this understanding is often implicit rather than explicitly stated. While health inequalities research has focused mainly on socioeconomic differences, increasing attention also has been given in the international literature to health inequalities by gender, ethnic group, or immigration status. By contrast, the term health disparities as used in the United States is most often assumed to refer to racial or ethnic differences. Because information on health in the U.S. has routinely been disaggregated by race or ethnic group and not by class, this has often contributed to ill-founded but widespread assumptions that racial or ethnic differences in health were genetically based. These assumptions tend to reinforce racial stereotypes and distract attention from structural barriers to economic opportunity that persist, despite the fact that racial discrimination is illegal.

A Working Definition of Health Inequalities

The dictionary defines inequality as 'the quality of being unequal or uneven' and disparity as 'difference,' without specifying the nature of the difference or to whom it may apply. Based on these definitions, health inequalities or disparities would encompass the entire discipline of epidemiology – in other words, the study of the distribution of diseases and risk factors compared across groups within populations, without restrictions on the kinds of groups considered relevant. For example, epidemiologists might study why residents of two equally affluent neighborhoods had very different rates of a particular disease, or why breast cancer occurred more frequently among women of European background than among women with family origins in Africa. Although each of these examples involves differences in health between different population groups, they reflect concerns much broader in scope than those motivating efforts to describe, understand, and/or reduce health inequalities or disparities. What do we really mean when we use these terms, and what is the basis for focusing on a particular subset of health differences?

In her seminal paper "The Concepts and Principles of Equity and Health" (Whitehead, 1992), Margaret Whitehead clearly and succinctly defined health inequalities as differences in health that are not only unnecessary and avoidable but also unfair and unjust; illustrative examples made it clear that the central concern was social justice, a desire to improve everyone's health with faster improvements for those groups that have faced economic and social disadvantages. Recognizing that concepts can affect policies, and that measurement, while never sufficient to guide action, is often necessary for accountability, an expanded definition was recently offered to complement, not to replace, Whitehead's (Braveman *et al.*, 1996; Braveman, 1998, 2006; Braveman and Gruskin, 2003a, 2003b). Its purpose is to make explicit a number of key concepts that experience has shown may require clarification under certain circumstances. That definition, further updated here, is as follows:

> A health inequality or disparity is a particular type of difference in health (or in the most important influences on health) that could potentially be shaped by policies. It is a systematic difference in health (or in modifiable health risks) according to social advantage, meaning one's relative position in a social hierarchy determined by wealth, power, and/or prestige. It is a difference in which disadvantaged social groups (such as the poor, racial/ethnic minorities, women, or other groups that have persistently experienced social disadvantage or discrimination) systematically experience worse health or greater health risks than more advantaged social groups. Health inequalities or disparities include comparisons not only between the best- and worst-off groups in a given category (e.g., the richest versus the poorest), but between the most socially advantaged group and all others.
>
> (Braveman, 2006: 180–182)

According to this definition, a 'health inequality' does not refer generically to any health difference but is a particular type of potentially avoidable difference in health or in important influences on health that can be shaped by policies. It is a difference in which disadvantaged social groups systematically experience worse health or greater health risks than the most advantaged social groups. The criterion of being systematic, first articulated by Starfield (2007), restricts the possibilities to those health differences that are routinely and persistently patterned across social groups; an occasional or random association between a given social characteristic and ill health would not qualify as a health inequality. The restriction to differences that could – at least in the presence of sufficient political will – be influenced by policy is based on practical rather than ethical or human rights considerations.

This definition does not simply specify that health inequalities involve comparisons among different social groups. It further restricts relevant differences to those seen across groups with different levels of underlying social advantage/disadvantage or social position, that is, one's position relative to others within social hierarchies. Virtually everywhere in the world, social position varies according to economic resources, power or control over resources, and prestige or social standing, which are often reflected by measures including: income or expenditures; accumulated wealth; education; occupational standing; residential location (e.g., rural/urban; slum/nonslum; less/more advantaged neighborhoods, villages, districts, and/or provinces); racial/ethnic, tribal, or religious group or national origin; and gender (with women disadvantaged on power, wealth, and/or prestige to varying degrees almost everywhere). Disadvantaged social groups include the poor, racial/ethnic minorities (or, as in South Africa, disenfranchised majorities), women, homosexuals, physically or mentally disabled persons, or other groups that have persistently experienced social disadvantage, discrimination, or exclusion. Age can be relevant as well; in many societies the elderly and/or children are disadvantaged by policies or traditions. The biological constraints posed by physical or mental disability are often compounded by social exclusion or marginalization. In most societies, sexual orientation is another basis for social advantage or disadvantage, with homosexuals often stigmatized. Social advantage and disadvantage are powerful determinants of health, both directly and indirectly, insofar as they determine the conditions in which people live and work, the resources they have, their relationships with others, and, potentially, how they view themselves (Marmot *et al.*, 1997).

Ethical Values and Human Rights Principles Underlying the Concept of Health Inequalities

Why would anyone want to replace Whitehead's crystal-clear, elegantly concise, and accessible definition with something so dense and lengthy? Why should the specific definition of health inequalities or disparities matter? Are we simply splitting academic hairs? Answering these questions requires us to discuss the values underlying a concern for health inequalities, to focus on important examples of disagreements about measurement that reflect differing values, and to consider the practical consequences that might result from pursuing different approaches.

Ethics and Health Inequalities

Ethical concerns regarding health inequalities generally focus on theories of justice, which – along with beneficence (doing good), nonmalfeasance (not doing harm), and autonomy (respect for individuals as agents) – is one of the four basic principles of ethics. Although medical ethicists generally have directed little attention to 'distributive justice,' a standard ethical principle (Peter and Evans, 2001) concerning the equitable allocation of resources in a society that might be expected to influence health, some ethicists and scholars from a range of fields have devoted considerable thought to this concept (Daniels, 1981, 1986; Mooney, 1987; Daniels et al., 1999; Powers and Faden, 2000; Peter and Evans, 2001; Anand, 2002; Chang, 2002). Peter and Evans (2001), Daniels (2001, 2006), and Ruger (2006) have critically reviewed a range of ethical concepts relevant to health inequalities. A common ethical thread is the notion that, given that health is a necessity of life rather than a luxury, justice requires that there should be equitable opportunities to be healthy. Many writers have stated that equitable health care is based on need rather than ability to pay or one's relative position in society; there also has been wide acknowledgment of the difficulty of defining need.

The late political philosopher Rawls (1971, 1985) argued that priority should be given to improving the situation of the most disadvantaged in a society. Although he did not explicitly address health, he reasoned that an egalitarian distribution of the resources needed for the essentials of life was justified by considering what one would want to be the prevailing rules for distribution of essential goods and services if those rules were to be chosen behind a "veil of ignorance" about whether individuals had been born into socially advantaged or disadvantaged families. Based on the principle of fair equality of opportunity for everyone to be healthy, American philosopher Norman Daniels (1982) developed a series of criteria for assessing systematically the fairness or equity of health-care systems. Originally developed for the United States, Daniels' framework has been adapted through a series of in-depth discussions involving a range of stakeholders in several developing countries (Daniels et al., 2000). His approach identifies explicit criteria to guide policy decisions; it has attracted considerable interest in part because the process of developing the criteria in a given country is in itself an important tool for building the societal consensus needed to ensure the necessary political will to implement equitable policies. Daniels and others have also explored ethical and pragmatic arguments for justice or equity in all the fundamental factors influencing health, including but not limited to health care (Daniels et al., 1999). Nobel Prize-winning economist Amartya Sen has written that human development should be measured not just in economic terms, which has been the rule, but in terms of indicators of human capability to freely pursue quality of life, with health and education being among the best indicators of that capability (Sen, 1999).

Health Inequalities and Human Rights

In addition to ethical concepts, international human rights principles can provide both a valuable theoretical basis for understanding and defining health inequalities and a rationale for reducing them. Human rights are a set of entitlements of all people in the world, regardless of who they are or where they live. When human rights are mentioned, most of us think about civil and political rights, such as freedom of speech, freedom of assembly, and freedom from torture or cruel or arbitrary punishment. However, there also are economic, social, and cultural rights, such as the right to a decent standard of living, which in turn includes rights to adequate food, water, shelter, and clothing requisite for health, as well as the right to health itself. International human rights agreements also include the right to participate in one's society and the right to dignified and safe working and living conditions. By now, almost every country in the world has signed one or more agreements that include important health-related rights. Sadly, in many places in the world, agreed-upon human rights generally are honored more in the breach than in the enforcement, and it would thus be naïve to think that human rights laws, as legal instruments, ensure the reduction of health inequalities. Nevertheless, human rights principles, as articulated in international agreements and laws, provide a key reference point in that they reflect a global consensus about values, reached thoughtfully among representatives of virtually all countries in the world. As Sofia Gruskin and colleagues have articulated, the analytic frameworks of human rights can be a powerful source of conceptual and practical guidance for social policies (Braveman and Gruskin, 2003b; Gruskin, 2002; Mann et al., 1999b). Gruskin coauthored earlier papers in which these ideas were developed (Braveman and Gruskin, 2003a, 2003b), and she has played the lead role in developing the concepts related to human rights.

One cross-cutting human rights principle with particular relevance to concepts of health inequalities is nondiscrimination – an individual's right to be treated equally as a person, without discriminatory treatment based on his or her social group. Specific international human rights agreements have explicitly focused on what we refer to here broadly as 'racial/ethnic' discrimination, encompassing discrimination not only by racial or ethnic group but also based on religion, tribe, national origin, or refugee status; other human rights agreements address women and children (Mann et al., 1999a). Because groups in power – the dominant racial/ethnic group, men, or adults, for example – have sometimes questioned or failed to acknowledge the disadvantaged status of the minority racial/ethnic groups, women, and/or children and their resulting need for special measures to protect their rights, agreements have been developed that explicitly recognize these groups as historically disadvantaged. Globally, such agreements have been very important in practice. Human rights principles such as nondiscrimination provide a universally recognized frame of reference for initiatives to reduce health disparities between more and less advantaged social groups. This frame of reference could be important in the United States as well, for example, in defending the rationale for affirmative action to rectify historic racial/ethnic and gender disparities that impact health and/or health care.

Economic, Social, and Cultural Rights

The economic, social, and cultural rights codified in international human rights agreements and laws also provide a powerful tool for conceptualizing health inequalities and justifying action to reduce them. The public, policy makers, and medical professionals often assume that the key to resolving health inequalities is eliminating disparities in medical care. Medical care can be an important determinant of health, particularly for those who have become ill; even when it cannot cure disease or extend life, medical care can improve functional status and relieve suffering. Inequalities in all aspects of medical care should be addressed, including the allocation of resources for health care as well as the utilization, quality, and financing (particularly with respect to the burden of payment on individuals or households) of services.

Medical care, however, is neither the sole determinant of health nor the most powerful determinant of whether one becomes sick or dies prematurely. The most powerful influences on health are the physical and social environments in which one lives and works, including conditions in homes, neighborhoods, workplaces, and communities. In developing countries, factors such as adequate and safe food supply, clean water, sanitation, exposure to known biological pathogens and environmental toxins, and grossly unsafe conditions at work and in transportation are obvious major factors. In affluent countries, poor quality (rather than quantity) of nutrition, inadequate physical activity, tobacco use, and excessive alcohol consumption feature more prominently (McGinnis and Foege, 1993; Mokdad et al., 2004). These behavioral risks and other risk factors are powerfully shaped by socioeconomic resources and opportunities.

Ethical and human rights principles provide a strong rationale for addressing inequalities in the nonmedical determinants of health along with medical care. Human rights call for a decent standard of living for all and for safe and dignified working conditions. Both ethical and human rights principles call for equal opportunities for all people to be as healthy as possible. Opportunities to be healthy extend far beyond the availability of medical care to buffer the health-damaging effects of underlying unjust living conditions; the underlying unjust determinants themselves also need to be addressed. Thus, based on human rights principles, the definition of health inequalities proposed at the beginning of this article refers to differences not only in health itself, but also in the most important determinants of health that could at least in theory be influenced by policies.

As one of the economic, social, and cultural rights addressed by international human rights agreements, the right to health is a cornerstone underlying efforts to reduce health inequalities. The World Health Organization's constitution (1946) defined the right to health as the right of everyone to enjoy the highest possible level of health. While this definition has been criticized for being vague and difficult to operationalize, Braveman and Gruskin (2003a) have proposed that the right to health can be defined operationally as the right of all social groups (defined by social position) to attain the level of health enjoyed by the most privileged group in society. The right to health thus provides the basis for comparing the health experienced by different social groups, always using as the reference group the most privileged group in a given category, that is, the group with the highest position in a social hierarchy based on wealth, power, and/or prestige. Drawing upon human rights concepts, pursuing health equity means removing obstacles for groups of people – such as the poor, disadvantaged racial/ethnic groups, women, or homosexuals – who have historically had more obstacles preventing them from realizing their rights to health and other human rights.

What Difference Could a Definition Make for How We Understand, Measure, and Act on Health Inequalities?

In many, if not most, nonacademic settings, Whitehead's clear and straightforward definition of health inequalities as differences in health that are avoidable, unjust, and unfair, or equal opportunities for everyone to be as healthy as possible, is likely to convey the key concepts. However, the terms 'injustice,' 'unfairness,' and 'avoidability' are open to widely varying interpretations, and this ambiguity can be problematic. For example, while most people in the United States and Europe believe it is unjust and unfair for women to not be able to vote, to be required to have their faces veiled in public, and to be forbidden to work outside the home, in some other countries these circumstances are viewed by the ruling groups as appropriate, just, and fair in light of women's unique (and, they would say, valued) role in society. Given a long history of racial/ethnic discrimination that has systematically put people of color at a disadvantage in multiple spheres of life, many in the United States and South Africa believe that justice and fairness are served by affirmative action to increase racial/ethnic diversity in professional positions; others, including some vocal members of the underrepresented groups, feel that such efforts are unjust, constituting 'reverse discrimination' that unfairly disadvantages people of European origin.

Measuring Health Inequalities

A range of methods has been used to quantify health inequalities, each reflecting implicit assumptions about definitions (World Bank, n.d.; Wagstaff *et al.*, 1991a, 1991b; Kunst and Mackenbach, 1994; Galal and Qureshi, 1997; Kakwani *et al.*, 1997; Mackenbach and Kunst, 1997; Manor *et al.*, 1997; Carr-Hill and Chalmers-Dixon, 2002; Wagstaff, 2002), which are discussed in an earlier paper (Braveman, 2006). Perhaps the most compelling example illustrating the need for a definition that can guide measurement and accountability is the approach taken by the authors of WHO's *World Health Report 2000* (WHO, 2000). That report made a welcome argument – consistent with the ethical principle of distributive justice, without articulating that principle – for the importance of assessing health not only by average levels but also by examining its distribution. At the same time, however, it recommended that 'health inequalities' be measured by examining the distribution of health indicators across ungrouped individuals, as is done by the Gini coefficient – not across preselected social groups. At first glance this may not seem unreasonable, partly because one might assume that the socially disadvantaged individuals in a society are always the sickest. Despite doing worse on the vast majority of important health outcomes, however, members of a particular disadvantaged group may do as well as or better than their more advantaged counterparts on particular outcomes. Selecting those particular outcomes could then be used to justify directing more resources toward better-off groups that already have more resources.

Thus, although surely this was not the report's authors' intention, this measurement can be used to justify neglecting health differences between more and less advantaged social groups while claiming to be reducing 'health inequalities.' In the debates that the measurement approach generated, it became clear that simpler definitions of health equity or health inequalities – which do not explicitly specify the importance of closing gaps that systematically and adversely affect the health of socially disadvantaged groups – could not provide a basis for refuting the approach advocated by the authors of the *World Health Report 2000*.

More importantly, the most problematic aspect of the measurement approach used in that report was that it in fact removed comparisons among social groups from the agenda. The proposal by the report's authors was not to use the new measurement approach as a supplement to other approaches – specifically, approaches comparing more and less advantaged social groups – but to replace those group-based approaches with the new method, dispensing with consideration of social groups selected on *a priori* grounds. The *a priori* grounds for selecting more and less socially advantaged groups are ethical and human rights values. The implications of the proposal to cease making social group comparisons were particularly striking because the proposal emerged at a time when consensus was building and technical work had paved the way for increased examination of health differences among more and less socially advantaged groups – particularly according to wealth – in routine public health monitoring by national governments and international agencies (Braveman *et al.*, 1996; Braveman, 1998; WHO, 1999; Gwatkin *et al.*, 2000; Evans *et al.*, 2001).

Inequity Versus Inequality

Why not use the term 'health inequity' rather than 'health inequality,' if health inequalities are a subset of health differences that are particularly unfair? If the causes of a given health inequality are known, and are due to social disadvantage/advantage, it would be appropriate to call it a health inequity. However, it may not always be possible to determine whether a given difference in health or health risks that is systematically associated with social disadvantage is unfair or unjust in itself. Such a determination may not be possible in some cases; for example, the causes of the black/white disparity in low birth weight and premature birth in the United States are mostly unknown, so we cannot say whether it is unfair or unjust. However, on the definition proposed here, that difference qualifies as a health inequality deserving attention because it is an important health difference adversely affecting an *a priori* disadvantaged social group, resulting in further disadvantage for that group in terms of health. Since the causes are unknown, intensive research to uncover them would be a high priority consistent with the goal of equity. In trying to raise awareness of health inequalities and support for reducing them among the general public, it may be wise to use the term 'health inequities' sparingly, because 'inequity' sounds strongly judgmental; it should be used when it is needed to convey the injustice reflected by a given inequality. However, in some situations, using the term 'inequity,' especially repeatedly, may make it more difficult for some people to be receptive to messages about health inequalities, and hence may make it more difficult to build consensus toward action. This is a decision about communication, however, not about the concept.

Avoidability

The proposed definition specifies that differences need only be potentially or theoretically avoidable through policy interventions. One might argue, particularly in the era of gene therapy and genomics, that virtually all states of ill health could be avoided if sufficient resources were invested in deciphering and manipulating their genetic codes. It would be a mistake to require empiric evidence of avoidability as a prerequisite for judging a given difference to qualify as an inequality. The modifiability in practice of a given difference in health – or in health determinant – may often be questionable, depending largely on the degree of political will to make the necessary policy changes.

For example, in the United States, the causes of large racial/ethnic disparities in low birth weight and premature birth rates are; poorly understood they are not explained by the socioeconomic characteristics that have been included in existing research (Institute of Medicine *et al.* 2007). Inadequate measurement of socioeconomic experiences across women's entire lifecourses, including childhood socioeconomic experiences, may account completely or partially for the unexplained disparities. In addition, many scientists believe that lifecourse experiences of chronic stress related to experiences of racial discrimination could be contributing factors. One would not want to argue that because the causes are currently uncertain (and therefore one cannot be certain about avoidability), this is not an appropriate health inequalities concern. Low birth weight (being born too small) and premature birth (being born too early) are among the strongest predictors of health not only in infancy and childhood but across the life course. According to the proposed definition, the large and persistent inequality in birth outcomes between African-Americans and European-Americans would be considered a health inequality/disparity warranting focused attention. The reason is that it is an important health difference that puts a historically disadvantaged social group, African-Americans, at further disadvantage with respect to their health. Giving priority to this inequality would involve allocating resources for research to uncover the causes. The proposed definition specifies that the differences in health or health determinants need only be theoretically avoidable; it must be reasonable to believe, based on current knowledge, that the differences could be avoidable, but evidence does not have to be provided empirically demonstrating avoidability.

Why restrict the relevant differences in health (or in its determinants) to those that could be influenced by policies? This corresponds to Whitehead's criterion that health inequalities are avoidable or unnecessary, and, like it, is based on common sense. However, the extent to which a given condition could be influenced by policies is often a matter of debate. For example, some people might argue that it is impossible to enact policies in the United States that redistribute resources in favor of less advantaged groups, given that country's deep-rooted ethos regarding individual responsibility and entrepreneurship. Also often cited as a barrier to redistribution is the relative lack of a tradition of social solidarity in the United States, as reflected for example by the absence of the universal health-care coverage that is the norm in Western European nations. It is reasonable to maintain that the relevant differences are those that could be influenced by policies given political will, assuming that such political will is at least theoretically possible in the future.

Implications for Resource Allocation

Additional illustrations also indicate the need for clarity about the concept of health inequalities. For example, at a recent meeting to discuss planning for a nationally funded center on oral health inequalities in a certain country, it was suggested that efforts be broadened to include addressing needs for oral health services among middle-class populations rather than focusing only on lower-income populations as it had been doing; many of those participating in the meeting appeared to feel uneasy but ill-equipped to argue that this was inappropriate, given the center's mandate to reduce oral health inequalities. The proposed clarification of the concept may have helped resolve the confusion, because middle-class populations would not be seen as socially disadvantaged; on the other hand, one might argue that they have fewer advantages than the wealthy. Referral to principles of distributive justice may have been helpful at that point in the discussion, had it arisen.

Another example is the suggestion that the longstanding gender disparity in life expectancy in affluent countries, with women generally living on average several years longer than men, should become a focus for initiatives on health inequalities. Like the previous examples, this illustrates a very important public health issue that deserves attention as part of a broad public health agenda, but it is not a health inequalities issue, because men have more social advantage (wealth, power, prestige) than women in almost all societies. The proposed definition specifies that in order to be a 'health inequality', a health difference not only must be observed among groups with different levels of underlying social advantage; it must put the disadvantaged groups at further disadvantage with respect to their health, that is, the *a priori* disadvantaged groups must do worse on that health indicator. If the disadvantaged group does better on a particular indicator, that particular comparison is not a relevant health inequality – although it certainly may be an important public health issue of a different kind.

Health (or health risk) differences in which socially disadvantaged groups systematically fare worse than their more socially advantaged counterparts are particularly unjust. This is because they place groups of people who are already at an underlying disadvantage in society – for example, because they were born into poor families, belong to a particular racial/ethnic group, or are women – at further disadvantage with respect to their health, and health in turn is essential for well-being and for escaping from social disadvantage. This element reflects the ethical principle of distributive justice. It is consistent with the concern developed in Sen's work regarding human capabilities. If health – along with education – is a basic human capability and is essential to fulfill one's human potential, then being doubly disadvantaged – first in virtue of one's social group and then in virtue of having worse health – is particularly unacceptable from an ethical perspective.

Yet another example to illustrate the need for specificity in the definition of 'health inequalities' is that in the United States, although African-American women with breast cancer have higher rates of mortality and shorter survival times, affluent women of European-American ancestry have higher incidence rates, and some have suggested that health disparity initiatives should address this health difference as well. A further illustration comes from a recent national workshop on health inequalities in which one lecturer repeatedly referred to an environmental health problem in a particular region as reflecting a "disparity"; although certain areas within the region were more affected than others, the regions did not differ in terms of social conditions of the populations.

In each of these (real) examples, a simpler and more intuitive definition of health inequalities or disparities provides no basis for rejecting a course of action that would significantly redirect resources earmarked for reducing inequalities between more and less advantaged social groups toward groups with more underlying advantage to start with (affluent groups, men, European-background women). By contrast, the proposed more complex definition dictates that resources to address health disparities be selectively directed toward the needs of disadvantaged groups. This would not preclude using other available resources to address the unmet needs of more advantaged segments of the population. This illustrates what Whitehead has called "leveling up" (Whitehead, 1992) – seeking improvements for everyone, but focusing on bringing up those who started off furthest behind. In the above examples, the proposed definition would specifically indicate that the gender disparity in life expectancy is not an appropriate health disparities issue, because in this particular case the *a priori* disadvantaged group – women – experience better health. Similarly, the higher incidence of breast cancer among European-Americans, the most advantaged racial/ethnic group in the United States, is an important general public health issue but not a health inequalities issue. A talk on avoidable environmental health problems in a region, without reference to more and less privileged groups, might be of interest as part of a workshop on environmental health or environmental epidemiology but not in a workshop on health disparities; by contrast, because it focuses on unnecessary errors that should have been prevented by more responsible planning and supervision, such a talk might be considered relevant to health disparities or inequalities if 'fairness' and 'avoidability' are the primary criteria. Health disparities/equity should not displace all other concerns, but they deserve particular attention highlighted by explicit criteria.

Final Remarks

At times, defining terms can be largely a semantic matter, without practical consequences. At other times, however, definitions can indeed matter. In the case of defining health inequalities or disparities, experience has shown how much difference a definition can make. Definitions determine what will be measured and monitored by local, provincial/state, national, and international governments and nongovernmental organizations; and measurement is crucial for accountability. Definitions also can matter insofar as they clarify – or obscure – key concepts such as distributive justice and the concept of equal opportunities to be healthy as a fundamental human right. The concept of health inequalities draws heavily from epidemiologic notions, but it is not just a technical concept. It inherently reflects social values from the fields of ethics and human rights.

If we do not understand a concept, we are likely to be less effective in pursuing its fulfillment; in the case of health inequalities, we can more easily be detoured by attempts to pull the agenda away from social justice concerns. How one understands and defines health inequalities can determine how resources earmarked for health equity are allocated across different social groups. Concepts can determine what will get the attention and support of the public and policy makers, and whether that attention and support will be sustained on policy agendas from local up to international levels.

A technically adequate definition of health inequalities needs to specify explicitly the relevance of social position, in other words, relative advantage and disadvantage in social hierarchies; it also must specify the kinds of comparisons that are relevant, that reflect distributive justice concerns. These are sensitive issues politically, because they raise the specter of potential redistribution of resources in favor of those who have been the 'have-nots,' that is, those less wealthy, powerful, and influential in a society. It may not always be essential to spell out all of these concerns in an explicit and detailed manner, but it is essential for public health professionals who are committed to reducing health inequalities to be absolutely clear about the concept, and to find ways to communicate the essence of the concept that will work within their particular societal contexts. It is hard to find a better definition than Whitehead's for this purpose in many societies.

If needed, further clarifications of Whitehead's definition on specific points could be drawn from the longer and more technical definition proposed here, without using the entire definition. Examples include:

- Health inequalities reflect unequal opportunities to be healthy, making socially disadvantaged groups (e.g., the

poor or racial/ethnic minorities) even more disadvantaged with respect to their health.
- Reducing health inequalities means trying to give disadvantaged social groups equal opportunities to be healthy.
- Social advantage refers to differences in relative social position determined by wealth, power, and prestige.
- Health inequalities are differences in health (or differences in important influences on health) that are systematically associated with being socially disadvantaged (e.g., being poor, a member of a disadvantaged racial/ethnic group, or female) and that put already disadvantaged groups at further disadvantage.
- Pursuing health equity – that is, striving to eliminate health inequalities/disparities associated with social disadvantage – means striving for equal opportunities for all social groups to be as healthy as possible, selectively focusing on those groups that have had fewer opportunities.

Clarity about concepts is needed to inform measurement approaches that will be adequate not only for studying specific research questions but also for ongoing surveillance to assess the magnitude of the health gaps and how they change over time in relation to policies in all sectors that influence health. Public health surveillance alone is certainly not sufficient to reduce health disparities, but without monitoring how the size of inequalities between more and less advantaged social groups changes over time in relation to policies, there is a lack of accountability for the differential effects of policies on vulnerable groups. We need to be clear about what we should measure and monitor and why. Epidemiology – the study of the distribution of diseases and risk factors across different populations – is concerned with health differences in general. In contrast, the term health inequalities or health disparities refers to a very specific subset of differences deemed worthy of special attention because of widely held social values. These values include the ethical concepts of distributive justice and equal opportunities to be healthy; they also reflect core human rights principles, including nondiscrimination and the obligation to remove obstacles some individuals have to realizing their human rights, which includes the right to be as healthy as possible. All potentially avoidable health differences should be of public health concern, health inequalities are a subset of health differences warranting special – although not exclusive – attention.

See also: Resource Allocation: International Perspectives on Resource Allocation; Resource Allocation: Justice and Resource Allocation in Public Health.

Citations

Anand S (2002) The concern for equity in health. *Journal of Epidemiology and Community Health* 56(7): 485–487.
Badan Pusat Statistik-Statistics Indonesia and ORC Macro (2003) Indonesia: Demographic and Health Survey 2002–2003. *Report of Demographic and Health Surveys.* Calverton, MD: Badan Pusat Statistik-Statistics Indonesia and ORC Macro.
Bellamy C (2004) The state of the world's children 2005: Childhood under threat. *Report for UNICEF.* New York: United Nations Children's Fund.
Braveman P (1998) Monitoring equity in health: A policy-oriented approach in low- and middle-income countries. *WHO/CHS/HSS/98.91 Equity initiative paper number 3*, pp. 2–3. Geneva, Switzerland: World Health Organization Department of Health Systems.
Braveman P (2006) Health disparities and health equity: Concepts and measurement. *Annual Review of Public Health* 27: 167–194.
Braveman P and Gruskin S (2003a) Defining equity in health. *Journal of Epidemiology and Community Health* 57(4): 254–258.
Braveman P and Gruskin S (2003b) Poverty, equity, human rights and health. *Bulletin of the World Health Organization* 81(7): 539–545.
Braveman P, Tarimo E, Creese A, Monasch R, and Nelson L (1996) Equity in health and health care: A WHO/SIDA initiative. *Report of the World Health Organization.* Geneva, Switzerland: World Health Organization.
Carr-Hill RA and Chalmers-Dixon P (2002) *A Review of Methods for Monitoring and Measuring Social Inequality, Deprivation, and Health Inequality.* York, UK: Center for Health Economics, University of York.
Chang WC (2002) The meaning and goals of equity in health. *Journal of Epidemiology and Community Health* 56(7): 488–491.
Daniels N (1981) Health-care needs and distributive justice. *Philosophy and Public Affairs* 10(2): 146–179.
Daniels N (1982) Equity of access to health care: Some conceptual and ethical issues. *Milbank Memorial Fund Quarterly/Health and Society* 60(1): 51–81.
Daniels N (1986) Why saying no to patients in the United States is so hard: Cost containment, justice, and provider autonomy. *New England Journal of Medicine* 314(21): 1380–1383.
Daniels N (2001) Justice, health, and healthcare. *American Journal of Bioethics* 1(2): 2–16.
Daniels N (2006) Equity and population health: Toward a broader bioethics agenda. *Hastings Center Report* 36(4): 22–35.
Daniels N, Bryant J, Castano RA, Dantes OG, Khan KS, and Pannarunothai S (2000) Benchmarks of fairness for health care reform: A policy tool for developing countries. *Bulletin of the World Health Organization* 78(6): 740–750.
Daniels N, Kennedy BP, and Kawachi I (1999) Why justice is good for our health: The social determinants of health inequalities. *Daedalus* 128(4): 215–251.
El-Zanaty F and Way A (2006) Egypt: Demographic and health survey 2005. *Report of Demographic and Health Surveys.* Cairo, Egypt: Ministry of Health and Population, National Population Council, El-Zanaty and Associates, and ORC Macro.
Evans T, Whitehead M, Diderichsen F, Bhuiya A, and Wirth M (2001) *Challenging Inequities in Health: From Ethics to Action.* New York: Oxford University Press.
Galal OM and Qureshi AK (1997) Dispersion index: Measuring trend assessment of geographical inequality in health – the example of under-five mortality in the Middle East/North African region, 1980–1994. *Social Science and Medicine* 44(12): 1893–1902.
Gruskin S (2002) Ethics, human rights, and public health. *American Journal of Public Health* 92(5): 698–699.
Gwatkin DR, Rutstein S, Johnson K, Pande RP, and Wagstaff A (2000) Socio-economic differences in health, nutrition, and population in Morocco [and comparable publications covering 40 additional countries]. *Report of the HNP/Poverty Thematic Group of the World Bank.* Washington, DC: World Bank.
Institute of Medicine, Committee on Understanding Premature Birth and Healthy outcomes, et al. (2007) *Preterm Birth: Causes, consequences, and Prevention.* Washington D.C.: The National Academies Press.
Kakwani N, Wagstaff A, and van Doorslaer E (1997) Socioeconomic inequalities in health: Measurement, computation, and statistical inference. *Journal of Econometrics* 77(1): 87–103.
Kunst AE and Mackenbach JP (1994) International variation in the size of mortality differences associated with occupational status. *International Journal of Epidemiology* 23(4): 742–750.
Mackenbach JP and Kunst AE (1997) Measuring the magnitude of socio-economic inequalities in health: An overview of available measures illustrated with two examples from Europe. *Social Science and Medicine* 44(6): 757–771.

Mann J, Gruskin S, Grodin M, and Annas GJ (1999a) *Health and Human Rights: A Reader*. New York: Routledge.
Mann J, Gruskin S, Grodin M, and Annas GJ (1999b) Introduction. In: Mann J, Gruskin S, Grodin M, and Annas GJ (eds.) *Health and Human Rights: A Reader*, pp. 1–3. New York: Routledge.
Manor O, Matthews S, and Power C (1997) Comparing measures of health inequality. *Social Science and Medicine* 45(5): 761–771.
Marmot M, Ryff CD, Bumpass LL, Shipley M, and Marks NF (1997) Social inequalities in health: Next questions and converging evidence. *Social Science and Medicine* 44(6): 901–910.
McGinnis JM and Foege WH (1993) Actual causes of death in the United States. *Journal of the American Medical Association* 270(18): 2207–2212.
Mokdad AH, Marks JS, Stroup DF, and Gerberding JL (2004) Actual causes of death in the United States, 2000. *Journal of the American Medical Association* 291(10): 1238–1245.
Mooney G (1987) What does equity in health mean? *World Health Statistics Quarterly* 40(4): 296–303.
Peter F and Evans T (2001) Ethical dimensions of health equity. In: Evans T, Whitehead M, Diderichsen F, Bhuiya A, and Wirth M (eds.) *Challenging Inequities in Health: From Ethics to Action*, pp. 24–33. New York: Oxford University Press.
Powers M and Faden R (2000) Inequalities in health, inequalities in health care: Four generations of discussion about justice and cost-effectiveness analysis. *Kennedy Institute of Ethics Journal* 10(2): 109–127.
Rawls J (1971) *A Theory of Justice*. Cambridge, MA: Harvard University Press.
Rawls J (1985) Justice as fairness: Political not metaphysical. *Philosophy and Public Affairs* 14(3): 223–251.
Ruger JP (2006) Ethics and governance of global health inequalities. *Journal of Epidemiology and Community Health* 60(11): 998–1003.
Sardán MG, Ochoa LH, and Guerra WC (2004) Bolivia: Demographic and health survey 2003. *Report of Demographic and Health Surveys*. Miraflores, Bolivia: INE.
Sen A (1999) *Development as Freedom*. New York: Random House.
Starfield B (2007) Pathways of influence on equity in health. *Social Science and Medicine* 64(7): 1355–1362.
United Nations Office of the High Commissioner for Human Rights (1999) International covenant on economic, social, and cultural rights. In: Mann JM, Gruskin S, Grodin MA, and Annas GJ (eds) *Health and Human Rights: A Reader*, Appendix B, pp. 458–465. New York: Routledge.
Wagstaff A (2002) Inequality aversion, health inequalities, and health achievement. *Journal of Health Economics* 21(4): 627–641.
Wagstaff A, Paci P, and van Doorslaer E (1991a) On the measurement of inequalities in health. *Social Science and Medicine* 33(5): 545–557.
Wagstaff A, van Doorslaer E, and Paci P (1991b) Horizontal equity in the delivery of health care. *Journal of Health Economics* 10: 251–256.
Whitehead M (1992) The concepts and principles of equity and health. *International Journal of Health Services* 22(3): 429–445.
WHO (1999) World health report 1999: Making a difference. *Report of the World Health Organization*. Geneva, Switzerland: World Health Organization.
WHO (2000) World health report 2000: Health systems; improving performance. *Report of the World Health Organization*. Geneva, Switzerland: World Health Organization.
WHO (2004) Maternal mortality in 2000: Estimates developed by WHO, UNICEF and UNFPA. *Report of the World Health Organization*. Geneva, Switzerland: World Health Organization, Department of Reproductive Health and Research.
World Bank (2008) *Quantitative Techniques for Health Equity Analysis: Technical Notes*. http://sitesources.worldbank.org/INTPAH/Resources/Publications/459843-1195594469249/HealthEquityFINAL.pdf.
World Health Organization (1946) Constitution of the World Health Organization. *Basic Documents*. New York: WHO.

Resource Allocation: Justice and Resource Allocation in Public Health

R Rhodes, Mount Sinai School of Medicine, New York, NY, USA

© 2008 Elsevier Inc. All rights reserved.

Public health measures have contributed dramatically to reducing the death rate and extending life expectancy in populations. Because of their success, their value is broadly acknowledged, at least in public discussion. Nevertheless, claims for the allocation of societal funds to public health projects are always in competition with claims for projects of other sorts. Ideally, broad considerations of justice should determine how a society's funds are allocated among the important needs for expenditures on social goods such as public health, education, defense, safety, transportation, law enforcement, the arts, and clinical medicine. Yet, the issues of justice persist even when we focus solely on a single domain. Within public health, we are challenged to decide how limited funding resources should be sorted out: Which projects should be addressed first? How much should be allocated to which efforts? What sorts of considerations should be taken into account and which factors should be ignored? Should all of the funds be directed at providing immediate benefits, or should some resources be allotted to prepare for future possible public health needs or to public health research? In times of urgency and need, how should limited supplies be allocated? Which populations should be rescued when all cannot be? How should the multitude of competing claims be prioritized?

In developing an understanding of justice in public health, focus on disasters and emergencies can be instructive because the circumstances make the importance of resource allocation vivid and pressing. Such circumstances dramatize the need for thinking clearly about justice in setting public policy and they can teach us how to conceptualize public health allocations even when there is no imminent disaster. This article reviews the leading theories of justice in medicine and then goes on to explain some principles of justice in public health by focusing on recent disasters that are familiar to everyone: The allocation of public health resources after the attack on the World Trade Center in New York City in September 2001, the flu vaccine shortage in the fall of 2004, and Hurricane Katrina in September 2005. A careful analysis of these dramatic examples explains the factors that make some allocations and policies just and others unjust. When public health resources are well allocated, the principles that underlie the decisions are assumed with relatively little contention. Implicit in this silent agreement are the presumptions (1) that everyone knows 'the' guiding principle of justice and (2) that 'the' principle has the solid endorsement of a broad majority of the population. Yet, a comparison of the principles most commonly invoked in discussions of justice reveals that there is no single principle that supports all of the relevant policies. No simple formula can tell us what justice requires in all circumstances. Rather, careful investigation and examination of the situation, and thoughtful reflection on the array of problems involved and the consequences of choosing one path or another suggest that justice requires distributions based on different principles in different contexts.

Prominent Conceptions of Justice

In his lengthy discussion of justice in book 5 of the *Nicomachean Ethics*, Aristotle equates justice to the entirety of interpersonal virtue while also acknowledging its complexity and contextuality. Aristotle defined justice as giving each his due and treating similarly situated individuals similarly. Yet, he acknowledged the complexity involved in determining which features should be taken into account in deciding that individuals are similarly situated and which of the generally important factors should be given priority in a particular situation. According to Aristotle, factors such as relationship, history, consequences, and feasibility are all considerations that may determine which allocation is just in a situation, but justice does require equality in the treatment of equals.

Although some contemporary philosophers follow Aristotle's insights and recommend an account of justice that draws on an array of reasons, those who write on issues of justice and health care appear to prefer a more Platonic approach and attempt to articulate a singular comprehensive account of justice. Consider the following competing contemporary accounts of justice that enter discussions of medicine and public health.

Utilitarianism

Utilitarianism has a long history in ethics, tracing back to the writings of Jeremy Bentham and John Stuart Mill. Today utilitarianism appears to be the dominant view of justice in medical and public health policy. It is the view that justifies policies that produce the best outcomes. For example, policies that aim at the maximization of quality-adjusted life years (QALYs), disability-adjusted life years (DALYs), or disability-adjusted life expectations (DALEs) are all utilitarian.

Utilitarian allocations aim at maximizing an outcome over a population. A utilitarian conception of justice is committed to treating people as equals and to deliberately ignoring relational and relative differences between individuals. Hence, utilitarians aim at producing the most of the desired results for the entire population that is to be governed by the policy. Utilitarians identify an objective standard for calculating outcomes, and employ that standard in policy decision. A policy is just on utilitarian grounds when it is the most likely to produce the greatest amount of the specified end, that is, it is efficacious. In the domain of medicine, utilitarians focus on measurements of health or life span. A cost–benefit analysis of the same considerations is employed to determine the policy for a population.

John Rawls

Since 1971, many of the positions on justice espoused by philosopher John Rawls, first in *A Theory of Justice* (1971) and later in *Political Liberalism* (1993) and other works, have come to play a significant role in public deliberation about nonutilitarian criteria for justice in society and the allocation of medical resources. One Rawlsian concept that has received especially broad endorsement in the medical ethics literature is fair equality of opportunity. The other concept that has been widely adopted is the difference principle, and people who have embraced some version of that principle now refer to such views as prioritarianism. These principles exemplify features of Rawls's view of what a liberal political conception of justice should include.

Rawls's two principles of justice provide "guidelines for how basic [political] institutions are to realize the values of liberty and equality" and assure all citizens "adequate all-purpose means to make effective use of their liberties and opportunities," as he writes in *Political Liberalism* (Rawls, 1993: 4). Together these principles specify certain basic rights, liberties, and opportunities and assign them priority against claims of those who advocate for the general good or the promotion of perfectionism (i.e., the best possible society).

Rawls (1993: 184) himself does not extend his principles of justice to health and medical care. In fact, he specifically maintains that "variations in physical capacities and skills, including the effects of illness and accident on natural abilities" are not unfair and they do not give rise to injustice so long as the principles of justice are satisfied. Yet, several prominent authors who write about justice and medicine discuss medical allocations by invoking Rawls's principles and they extend particular Rawlsian concepts to medicine.

According to Rawls's first principle, justice requires a liberal democratic political regime to assure that its citizens' basic needs for primary goods are met and that citizens have the means to make effective use of their liberties and opportunities. Rawls's second principle regulates the basic institutions of a just state so as to assure citizens fair equality of opportunity. The first principle has priority over the second in that it requires political institutions to provide whatever citizens must have in order to understand and to exercise their rights and liberties. According to Rawls, his two principles taken together assure such basic political rights and liberties as liberty of conscience, freedom of association, freedom of speech, voting, running for office, freedom of movement, and free choice of occupation. They also guarantee the political value of fair equality of opportunity in the face of inevitable social and economic inequalities. Both principles, therefore, express a commitment to the equality of political liberties and opportunities.

In Rawls's account, the difference principle is the second condition of the second principle of justice. Recognizing that economic and social inequalities are an unavoidable feature of any ongoing social arrangement, his second principle expresses the limits on unequal distributions. He holds that equal access to opportunities is a necessary feature of a just society, and then, so as to compensate for eventual disparities and to promote persisting equality of opportunity, he calls for corrective distribution measures through application of the difference principle. As Rawls (1993: 6) states the principle, "Social and economic inequalities ... are to be to the greatest benefit of the least advantaged members of society." In other words, governmental policies that distribute goods between citizens must be designed to rectify inequality by first advancing the interests of those who are otherwise less well off than their fellow citizens.

Norman Daniels and Fair Equality of Opportunity

Norman Daniels has used the Rawlsian concept of fair equality of opportunity to argue that health care should be treated as a basic need. He maintains that "[h]ealth care is of special moral importance because it helps to preserve our status as fully functioning citizens" (Daniels, 2002: 8). Daniels wants us to count at least some medical services as primary goods so that they are "treated as claims to special needs." From Daniels's point of view, therefore, the allocation of health-care resources should aim at equalizing social opportunity.

Daniels expects his claim to lead to the conclusion that a just society should provide its members with universal health care, including public health and preventive measures. Yet, recognizing that a society will limit the amount of health care it provides, Daniels proposes "normal species function" as the benchmark for deciding which care to provide. He holds that health care that will restore or maintain normal species function should be provided. Nothing has to be provided, however, for those who are already within the normal range. Furthermore, Daniels points to the many social determinants of health inequalities and invokes Rawls's difference principle to claim that a just society should provide the most health care to those who are most disadvantaged with respect to health.

Prioritarianism

Prioritization, which builds on Rawls's difference principle, stands in opposition to utilitarian approaches to the distribution of scarce resources. Whereas utilitarian allocations aim at the maximization of an outcome over a population and deliberately ignore the relational and relative differences between individuals, prioritarian allocations aim at the identification of unwanted inequalities and then distribute resources so as to compensate for or correct them. Prioritarian allocations reflect a concern for how individuals fare in relation to each other and attempt to advantage those whose position is worse than others'.

Numerous papers in the bioethics literature address the conflict between prioritarian concerns and utilitarian cost-effectiveness analysis in the allocation of medical resources. For instance, Dan Brock (1998, 2002), Frances Kamm (1993, 2002), and David Wasserman (2002) argue the merits of one approach over the other in a variety of vexing cases. They reflect on the difference between policies that will save the lives of some people or save an arm for some other people. They are concerned with whether public policies should provide a greater advantage to some who are already well off (e.g., save the lives of the able-bodied), or provide a smaller advantage to some who are worse off (e.g., save the use of an arm for a group with some other preexisting disability). These tragic choices discussions aim at discovering a principled basis for making decisions by sometimes focusing on identifiable individuals, and sometimes not. They sometimes address trade-offs of future significant harms against present small harms or more certain imminent harms against more hypothetical distant harms. Typically, these discussions favor policies that will allocate resources to immediate needs over future needs and benefits to identifiable individuals over benefits to those who cannot be currently identified.

Public Health Models that Challenge Popular Theories of Justice

In light of these competing theories of justice, it is illuminating to scrutinize some of the public health policies that were implemented in the fall of 2001. Consider two examples.

Medical Emergencies

Triage is the broadly endorsed approach for responding to medical emergencies. It is the approach that was immediately adopted by health-care workers on September 11, 2001 for dealing with the medical needs that were expected once the Twin Towers of the World Trade Center collapsed, and its appropriateness has not been challenged in any of the subsequent literature. Triage is the public health model for responding to domestic medical emergencies that requires health-care professionals to make judgments about the likely survival of patients who need medical treatment. Recognizing that some people have urgent needs (i.e., they will die or suffer significant harm if not treated very soon) and that the resources available are scarce (e.g., supplies, facilities, trained personnel), patients are sorted into three groups and they are either treated, put aside, or asked to wait according to their group classification. Those who are not likely to survive are deprived of treatment so that the available resources can be used to save the lives of those who are more likely to live. Those who are likely to die without treatment but who are likely to live if treated promptly are treated first. Those who are in need of treatment but who can wait longer without dying are treated after those who are urgently ill. On the morning of 9/11, the disaster plan that had previously been developed and practiced was implemented at hospitals in the New York vicinity. Many beds in intensive care units (ICUs) were emptied. Elective surgery was canceled. Patients who could have been sent home were discharged. Collection activities in blood banks went into high gear, but they were only accepting type O− donors.

In medical emergencies, health-care professionals deliberately disregard the concepts of giving everyone a fair equal opportunity to receive medical treatment, and they also pointedly ignore relative differences in economic and social standing. Instead, they focus exclusively on the medical factors of urgency of need and the likelihood of survival. No one presumes to measure whether or not each patient has previously received a fair or equal share of available resources, and no one stops to assess who has been more or less advantaged. No one sorts out the small differences between individuals that would provide somewhat greater utility from one allocation rather than another. And no one criticizes medicine for not attending to those differences (Rhodes, 2001). (I have argued generally that physicians have a role-related responsibility to avoid making judgments about patients' worthiness and that they must treat all patients similarly based on medical considerations.) In fact, the long tradition of medical ethics, dating back at least to the Hippocratic tradition, requires physicians to provide treatment based on need. Hence the ethics of medicine appears to require physicians to commit themselves to unequal treatment (since need is unequal) and also to the nonjudgmental regard of each patient's worthiness.

Research and Public Health

Biomedical research and public health policies typically focus on populations. Biomedical research attempts to disconfirm hypotheses about predicted outcomes and thereby to develop facts about the response of organisms with certain common characteristics. With respect to human-subject research, groups of people are selected for study because of some relevant biological or environmental similarities. Any knowledge gained from the process is useful to the extent that it is applicable to all of those who share the common condition.

Public health policies are also designed to have an impact on all, and only, those individuals who are similarly impacted by a disease or a health-related condition. In deliberately focusing on one affected group or another, biomedical research and public health policies typically provide benefits only to the target group. The goals of biomedical research and public health are pointedly directed at everyone in the group that might benefit from them. By looking back at outcomes, researchers attempt to develop knowledge about biological or psychological reactions. By looking toward the future, public health officials attempt to develop a generalizable approach to the prevention, reduction, or treatment of biological or psychological problems. (Although a subject for biomedical research may disproportionately affect a relatively disadvantaged population (e.g., the effect of lead paint on child development), the study findings and the subsequent public health policies will have implications for all of those who have been or who may be affected.) As with medical triage in the emergency setting, biomedical research and public health have not been criticized for holding to these agendas.

Because ideas about justice and medicine are typically discussed singly, in artificially isolated contexts and with a focus on carefully selected examples, it is hard to notice when and how their underlying conceptions clash. Yet, the broad consensus on emergency triage, public health research, and public health policy provide an occasion to consider justice across a broad spectrum of medical contexts. These examples also challenge the assumption that a consensus supports a single principle of justice in medicine and public health. As Ronald Green has noted in his criticism of Daniels, the "mistake ... is trying to decide such matters by reference to a single consideration – and not necessarily the most important one" (Green, 2001).

Consequentialist considerations of efficacy and equality support well-accepted views on emergency triage. When the time constraints of an emergency and the needs for medical resources significantly outstrip the available resources, responses should be based on efficacy and treating all with similar medical needs similarly. The sweeping exclusions of triage represent the goal of avoiding the worst outcome more than the utilitarian aim of maximizing the greatest utility, particularly when utility might require fine-grained sorting and ranking. Triage, therefore, is not entirely compatible with utilitarianism, nor is it consistent with either fair equality of opportunity or prioritarianism. These different principles (avoid the worst outcome, maximize utility, fair equality of opportunity, and prioritarianism) cannot all be appropriate for guiding the same allocation decisions.

The intuitions supporting the view that priority should be given to equalizing social opportunities or to providing the greatest benefit to the least advantaged are undermined by the strong sense that nonmedical relative differences should not come into play in decisions about emergency responses. This invites questions about the appropriate framework for policy decisions about public health needs and setting the research agenda. Emergency triage allocates resources by taking everyone's prognosis and expected outcome into account. Individuals certainly get unequal lots and no priority is allowed to those who are more generally worse off.

Similarly, public health research sometimes has no impact on the social participation, health, or longevity of the entire population. If it turns out that we never have another disaster similar to what occurred on September 11th, if we never again experience a catastrophe that creates enormous amounts of pulverized concrete and incinerated computers and office furniture, research on their effects may never promote the social participation or health of anyone. Or, if the burdens of the interventions that the studies support turn out to be prohibitively costly (e.g., give up skyscrapers and computers), they will not be adopted and no one's fair equality of opportunity will be advanced. Public health research involves a quest for information that may or may not be useful. It also sometimes directs resources to the needs of the relatively few affected individuals. So, the standards of promoting fair equality of opportunity or maximizing health may not quite fit. If fair equality of opportunity was the only consideration to be taken into account, many other uses of resources would always have preference over public health research. Yet, the consensus in favor of such research suggests that other reasons support its broad endorsement.

Furthermore, while public health policies sometimes meet the standard of promoting utility, or fair equality of opportunity, or priority for the worse off, sometimes they do not. In sum, broadly endorsed public health policies suggest that emergency triage, public health research, and public health policy rely on more than a single principle of justice.

A Lesson from Experience

The incongruity between policy consensus on the one hand and lauded principles of justice on the other suggests that there is a mistake in our search for 'the' ruling principle of justice. It also suggests an alternative for looking at the problem of justice. When we stop to examine our own thinking about these issues, we notice that we actually invoke different reasons to support different principles and different rankings of considerations in different contexts. That insight suggests that there is no obvious reason to presume that a single principle defines justice. With sensitivity to the complexity of human values and to the different contexts of medical and public health policies, we can appreciate that a variety of reasons justify public health resource allocations. Even though such a contextual approach to determining the just distribution of resources will sometimes favor one principle and at other times rely upon another, decisions can express a widely shared view about the primacy of one consideration over another and reflect reasons that no one can reasonably reject. In this sense, a contextual view of justice is not random and not idiosyncratically subjective. Rather, it expresses deep similarities in human concerns and shared priorities that relate to our human mortality and vulnerability.

The Flu Vaccine Shortage and Hurricane Katrina

Before enumerating a list of principles of justice for guiding public health allocations, consider the flu vaccine shortage in the fall of 2004 and Hurricane Katrina in the fall of 2005. In 2004, people recognized that it was important to find a better way to allocate the limited supply of flu vaccine than to allow it to go to those with good connections, the aggressive, and the lucky. Communities and then the U.S. Centers for Disease Control promulgated distribution policies that allotted the vaccine to those who were likely to die or suffer serious harm if they contracted the disease, and then they implemented schemes to restrict distribution accordingly. The supply was therefore directed to the immunocompromised, the very young, pregnant women, the elderly, and health-care providers who would be called upon to treat affected individuals.

These policies were very broadly endorsed and achieved excellent compliance. The almost total absence of debate over their implementation was evidence of the extent of the consensus. Aside from the advocates for children and the elderly who each argued that their constituent group should have even more priority over others in the vaccine target group, the U.S. population accepted the plans that were implemented.

The principle supporting the flu vaccine allocation was not utilitarian because utility alone would have disqualified those with only a short remaining life span because vaccination for the elderly and the immunocompromised could be expected to provide a low QALY payoff. Neither did the policy consider previous injustices or disadvantages in the allocation so as to give priority to the least well off, nor did it try to equalize opportunities in some wider sense. The principle inherent in the vaccine distribution policy was avoid the worst outcome, that is, avoid the most deaths and serious illnesses. The consensus of support and the lack of opposition speaks to how the importance of one particular goal can be apparent.

Reaction to what happened before, during, and after Hurricane Katrina illustrates a broad consensus at the other end of the spectrum. In the case of Katrina, there was general agreement that the U.S. government had failed to adequately prepare for the disaster, failed to warn and protect Gulf Coast residents, failed in its attempts at rescue and meeting the tremendous needs of affected communities in the aftermath, and failed in providing honest and timely communication about the formaldehyde risk of the trailers later provided to shelter some of those left homeless. These realizations point us to further broad agreement on the importance of investment in disaster preparedness, of meeting the urgent needs of all citizens, of making leadership appointments based on qualifications rather than cronyism and politics, of timely and honest communication. Again, this consensus on values is not a matter of chance coincidence, it reflects the central importance of key human concerns.

Justice in Allocations for Public Health

We all are vulnerable to death, pain, illness, and disability, and we all want to avoid those consequences for ourselves and our loved ones. We also all have to acknowledge that there are not enough resources to provide for all of the public health projects that we would like. Hence, we recognize the necessity of prioritizing our values and sacrificing some of what we would like to have so that we can be more likely to secure those things that are more important to us. Because the achievement of certain goals is essential to our enjoying others, because certain hardships are more enduring and painful than others, and because this is so for almost everyone almost always, people tend to agree on the primacy of some important concerns. These features of our shared human nature make the concordance on some matters of public health not contingent and coincidental, but a genuine agreement expressing the human importance of some feature of a situation. This natural consensus provides us with an array of principles of justice that are relevant to any consideration of justice and public health (see **Table 1**).

Triage may be the appropriate guiding conception of justice for policies that respond to large-scale emergency situations. The justification for triage is that it is the policy most likely to avoid the worst outcome and to save the greatest number of lives. Reasonable people would want to survive a disaster and they would want their loved ones to survive. Foregoing treatment for those who are least likely to survive so as to provide the best chance of survival to the most people yields the result that everyone wants most. (In this analysis I am drawing freely on T.M. Scanlon's conception of justice (Scanlon, 1998)). So long as the same criteria for treatment are applied to everyone, the loved ones of those from whom treatment is withheld should not complain of injustice. Because hypothetical consent to triage policies can be legitimately presumed, a triage allocation of emergency services is not likely to undermine social stability.

Disaster preparedness requires the allocation of communal resources for research, training, and equipment. Policies to allocate resources for preparedness and research are justified because the ability to respond efficiently could crucially depend on preparedness and the information learned from studies. The goods that can be had would not be available without the prior contribution from a common pool. Hence, it is reasonable to provide some resources for preparedness and research to increase the chance for a good outcome and to minimize the chance for the worst outcome (i.e., maximin).

In the face of a credible risk of biological warfare, mandatory inoculation against a serious contagious disease is an appropriate policy when a reasonably safe and effective vaccine is available. Reasonable people would endorse such required inoculation because it provides protection from the disease, that is, it provides a public good that everyone values. Everyone should, therefore, bear a fair share of the burden of safety. Those who might refuse to

Table 1 Justifications for public health policies and allocations

Principles of justice	Examples of public health policies
Avoid free-riders	Mandatory inoculation and quarantine; Safe disposition of corpses
Avoid undue burdens	Inoculation exemption; Environmental protection
Avoid worst outcomes	Medical triage; Danger alert
Advance the worst off	Education; Clean air, clean water, and sewage treatment
Promote efficacy	Access to health care; Clean air, clean water, and sewage treatment
Promote equality	Access to health care; Disaster relief
Maximin	Disaster preparedness; Epidemiological screening and research
Preserve trust	Honest and timely disclosure; Qualified leadership
Provide public goods	Education; Health research
Provide services of vital importance to well-being	Provide primary goods (shelter, food, clothing); Dispense safe and effective vaccines

comply would be free-riders, ready to treat others unjustly by taking advantage of their good will and sense of communal responsibility. Public health measures are similarly justified by the public good of protection against disease that they provide and by the anti free-rider principle that would prohibit unsafe practices. And when it comes to actually dispensing vaccine in the face of a credible risk, because the relative differences between individuals may not be significant enough to be taken into account, a distribution scheme based on equality, such as a lottery or first come first serve, may be required.

Furthermore, with respect to public health measures like vaccination, there may be good reasons for allowing a few to be exempt. Those who are especially vulnerable to the inherent dangers of immunization – for example, those with impaired immune systems – would bear more than the typical burden of being vaccinated. If everyone else in the society was inoculated, exempting those few who would otherwise bear an undue burden, would not increase the risk for others.

The public health concerns after September 11th and Hurricane Katrina reflect three slightly different principles. Clean air, clean water, and sewage treatment are the kinds of public goods that everyone needs constantly. Their vital and constant importance to everyone's well-being is a justification for policies to provide and protect them. In many settings, clean air, clean water, and sewage treatment are also the kinds of benefits that no one can have unless everyone has them, and making them available or unavailable at all makes them available or unavailable to everyone in the society. In many situations, these are also services that can be provided with greatest efficacy by providing them for everyone.

Another important consideration is also relevant to the endorsement of public health interventions that provide for everyone's vital and constant needs. Such interventions are likely to make the greatest difference in health and well-being for the economically and socially least advantaged. The well-to-do could leave town for the clean air of the country or simply purchase gas masks to protect themselves from air pollution. They would also have the wherewithal to purchase bottled water, to dig private wells, and to install private sewage systems. The well-to-do would be better off with the general availability of clean air, clean water, and sewage treatment. Yet, the underlying interrelation between poverty and disease and the consequent disparity between the well-to-do and the poor with respect to health status and life expectancy (Daniels, 2002; Sheehan, 2002; Smith, 2002) suggest that the economically and socially disadvantaged would enjoy an even greater benefit from policies that made these benefits generally available. Furthermore, the continuous lack of such basic goods as clean air, clean water, and sewage treatment for some, while others enjoy them as private resources, could promote social instability. The difference principle is, therefore, an additional reason for adopting public health measures to provide these services.

It justifies the same policies that would be supported by the vital importance of the services and the fact that such services are most feasibly supplied to all at once (i.e., efficacy). This example, therefore, illustrates how different principles can be just and converge in support of public health policies.

Overview

To the extent that policy domains covered by different principles can be legitimately distinguished, a variety of appropriate and compelling principles can express the complex and varied considerations that make different policies just. The just allocation of medical and public health resources is and should be governed by a variety of considerations that reasonable people endorse for their saliency.

Several principles of justice have a legitimate place in medical and public health allocation, and the just solution to practical problems in public health should be guided by meeting mutually supported and compelling concerns. The principles of justice include: the anti free-rider principle, avoid undue burdens, avoid the worst outcome, the difference principle, efficacy, equality, maximin, provide public goods, and the vital and constant importance to well-being. (I do not claim that this list is a full elaboration of the relevant considerations for justice in medicine and public health.) To the extent that the scarcity of resources makes it impossible to fulfill all of the legitimate claims for a society's allocation of resources, some principle(s) will have to be sacrificed and some projects that are supported by compelling reasons will have to be scaled down from an ideal level, delayed, or abandoned. When these hard choices have to be made, they too should be made for good reasons that reasonable people would support. Daniels's relevance condition appears to capture this aspect of policy setting (Daniels, 2002: 16). In making difficult choices about the ranking of projects and priorities and the design of policies, different considerations will have different levels of importance in different kinds of situations. There is no obvious reason to presume that one priority will always trump the others. When the priority of a principle reflects the endorsement of an overlapping consensus of reasonable people, the justice of the policy is clear. When large groups of people rank the competing considerations differently, a significant consensus on the principles that are irrelevant may emerge and that consensus can serve as the basis for just policy. To the extent that flexibility can be supported by the available resources, policies should show tolerance for different priorities.

As a general caution, however, public health policy makers need to be alert to the kinds of illegitimate considerations that can distort and pervert any policy. Common psychological tendencies can interfere with judgment. For example, human psychology inclines people to exaggerate the impact of a loss and also inclines people to underappreciate the value of future goods. Prejudice, stereotyping, the desire to do something, pressing needs made vivid by individual cases, lack of insight, and lack of foresight are other common psychological inclinations that can distort judgment and lead to unjust public health policies. Furthermore, politics and personal gain may be motivating elements, but they do not promote reasonable public health policy. And then there is greed, which can be camouflaged under seemingly acceptable justifications.

Our recent experience has also taught us lessons about communication and trust and their importance in the design and implementation of just public health policies. After the fall of the World Trade Center Twin Towers, public health officials from the Environmental Protection Agency and government representatives failed to honestly communicate about the danger and misled the public about the air quality and the need for protection from the toxic environment. Today, thousands of people who worked at the site are ill and dying, at least in part because of the failures to provide full and honest disclosure (DePalm, 2006, 2007). Apparently, those who made the decisions to withhold information and to promulgate false reports were more concerned with promoting political ends than with promoting the goal of safety – a truly central human value. Similarly false and misleading reports before, during, and after Hurricane Katrina cost lives and exaggerated the tragedy for many. These inaccurate and misleading communications undermined trust in government, in public health pronouncements, and in public health policy. When people believe that they are being deceived and that the reasons for policies are personal or political advantage rather than the public good, they are less inclined to accept the pronouncements and cooperate with the policy.

In contrast, the honest communication about the flu vaccine shortage, the clear communication about justification for the policies that governed vaccine distribution, and the efforts to communicate crucial information about distribution to the public, all contributed to cooperation with the policy and the success it achieved in avoiding deaths and serious illness. These examples highlight the need for full and honest communication and education about matters of public health and their importance in promoting justice.

Conclusion

In sum, it is difficult to achieve justice in public health policy because there is neither a single ideal governing principle nor a simple formula for success. A variety of considerations can legitimately support good policy. For public health policies to be just, the description of the situations they aim to address must be accurate and the reasons behind them must be the ones that reasonable people would find most compelling and most appropriate. Policies must reflect the choices that reasonable people would make and the priorities that reasonable people find most pressing.

See also: Corruption and the Consequences for Public Health; Demand and Supply of Human Resources for Health; Health Finance, Equity in; Resource Allocation: International Perspectives on Resource Allocation.

Citations

Brock DW (1998) Aggregating costs and benefits. *Philosophy and Phenomenological Research* 58: 963–968.
Brock DW (2002) Priority to the worse off in health-care resource prioritization. In: Rhodes R, Battin MP and Silvers A (eds.) *Medicine and Social Justice: Essays on the Distribution of Health Care*, pp. 362–372. New York: Oxford University Press.
Daniels N (2002) Justice health, and health care. In: Rhodes R, Battin MP and Silvers A (eds.) *Medicine and Social Justice: Essays on the Distribution of Health Care*, pp. 6–23. New York: Oxford University Press.
DePalm A (2006) Illness persisting in 9/11 workers, big study finds. *The New York Times,* September 6.
DePalm A (2007) As a way to pay victims of 9/11, insurance fund is problematic. *The New York Times,* February 15.
Green RM (2001) Access to healthcare: Going beyond fair equality of opportunity. *American Journal of Bioethics* 1(2): 22–23.
Kamm FM (1993) *Morality, Mortality, Vol I: Death and Who to Save from It.* New York: Oxford University Press.
Kamm FM (2002) Whether to discontinue nonfutile use of a scarce resource. In: Rhodes R, Battin MP and Silvers A (eds.) *Medicine and Social Justice: Essays on the Distribution of Health Care*, pp. 373–389. New York: Oxford University Press.
Rawls J (1971) *A Theory of Justice.* Cambridge, MA: Harvard University Press.
Rawls J (1993) *Political Liberalism.* New York: Columbia University Press.
Rhodes R (2001) Understanding the trusted doctor and constructing a theory of bioethics. *Theoretical Medicine and Bioethics* 22(6): 493–504.
Scanlon TM (1998) *What We Owe to Each Other.* Cambridge, MA: The Belknap Press of Harvard University Press.
Sheehan M and Sheehan P (2002) Justice and the social reality of health: the case of Australia. In: Rhodes R, Battin MP and Silvers A (eds.) *Medicine and Social Justice: Essays on the Distribution of Health Care*, pp. 169–182. New York: Oxford University Press.
Smith P (2002) Justice, health, and the price of poverty. In: Rhodes R, Battin MP and Silvers A (eds.) *Medicine and Social Justice: Essays on the Distribution of Health Care*, pp. 301–318. New York: Oxford University Press.
Wasserman D (2002) Aggregation and the moral relevance of context in health-care decision making. In: Rhodes R, Battin MP and Silvers A (eds.) *Medicine and Social Justice: Essays on the Distribution of Health Care,* ch. 5 New York: Oxford University Press.

Further Reading

Aristotle (1971) *The Nichochean Ethics of Aristotle,* David Ross W (trans.). London: Oxford University Press.
Bentham J (1982) *An Introduction to the Principles of Morals and Legislation.* Burns JHL, Hart HLA (eds.) London: Methuen.
Boylan M (ed.) (2004) *Public Health Policy and Ethics, Vol. 19.* Amsterdam the Netherlands: Kluwer Academic Publishers.

Brock DW (1998) Aggregating costs and benefits. *Philosophy and Phenomenological Research* 58: 963–968.

Daniels N and Sabin JE (1997) Limits to health care: Fair procedures, democratic deliberation, and the legitimacy problem for insurers. *Philosophy and Public Affairs* 26: 303–350.

Mill JS (1979) *Utilitarianism*. Sher G (ed.) Indianapolis, IN: Hacket Publishiing.

Rhodes R, Battin MP and Silvers A (eds.) (2002) *Medicine and Social Justice: Essays on the Distribution of Health Care.* New York: Oxford University Press.

Human Rights Approach to Public Health Policy

D Tarantola, School of Public Health and Community Medicine, Sydney, NSW, Australia
S Gruskin, Harvard School of Public Health, Boston, MA, USA

© 2008 Elsevier Inc. All rights reserved.

Introduction

The origin and justification for human rights, whether anchored in natural law, positive law, or other theories and approaches laid out by various authors, as well as their cultural specificity and actual value as international legal commitments, remains subject to ongoing lively debate. Theoretical and rhetorical discourses continue to challenge and enrich current understanding of the relevance of human rights for policy and governance. Nonetheless, human rights have found their way into public health and play today an increasing role in the shaping of health policies, programs, and practice.

Health and human rights are not distinct but intertwined aspirations. Viewed as a universal aspiration, the notion of health as the attainment of physical, mental, and social well-being implies its dependency on and contribution to the realization of all human rights. From the same perspective, the enjoyment by everyone of the highest attainable standard of physical and mental health is in itself a recognized human right. From a global normative perspective, health and human rights are closely intertwined in many international treaties and declarations supported by mechanisms of monitoring and accountability (even as their effectiveness can be questioned) that draw from both fields.

With respect to health specifically, it is arguably viewed as an important prerequisite for and desirable outcome of human development and progress. Health is

> ...directly constitutive of the person's wellbeing and it enables a person to function as an agent – that is, to pursue the various goals and projects in life that she has reason to value. (Anand, 2004: 17–18)

Health is also the most extensively measured component of well-being; it benefits from dedicated services and is commonly seen as a *sine-qua-non* for the fulfillment of all other aspirations. It may also be... "a marker, a way of keeping score of how well the society is doing in delivering well-being" (Marmot, 2004: 37).

Health and human rights individually occupy privileged places in the public discourse, political debates, public policy, and the media, and both are at the top of human aspirations. There is hardly a proposed political agenda that does not refer to health in its own right, as well as justice, security, housing, education, and employment opportunities – all with relevance to health. These aspirations are often not framed as human rights but the fact that they are contained in human rights treaties and often translated into national constitutions and legislations provides legal support for efforts in these areas.

Incorporating human rights in public health policy therefore responds to the demands of people, policy makers, and political leaders for outcomes that meet public aspirations. It also creates opportunities for helping decipher how all human rights and other determinants of well-being and social progress interact. It allows progress toward these goals to be measured and shapes policy directions and agendas for action.

This article highlights the evolution that has brought human rights and health together in mutually reinforcing ways. It draws from the experience gained in the global response to HIV/AIDS, summarizes key dimensions of public health and of human rights and suggests a manner in which these dimensions intersect that may be used as a framework for health policy analysis, development, and evaluation.

Human Rights as Governmental Obligations

Human rights constitute a set of normative principles and standards which, as a philosophical concept can be traced back to antiquity, with mounting interest among intellectuals and political leaders since the seventeenth century (Tomushat, 2003). The atrocities perpetrated during World War II gave rise, in 1948, to the Universal Declaration of Human Rights (United Nations, 1948) and later to a series of treaties and conventions that extended the aspirational nature of the UDHR into instruments that would be binding on states under international human rights law. Among these are the International Covenant on Civil and Political Rights (ICCPR) and the International Covenant on Economic, Social, and Cultural Rights (ICESCR), both of which came into force in 1976.

Human rights are legal claims that persons have on governments simply on the basis of their being human. They are "what governments can do to you, cannot do to you and should do for you" (Gruskin, 2004). Even though people hold their human rights throughout their lives, they are nonetheless often constrained in their ability to fully realize them. Those who are most vulnerable to violations or neglect of their rights are also often those who lack sufficient power to claim the impact of the lack of enjoyment of their rights on their well-being, including their state of personal health. Human rights are intended to be inalienable (individuals cannot lose these rights any more than they can cease being human beings); they are indivisible (individuals cannot be denied a right because it is deemed less important or nonessential); they are interdependent (all human rights are part of a complementary framework, one right impacting on and being impacted by all others) (United Nations, 1993). They bring into focus the relationship between the State – the first-line provider and protector of human rights – and individuals who hold their human rights simply for being human. In this regard, governments have three sets of obligations toward their people (Eide, 1995):

- They have the obligation to respect human rights, which requires governments to refrain from interfering directly or indirectly with the enjoyment of human rights. In practice, no health policy, practice, program, or legal measure should violate human rights. Policies should ensure the provision of health services to all population groups on the basis of equality and freedom from discrimination, paying particular attention to vulnerable and marginalized groups.
- They have the obligation to protect human rights, which requires governments to take measures that prevent non-state actors from interfering with human rights, and to provide legal means of redress that people know about and can access. This relates to such important non-state actors as private health-care providers, pharmaceutical companies, health insurance companies and, more generally, the health-related industry, but also national and multinational enterprises whose actions can impact significantly on lifestyle, labor, and the environment such as oil and other energy-producing companies, car manufacturers, agriculture, food industry, and labor-intensive garment factories.
- They have the obligation to fulfill human rights, which requires States to adopt appropriate legislative, administrative, budgetary, judicial, promotional, and other measures toward the full realization of human rights, including putting into place appropriate health and health-related policies that ensure human rights promotion and protection. In practice, governments should be supported in their efforts to develop and apply these measures and monitor their impact, with an immediate focus on vulnerable and marginalized groups.

Government responsibility for health exists in several ways. The right to the highest attainable standard of health appears in one form or another in most international and regional human rights documents, and equally importantly, nearly every article of every document can be understood to have clear implications for health.

The Right to Health

The right to the highest attainable standard of health builds on, but is by no means limited to, Article 12 of the ICESCR (**Table 1**). Rights relating to autonomy, information, education, food and nutrition, association, equality, participation, and nondiscrimination are integral and indivisible parts of the achievement of the highest attainable standard of health, just as the enjoyment of the right to health is inseparable from all other rights, whether they are categorized as civil and political, economic, social, or cultural. This recognition is based on empirical observation and on a growing body of evidence that establishes the impact that lack of fulfillment of any and all of these rights has on people's health status: Education, nondiscrimination, food and nutrition epitomizing

Table 1 The right to highest attainable standard of health, Article 12 of the International Covenant on Economic, Social and Cultural Rights

1. The States Parties to the present Covenant recognize the right of everyone to the enjoyment of the highest attainable standard of physical and mental health
2. The steps to be taken by the States Parties to the present Covenant to achieve the full realization of this right shall include those necessary for:
    a. The provision for the reduction of the stillbirth rate and of infant mortality and for the healthy development of the child
    b. The improvement of all aspects of environmental and industrial hygiene
    c. The prevention, treatment, and control of epidemic, endemic, occupational and other diseases
    d. The creation of conditions which would assure to all medical service and medical attention in the event of sickness

From United Nations (1966a) *Article 2, International Covenant on Economic, Social and Cultural Rights*. United Nations General Assembly Resolution 2200A [XX1], 16/12/1966, entered into force 03/01/1976 in accordance with Art 17. New York: United Nations.

this relationship (Gruskin and Tarantola, 2001). Conversely, ill-health constrains the fulfillment of all rights as the capacity of individuals to claim and enjoy all their human rights depends on their physical, mental, and social well-being.

The right to health does not mean the right to be healthy as such, but the obligation on the part of the government to create the conditions necessary for individuals to achieve their optimal health status. In addition to the ICESCR, the right to health is further elaborated in CERD (Convention on the Elimination of all forms of Racial Discrimination, 1965); in CEDAW (Convention on the Elimination of all forms of Discrimination against Women, 1979), and CRC (Convention on the Rights of the Child art 24 1989) and in a range of regional human rights documents.

In May 2000, the United Nations Committee on Economic, Social, and Cultural Rights adopted a General Comment further clarifying the substance of government obligations relating to the right to health (UN Committee on Economic, Social and Cultural Rights, 2000). In addition to clarifying governmental responsibility for policies, programs and practices impacting the underlying conditions necessary for health, it sets out requirements related to the delivery of health services including their availability, acceptability, accessibility, and quality. It lays out directions for the practical application of Article 12 and proposes a monitoring framework. Reflecting the mounting interest in determining international policy focused on the right to health, the UN Commission on Human Rights appointed in 2002 a Special Rapporteur whose mandate concerns the right of everyone to the enjoyment of the highest attainable standard of physical and mental health. The Special Rapporteur's role is to undertake country visits, transmit communications to states on alleged violations of the right to health, and submit annual reports to the Commission and the UN General Assembly. Accordingly, through publication review and country visits, the Special Rapporteur has explored policies and programs related to such issues as maternal mortality, neglected medicines, and reproductive health as they connect to human rights (Hunt, 2007).

All international human rights treaties and conventions contain provisions relevant to health as defined in the preamble of the Constitution of the World Health Organization (WHO), repeated in many subsequent documents and currently adopted by the 191 WHO Member States: Health is a "state of complete physical, mental, and social well-being, and not merely the absence of disease or infirmity." The Constitution further stipulates that "The enjoyment of the highest attainable standard of health is one of the fundamental rights of every human being without distinction of race, political belief, economic or social condition." The Constitution was adopted by the International Health Conference held in New York from 19 June to 22 July 1946, signed on 22 July 1946 by the representatives of 61 States (World Health Organization, 1946), and entered into force on 7 April 1948. Amendments adopted by the Twenty-sixth, Twenty-ninth, Thirty-ninth and Fifty-first World Health Assemblies (resolutions WHA26.37, WHA29.38, WHA39.6 and WHA51.23) came into force on 3 February 1977, 20 January 1984, 11 July 1994 and 15 September 2005, respectively, and are incorporated in the present text.

The Emergence of a New Public Health

The focus of public health from its inception in the eighteenth century through the mid-1970s remained on combating disease and some of its most blatant social, environmental, and occupational causes. The state acted as a benevolent provider of services and the source of policies, laws, regulations, and practices generally based on the disease prevention and control model emphasizing risk- and impact-reduction strategies through immunization, case finding, treatment, and changes in domestic, environmental, and occupational hygiene.

In 1978, the Alma Ata conference solidified a new international health agenda (Litsios, 2002). The aim of achieving Health for All by the Year 2000 was put forward, and this was to be achieved through a Primary Health Care (PHC) approach. Invoking the human right to the highest attainable standard of health, the Declaration of Alma Ata called on nations to ensure the availability of the essentials of primary health care, including education concerning health conditions and the methods for preventing and controlling them; promotion of food supply and proper nutrition; an adequate supply of safe water and basic sanitation; maternal and child health care, including family planning; immunization against major infectious diseases; prevention and control of locally endemic diseases; appropriate treatment of common disease and injuries; and provision of essential drugs (Declaration of Alma Ata, 1978).

The 1980s also witnessed the recognition that health was not merely determined by social and economic status but was dependent on dynamic social and economic determinants that could be acted upon through policy and structural changes. In 1986, the Ottawa Charter on Health Promotion helped sharpen the vision of the relationships between individual and collective health and its social, economic, and other determinants (Ottawa Charter for Health Promotion, 1986). The Charter spelled out the fundamental conditions and resources for health as peace, shelter, education, food, income, a stable ecosystem, sustainable resources, social justice, and equity. All of these prerequisites could have been framed as human rights. Probably to stay clear from political controversy that could have been divisive and best been addressed in a United Nations forum, however, the Charter did not explicitly bring human rights or state obligations into play.

The late 1980s and the 1990s saw growing attention being directed in the policy discourse to human rights and to their particular implications for health, and this resulted from several factors. First, the ICCPR and IESCR entered into force in 1976, and in the 1980s the UN Committees responsible for the monitoring of their implementation had begun to decipher their actual meaning and core contents, making the obligations of governments explicit and measurable. Second, the decay of the world geopolitical block ideologies of the late 1980s and the advent of economic neoliberalism created a space for alternate paradigms to help shape public policy and international relations. Human rights entered the scene of geopolitical reconstruction and became common parley after the Glasnost and the fall of the Berlin Wall, in 1989, regardless of whether in reality they were used or abused by new political leaders. Third, the connection between human rights and health was increasingly being shaped around focal causes in various social and political movements. This resulted in the creation of NGOs, some of which engaged in human rights work (responding to torture in particular), others in advocacy around reproductive health and rights issues, while others provided health assistance in armed conflicts and natural disasters, all with the intent of positively impacting on policy and practice. Fourth, and particularly important for the ways this contributed to the integration of human rights concepts into health policy, the emergence of AIDS in 1981, and the recognition of HIV as a global pandemic, resulted in a variety of human rights violations by those seeking to address this mounting public health problem. As traditional disease control policies that had marked the earlier history of public health were put in place by state authorities, with a few exceptions, community-based and advocacy organizations, supported by academic groups, voiced the necessity for policies that afforded greater protections for the rights of people living with or vulnerable to HIV.

Until this time, the focus of public health had generally been to promote the collective physical, mental, and social well-being of people, even if in order to achieve public health goals, policies had to be implemented that sacrificed individual choice, behavior, and action for the common good. This was, and continues to be, exemplified by the principles and practices that guide the control of such communicable diseases as tuberculosis, typhoid, or sexually transmitted infections, where quarantine or other restrictions of rights are imposed on affected individuals. In a number of instances, in particular where health policy addressed communicable diseases and mental illness, restrictions of such rights as privacy, free movement, autonomy, or bodily integrity have been imposed by public health authorities with the commendable intention to protect public health even without valid evidence of their intended public health benefit. The current resurgence of this issue in the context of systematic testing for HIV in health facilities or within entire populations, advocated by some in order to enhance the early access to care and treatment by people found infected, illustrates that disease control methods blind to human rights have by no means vanished. Insufficient attention has been devoted to assessing and monitoring the impact of such policies on the life of people whose rights were being restricted or denied, and to the negative consequences such impositions can have on their willingness to participate supportively in public health efforts that concern them. Public health abuses have also been exemplified by policies which result in the excessive institutionalization of people with physical or mental impairments where alternate care and support approaches have not been adequately considered. In the fields of disability and in mental health, in a number of countries national policies have been found to be discriminatory and, in the case of mental health, at times when carried out in practice to amount to inhuman and degrading treatment. And far from uncommon was – and remains – something often invisible to policy but invidious if not adequately addressed, discrimination in the health-care setting on the basis of health status, gender, race, color, language, religion, or social origin, or any other attribute that can influence the quality of services provided to individuals by or on behalf of the State.

HIV and Genesis of the Integration of Human Rights into Health Practice

Cognizant of the need to engage HIV-affected communities in the response to the fast-spreading epidemics in order to achieve their public health goals, human rights were understood as valuable by policy makers not for their moral or legal value but to open access to prevention and care for those who needed these services most, away from fear, discrimination and other forms of human rights violations, and as a way to ensure communities that needed to be reached did not go underground. The deprivation of such entitlements as access to health and social services, employment, or housing imposed on people living with HIV was understood to constrain their capacity to become active subjects rather than the objects of HIV programs, and this was recognized as unsound from a public health perspective.

The evolution of thinking about HIV/AIDS moved from the initial recognition of negative effects of human rights violations among people living with HIV to principles that guided the formulation of a global strategy on HIV/AIDS and, beyond, to the application of these principles to other health issues. In the decade that followed the emergence of AIDS, tremendous efforts were made to induce behavior change through policies that supported intensified, targeted prevention efforts. Everywhere, the initial approaches to HIV had been focused on the reduction of risk of acquiring HIV infection through policies that supported the creation of protective barriers: The use of condoms, early diagnosis and treatment of sexually transmitted infections, and reduction in the number of sexual partners. Some of these efforts were successful on a small scale, in particular where communities were educated and cohesive, as was the case for communities of gay men on the East and West Coasts of the United States, Western Europe, and Australia. Less immediately successful were interventions in communities under immediate social or economic stress and those hampered in their ability to confront HIV/AIDS as a result of strong cultural and other barriers. In sub-Saharan African countries, for example, early interventions related to condoms and other prevention methods, even when supported by national-level policy, were confronted with denial and rejection. Gender-related discrimination was often at the core of resistance to change. Stigma and discrimination directed toward people living with HIV or people whose behaviors were associated with a risk of acquiring and transmitting infection (sex workers, injecting drug users, as well as people defined by their racial or ethnic characteristics) also created obstacles to reaching those who, even perhaps more than others, needed open access to prevention and care. For these reasons, the protection of human rights and combating discrimination became important underlying principles of the first Global Strategy on HIV/AIDS formulated by WHO in 1987 (World Health Organization, 1987).

The risk-reduction strategies of the late 1980s confronted several obstacles in implementation. One was the practical difficulty of scaling up successful approaches to national or international levels. Another was the poor results achieved from applying models proven successful in some settings to different social and cultural environments: Clearly, one size did not fit all. Empirical evidence showed that even as the capacity of individuals to minimize or modulate their risk of exposure to HIV was closely related to specific behaviors or situations, these were in turn influenced by a variety of other factors. In 1992, a risk-vulnerability analysis and reduction model was put forward, positing that in order to successfully impact on risk-taking behaviors, it was necessary to recognize and act on factors that determined the likelihood of individuals engaging in such behaviors (Mann and Tarantola, 1992). A broader perspective suggesting the need for an expanded response to HIV began to emerge, bridging risk, as measured by the occurrence of HIV infection, to risk-taking behaviors, and to their vulnerability determinants. Vulnerability factors could be categorized for simpler analysis as individual (linked to personal history and status, agency, knowledge, or skills); societal (linked to social, economic, and cultural characteristics of the community within which people lived or had lived, including the policy and legal environment); and program-related (dependent on the capacity and approach of programs – health and social in particular) and the extent to which they responded appropriately to people's needs and expectations and assured their participation (Mann and Tarantola, 1996).

While the linkages between health outcomes and health determinants was already very present in the public health discourse, the mounting HIV epidemic made clear the need for policy to simultaneously address a wide and complex assembly of health outcome and determinants touching many facets of society. Simply listing these determinants born out of the established and empirical evidence was overwhelming. There was a need to categorize these determinants in a logical fashion and in a way that would allow them to be taken up by different sectors engaged in human development. The human rights framework was very well suited to this purpose in that it allowed vulnerability factors to be categorized as civil, political, social, economic, or cultural, and each of these factors, recognized through research or empirical evidence, could be easily linked to one or more specific human rights. This expanded approach helped clarify the related responsibilities of different sectors, thereby expanding the scope of public policy change and possible interventions. Importantly, these interventions could build on commitments already expressed, and obligations subscribed to, by governments under international human rights law. From an initial focus on nondiscrimination toward people known or assumed to live with HIV/AIDS, human rights was now helping guide the analysis of the roots, manifestations, and impacts of the HIV epidemics. Stemming from an instrumental approach rather than moral or legal principles, the response to HIV had exposed the congruence between sound public health policy and the upholding of human rights norms and standards (Mann et al., 1994).

The analytical and action-oriented risk and vulnerability framework that linked HIV to the neglect or violations of human rights and the call for needed structural and societal changes grounded in solid policy were important features of the 1994 Paris Summit Declaration on HIV/AIDS (UNAIDS, 1999) and later served as one of the founding principles of the 1996 UNAIDS global strategy and its subsequent revisions (UNAIDS, 1996). These ideas are also apparent in the Declaration of Commitment which emerged from the 2001 United Nations General Assembly.

International activism and a series of international political conferences that took place in this period facilitated similar changes in the approach taken to a wide range of diseases and health conditions, in particular with respect to reproductive and sexual health issues (Freedman, 1997). The 1994 Cairo International Conference on Population and Development was a watershed in recognizing the responsibility of governments worldwide to translate their international-level commitments into national laws, policies, programs, and practices that promote and do not hinder sexual and reproductive health among their populations. National laws and policies were thus open to scrutiny to determine both the positive and negative influences they could have on sexual and reproductive health programming, information, services, and choices. Human rights concerns, including legal, policy, and practice barriers that impact on the delivery and use of sexual and reproductive health services thereafter became a valid target for international attention.

Human Rights and Health Policy in the New Millennium: Key Concepts

As, from a theoretical perspective, the interaction between health and human rights was drawing increased attention from policy makers in an expanding array of health-related domains, two issues were and continue to be cited as creating obstacles to the translation of theory into practice. The first is that the realization of the right to health cannot be made real in view of the structures, services, and resources it requires. The second, often cited by those concerned with communicable disease control, is that the protection of human rights should not be the prime concern of policy makers when and where such public health threats as emerging epidemics call for the restriction of certain individual rights. As these two obstacles are often used and misused to question the validity of the health and human rights framework, they are discussed briefly below.

Progressive Realization of Health-Related Human Rights

In all countries, resource and other constraints can make it impossible for a government to fulfill all rights immediately and completely. The principle of progressive realization is fundamental to the achievement of human rights as they apply to health (United Nations, 1966a), and applies equally to resource-poor countries as to wealthier countries whose responsibilities extend not only to what they do within their own borders, but also their engagement in international assistance and cooperation (United Nations, 1966b).

Given that progress in health necessitates infrastructure and human and financial resources that may not match existing or future needs in any country, the principle of progressive realization takes into account the inability of governments to meet their obligations overnight. Yet, it creates an obligation on governments to set their own benchmarks, within the maximum of the resources available to them, and to show how and to what extent, through their policies and practices, they are achieving progress toward the health goals they have agreed to in international forums such as the World Health Assembly, as well as those they have set for themselves. In theory, States account for progress in health (or lack thereof) through a variety of mechanisms that include global monitoring mechanisms, as well as national State of the Health of the Nation reports or similar forms of domestic public reporting.

Human Rights Limitations in the Interest of Public Health

There remains a deeply rooted concern of many in the health community that application of a health and human rights approach to health policy will deprive the State from applying such measures as isolation or quarantine or travel restrictions when public health is at stake. Public health and care practitioners alike, acting on behalf of the State, are used to applying restrictions to individual freedom in cases where the enjoyment of these rights creates a real or perceived threat to the population at large. Recently, the SARS and Avian flu epidemics have demonstrated that such restrictions can also be applied globally under the revised International Health Regulations (IHR), the only binding agreement thus far under the auspices of WHO (World Health Organization, 2005). They stipulate that WHO can make recommendations on an *ad hoc*, time-limited, risk-specific basis, as a result of a public health emergency of international concern, and that implementation of these Regulations "shall be with full respect for the dignity, human rights and fundamental freedoms of persons." The human rights framework recognizes that these are situations where there can be legitimate and valid restriction of rights, and this under several circumstances relevant to the creation of health policies: Public emergencies and public health imperatives. Public emergencies stipulate that in time of a public emergency that threatens the life of the nation and the existence of which is officially proclaimed, the States Parties to the present Covenant may take measures derogating from their obligations under the present Covenant to the extent strictly required by the exigencies of the situation, provided that such measures are not inconsistent with their other obligations under international law and do not involve discrimination solely on the ground of race, color, sex, language, religion, or social origin (Art 49, ICCPR). Public health imperatives give governments the right to take the steps they deem necessary for the prevention, treatment, and control of epidemic, endemic, occupational, and other diseases (Art 16, ICCPR).

Public health may therefore justify the limitation of certain rights under certain circumstances. Policies that interfere with freedom of movement when instituting quarantine or isolation for a serious communicable disease – for example, Ebola fever, syphilis, typhoid, or untreated tuberculosis, more recently SARS and pandemic influenza – are examples of limitation of rights that may be necessary for the public good and therefore may be considered legitimate under international human rights law. Yet arbitrary restrictive measures taken or planned by public health authorities that fail to consider other valid alternatives may be found to be both abusive of human rights principles and in contradiction with public health best practice. The limitation of most rights in the interest of public health remains an option under both international human rights law and public health laws, but the decision to impose such limitations must be achieved through a structured and accountable process. Increasingly, such consultative processes are put in place by national authorities to debate over the approach taken to public health issues as they arise, such as in the case of immunization, disability, mental health, HIV, smoking, and more recently pandemic influenza preparedness.

Limitations on rights are considered a serious issue under international human rights law – as noted in specific provisions within international human treaties – regardless of the apparent importance of the public good involved. When a government limits the exercise or enjoyment of a right, this action must be taken only as a last resort and will only be considered legitimate if the following criteria are met:

1. The restriction is provided for and carried out in accordance with the law.
2. The restriction is in the interest of a legitimate objective of general interest.
3. The restriction is strictly necessary in a democratic society to achieve the objective.
4. There are no less intrusive and restrictive means available to reach the same goal.
5. The restriction is not imposed arbitrarily, i.e., in an unreasonable or otherwise discriminatory manner (United Nations, 1984).

The restriction of rights, if legitimate, is therefore consistent with human rights principles. Both principles of progressive realization and legitimate limitations of rights are directly relevant to public health policy as they can inform decisions on how to achieve the optimal balance between protecting the rights of the individual and the best interest of the community. Examples of the impact of human rights violations and protection on public health are set out below. Discrimination – a frequent, severe, and persistent issue confronted both in society and in the health-care setting – has been chosen to illustrate how public health can be hampered by the neglect of human rights and enhanced by their incorporation in public health policy.

Public Health Policy and Nondiscrimination

Discrimination can impact directly on the ways that morbidity, mortality, and disability – the burden of disease – are both measured and acted upon. In fact, the burden of disease itself discriminates: Disease, disability, and death are not distributed randomly or equally within populations, nor are their devastating effects within communities. Tuberculosis, for example, is exploding in disenfranchised communities, in particular among prison inmates and people already affected by HIV and subjected to dual discrimination both in their communities and in the health-care setting.

Far from uncommon, discrimination in health systems, including health centers, hospitals, or mental institutions, may further contribute to exacerbating disparities in health. A few examples of myriads that could be cited are named here. Undocumented migrant workers receive poor or no treatment for fear of having to justify their civil status. Documented migrant workers, refugees, and asylum seekers and their families may not avail themselves of services that have not been designed to suit their culture and respond to their specific needs. People with hemophilia have been given unsafe blood products on the premise that this adds only a marginal risk to their lives. People with physical or mental disabilities receive substandard care; they are unable to complain or if they do, they fare poorly in legal action (Moss et al., 2007). Discrimination in health systems concerns not only diseases that are already stigmatized, such as AIDS, hepatitis B and C, tuberculosis, and cancer, but also others, such as diabetes and cardiovascular diseases, which could be alleviated if equal treatment within societies and within health-care settings became the norm. A health and human rights approach to policy development concerning health systems requires that state authorities refrain from enacting discriminatory policies and provide information, education, training, and support to their staff toward eliminating discrimination in public health practice and within the workforce.

Discrimination can also be at the root of unsound human development policies and programs that may impact directly or indirectly on health. For example, an infrastructure development project may require the displacement of entire populations and fail to pay sufficient attention to the new environment to which these populations will have to adjust. In the developing world, when the health impact of large-scale development programs at the local level is considered, it is often from the perspective of the possible further spread of such infectious diseases as malaria and other waterborne diseases. The psychological capacity of displaced communities to relocate and rebuild new lives or the long-term physical and social consequences of such displacement are seldom factored into the equation.

The ongoing international movement toward poverty alleviation has emphasized the critical importance of health in the fight against poverty. The eight Millennium Development Goals (MDGs) – which set targets for 2015 to halve extreme poverty, halt the spread of HIV/AIDS, and improve health and education – have been agreed to by all the world's countries and all the world's leading development institutions (United Nations, 2005). Arguably, all MDGs have a linkage to health either by their direct bearing on health outcomes and the needed services (e.g., through efforts to reduce child and maternal mortality, HIV, malaria, and other diseases) or by underscoring principles central to public health policy (e.g., gender equality) or else by calling for the creation of policies addressing the underlying conditions for progress in health (e.g., education, environmental sustainability, and global partnerships).

Public Health Policy and the Value of Health and Human Rights

Human rights and public health policy intersect in a number of ways, which, for practical purposes, can be regrouped into three broad categories: The national and international context within which policy is developed; the outcome of public policy; and the process through which it is developed, applied, and monitored.

Context

A distinction exists between public policy affecting health (most of them do) and public health policy (often emerging from public health governmental authorities or on their initiative). Policies affecting health – for example, those related to gender, trade, intellectual property, the environment, migration, education, housing, or labor – are contingent upon national laws and international treaties or agreements which often overlook – by omission or commission – their potential health consequences. As the Health Impact Assessment of development and social policies gained credence in the 1990s, the development of a human rights assessment for the formulation and evaluation of public health policies emerged (Gostin and Mann, 1999). Health Impact Assessment (HIA), applying different methods, has become more frequently practiced to guide policy options both nationally and internationally. While the aim of such exercises is to forecast the health impact of a single or alternative policies or programs (including those related to infrastructure, financing, service delivery, transportation, or production and many others), the impact of such policies and programs on both health and human rights remains to be adequately tested. Much work is currently ongoing toward the development of a Health and Human Rights Impact Assessment for which assessment methods and health and human rights indicators are required.

An example where such an impact assessment might have been useful was when a number of countries – industrialized and developing alike – applied for membership of the World Trade Organization when such a membership implied for the signatory country to become party to the Agreement on Trade Related Aspects of Intellectual Property Rights (TRIPS). The constraints imposed by TRIPS on developing countries with regards to intellectual protection of pharmaceuticals in particular only became evident in the late 1990s as new, proven therapies for HIV-AIDS were reaching the international market. Civil society movements and some international organizations embarked on an active campaign to overcome the constraints set by TRIPS to the production or importation of generic medicines by developing countries needing them most. It was not until 2002, however, that WHO and WTO jointly produced a document on WTO agreements and public health (World Health Organization and World Trade Organization, 2002). In most developing countries, Ministries of Health had not been consulted, been equipped to assess, or had underestimated, the possible health impacts of the new trade and intellectual property agreement they were signing on to as new members of the WTO. This was and continues to be a painful reminder of the oversight or deliberate neglect of the possible health consequences of public policy guided by other agendas, international trade in this case.

Public health policy should seek the optimal synergy between health and human rights, building on the premise that the optimal quality of a public health policy is attained when the highest possible health outcome and the fullest realization of human rights are both attained. This requires a close interaction between public health professionals, human rights practitioners and representatives of affected communities. The response to HIV has been shaped by such an interaction with significant positive impact – at least in the short term – in such countries as Australia, Sweden, Thailand, Brazil, or Uganda. Where misconceptions about either sound public health or human rights have distorted HIV policies and programs, the epidemic has continued to strive, as illustrated by the situation in South Africa or China.

As it is generally formulated and monitored by the State, public health policy should operate in the context of the obligations the State has subscribed to under international human rights treaties and national law. Central to these obligations are those to respect, protect, and fulfill all human rights, including the rights to participate in public affairs and policy making, equality, nondiscrimination, and dignity.

Outcome and Impact

Both public health policy and human rights emphasize the importance of outcome and impact, crudely measured in public health terms by the reduction of mortality, morbidity and disability, and the improvement of quality of life, along with economic measurement enabling an assessment of the value for money of particular policies or programs that can guide priority setting. The extent to which outcome includes the fulfillment of human rights is seldom factored in. For example, one would like to see the value of policies that promote sex education in school measured not only in terms of reduction of teenage pregnancy or the incidence of sexually transmitted diseases, but how the right of the child to information is fulfilled in this way and how it impacts on further demands for other health-related, life-saving information. Likewise, when assessing the outcome and impact of policies that prioritize childhood immunization programs, one would want to know not only how immunization makes people healthier, both early and later in their childhood, but also how such public health policies will advance the right of the child to growth and development and her right to education by improving her attendance to and performance at school.

Measuring the outcome and impact of health and health-related policies from a combined health and human rights perspective implies measurement indicators that are neither fully developed nor tested. One of the constraints is that measuring health and human rights on the national, aggregate level is not sensitive to disparities that may exist within the nation, for example as a result of discrimination.

Process

The human rights to information, assembly, and participation in public affairs – including policy making – imply, among other practical steps, the engagement of communities in decisions affecting their health. As highlighted earlier, the history of health and human rights has amply established that community representation in decision-making bodies increases the quality and impact of public health measures. An important issue is to determine who can legitimately speak on behalf of concerned communities. In the last two decades, stimulated by the response to HIV in particular, nongovernmental organizations, and more broadly civil society, have played key roles in drawing attention to policies that were or could be detrimental to health (e.g., restrictions in access to medicines, denial of sex education of young people, access to harm reduction methods among substance users, promotion of tobacco products in young people, marginalized communities and low-income countries, environmental degradation, marketing of unhealthy foods). While state machineries are increasingly cognizant of the growing need for transparency in policy development, civil society is likely to sustain its contribution to such a process, and this through active monitoring by national-level NGOs and such international groups as Amnesty International, Human Rights Watch, or Physicians for Social Responsibility.

Conclusion

This article has attempted to lay out the principles underlying the application of health and human rights principles to public health policy, and it has done so by recalling the historical emergence of these concepts and the opportunities they provide for new approaches to policy development.

Health and human rights, together and independently from each other, have achieved today a degree of prominence in the political and public discourse never witnessed before. The fields of health and rights are illuminated today by their commonalties, no longer by their differences. Both are obligations of governments toward their people; and each supports and requires the fulfillment of the other.

Overall, health and human rights provide a framework for all aspects of policy and program development. In practice, human rights considerations are often built into public health policy through the application of what are today called rights-based approaches. The practical application of these principles is a subject of active and rich debates. Rights-based approaches to health are but some of the attempts currently being made to offer practical guidance to health policy makers and other stakeholders in health and human rights toward translating these principles into health policies, programs, and interventions. Through further reflection, practice and research, public health and human rights practitioners can further establish how and to what extent the promotion and protection of health and human rights interact. In the search for a world where the attainment of the highest standard of physical, mental, and social well-being necessitates, and reinforces, the dignity, autonomy, and progress of every human being, the broad goals of health and human rights are universal and eternal. They give us direction for our understanding of humanity and practical tools for use in our daily work.

See also: Global Health Initiatives and Public Health Policy; Health Policy: Overview; The State in Public Health, The Role of.

Citations

Anand S (2004) The concerns for equity in health. In: Anand S, Peter F and Sen A (eds.) *Public Health and Ethics*, pp. 17–18. Oxford, UK: Oxford University Press.

Anonymous (1978) Declaration of Alma Ata, International Conference of Primary Health Care. Alma Ata: USSR, 6–12 September 1978. http://www.who.int/hpr/NPH/docs/declaration_almaata.pdf (accessed December 2007).

Burris SC, Swanson JW, Moss K, Ullman MD, and Ranney LM (2006) *Justice Disparities: Does the ADA Enforcement System Treat People with Psychiatric Disabilities Fairly?* Maryland Law Review. http://ssrn.com/abstract=905118 (accessed March 2008).

Eide A (2001) Economic, social and cultural rights as human rights. In: Eide A, Krause C and Rosas E (eds.) *Economic, Social, and Cultural Rights: A Textbook*, pp. 9–28. The Hauge, The Netherlands: Kluwer Law International.

Freedman L (1997) Human rights and the politics of risk and blame: Lessons from the international reproductive health movement. *Journal of the American Medical Women's Association* 52(4): 165–168.

Gostin L and Mann J (1999) Toward the development of a human rights impact assessment for the formulation and evaluation of public health policies. In: Mann J, Gruskin S, Grodin M and Annas G (eds.) *Health and Human Rights: A Reader*, pp. 54–71. New York: Routledge.

Gruskin S (2004) Is there a government in the cockpit: A passenger's perspective or global public health: The role of human rights. *Temple Law Review* 77: 313–334.

Gruskin S and Tarantola D (2001) Health and human rights. In: Detels R, McEwen J, Beaglehole R and Tanaka H (eds.) *The Oxford Textbook of Public Health*, 4th edn. Oxford, UK: Oxford University Press.

Hunt P (2007) *Report of the Special Rapporteur on the Right of Everyone to the Enjoyment of the Highest Attainable Standard of Physical and Mental Health*. Human Rights Council 4th session, A/HRC/28, 17 January 2007. pp. 15–21.

Litsios S (2002) The long and difficult road to Alma-Ata: A personal reflection. *International Journal of Health Services* 32: 709–732.

Mann J and Tarantola D (1992) Assessing the vulnerability to HIV infection and AIDS. In: Mann J, Tarantola D and Netter T (eds.) *AIDS in the World*, pp. 557–602. Cambridge, MA: Harvard University Press.

Mann J and Tarantola D (1996) Societal vulnerability: Contextual analysis. In: Mann J and Tarantola D (eds.) *AIDS in the World II*, pp. 444–462. London: Oxford University Press.

Mann JM, Gostin L, Gruskin S, Brennan T, Lazzarini Z, and Fineberg H (1994) Health and human rights. *Health and Human Rights* 1(1): 58–80.

Marmot M (2004) Social causes of inequity in health. In: Anand S, Peter F and Sen A (eds.) *Public Health and Ethics*, p. 37. Oxford, UK: Oxford University Press.

Ottawa Charter for Health Promotion (1986) *First International Conference on Health Promotion: The Move Towards a New Public Health*. November 17–21, 1986, Ottawa, Ontario, Canada. WHO/HPR/HEP/95.1. http://www.who.int/hpr/NPH/docs/ottawa_charter_hp.pdf (accessed December 2007).

Tomuschat C (2003) *Human Rights, Between Idealism and Realism*. New York: Oxford University Press.

UNAIDS (1996) *Global Strategy, 1996/2001*. Geneva, Switzerland: United Nations Joint Programme on HIV AIDS.

UNAIDS (1999) *From Principle to Practice: Greater Involvement of People Living with or Affected by HIV/AIDS (GIPA) UNAIDS/99.43E*. http://data.unaids.org/Publications/IRC-pub01/JC252-GIPA-i_en.pdf (accessed December 2007).

United Nations (1948) *Universal Declaration of Human Rights. G.A. Res. 217A (III) UN GAOP, Res 71, UN Doc.A/810*. New York: United Nations.

United Nations (1966a) *Article 2, International Covenant on Economic, Social and Cultural Rights. United Nations General Assembly Resolution 2200A [XX1], 16/12/1966, entered into force 03/01/1976 in accordance with Art 17*. New York: United Nations.

United Nations (1966b) *Article 2, International Covenant on Civil and Political Rights. United Nations General Assembly Resolution 2200A [XX1], 16/12/1966, entered into force 23/03/1976 in accordance with Article 49*. New York: United Nations.

United Nations (1984) The Siracusa principles on the limitation and derogation provisions. In: *The International Covenant on Civil and Political Rights*. Annex to UN Document E/CN.4/1985/4 of 28/09/1984. New York: United Nations.

United Nations (1993) *Vienna Declaration and Programme of Action (A/CONF.157/23)*. http://www.unhchr.ch/huridocda/huridoca.nsf/(Symbol)/A.CONF.157.23.En (accessed December 2007).

United Nations (2001) *Declaration of Commitment on HIV/AIDS: Global Crisis-Global Action*. Resolution adopted by the General Assembly. United Nations. New York (A/S-26/L.2). http://www.un.org/ga/aids/docs/aress262.pdf (accessed December 2007).

United Nations (2005) *UN Millennium Project 2005. Investing in Development: A Practical Plan to Achieve the Millennium Development Goals*. New York: United Nations Development Programme.

United Nations Committee on Economic, Social and Cultural Rights (2000) *General Comment 14 on the Right to the Highest Attainable Standard of Health*. New York: United Nations.

World Health Organization (1946) *Constitution of the World Health Organization*. Off. Rec. Wld Hlth Org., 2, 100. Geneva, Switzerland: World Health Organization. http://www.who.int/governance/eb/who_constitution_en.pdf (accessed December 2007).

World Health Organization (1987) *The Global Strategy for AIDS Prevention and Control*. Geneva, Switzerland: World Health Organization; unpublished document SPA/INF/87.1.

World Health Organization (2005) *Revisions of the International Health Regulations*, endorsed by the Fifty-eighth World Health Assembly in Resolution 58.3. Geneva, Switzerland: World Health Assembly 23/05/2005.

World Health Organization (2006) *Constitution of the World Health Organization Basic Documents*. Forty-fifth edition. Supplement, October 2006. http://www.who.int/governance/eb/who_constitution_en.pdf (accessed December 2007).

World Health Organization and World Trade Organization (2002) *WTO Agreements and Pubic Health, a joint study by the WHO and the WTO Secretariat, World Health Organization and World Trade Organization*. Geneva, Switzerland: World Health Organization. http://www.wto.org/english/news_e/pres02_e/pr310_e.htm (accessed December 2007).

Further Reading

Lee K, Buse K, and Fustukian S (2002) *Health Policy in a Globalizing World*. Cambridge, UK: Cambridge University Press.

Mann JM, Gostin L, Gruskin S, Brennan T, Lazzarini Z, and Fineberg H (1994) Health and human rights. *Health and Human Rights* 1: 6–23.

World Health Organization (2002) *25 Questions and Answers on Health and Human Rights*. Health and Human Rights Publications, Issue No. 1. Geneva, Switzerland: World Health Organization.

Interest Groups and Civil Society, in Public Health Policy

N Mays, London School of Hygiene and Tropical Medicine, London, UK

© 2008 Elsevier Inc. All rights reserved.

Introduction: From Government to Governance

Put simply, public policy is 'what governments do and neglect to do' (Klein and Marmor, 2006: 890). To understand how and why governments do as they do, Klein and Marmor argue that three basic tools suffice:

- an understanding of the ideas, assumptions and theories policy actors bring to assessing problems, their causes, and their solutions
- analysis of the institutions within which governments operate (i.e., the 'rules of the game')
- an analysis of the interests operating in a particular political arena.

This article looks at interest groups and, particularly, those drawn from civil society.

The public policy process has changed profoundly in most countries since World War II in a gradual shift from 'government' to 'governance' (Rhodes, 1997). A relatively simple policymaking process in which the government of each nation state was central, working with a small number of professional groups and with civil servants largely monopolizing policy advice, has gradually given way to a more complex, messy process in which government shares power with, and is influenced by, a wider range of national and even global actors located outside formal political structures (Pierre and Peters, 2000). The 'core' of the state is said to have lost power due to developments within countries and internationally as a result of the forces of globalization. Rhodes refers to the latter as the 'external hollowing out of the nation state' (Rhodes, 1997: 18). At its extreme, the governance literature portrays the central government of a typical nation state as, 'now only one actor among many in the policy-making process...the process of governing today involves a much more pluralistic conceptualization of power...' (Richards and Smith, 2002; 19).

This trend means that a range of interest groups, including so-called 'civil society organizations,' operating within and across countries (see discussion that follows for definitions of various types of interest group), have greater salience in making and delivering public health policy than was the case 50 years ago. Although business interest groups, especially transnational corporations, and international donors currently exert considerable influence on national governments, transnational nongovernmental organizations (NGOs), civil society organizations, and related social movements can also successfully put pressure on governments, as well as supporting them on occasions in the face of demands from business (e.g., to reduce social protection).

The extent to which the power of the central state has diminished in the face of the rise of civil society varies from country to country and from issue to issue. In many low-income countries there was little sign until comparatively recently of the policy process becoming more directly permeable to nongovernmental influences except externally to big business and international donors and internally to well-organized professional groups such as doctors. However, in the 1980s and 1990s there was growing evidence of broader interest-group activity in many poor countries. In part, this growth resulted from the emergence of less authoritarian and elitist forms of government and, in part, from a growing recognition by donor agencies of the useful role which organizations outside government could play in delivering services, supporting policy and institutional reform, and encouraging governments to be more accountable to their people. As a result, donors provided more funds to nongovernmental organizations in low-income countries, and their number and importance grew.

In many settings today, particularly in more democratic and higher-income countries, public health policy is developed and sometimes implemented through complex, largely self-organizing networks of actors that involve public, private, and civil society organizations (e.g., NGOs and other voluntary bodies) that enjoy considerable autonomy from central government. Although these developments make public health policymaking more complicated and less predictable, they also offer public health professionals and advocates new resources and alternative channels by which to promote their messages and deliver services. For example, it is generally the case that public health initiatives and services that involve NGOs and end users tend to be seen by the public as more trustworthy and worthwhile than those led exclusively by government agencies.

Interest Groups and Civil Society Organizations

There is a potentially confusing range of terms used to describe organizations outside the formal system of government, but which can from time to time contribute to and shape public health policy, such as 'interest group',

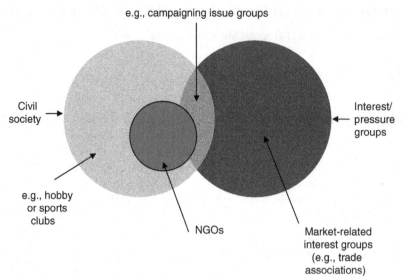

Figure 1 Civil society organizations, interest and pressure groups, and NGOs. Note: not to scale. From Buse K, Mays N, and Walt G (2005) *Making Health Policy*. Maidenhead: Open University Press, Figure 6.1, page 103, adapted with permission.

'pressure group' 'civil society organization' and 'nongovernmental organization' (**Figure 1** attempts to clarify the distinctions between different types of organizations outside the government sphere). Generally, 'interest group' and 'pressure group' can be used synonymously. At its simplest, an 'interest group' promotes or represents the demands of a particular part of society (e.g., people suffering from blindness or manufacturers of pharmaceuticals) or stands for a particular cause (e.g., environmentalism or free trade). Different types of interest group involved in public health policy typically include bodies representing:

- staff, such as the medical, nursing, and allied health professions (e.g., physiotherapy, speech therapy)
- providers, such as hospital associations
- insurers, such as sickness funds and private insurance companies
- payers, such as employers' associations
- different groups of patients and users (e.g., people with mental health problems or those who are HIV-positive), as well as citizens and consumers
- suppliers of goods and services to the health system, such as pharmaceutical companies and medical equipment manufacturers
- other commercial interests whose activities bear on public health and the environment, such as the food and drink industry, supermarket chains, motor manufacturers, and airlines.

Although there are varying definitions of interest or pressure groups, they tend to:

- be voluntary – people or organizations choose to join them
- aim to achieve some desired goals
- stay outside the formal government process while striving to influence it.

Unlike political parties that are also voluntary and goal-oriented, pressure groups do not plan to take formal political power but wish to be involved in decisions affecting their interests. Sometimes pressure groups evolve into political parties and then become involved in policymaking from within government – such as the German Green Party, which began life as an environmental pressure group – but most remain as organized groups outside government, even if some of them have very close relationships with government (see the discussion of 'policy communities' that follows).

Today it is common to describe interest groups as existing in civil society. Heywood (2000: 17, cited in Richards and Smith, 2002: 171) defines civil society as 'a realm of autonomous groups and associations such as businesses, pressure groups, clubs, families and so on. . . .; civil society encompasses institutions that are "private" in that they are independent from government and organized by individuals in pursuit of their own ends.' Others see civil society slightly less broadly as lying between the private space of the family or household and the public sphere of the government, thereby excluding families. Either way, this explains why the term 'civil society group' is sometimes used interchangeably with 'interest group,' although public policy issues can be very peripheral to the identity of some civil society groups. For example, sports clubs will only very occasionally take a position on an issue of public policy when it risks impinging on their sporting activities, whereas the raison d'être of other groups lies in political campaigning.

As a result, not all civil society groups are necessarily interest groups. Civil society organizations represent a wider range of organizations (**Figure 1**).

NGOs form the most familiar part of civil society. The term NGO originally referred to any not-for-profit organization outside government but more recently has taken on a more specific meaning, particularly in the fields of public health and international development, of a relatively highly structured organization with a headquarters and paid staff working in client advocacy and/or service delivery, in many cases providing a service that might previously have been provided directly by the state. Many NGOs also retain a desire to influence public policy and can thus act as pressure groups.

If not all civil society groups are necessarily to be seen as interest groups, then there is also some debate as to whether it is accurate to call all interest groups civil society groups. It is increasingly common analytically to exclude interest groups related to market activities (i.e., business organizations such as trade associations) from civil society, on the basis that civil society is 'a sphere located between the state and market: a buffer zone strong enough to keep both state and market in check, thereby preventing each from becoming too powerful and dominating.' (Giddens, 2001: iii). **Figure 1** is drawn from this perspective. In this article, 'civil society' is defined as the social space not occupied by the family and household, the state, or the market.

Resources of Interest Groups

The resources that interest groups can mobilize vary widely, but include the following:

- Their members – the larger the number of members, all other things equal, the more influence an interest group is likely to have.
- Their level of funding and resources – funding affects all aspects of an interest group's activities, such as the ability to hire professional staff to organize campaigns, prepare critiques of government policy, contribute to political parties, and organize demonstrations.
- Their knowledge about their area of concern – some of this information and understanding may be unavailable from any other source. For example, a government may be dependent on a pharmaceutical company for the first trial evidence of the effectiveness of a new drug.
- Their persuasive skills in building public support for particular positions or policies by stimulating activity by others, such as the mass media.
- Their contacts and relations with policymakers, officials, ministers, opposition parties, and the media.
- The sanctions, if any, at their disposal – these could range from embarrassing the government in international fora or the mass media to organizing consumer boycotts harming the domestic economy or protracted industrial action.

Interest groups are also increasingly involved in legal action or the threat of legal action against governments and transnational corporations to promote their point of view and force change in policy. For example, national and international civil society organizations played an important part in the legal action against the South African government which forced the government to concede the principle that antiretroviral drugs should be made available universally.

Strategies and Relations to the State: 'Insider' and 'Outsider' Groups

Interest groups can also be analyzed in terms of how far they are recognized or legitimized by governments which, in turn, relates to their aims and their strategies. Grant (1995) distinguishes two basic categories in this respect – 'insider' and 'outsider' groups. Insider groups are groups which are still not officially part of the machinery of government but are regarded as legitimate by government policymakers, are consulted regularly, and are expected to play by the 'rules of the game.' For example, if they accept an invitation to sit on a government committee, they will respect the confidentiality of the discussions that take place there until ministers are ready to make a statement about the direction of policy. Insider groups thus become closely involved in testing policy ideas and in the development of their field. Typically, in health policy, producer groups such as medical and nursing associations expect to be consulted or directly involved in policy developments and frequently are, even if they do not always get their own way.

In the UK, the Association of the British Pharmaceutical Industry (ABPI) has insider status with the Department of Health on the grounds that the government is both concerned to promote the UK pharmaceutical industry and to ensure that safe and effective medicines are available at the earliest opportunity to patients. There are regular meetings between the industry, senior officials, and ministers. The ABPI has also recruited retired civil servants to help it negotiate with government over drug regulation and prices.

Outsider groups, by contrast, are either organizations that reject a close involvement in government processes on strategic grounds or have been unable to gain a reputation as legitimate participants in the policy process. Perhaps the most high-profile outsider groups in the contemporary health field are so-called 'new social movements' such as radical antiabortion and antivivisection organizations because of the vehemence of their views and their reputation for taking direct action against clinics, laboratories, and sometimes those who work in them. One of the best-known direct action groups in public health was BUGA UP (Billboard Utilising Graffitists Against Unhealthy Promotions). Founded in 1979 in Sydney, Australia, it was notorious (or celebrated, depending on your point of view) for illegally defacing outdoor advertising of unhealthy products, particularly tobacco and alcohol. Its tactic was to alter advertisements to provide a critical commentary on the industry's promotions. 'Anyhow, Have a Winfield' was changed to 'Anyhow, it's a Minefield' or 'Man how I hate Winfield.' When members of BUGA UP were charged, they defended themselves by arguing that their actions were essential to prevent a greater harm from occurring (Chapman, 1996).

Interest groups may shift their strategies over time. For example, in its early life Greenpeace favored direct action as a way of drawing attention to conservation issues. Most notably it disrupted the activities of whaling vessels. More recently, Greenpeace has adopted a less flamboyant and less confrontational strategy through scientifically based advocacy, but still uses confrontational tactics on occasions. In the process, it has developed closer relations with governments, although it has yet to attain full insider group recognition. Groups that shift their strategies or positions are known as 'thresholder' groups. Studies of the evolution of policy in the field of human immunodeficiency virus/acquired immunodeficiency syndrome (HIV/AIDS) in the United States and Britain clearly show how outsider groups played a key role in the early stages of the epidemic by using their knowledge about the syndrome to pressure governments to take the topic seriously. Some of these same organizations became more closely involved in both policy and service delivery as circumstances changed, and they were able to accept insider status. Often an outsider group becomes an insider group through taking responsibility for delivering services paid for by government or international donors.

Contribution of Interest Groups to the Policy Process

Taken together, the different types of interest groups fulfill a range of functions in policymaking, particularly as the scope of the modern state has widened since World War II. Peterson (1999) argues that interest groups can provide opportunities for the following:

- Participation: Given that elections in democracies are both an infrequent and a highly indirect way for citizens to involve themselves in public issues, interest groups provide an alternative way for voters to get involved in politics and register their opinions to politicians.
- Representation: When policymakers take into account the views of a range of interest groups, the range of opinion under consideration normally widens.
- Political education: Members learn about the political process, for example, if they become office holders in an interest group.
- Motivation: Interest groups can draw new issues to the attention of governments, provide more information, change the way governments view issues, and even develop new policy options through their scientific and political activities.
- Mobilization: Interest groups build pressure for action, and support for, or opposition to, new policies (e.g., by stimulating media interest in a topic or by blocking implementation of a policy).
- Monitoring: Interest groups assess the performance and behavior of governments, thereby contributing to the public accountability of leaders, for example, by seeing whether political promises are implemented. They are also increasingly involved in holding private corporations to account as national governments struggle to deal with the power of transnational businesses.
- Provision: Interest groups can use their knowledge of a particular patient group or area of policy to deliver services with or without government funding (e.g., missionary societies).

Richards and Smith (2002: 173) identify four further benefits for governments, in particular, from involving pressure groups or interest groups in the policy process:

1. Legitimacy: State intervention is generally seen as more appropriate if policies have been developed with the involvement of key groups affected.
2. Information: Interest groups often represent experts in a particular field (e.g., health professionals) whose advice may be helpful to the state.
3. Implementation: Policy implementation is enormously easier and less costly if the state can rely on key interest groups to cooperate, perhaps by making some concessions to the self-interest of the groups (e.g., allowing doctors to continue their private practice along with their commitment to a public health-care system).
4. Order: Policy uncertainty can be reduced by placating groups with coherent memberships and resources (this can also be a way of marginalizing more unpredictable, potentially disruptive groups).

Larger interest groups tend to have a wider range of functions and ways of operating. For example, Oxfam, the British-based international antipoverty NGO, describes itself as 'a development, advocacy and relief agency working to put an end to poverty world-wide.' Its activities cover 'motivation,' 'mobilization,' 'monitoring,' and 'provision' according to Peterson's typology, as well as 'representation' in some of the 70 countries in which it works. Smaller NGOs tend to have more focused goals and activities. For example, the Fred Hollows Foundation, based in Australia, is an NGO devoted to working with local blindness prevention agencies in 29 countries to reduce unnecessary and avoidable blindness, with a primary focus on cataract. Thus, as with many NGOs, its main function is 'provision,' including training local staff to deliver services and developing high-quality, low-cost technologies for eye care. However, in its work with indigenous Australians, it has extended its role to include advocacy ('motivation' and 'mobilization').

From Policy Communities to Issue Networks

Political scientists have observed that when it comes to policy formulation in public health (as opposed to getting an issue onto the agenda in the first place), the most influential participants are usually individuals and organizations with an enduring interest and knowledge of the field.

One way of understanding the formal and informal relationships between government and nongovernment (interest group) actors is to identify the various policy subsystems or policy communities in which they interact. At its simplest, a policy subsystem or community is a recognizable subdivision of public policymaking. In health policy, for example, mental health policy formulation is distinctively different from policy on environmental health issues and involves different actors. Some subsystems, known as 'iron triangles,' are small, very stable, and highly exclusive three-way sets of relationships, usually among politicians, bureaucrats, and a commercial interest. In the case of defense procurement, the triangle is constituted by government, suppliers, and end users in the military. Other subsystems are typically larger (i.e., involving more entities) and more fluid, with less clear boundaries (e.g., family policy).

The challenges in the 1980s and 1990s to the dominant position of the medical profession in health policy in Britain and other Western countries led to a shift from more to less closed policy communities in health, with a conscious attempt by governments to develop new networks, including groups representing users, business, and free market-oriented think tanks, although consumer groups remained relatively weaker than professional groups.

Marsh and Rhodes (1992) distinguished between 'policy communities' – which they saw as highly integrated networks in which all participants had resources to exchange, relationships were stable, and exclusive narrow interests predominated – and 'issue networks,' which they saw as loosely interdependent, less predictable, with unstable networks of a large number of members, usually serving a consultative function in relation to policy development. The main feature of a policy community is sustained interaction between the participants through a web of formal and informal relationships (Lewis, 2005). In health policy, organizations and individuals representing practitioners (health professionals), users, the public, researchers (from laboratory sciences to the social sciences), commentators (journalists and policy analysts), businesses (e.g., drug companies, medical equipment manufacturers, the food industry), hospitals and clinics, insurers, government officials, politicians, and international organizations will be involved to differing degrees depending on the issue at stake. Policy communities are not necessarily consensual networks. Increasingly, health policy communities in Western countries are marked by conflicts between a range of powerful interests representing professional and commercial providers, the community, and government as new groups make their presence felt.

The Emergence of New Social Movements

Beginning in the 1970s but gathering global force in the 1990s as part of the shift from 'government' to 'governance,' the relatively closed systems of decision making in public policy, including public health, were challenged by the emergence of what were dubbed new social movements (NSMs). These organizations were very different from conventional NGO bureaucracies and, unlike political parties, were frequently single-issue movements in civil society, focusing on problems traditionally not well represented in mainstream politics, such as the environment, human rights, peace, and animal welfare.

They have a number of other distinctive features:

- They tend to be nonhierarchical and have flat, fluid structures.
- They predominantly use 'outsider' tactics (see above) that emphasize direct action, including illegal acts, demonstrations, and occupations.
- They tend not to be class-based, instead promoting issues that cut across economic and sectional interests.
- They are increasingly not confined to a single country; rather, they are often international or even global (e.g., Amnesty International).
- They focus on introducing new ideas and information into the policy debate by attracting media coverage of their activities rather than working through conventional governmental consultative channels.
- They tend to focus on high-profile, single-issue campaigns (e.g., campaigns against genetically modified organisms or the indebtedness of poor countries).

Social scientists generally see the rise of NSMs as a response to, and enabled by, developments such as postindustrialism, the rise of knowledge-based rather than industrial societies in high-income countries, the acceleration of globalization, and the increasing diffusion of political power with the weakening of the nation-state in favor of the interests of transnational corporations (Melucci, 1996; cited in Hudson and Lowe, 2004: 106). For example, flexible, low-cost protest movements against the perceived harmful consequences of economic globalization are enabled by the same technologies (the Internet, e-mail, text messaging, etc.) that enable the global financiers whom they oppose to move capital between countries by using a few computer key strokes. According to Peterson's typology of roles fulfilled by interest groups (discussed previously), NSMs have provided increased opportunities for public participation in policy, allowed a wider range of opinion to enter the policy debate (representation), offered fora for political education, pressured for change (motivation), and monitored the actions of governments. The only role they have not typically occupied is provision of services.

International and Global Civil Society Organization Activity

The emergence of global social movements, international NGOs (e.g., Greenpeace, Amnesty International and Help the Aged), transnational public health advocacy (most notably in the field of HIV/AIDS), and most recently global philanthropic organizations such as the Bill and Melinda Gates Foundation, have inevitably led to the question of whether it is meaningful to talk of a global civil society, defined as: 'the sphere of ideas, values, institutions, organisations, networks, and individuals located between the family, the state and the market and operating beyond the confines of national societies, polities and economies' (Anheier et al., 2001: 17). Although arguments continue about the appropriateness of the term, there has undoubtedly been a dramatic increase in transnational interactions between civil society organizations. Normatively, this can be seen as a strategic, grassroots response to globalization, providing much needed global consciousness raising and resistance to global capitalism in the face of the declining capacity of nation states to regulate transnational corporations. Global civil society has also cohered in response to the emergence of a range of other global political issues such as global warming (climate change), environmental degradation, infectious disease epidemics, human trafficking, and international terrorism when it is clear that nation-states acting singly can do relatively little.

Regulating transnational corporations has become an increasing focus of networked civil society action as business has become increasingly globalized and beyond the reach of national jurisdictions. To this end, civil society organizations use both cooperative (e.g., eco-consumerism, collaborations with business, promotion of voluntary codes of conduct and stewardship) and confrontational strategies such as consumer boycotts, public relations wars, surveillance and exposure of corporate malpractice, and shareholder activism.

There are also new official venues for civil society activity in public health at the international level, for instance, through the European Union, around the meetings of the World Trade Organization, the Group of 8 (G8), and United Nations bodies. As a result, civil society organizations have been able to open new channels of access to official policymakers and develop new forms of policy network at the European and global levels, thus reducing their dependence on nation-states as the main sites for decision making. Interest groups can shift their attention back and forth between individual countries and internationally, depending on the progress they are making at each level.

What Impact Do Civil Society Organizations Have in Public Health Policy?

Despite the obvious increase in civil society activity at national and international levels in the public health field, questions inevitably arise as to whether this activity makes a detectable difference to policy and how influential such groups are compared with others involved in the policy process. The effectiveness of civil society organizations can be appraised across different stages and levels of policy. Thus civil society may generate new information, frame debates, and set the policy agenda; it may secure the support of key actors and establish new norms; it may produce procedural change (e.g., establish an international code or treaty); it may influence the behavior and decisions of state and nonstate actors; and finally, it may be credited with having made a direct and major contribution to policy change.

Among interest groups, business interests are generally still the most powerful in most areas of public policy, followed by labor interest groups. This is because both capital and labor are vital to the economic production process. In capitalist societies, ownership of the means of production is concentrated in the hands of business corporations rather than the state. As a result, business has huge power vis-à-vis government, particularly in the current globally interconnected environment in which corporations can potentially shift their capital and production relatively easily between countries if their interests are being harmed by government policies.

Even in health-care systems in which most services are provided in publicly owned and managed institutions, there will still be extensive links with private-sector actors who bring new ideas, demands, and practices into the public sector. Provider professionals and workers have an important influence on policy, in addition to business interests. In the case of the doctors, this influence results from a medical monopoly over a body of esoteric knowledge that is allied to the control that doctors are able to exert over the market for their services. Governments continue to have a strong influence because of the large contribution of public finance and provision in most (particularly high-income) countries.

However, consumer and citizen interests are also increasingly heard and responded to. Although it is hard to generalize, civil society organizations' main impact appears to lie in championing new ideas and pushing issues onto the policy agenda of governments and corporations rather than in determining the contours of the eventual policy response. It is increasingly apparent that interest groups such as patient organizations are playing a more influential role in health policy even in low-income countries, where they have traditionally been weak or absent. Of course, the extent of influence on policy from outside government and the immediate impact of party politics will vary from place to place and from issue to issue.

The Jubilee 2000: Drop the Debt campaign was one of the most high-profile and arguably relatively effective civil society campaigns of the last decade and highlights many of the strengths and limitations of global civil society. It coordinated over 60 national campaigns worldwide, including 17 in Latin America, 15 in Africa, and 10 in Asia, and raised 17 million signatures, including 1 million from Bangladesh and one-quarter of the 4 million population of the Republic of Ireland. The campaign had an impact on key bilateral negotiations relating to the debt of poor countries, as well as offering unprecedented scrutiny and media coverage of the impact of global macroeconomic policies and institutions.

However, the campaign faced major difficulties in achieving global coherence. The U.S. campaign focused only on the very poorest states for domestic political reasons, and this led to tensions with many southern activists. In addition, some of the global legitimacy of the campaign was undermined by the North–South imbalance in funding and access to decision makers. Despite the disproportionate share of resources deployed by northern activists, which reflected what the campaign was criticizing, the campaign did succeed in giving voice to and empowering southern groups. The international connections boosted the credibility of southern groups in their own countries.

The history of the response to HIV/AIDS across the globe is noteworthy for the very high level of involvement and influence of civil society organizations. 'Never before have civil society organizations – here defined as any group of individuals that is separate from government and business – done so much to contribute to the fight against a global health crisis, or been so included in the decisions made by policy-makers' (Zuniga, 2006). The HIV/AIDS history is also notable for the diversity of interest group activities which together redefined the policy agenda, the large number of HIV/AIDS organizations involved with strong transnational linkages

Table 1 Possible advantages and drawbacks of involving interest groups in shaping health policy

Potential advantages of 'open' policy processes	*Potential negative consequences of 'open' policy processes*
Wide range of views is brought to bear on a problem, including a better appreciation of the possible impacts of policy on different groups	Difficult to reconcile conflicting and competing claims for attention and resources of different interest groups
Policymaking process includes information that is not accessible to governments	Adds to complexity and time taken to reach decisions and implement policies
Consultation and/or involvement of a range of interests gives policy greater legitimacy and support so that policy decisions may be more likely to be implemented	Concern to identify whom different interest groups 'truly' represent and how accountable they are to their members or funders
New or emerging issues may be brought to governments' attention more rapidly than if process is very 'closed,' thereby allowing a rapid response	Risk of token involvement of civil society in policy decision rather than genuine engagement
	Less well resourced, less well connected interests may still be disadvantaged by being overlooked or marginalized
	Interest groups may not be capable of providing the information or taking the responsibility allocated to them
	Activities of interest groups may not be transparent
	Under pressure to raise their media profile to help with fund-raising, organizations may adopt irresponsible, extreme positions
	Proliferation of 'front' groups enables corporate interests to develop multiple, covert channels of influence
	Interest groups can be bigoted, self-interested, badly informed, abusive, and intimidatory – being in civil society does not confer automatic virtue

Source: Buse K, Mays N, and Walt G, *Making Health Policy*. Maidenhead, UK: Open University Press, 2005, Table 6.2, p. 117, adapted with permission.

(currently over 3000 in 150 countries), and the gradual shift of activism from the high- to low-income countries. In the United States and Western Europe in the 1980s, the most affected population group was homosexual men who had recent experience of the gay rights movement of the 1970s. They used some of the same civil rights strategies and refused to play the passive role of 'patients.' Similarly, in low-income countries subsequently, HIV/AIDS activism has been inspired by, and allied itself to, wider social justice movements such as those for debt relief, as well as building alliances with established groups in the North.

Is Interest Group Participation a Good Thing in Policy Terms?

Generally, in democratic societies, the involvement of organizations outside the government in policy processes is seen as a good thing. However, there are potential drawbacks. After all, organized criminal gangs are technically part of civil society. **Table 1** summarizes the possible advantages and drawbacks.

One of the most striking features of recent times has been the proliferation of 'front' organizations for big business masquerading as civil society organizations to disguise commercial lobbying as grassroots democratic debate (Buse and Lee, 2005). In 2006, Cancer United was set up ostensibly to campaign for equal access to cancer care across the European Union. It was presented to prospective celebrity supporters as a coalition of doctors, nurses, and patients, but was funded by Roche with Roche's public relations arm acting as its secretariat. A related trend is for the pharmaceutical industry to fund patients' groups such as the English Fight for Herceptin Campaign, a web-adept, media-friendly, apparently grassroots women's action group, but in fact supported by the manufacturer's public relations firm.

Conclusion

Public policymaking, including in public health, has become more complex, involving a wider, less predictable range of interest groups, including civil society organizations. National governments are also increasingly subject to external and transnational pressure not just from transnational corporations but also from emerging global civil society. Despite the widely identified shift from 'government' to 'governance' since World War II, it is important to keep a sense of perspective. Although the unfettered power of many nation-states has diminished appreciably, the state remains influential, particularly in Western countries, in initiating, structuring, and managing the relations between the government and civil society actors, including nongovernmental organizations. As a result, public health practitioners and advocates need to become expert in the political skills of stakeholder analysis and develop strategic alliances with government officials, professional groups, civil society organizations, donors, and the research community if they wish their policies to be taken up and implemented (Buse et al., 2006). Public health policy has always been inherently political, never more so than today.

See also: Agenda Setting in Public Health Policy; Global Health Initiatives and Public Health Policy; Human Rights, Approach to Public Health Policy; The State in Public Health, The Role of.

Citations

Anheier H, Glasius M, and Kaldor M (2001) Introducing global civil society. In: Anheier H, Glasius M, and Kaldor M (eds.) *Global Civil Society 2001*, pp. 3–17. Oxford, UK: Oxford University Press.

Buse K and Lee K (2005) *Business and Global Health Governance*. Discussion Paper No. 5. WHO Department of Ethics, Trade, Human Rights and Law and LSHTM Centre on Global Change and Health. Working Papers on Globalization and Health.Geneva, Switzerland: WHO.

Buse K, Martin-Hilber A, Widyantoro N, and Hawkes SJ (2006) Management of the politics of evidence-based sexual and reproductive health policy. *The Lancet* 368: 2101–2103.

Buse K, Mays N, and Walt G (2005) *Making Health Policy*. Maidenhead, UK: Open University Press.

Chapman S (1996) Civil disobedience and tobacco control: The case of BUGA UP. Billboard Utilising Graffitists Against Unhealthy Promotions. *Tobacco Control* 5: 179–185.

Giddens A (2001) Foreword. In: Anheier H, Glasius M, and Kaldor M (eds.) *Global Civil Society 2001*, p. iii. Oxford, UK: Oxford University Press.

Grant W (1995) *Pressure Groups, Politics and Democracy*. London: Harvester Press.

Heywood A (2000) *Key Concepts in Politics*. Basingstoke, UK: Palgrave.

Hudson J and Lowe S (2004) *Understanding the Policy Process: Analysing Welfare Policy and Practice*. Bristol, UK: The Policy Press.

Klein R and Marmor TR (2006) Reflections on policy analysis: Putting it together again. In: Moran M (ed.) *The Oxford Handbook of Public Policy*, pp. 890–910. Oxford, UK: Oxford University Press.

Lewis J (2005) *Health Policy and Politics: Networks, Ideas and Power*. Melbourne: IP Communications.

Marsh D and Rhodes RAW (1992) Policy communities and issue networks: Beyond typology. In: Marsh D and Rhodes RAW (eds.) *Policy Networks in British Government*, pp. 1–26. Oxford, UK: Clarendon Press.

Melucci A (1996) *Challenging Codes: Collective Action in the Information Age*. Cambridge, UK: Cambridge University Press.

Peterson MA (1999) Motivation, mobilisation and monitoring: The role of interest groups in health policy. *Journal of Health Politics, Policy and Law* 24: 416–420.

Pierre J and Peters BG (2000) *Governance, Politics and the State*. Basingstoke, UK: Macmillan.

Rhodes RAW (1997) *Understanding Governance: Policy Networks, Governance, Reflexivity and Accountability*. Buckingham, UK: Open University Press.

Richards D and Smith MJ (2002) *Governance and Public Policy in the UK*. Oxford, UK: Oxford University Press.

Zuniga J (2006) Civil society and the global battle against HIV/AIDS. In: Beck E, Mays N, Whiteside A, and Zuniga J (eds.) *The HIV Pandemic: Local and Global Implications*, pp. 706–719. Oxford, UK: Oxford University Press.

Further Reading

Buse K, Mays N, and Walt G (2005) *Making Health Policy*, pp. 137–156. Maidenhead, UK: Open University Press.

Hudson J and Lowe S (2004) *Understanding the Policy Process*, pp. 127–144. Bristol, UK: The Policy Press.

Kuruvilla S (2005) *CSO Participation in Health, Research and Policy: A Review of Models, Mechanisms and Measures.* Working Paper 251. London: Overseas Development Institute. http://www.odi.org.uk/RAPID/Publications?RAPID_WP_251.html (accessed August 2007).

Lee K, Buse K, and Fustukian S (eds.) (2002) *Health Policy in a Globalizing World.* Cambridge, UK: Cambridge University Press.

Reich MR (2002) Reshaping the state from above, from within, from below: Implications for public health. *Social Science and Medicine* 54: 1669–1675.

Richards D and Smith MJ (2002) *Governance and Public Policy in the UK*, pp. 171–198. Oxford, UK: Oxford University Press.

Seckinelgin H (2002) Time to stop and think: HIV/AIDS, global civil society and people's politics. In: Glasius M, Kaldor M, and Anheier H (eds.) *Global Civil Society 2002*, pp. 109–136. Oxford, UK: Oxford University Press.

Walt G (1994) *Health Policy: An Introduction to Process and Power.* Johannesburg, London, and New Jersey: Witswatersrand University Press and Zed Books Chap. 6, 7.

Relevant Websites

http://ec.europa.eu/civil_society/index_en.htm – European Union and Civil Society.

http://www.jhu.edu/ccss – Johns Hopkins Institute for Policy Studies, Center for Civil Society Studies.

http://www.lse.ac.uk/collections/ccs – London School of Economics and Political Science, Centre for Civil Society.

http://www.dfid.gov.uk – UK Department for International Development (DfID) Working with Civil Society.

http://www.unaids.org/en/GetStarted/CivilSociety.asp – UNAIDS and Civil Society.

http://www.undp.org/partners/cso – UN Development Program and Civil Society Organizations.

http://www.uncp.org.org/civil_society/gcsf – UN Global Civil Society Forum.

http://www/unglobalcompact.org/ParticipantsAndStakeholders/civil_society.html – UN Global Compact.

http://www.un.org/issues/ngo/ngoindex.html – UN Relations with Civil Society.

http://web.worldbank.org/WEBSITE/EXTERNAL/TOPICS/CSO.html – World Bank and Civil Society.

http://www.who.int/civilsociety/en/ – World Health Organization and Civil Society.

People's Health Movement

R Narayan, Bangalore, India
C Schuftan, Ho Chi Minh City, Vietnam

© 2008 Elsevier Inc. All rights reserved.

Background

In 1978, in Alma Ata, the universal slogan 'Health for All' by the year 2000 was coined. At the same time, the famous Alma Ata Declaration was overwhelmingly approved, putting people and communities at the center of health planning and health-care strategies, as well as emphasizing the role of community participation, appropriate technology and intersectoral coordination. The Declaration was endorsed by most of the governments of the world and symbolized a significant paradigm shift in the global understanding of Health and Health Care (WHO, UNICEF, 1978).

Twenty-five years later, after much policy rhetoric, some concerted but mostly ad-hoc action, quite a bit of misplaced euphoria, distortions brought about by the growing role of the market economy as it has affected health care, and a fair dose of governmental and international health agencies' amnesia, this Declaration remains unfulfilled and mostly forgotten, as the world comes to terms with the new economic forces of globalization, liberalization, and privatization that have made Health for All a receding dream.

The People's Health Assembly in Savar, Bangladesh, in December 2000, and the People's Health Movement that evolved from it are both a civil society effort to counter this global *laissez-faire* and to challenge health policy makers around the world with a Peoples Health Campaign for Health for All-Now! (Narayan, 2000).

The first People's Health Assembly

The first People's Health Assembly brought together 1450 people from 92 countries and resulted in an unusual 5-day event in which grassroots people shared their concerns about the unfulfilled Health for All challenge. The Assembly's program included a variety of interactive dialogue opportunities for all health professionals and activists who gathered for this significant event. These included:

- a rally for Health for All Now!;
- meetings in which the testimonies on the health situation from many parts of the world and the struggles of people were shared and commented upon by multidisciplinary resource groups (People's Health Movement, 2002);
- parallel workshops to discuss a range of health and health-related challenges;
- cultural programs to symbolize the multicultural and multiethnic diversity of the people of the world;

- exhibitions and video/film shows;
- an abundance of dialogue, in small and large groups, using formal and informal opportunities.

This People's Health Assembly was preceded by a long series of preassembly events all over the world. The most exceptional of these was the mobilization in India. For nearly 9 months preceding the assembly, there were grassroots local and regional initiatives of people's health enquiries and audits, sensitization including health songs and popular theater, subdistrict- and district-level seminars, policy dialogues and translations of national consensus documents on health into regional languages, as well as campaigns to challenge medical professionals and the health system to become more Health-for-All-oriented. Finally, over 2000 delegates traveled to Kolkata (Calcutta), mostly riding on five converging people's health trains. Here, they brought their ideas and felt needs first elaborated in 17 state and 250 district conventions. In Kolkata, after 2 days of conferences, parallel workshops, exhibitions, two public rallies for health and a myriad of cultural programs, the Assembly endorsed the Indian People's Health Charter. Approximately 300 delegates from this assembly then traveled to Bangladesh, mostly by bus, to attend the Global Assembly. Similar preparatory initiatives, though less intense, took place in Bangladesh, Nepal, Sri Lanka, Cambodia, Philippines, Japan, and other parts of the world, including Latin America, Europe, Africa, and Australia.

The People's Charter for Health

As a result of a full year's mobilization and 5 days of very intense and interactive work in Savar, a Global People's Health Charter emerged, which was endorsed by all participants (People's Health Assembly, 2000a). This charter has now become:

- an expression of the movement's common concerns;
- a vision for a better and healthier world;
- a call for more radical action;
- a tool for advocacy for people's health;
- a worldwide rallying manifesto for global health movements, as well as for networking and coalition building.

The significance of this Global People's Health Charter is multiple:

- It endorses health as a social, economic and political issue and as a fundamental human right.
- It identifies inequality, poverty, exploitation, violence, and injustice as the roots of preventable ill health.
- It underlines the imperative that Health for All means challenging powerful economic interests, opposing globalization as the current iniquitous development model; it thus drastically changes our political and economic priorities.
- It brings in a new perspective and the voices from the poor and the marginalized (the rarely heard) encouraging people to develop their own local solutions.
- It encourages people to hold accountable their own local authorities, national governments, international organizations and national and transnational corporations.

The vision and the principles of the charter, more than any other document preceding it, extricates health from the myopic biomedical-techno-managerialist approach it has seen in the last two decades – with its vertical, selective magic-bullets-approach to health – and centers it squarely in the more comprehensive context of today's global socioeconomic-political-cultural-environmental realities. However, the most significant gain of the People's Health Assembly 1 and the charter is that for the first time since Alma Ata, a Health For All plan of action unambiguously endorses a call for action that tackles the broader determinants of health, which include:

- the violations of people's right to health;
- the economic, social and political determinants of health;
- the environmental determinants of health;
- war, violence, conflict, and natural disasters as the cause of preventable mortality and ill health;
- the lack of a people-centered health sector reform with poor people participating in fostering a healthier world.

In a nutshell, the People's Health Movement started promoting a wide range of approaches and initiatives which combated the ill effects of the triple assault by the forces of globalization, liberalization, and privatization on health, health systems, and health care. In more detail, the PHM initiatives still today call for:

- combating the negative impacts of globalization as a worldwide economic and political ideology and process;
- significantly reforming the international financial institutions and the WTO to make them more responsive to poverty alleviation and the Health for All-Now! movement;
- writing off of the foreign debt of the least developed countries and the use of its equivalent for poverty reduction, health, and education activities;
- greater checks on and restraints of the freewheeling powers of transnational corporations, especially pharmaceutical companies (and mechanisms to ensure their compliance);
- greater and more equitable household food security;
- caps on the runaway international financial transfers;
- unconditional support of the emancipation of women and the respect of their full rights;

- putting health higher in the development agenda of governments;
- promoting the health (and other) rights of displaced and minority people;
- halting the process of privatization of public health facilities and working toward greater controls of the already installed private health sector;
- more equitable, just, and empowered people's participation in and greater influence on health and development matters;
- a greater focus on poverty alleviation in national and international development plans;
- greater and unconditional access of the poor to health services and treatment regardless of their ability to pay;
- strengthening public institutions, political parties, and trade unions involved, as the movement is, in the struggle of the poor;
- challenging restricted and dogmatic fundamentalist views of the development process;
- exerting greater vigilance and activism in matters of water and air pollution, the dumping of toxics, the disposal of water, climate changes and CO_2 emissions, soil erosion, and other attacks on the environment;
- protecting biodiversity and opposing biopiracy and the indiscriminate use of genetically modified seeds;
- holding violators of environmental crimes accountable;
- systematically applying environmental and health assessments and people-centered environmental audits of development projects;
- opposing war in all its forms, as well as the misdirected anti-terrorist-focused thrust of many global policies;
- categorically opposing the Israeli occupation of Palestinian territory (having, among other, a sizeable negative impact on the health of the Palestinian people);
- the democratization of the UN bodies and especially of the Security Council;
- becoming more actively involved in actions addressing the silent epidemic of violence against women;
- more prompt responses and preparedness and rehabilitation measures in cases of natural disasters; recognizing the politics of aid;
- making a renewed call for more democratic primary health care that is given the resources needed and holding governments accountable in this task;
- vehemently opposing the commoditization and privatization of health care (and the sale of public health facilities);
- promoting independent national drug policies centered around essential, generic medicines;
- calling for the transformation of WHO, supporting and actively working with its new Commission on the Social Determinants of Health and making sure WHO remains accountable to civil society;
- assuring that WHO stays staunchly independent from corporate interests;
- sustaining and promoting the defense of effective patient's rights;
- expanding and incorporating traditional medicine into people's health care;
- working for changes in the training and retaining of health personnel to assure they cover the great issues of our time as depicted in the People's Charter for Health;
- defending and fostering public health-oriented (and not-for-profit) health research worldwide;
- building strong people's organizations and a global movement working on health issues;
- more proactively and effectively countering of the media that are at the service of the globalization process;
- empowering people leading to their greater control of the resources needed for the health services they need and obtain;
- creating the bases for a better analysis and better concerted actions by its members through greater involvement of them in the PHM's website and list-server;
- fostering a global solidarity network that can actively support fellow members when facing disasters, emergencies, or acute repressive situations.

This comprehensive view of actions for health was probably the most significant contribution of the People's Health Assembly 1 (PHA1) and the evolving People's Health Movement as early as in the year 2000 (Schuftan, 2002). PHA1 was not without criticism. A critical analysis of it was analyzed by the leadership and taken into account in the preparation of PHA2 (Werner and Sanders, 2000).

Significant Gains Made by the People's Health Movement

The ongoing and growing mobilization process at local and global levels, and PHA1 as the historic first gathering that launched the movement are noteworthy. For the first time in decades, health and non-health networks have come together to work on global solidarity issues in health. These networks include the International People's Health Council (IPHC), Health Action International (HAI), Consumers International (CI), the Asian Community Health Action Network (ACHAN), the Third World Network (TWN), the Women's Global Network for Reproductive Rights (WGNRR), Gonoshasthya Kendra (GK), and the Dag Hammarskjold Foundation (DHF). From 2003 on, new networks such as the Global Equity Gauge Alliance (GEGA) and the Social Forum Network are further strengthening the Movement.

At the country level, in some regions, this coalescence is also under way. In India, for instance, the national collective includes the science movements, the women's movements, the alliance of people's movements, environmental groups, the health networks and associations, some research and policy networks, and even some trade unions.

Another significant development has been the evolving solidarity that PHM has found for its various collective documents at the global level (People's Health Assembly, 2000b, c). These have included themes such as:

- health in the era of globalization: From victims to protagonists;
- the political economy of the assault on health;
- equity and inequity today: some contributing social factors;
- the medicalization of health care and the challenge of Health for All;
- the environmental crisis: Threats to health and ways forward;
- communication as if people mattered: Adapting health promotion and social action to the global imbalances of the twenty-first century.

Taken together, these documents represented an unprecedented, emerging, global consensus. At the country level, consensus documents that support public education and public policy advocacy have been produced. In India, for instance, five short booklets, translated into most Indian languages, are available on the following five themes:

- what globalization means to people's health;
- whatever happened to Health for All by the year 2000;
- making life worth living by meeting the basic needs of all;
- a world where we matter: Focus on the health-care issues of women, children, street kids, the disabled, and the aged;
- confronting the commercialization of health care.

These booklets have been published by 18 national networks that form the national coordinating committee in India, an unprecedented consensus, the first of its kind in five decades.

The People's Health Assembly 2 (PHA2) followed in July 2005 in Cuenca, Ecuador where 1492 participants from 80 countries attended (Latham, 2006). PHA2 dealt with issues concerning health in nine distinct but complementary tracks. The tracks covered nine streams of issues such as equity and people's health care, intercultural encounters on health, trade and health, health and the environment, gender, women, and health sector reform, training and communicating for health, the right to health for all in an inclusive society, health in the people's hands, and People's Health Movement affairs.

Again, it was an unusual international health meeting expressing and symbolizing an alternative health and development culture of dialogue and celebration. PHA2 was preceded by holding of the first session of the International People's Health University in which 52 young people were trained as PHM activists. This is an effort to bring young people into the leadership of the movement. The first forum of researchers for people's health was also held.

Another significant gain has been the translation of the People's Charter for Health into over 40 languages worldwide. These include Arabic, Bangla, Chinese, Danish, English, Farsi, Finnish, Flemish, French, German, Greek, Hindi, Indonesian, Italian, Japanese, Kannada, Malayalam, Ndebele, Nepalese, Tagalo, Portuguese, Russian, Shona, Sinhala, Spanish, Swahili, Swedish, Tamil, Urdu, Ukrainian, Vietnamese, and translation is now in progress in Tongan, Lithuanian, Norwegian, Welsh, Thai, Cambodian, Pastun, Dhari, Korean, and Creole. An audio tape in English with Braille titles is also available. All these have been translated by volunteers, committed to the People's Health Movement. PHA2 produced a new document called 'The Cuenca Declaration,' which reiterated and updated the principle enshrined in the charter. This declaration has already been translated into five languages. (People's Health Movement, 2006).

Audiovisual aids including videos for public education, exhibitions, slides, and other forms of communication are now also available. The BBC Life Series video on 'The Health Protesters' is a good example based on PHA1.

The movement itself has evolved a communications strategy, which importantly includes its website, the e-list server group for exchange and discussion, a series of news briefs (nine since January 2001), and a host of press releases on a wide variety of themes and on special events and crises on an as-needed basis.

Presentations of the People's Health Charter and the Cuenca Declaration take place repeatedly in national, regional, and international forums, which have included the World Health Organization (WHO), the Global Forum for Health Research (GFHR Forum 5 and 6), the World Health Assembly, and the International Conference on Health Promotion.

The development of a standing relationship between the PHM and WHO is particularly promising. In April 2001, the very effective and assertive in-house lobbying by PHM resulted in the formation of the WHO Civil Society Initiative announced at the World Health Assembly, in May 2001. In May 2002, WHO invited PHM to present the People's Charter for Health in the World Heath Assembly. In May 2003, over 80 PHM delegates from 30 countries attended the WHA, made statements on primary health care, TRIPS, and other issues and were invited to meet the then director general designate, who welcomed a greater dialogue with PHM members at all levels. The Assembly was preceded by a PHM Geneva meeting for the 25th anniversary of the Alma Ata Declaration, which was attended by some WHO staff, including the PAHO Regional Director. In 2004, PHM was instrumental in WHO's creation of the Commission on the Social Determinants of Health. One PHM member is a Commissioner in it and several PHM members actively participate in the nine knowledge networks that the CSDH appointed. These are all small, but incremental movements toward a critical collaboration of PHM with WHO.

In many countries of the world, emerging country-level PHM circles are organizing public meetings and campaigns that include taking health to the streets as a rights issue. Discussions on the charter by professional associations and public health schools, articles, and editorials in medical/health journals are also beginning to increase. In 2006, PHM launched a Global Right to Health Care Campaign, which is in an advanced organizational phase in over a dozen countries.

Policy dialogues and action research circles on WHO/WHA, poverty and AIDS, women's access to heath, the disabled, health research, disaster response, access to essential drugs, macroeconomics and health, public–private partnerships, and food and nutrition security issues are at different stages of work and progress. For instance, a People's Charter on HIV/AIDS, developed through several meetings at the country level, was launched in 2005 at the International AIDS conference in Bangkok.

Starting in February 2006, PHM is undergoing restructuring to decentralize its decision making more given the growth of the movement. The Global Secretariat is moving from Bangalore to Cairo, a small coordinating committee is being created to assist the Global Secretariat and a steering group, representing the world's regions and thematic circles of PHM is being restructured. Several future sessions of the People's Health University are in different planning stages.

In short, every day the list of follow-up actions at various levels increases.

Conclusion

To conclude, the People's Health Movement has been a rather unprecedented development in the journey toward the Health for All goal. The movement:

- now encompasses a multiregional, multicultural, and multidisciplinary mobilization effort;
- is bringing together the largest ever gathering of activists and professionals, civil society representatives, and the people's representatives themselves;
- is working on global issues to raise awareness, as well as the level of concrete actions;
- is involved in solidarity with the health struggles of people, especially the poor and the marginalized, affected by the current global economic and geographical order.

Recognizing that we need to carry out a continuous, sustained, and collective effort, the People's Health Movement process, through the People's Health Charter and the Cuenca Declaration, reminds us that a long road lies ahead in the campaign for Health for All-Now!

See also: Alma Ata and Primary Health Care: An Evolving Story.

Citations

Latham M (2006) *A Global Struggle for Health Rights: The PHA2 Story.* SCN News. No. 31.

Narayan R (2000) The People's Health Assembly – A people's campaign for health for all now. *Asian Exchange* 16: 6–17.

People's Health Assembly (2000a) *People's Charter for Health, People's Health Assembly.* Dhaka, Bangladesh: GK Savar 8 December 2000.

People's Health Assembly (2000b) Discussion papers prepared by PHA Drafting Group, PHA Secretariat. Dhaka, Bangladesh: GK Savar.

People's Health Assembly (2000c) *Health in the Era of Globalization: From Victims to Protagonists.* Dhaka, Bangladesh: GK Savar. A discussion paper by PGA Drafting Group, PHA Secretariat.

People's Health Movement (2002a) *Voices of the Unheard: Testimonies from the People's Health Assembly, December* 2000. Dhaka, Bangladesh: GK Savar.

People's Health Movement (2002a) *The Cuenca Declaration, December 2000.* Ecuador: Cuenca.

Schuftan C (2002) *The People's Health Movement (PHM) in 2002: Still at the Forefront of the Struggle for "Health for All Now"* issue paper-2 for World Health Assembly, May 2002.

Werner D and Sanders D (2000) Liberation from what? A critical reflection on the People's Health Assembly 2000. *Asian Exchange* 16: 18–30.

WHO, UNICEF (1978) *Primary Health Care. Report of the International Conference on Primary Health Care.* 6–12 September, 1978, Alma Ata, USSR. Geneva, Switzerland: World Health Organization.

Relevant Websites

http://www.phmovement.org – Health for All Now! People's Health Movement.
http://www.politicsofhealth.org – Politics of Health Knowledge Network.
http://www.iphcglobal.org.
http://www.pha-exchange@kabissa.org.

Global Health Initiatives and Public Health Policy

R Brugha, Royal College of Surgeons in Ireland, Dublin, Ireland

© 2008 Elsevier Inc. All rights reserved.

Introduction

The first decade of the new millennium has seen a rapid and remarkable change in the global development assistance architecture with the establishment of new aid mechanisms and new global partnerships, tasked with the achievement of specific disease control goals. Some, such as the Global Fund to Fight AIDS, Tuberculosis and Malaria (GFATM) and the Global Alliance for Vaccines and Immunization (GAVI), cut across traditional bilateral donor–recipient country relationships and occupy territory previously held by normative multilateral agencies. Others, which some commentators include under the umbrella term Global Health Initiatives (GHIs), are new disease-focused initiatives launched by longstanding multilateral and bilateral donors. The latter include the World Bank Multi-Country AIDS Program (MAP) and the U.S. President's Emergency Plan for AIDS Relief (PEPFAR).

In many ways, GHIs epitomize the cognitive, spatial, and temporal dimensions of globalization (Lee et al., 2002; Buse et al., 2005): New ideas and values are disseminated at a global level, for example, the value of adapting business models to fight global disease threats. Models for global action transcend state boundaries, and these new initiatives evolve rapidly. Some of the new Global Public Private Partnership entities, such as GFATM and GAVI, have introduced genuinely new forms of governance at global and country levels, and have facilitated and provided mechanisms for the empowerment of old and new actors in the global health arena – civil society and the private for profit sectors. The scale of funds channeled through these new global entities for the control of specific diseases has profoundly altered the relationship between global and country actors, in that GHIs can shape or distort national policy agendas and supplant longstanding actors (Buse et al., 2005). In response, the normative multilateral agencies of the United Nations (UN) system have striven and sometimes struggled to redefine their roles, in what are more pluralistic policy environments at the global and country levels (Organisation for Economic Cooperation and Development, 2004; Global Task Team, 2005; Lele et al., 2005; Shakow, 2006).

The new GHIs with the greatest financial resources, established since 2000, were put in place because of a generally recognized need to accelerate the scale-up of control of the major communicable diseases. Urgency – their rationale – called for rapid top-down financing, and perhaps inevitably they have conflicted with donor harmonization and alignment principles (Anonymous, 2005; Organisation for Economic Cooperation and Development, 2005). Harmonization refers to donors adopting a common set of procedures for providing aid; alignment occurs where donors adopt the recipient country's (usually government) procedures for managing aid and ensure that aid supports country priorities. This article offers a definition of GHIs, places their recent growth in an historical perspective and in the context of an evolving aid architecture, and identifies areas of concern from a recipient country perspective. Rather than debate the appropriateness of these new mechanisms for achieving health and HIV global control goals, the focus is on a description of how the global policy arena has changed; the shifts in the roles, relationships, and influence of global actors; the effects of new on old models of governance at global and country levels; and the complexity and uncertainties that this new aid architecture has created for global and country policy makers.

What Are Global Health Initiatives?

Recent reviews have used the term global health initiative interchangeably with global health program and global health partnership (Lele et al., 2005). The World Health Organization (WHO) website, under global health initiative, states:

> An emerging and global trend in health is a focus on partnerships – alongside public–private partnerships there are also a number of global health initiatives ... (which) are typically programs targeted at specific diseases and are supposed to bring additional resources to health efforts (http://www.who.int/trade/glossary/story040/en/index.html).

From a WHO perspective, therefore, the term GHI is not synonymous with new partnerships involving private actors, although it indicates a close relationship and overlap between the terms. WHO and recent reviews by the World Bank (World Bank, 2004) included, as a GHI, the Global Fund, which is a Global Health Partnership that operates with a high degree of independence, overlapping with but lying outside of the multilateral UN system. They also included Global Health Partnerships, which are more closely aligned with and are hosted by UN agencies: Roll Back Malaria (RBM), The Stop TB Partnership, and The GAVI Alliance. GAVI, while hosted by UNICEF, has a governance structure that is more independent of the UN system than is RBM and Stop TB.

Two new and related features in the global health initiative arena, especially over the last 10 years, have been (1) the new actors involved, especially the for-profit private sector, and the much greater power and importance of some longer-standing actors such as philanthropic trusts and (2) the mushrooming of new forms of public–private partnership that have been established to deliver on disease-control goals. It is the literature on these new partnerships – notably from Buse, Caines, and Widdus – that has provided most of the lessons and insights on the evolving global health initiative arena at the global level (Buse and Harmer, 2007; see also the section titled 'New global aid and governance mechanisms' below). The Global Public Private Partnership for Health field is now huge. By 2003, over 90 partnerships had been identified by the Geneva-based Initiative on Public Private Partnerships for Health. Arguably, many of these in the categories of improvement of access to health products and global coordination mechanisms can be considered to be GHIs (**Table 1**).

The World Bank has defined global programs as:

> partnerships and related initiatives whose benefits are intended to cut across more than one region of the world and in which the partners reach explicit agreement, agree to establish a new (formal or informal) organization, generate new products or services, contribute dedicated resources to the program. (World Bank, 2004:2)

However, more recent reviews have included two new initiatives, from a multilateral and a bilateral donor, as GHIs: the World Bank's MAP and PEPFAR. Their inclusion gives primacy to country experiences of new initiatives as driving a global agenda at the country level, irrespective of their global governance structures. PEPFAR and MAP are largely focused on sub-Saharan Africa, where most concerns about the effects of GHIs have arisen. Such a country perspective points to the need for a definition that is not limited to how GHIs are governed.

From the perspective of country policy makers, a much more complex range of global actors have been seeking to exert policy influence at the country level since the start of the new millennium. The pressure points they use include significant scaling-up of resources for disease control through new channels alongside traditional aid mechanisms; global expertise, where the new business models of public–private partnerships compete with the approach of the traditional normative UN agencies; and performance-based funding and the channeling of significant resources directly to civil society groups at the country level, where aid in the 1980s and 1990s was predominantly to governments.

Together, these different examples and uses of the term give rise to the broad definition of a global health initiative: a blueprint for financing, resourcing, coordinating, and/or implementing disease control across at least several countries in more than one region of the world. The term initiative suggests an approach that is (or purports to be) new, and blueprint implies a common approach that is applied across a range of different country and regional contexts. Defining a global initiative by its functions, rather than by its governance structure, makes for a widely inclusive definition.

Table 1 Global public private partnerships: Number by function

1. Product development	35
Partnerships involved in the discovery and/or development of new drugs, vaccines, or other health products addressing neglected diseases and conditions in low- and middle-income countries	
2. Improvement of access to health products	26
Collaborations focused on improving access and/or increasing the distribution of currently available drugs, vaccines, or other health products addressing neglected diseases and conditions in low- and middle-income countries. Can involve long-term donations, discounted, subsidized, or negotiated pricing on products	
3. Global coordination mechanism	12
Alliances serving as a mechanism for coordinating multiple efforts to ensure the success of global health goals, often for a particular disease/condition and involving some combination of the other approaches such as product development, increasing product access, health service strengthening, advocacy, education, research, regulation, and quality assurance	
4. Health services strengthening	9
Partnerships involved in improving the infrastructures or systems for delivery of health services in low- and middle-income countries. Can be international, national, regional, district, or community level and can include employer/workplace initiatives	
5. Public advocacy, education, and research	15
Collaborations focused on advocacy, education, or research around health issues predominately affecting poor populations in low- and middle-income countries. This includes fund raising, social mobilization, and social marketing efforts	
6. Regulation and quality assurance	3
Initiatives working toward improving the regulatory environment and product quality, appropriate use of and access to effective health products addressing neglected diseases and conditions in low- and middle-income countries	

Source: IPPPH (http://www.globalforumhealth.org/site/003_The%2010%2090%20gap/004_Initiatives%20&%20networks/004_IPPPH.php).

Global Fund and GAVI are (or claim to be) solely financing entities, whereas RBM and Stop TB have very broad remits to achieve their disease-specific aims, extending from raising funds to coordinating country-level implementation. **Figure 1** and **Table 2** illustrate how the concept includes initiatives that originate in and are driven by traditional multilateral and bilateral agencies, as well as new entities with hybrid governance structures, which usually include a strong voice for civil society and their philanthropic donors. The figure also illustrates the range of initiatives (actors), new and old, and the complexity of the global aid architecture faced by country-level policy makers. The structural, contextual factors that influence and determine global and thereby national health policy have been radically transformed in less than a decade.

Toward Coordinated Development Assistance Mechanisms

The bulk of development agency funding for health in developing countries up to the early 1990s came chiefly from two sources: From the World Bank in the form of loans and credits and through earmarked support from bilateral donor countries to time-limited projects and programs. These were vertical mechanisms, utilizing donor-specific planning, management, monitoring, and reporting systems (Cassels and Janovsky, 1998). By the mid 1990s, there was increasing recognition, especially among northern European bilateral donors and key individuals in WHO, that the uncoordinated and fragmented nature of development assistance was an obstacle to coherent country-led policy making and strengthening

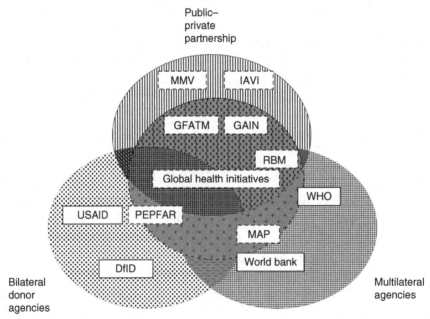

Figure 1 Selected global health initiatives by organizational type.

Table 2 Examples of selected global health initiatives by organizational type

Bilateral agencies	DfID (UK Department for International Development)
	USAID (United States Agency for International Development)
Multilateral agencies	WHO (World Health Organization)
	World Bank
Global Health Initiatives (public–private partnerships)	GFATM (Global Fund to Fight AIDS, Tuberculosis and Malaria)
	GAIN (Global Alliance for Improved Nutrition)
Global Health Initiatives (multilateral agencies)	WHO RBM (Roll Back Malaria)
	World Bank MAP (Multi-country AIDS Program)
Global Health Initiatives (bilateral agencies)	GFATM (Global Fund to Fight AIDS, Tuberculosis and Malaria)
	PEPFAR (US President's Emergency Plan for AIDS Relief)
Product development	MMV (Medicines for Malaria Venture)
Public–private partnerships	International AIDS Vaccine Initiative

of health systems. Concerns were expressed that the potential benefits of increased resources could be lost through lack of aid coordination, especially if – as described by Buse and Walt (1997) – donor initiatives were an unruly mélange.

From 1997, some (mainly European) donors began to shift from ear-marked funding to supporting the whole health sector in coordinated Sector Wide Approaches (SWAps), where donor and government funds are put into a common pool (Cassels and Janovsky, 1998). SWAps aim to forge coordinated planning, management, and reporting systems, under the stewardship of recipient governments. By 2000, health SWAps had been started or established in 22 countries worldwide, 19 of which were in Africa. After 2000, some European donors began to shift funds out of sector-specific SWAps to provide direct budget support to developing country governments. A parallel and largely compatible development, under the auspices of the World Bank, was the development and funding of Poverty Reduction Strategy Plans as part of the Highly Indebted Poor Country (HIPC) Initiative.

SWAps also contributed to the emergence of new processes for prioritizing and allocating the pooled funds of governments and bilateral donors. Partners in the SWAp meet annually or biannually, typically for periods of 1–3 weeks, to reach consensus on health sector priorities. However, these were new processes and new relationships among the same sets of policy actors. Some major donors (notably the United States) have been constrained by their agency rules from contributing funds to common pools, where accountability for – and attribution of outcomes to – specific donor funds would no longer be possible. There were efforts to engage these donors and bring on-board new country actors, notably faith-based and other civil society umbrella bodies, at annual health sector reviews. However, these agencies have often not had a seat at the table where the inner circle or elites, comprising government and SWAp donors, negotiated how pooled funds would be utilized and by implication which elements of the government's health policies would be implemented.

New Global Aid and Governance Mechanisms

Global development governance structures remained relatively stable up to the early 1990s, with the WHO as the normative technical and the lead global health agency. The publication of the World Bank's 1993 World Development Report was a seminal event. It heralded a period of dominance of the Bank over WHO in global health development policy making and, crucially, challenged the accepted preeminence of the public sector, in that it recommended a much greater role for the private sector. The appointment of Brundtland to head the WHO in 1998, following WHO's nadir under the direction of Nakajima, coincided with the establishment of new Global Health Partnerships, including Roll Back Malaria (RBM) in 1998 and the Stop TB Partnership in 1999. Rather than attempt to resist the tectonic shift in global health governance, Brundtland's strategic response was to commit WHO to be "more innovative in creating influential partnerships ... (because the) broad health agenda is too big for WHO alone" (Brundtland, 1999).

Global Health Partnerships (GHPs) represent a radical shift in global governance away from dominance by multilateral (UN) agencies and their member governments of the global health agenda. They mushroomed around 1998–2002, with an average of approximately 12 new partnerships annually (see **Figure 2**). Some of the large GHPs include representatives of philanthropic trusts and for-profit and nonprofit private sector actors on their governing boards, reflecting the growing role of these sectors in globalized approaches to addressing global health problems. Partnerships can be located within longstanding multilateral agencies, such as WHO and UNICEF, while – as in the case of GAVI – maintaining strong links to philanthropic trusts and the commercial private sector. There is also the Global Fund, within which all of the longstanding actors and other new voices (NGOs and representatives of people living with diseases) have struggled for influence. Donor and recipient country government representatives together form a majority of seats on the governing boards of GFATM and GAVI, two of the most influential GHPs. The traditional multilateral agencies (WHO, World Bank, and UNICEF) are represented but only have a minority voice. Power to influence the direction of global health policies has become distributed among a broader range of actors; some of these – notably civil society members of governing boards – often represent looser networks or interest groups, rather than institutions.

Buse and Walt (2000a, 2000b) provided one of the earliest and most systematic conceptual analyses of public–private partnerships as new global governance entities. Recent reviews have concluded that:

> the main concerns about Global Health Partnership institutional issues at the global level are generally amenable to relatively straightforward solutions ... (including) greater transparency, more appropriate partner representation on governing bodies, and business approaches.
> (Caines *et al.*, 2004)

GAVI, launched in late 1999, was the first of the new GHPs to disburse large amounts of funds to countries

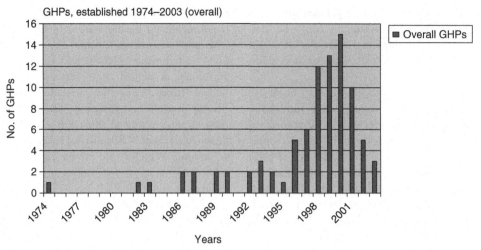

Figure 2 The annual number of new Global Health Partnerships, 1974–2003. Source: IPPPH (http://www.globalforumhealth.org/site/003_The%2010%2090%20gap/004_Initiatives%20&%20networks/004_IPPPH.php).

on a global scale, with the potential of affecting (positively and/or negatively) countries' health systems beyond their intended goals of improving immunization coverage (Stillman and Bennett, 2005). However, the most visible and transparent of all the GHIs is the Global Fund. GFATM's launch in January 2002 followed an 18-month period of high-level meetings, behind-the-scenes negotiations, and contestation over the focus and approach of a new mechanism to finance disease control in endemic countries, which would operationalize the commitment made by the G8 political leaders at Okinawa in July 2000. The attention of the G8 leaders was seen as an opportunity to be seized for pushing disease control in poor countries up on the global agenda; this new global initiative promised to be the vehicle to achieve this. However, the apparent consensus at the announcement of the Global Fund in Geneva in June 2001 masked a struggle for power over who would have access to funds and whether the Fund would use existing or establish new mechanisms for channeling funds.

Caines (2005) has summarized the attractiveness of GHIs to some stakeholders, especially donors. They offer opportunities to:

> channel resources into politically high profile areas; raise the profile of neglected issues and, in some cases, lead policy; attract new partners (e.g., the private sector) into the global fight against specific diseases; leverage additional funds and diversify the donor base; provide a means of supporting global public goods, secure substantial economies of scale (e.g., in drug procurement); and support a more coordinated international and national response by pooling resources to enhance aid effectiveness.
>
> (Caines, 2005)

Donors prefer these new channels because of a perception of poor past performance by UN agencies and the belief (or hope) that these new mechanisms will be more efficient (Caines et al., 2004). Global health initiatives also have the capacity to absorb and account for the use of large levels of development funds, easing the oversight burden on bilateral donors. They transfer the financial oversight and risk for how development funds are used (or misused) by countries away from the original donors and on to these initiatives.

The greater complexity in the global governance and aid architecture since 2000 and the consequent effects on countries has been exemplified in the efforts to scale up antiretroviral treatment in sub-Saharan Africa. WHO and UNAIDS continue to be the normative UN multilateral agencies with responsibility for coordinating global HIV/AIDS control policy and providing support to countries. In December 2003, the WHO launched its 3 by 5 initiative – 3 million people in poor and transitional countries who need antiretroviral treatment (ART) to be on ART by 2005. WHO's role in 3 by 5 was primarily to promote country partnerships, build national capacity, and provide technical guidance. Global Fund grants to countries would fund the strategy. A quotation from a senior Ministry of Health official in Tanzania in 2004 illustrates the effects of the crowded global arena and multiple initiatives on country-level policy priorities:

> Since the start of the (Global Fund) Tracking Study, so much has changed here in Tanzania. We had Clinton in August and September 2003, 3 by 5 landed like a bomb in December ... WHO have 40 people going around the world writing proposals for Round Four Global Fund ... they turn up here without any warning to write the ARV component of Round Four. Our CCM's priority was impact mitigation for orphans and vulnerable children ... the change in leadership in the UN and WHO have disturbed everything in Geneva for this round. Politically we will now only get money for care and treatment and this is wrong. Our priority in Tanzania is orphans.
>
> (Starling et al., 2005)

In 2005, the global health community was attempting to reach consensus on how to achieve greater coherence in division of responsibilities between global institutions and greater coordination of country-level activities. The Global Task Team (GTT) report (2005) on improving AIDS coordination among multilateral institutions and international donors called for a better understanding of the comparative advantages and roles of the different global institutions. The recommendation in a follow-up report was "to improve collaboration and division of labor, rather than major and radical reform of the overall architecture" (Shakow, 2006). Shakow highlighted and recommended a greater clarification in the functional division of roles between financing (Global Fund) and support to implementation (multilateral and bilateral agencies), with the World Bank straddling these functions and in particular undertaking strengthening of health systems. This can be seen as an effort to rationalize the global aid architecture, following a period of uncertainty that contributed to a struggle among global actors for turf.

A 2002–03 survey of donor practices in 11 recipient countries ranked the highest burdens for countries: Donor funds dictating country policies and priorities, difficulties with donor procedures, uncoordinated donor practices, excessive demands on time, and delays in disbursements (Organisation for Economic Cooperation and Development, 2003). These were the burdens that donors investing in SWAps were aiming to reduce. However, a limitation of donor harmonization initiatives up to 2005 was that they focused on the pratices of, and developed principles for, the traditional multilateral and bilateral donors, while neglecting the emerging Global health initiatives. The Three Ones principles were adopted at a UN meeting in April 2004, whereby donors and recipient governments committed to agreeing on, for each country, one HIV/AIDS Action Framework, one National AIDS Coordinating Authority, and one monitoring and evaluation system. In 2005, the focus of the harmonization agenda was widened to include GHIs – including Global Fund, MAP, and PEPFAR – because these were seen as, to a lesser or greater extent, a reversion to a project-oriented approach to planning and priority setting, where country policies were being dictated by powerful donors (Global Task Team, 2005; Anonymous, 2005).

The global health arena has changed profoundly over the last 6–10 years and what constitutes an appropriate international forum – which was once synonymous with the World Health Assembly, WHO, and other multilateral agencies of the UN system – is now contested. Competition for control of the UN system has been replaced by a resurgence in bilateral aid mechanisms (such as PEPFAR) plus powerful new global financial instruments that operate in parallel to multilateral agencies and compete for donor attention and resources. In 2005–07, representatives of recipient country governments, bilateral and multilateral agencies, and some of the large global partnerships (notably GFATM) focused on addressing the disruptive effects of some GHIs on donor alignment and harmonization efforts at the country level (Global Task Team, 2005; Anonymous 2005). Recommendations and experiences from the field contributed to the principles outlined in the 2005 Paris Declaration on Aid Effectiveness (Organisation for Economic Cooperation and Development, 2005). The consequences for health policy making in countries of a more complex set of global actors, each with its set of agendas and expectations, can be profound. Some of the few recent country studies on GHIs have reported that the level of resources and expectations that GHIs bring to the control of specific diseases are diverting health workers away from other health and health systems' priorities (Stillman and Bennett, 2005).

The Effects of Global Health Initiatives on Country Policy Making

The evidence in 2007 of the effects of Global health initiatives on recipient countries is patchy. The few available studies, some of which are found on GFATM's library website, have largely relied on interviews with relatively small numbers of global and country-level respondents: see Brugha *et al.* (2004), Stillman and Bennett (2005), and Wilkinson *et al.* (2006). The rapid evolution of the GHI arena has made tracking and reporting on it difficult in that new initiatives, notably GFATM, are adept at learning lessons and adapting their systems. Findings can rapidly become dated and new problems experienced by recipient countries are superimposed on and submerge earlier ones. Findings are often context-specific, with contrasting experiences of the same initiative across different countries. However, some early problems have been refractory and similar findings have been replicated in country studies from 2003 to early 2006. **Figure 3** provides a framework for considering the possible effects of GHIs on country policies and systems, where the earmarking of funds for specific disease can distort national policy priorities, distract attention from strengthening crosscutting systems, and promote parallel programs.

Table 3 summarizes findings from recent studies, focusing on what country respondents perceived to be the effects of GHIs on country policy and planning processes, notably on country ownership, alignment of donor support with country policies, and the greater opportunities for nongovernment actors that some of these initiatives bring. Neither the issues nor the cited studies can be exhaustive, given the rapid evolution in the global health initiative arena and the gray literature nature of most studies. Inevitably – given the importance, visibility, and transparency of the Global Fund and because the initiative started 2 years earlier than (for example) PEPFAR – the majority of the cited findings

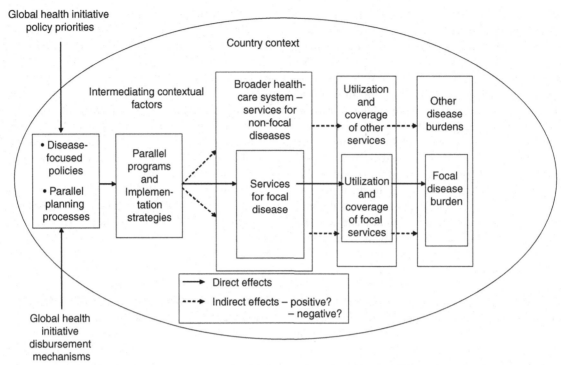

Figure 3 System-wide effects of global health initiatives. Adapted from Bennett S and Fairbank (2003) *The System-wide Effects of the Global Fund to Fight AIDS, Tuberculosis and Malaria: A Conceptual Framework*. Abt Associates Inc. Bethesda, MD: Partners for Health Reformplus. http://www.phrplus.org/Pubs/Tech031_find.pdf (accessed February 2008).

relate to GFATM. Some country-level effects are a re-presentation of issues reported decades earlier – around project approaches and parallel systems – while other effects are genuinely revolutionary and widely seen as positive. For example, both the Global Fund and PEPFAR have disbursed significant funds to civil society. However, their effects on national policy making have been quite different, reflecting different philosophies: PEPFAR is an illustration of the U.S. suspicion of government-led efforts, in that it bypasses government channels in disbursing funds to civil society groups, whereas GFATM has been grasped by civil society interest groups as an opportunity to become involved and shape national policy responses to HIV/AIDS.

It is the confluence of the failure of earlier donor efforts to adequately respond to HIV/AIDS and the emergence of these new models that has enabled GFATM to have what many commentators see as its most positive effect, which is to make policy making more pluralistic at the global and country levels (Buse *et al.*, 2005). In aid-recipient countries, national AIDS councils, and new governance structures such as GFATM country coordination mechanisms (the latter, unlike the former, attract significant funds) have enabled a wider set of actors to engage in and influence national policy. These structures and struggles for power reflect what has been happening at the global level. They also reflect the connectedness between global and national spheres of action, linking civil society as well as other actors across these levels in influencing policy.

Other effects, such as competition for scarce human resources, highlight intrinsic weaknesses in global governance, which extend beyond GHIs, due to the unwillingness of global policy makers to curb the migration of expensively trained staff from poor to wealthy countries. A common recommendation across most reviews of the global initiative terrain is for "donors to invest more in health system strengthening to complement resources brought in by GHPs" (Caines *et al.*, 2004), in view of the lack of synergies and lack of coordination in the effects of new and longstanding aid mechanisms on health systems. Given the anecdotal nature of country findings to date, there is clearly a need for investment by donors to obtain better evidence to substantiate, explore, or help to discount early fears about likely negative effects of GHIs on country systems. More importantly, there is a need for evidence to inform global and country policy makers on how to achieve greater coherence between aid mechanisms (Bennett *et al.*, 2006).

Conclusion

Polarization in disease control approaches reflects passionate beliefs – and sometimes different ideologies and political value systems – that have long competed for control of

Table 3 Effects of global health initiatives on country policy processes

Issues	Findings and sources
1. Country ownership	• GFATM and GAVI were initially perceived as devised in the north but offering funds that poor countries could not forego.[a,b] Perceptions differed by country and by type of respondent: GFATM seen as more country-owned than other donor funds in Zambia,[b] because countries could decide what to apply for,[b,h] and because it put countries, especially civil society, in the driver's seat.[e] • Where there was lack of ownership, it was due to GFATM's insistence on its own procedures in Malawi,[f] because rapid evolution in Global Health Initiative (GHI) processes prevented new systems bedding down at country level,[b] and lack of ownership at subnational levels because tight deadlines and short turn-around time prevented national consultation with districts and regions in Ethiopia[f]
2. Alignment with country policies, priorities, and strategic plans	• There was a perception early on that GFATM and GAVI had forced countries to revert to more top-down globally driven policy and priority setting.[a,b] Later studies reported improving alignment between GFATM-supported programs and national priorities[f] • MAP failed to engage high-level political support at the country level; a failure by countries to prioritize appropriate control activities within national HIV/AIDS control strategic plans was an impediment to MAP aligning with these plans[d] • In contrast to the major HIV/AIDS GHIs, smaller GHPs that focused on neglected diseases – onchocerciasis, filariasis, and trachoma – were perceived at the country level to be working well and addressing country priorities[c]
3. Alignment with country systems: • Planning	• GFATM requested countries to utilize an existing country partnership. However, the three-disease focus meant that countries applying for support for malaria as well as HIV/AIDS control needed to establish new partnerships – country coordination mechanisms (CCMs) – which duplicated the activities of the pre-existing national AIDS councils.[b] This reflected "weak coordination between GFATM and the Bank both at strategic institutional level and at the level of individual countries"[e]
• Management	• Most GHPs seen as wanting their own coordination mechanism and procedures, preventing countries from realizing potential economies of scale and integration across similar programs.[e,g] In contrast, countries applying for GAVI support were able to adapt and use existing Immunisation Coordination Committees[a]
• Management	• Failure to engage Ministry of Finance at an early stage – and in Tanzania riding roughshod over government systems – accounted for early obstacles to GFATM disbursement.[b] Countries had to accept new financial oversight systems – Local Fund Agents – even if they had established, functioning audit systems[b,f]
• Reporting	• In 2005, the GFATM round system was still entrenching a project approach,[h] vertical approaches[f] and parallel systems,[g] undermining efforts to incorporate support into coordinated national strategic planning, management, monitoring, and reporting systems.[h] In late 2006, the GFATM Board was taking on board recommendations of two independent 2005 studies[g,h] to show greater flexibility and allow countries with proven systems and good track records to use these systems to manage Global Fund grants
4. Public–private partnerships and governance	• GFATM seen as more effective than other donors in diversifying stakeholder participation and making involvement of civil society a reality, through enabling NGOs to gain direct access to financial resources.[b,e,h] New NGO umbrella bodies formed in response to the need for representation on CCMs. Private sector participation in planning was providing an opportunity for new collaborations and helping to overcome a long history of mistrust between the sectors[f] • In some countries (e.g., Uganda), competition between government and NGOs was a problem; in others (Zambia), government was willing to have a NGO and a faith-based body as Principle Recipients responsible for managing GFATM funds[b] • Weak CCM governance, ineffective representation of different constituencies, and dominance by government[b] were still a chronic and refractory problem across several countries in late 2005[h]

[a]Brugha R, Walt G, and Starling M (2002) GAVI, the first steps: lessons for the Global Fund. *Lancet* 359: 435–438.
[b]Brugha R, Donoghue M, Starling M, *et al.* (2004) The Global Fund: managing great expectations. *Lancet* 364: 95–100.
[c]Caines K and Lush L (2004) Impact of Public-Private Partnerships Addressing Access to Pharmaceuticals in Low and Middle Income Countries: A Synthesis Report from Studies in Botswana, Sri Lanka, Uganda and Zambia. Geneva: Initiative on Public Private Partnerships for Health.
[d]World Bank (2005) *Improving the Effectiveness of HIV/AIDS Assistance, An OED Evaluation of the World Bank's Assistance for HIV/AIDS Control.* Washington, DC: The World Bank. http://www.worldbank.org/oed/aids/docs/report/hiv_complete-report.pdf (accessed February 2008).
[e]Lele U, Ridker R, and Upadhyay J (2005) Health System Capacities in Developing Countries and Global Health Initiatives On Communicable Diseases. Background paper prepared for the International Task Force on Global Public Goods. April 22, 2005. http://www.umalele.org/publications/health_system_capacities.pdf (accessed November 2007).
[f]Stillman K and Bennett S (2005) *Systemwide Effects of the Global Fund: Interim Findings from Three Country Studies.* September 2005. Bethesda, MD: PHRPlus, Abt Associates. http://www.phrplus.org/Pubs/Tech080_fin.pdf (accessed November 2007).
[g]McKinsey & Company (2005) *Global Health Partnerships: Assessing Country Consequences.* http://www.hlfhealthmdgs.org/Documents/GatesGHPNov2005.pdf (accessed November 2007).
[h]Wilkinson D, Brugha R, Hewitt S, *et al.* (2006) *Assessment of the Proposal Development and Review Process of the Global Fund to Fight AIDS, Tuberculosis and Malaria: Assessment Report.* February 2006. Euro Health Group. http://www.theglobalfund.org/en/files/links_resources/library/studies/integrated_evaluations/EHG_Final_Report_Executive_Summary.pdf (accessed November 2007).

the global health arena. These factors are intertwined: European country donors tend to promote coordinated public sector aid models; the United States and Japan opt for private-sector models expressed through bilateral aid programs. However, the global aid arena is now different from what it was throughout the twentieth century in at least two respects. Firstly, whereas in the past global approaches tended to oscillate between selective, vertical disease control and horizontal, comprehensive approaches, now selective and comprehensive models are being implemented in parallel in aid-recipient countries. This hugely complicates the working lives of national policy makers and program managers in that the new global financing instruments seek to influence national policies in relation to the introduction of new commodities (GAVI) and types of control strategies (PEPFAR); most, at least in their early years, have tried to impose parallel systems and processes for strategic planning, management, and reporting.

Secondly, the array of actors at the global and country levels is broader and their relationships are less clear. Powerful donors represent and finance disease control through a range of different aid mechanisms. The policy arena at both levels is more pluralistic, especially since the advent of organized and vocal civil society representative bodies. There is overlap and competition – for resources and for control of the policy agenda – between global entities (WHO and GFATM) and between country bodies (National AIDS Councils and GFATM Country Coordination Mechanisms). However, policy elites can still transcend organizational boundaries. Individuals at the global and country levels represent the interests of different stakeholders. A UNICEF representative sitting on a country interagency coordination committee can be seen as supporting country-level decision making, representing his or her agency and representing GAVI, which is housed in UNICEF. Interests may conflict, for example in deciding on the introduction of a new and expensive vaccine. Consequently, the resultant aid and development architecture has become almost unmanageably complex for recipient countries, as governments and their partners have to negotiate and manage relationships with (Caines *et al.*, 2004):

- many bilateral donors funding individual programs and standalone projects;
- donors channeling funds through common funding mechanisms, including SWAps, poverty action funds, and budget support;
- powerful new global partnerships, notably Global Fund and GAVI, as well as a wide variety of more focused drug access partnerships;
- new HIV/AIDS global health initiatives (MAP and PEPFAR), parallel to existing programs sometimes funded by the same donors – i.e., World Bank loans and USAID bilateral funding;

- normative multilateral UN agencies – closely linked with Global Health Partnerships such as RBM, Stop TB, and UNAIDS – all with expectations of engaging intensively with recipient governments, despite their bringing limited funds.

The findings from once-off studies may misrepresent the nature and effects of GHIs, which evolve over time. An entity such as the Global Fund can be experienced as a top-down imposition of global approaches in its early years and yet be seen as more country-owned in many respects in studies conducted in 2004–05, as country stakeholders learn to work the new systems (see **Table 3**). Distinctions between different GHIs may become apparent over time, between those that are willing to adapt their procedures to fit with country systems and those that prioritize their needs for attribution so as to serve the interests of northern hemisphere politicians. The latter may be seen as distorting country policy making by using performance-based approaches to put pressure on countries to pursue low-hanging fruit and focus on more easily reached target populations. Empirical cross-country studies, including policy analyses, are needed to track, assess, and obtain a pluralistic perspective on their effects on national policy making, as GHIs evolve and adapt their approaches in the coming years.

Citations

Anonymous (2005) *Best Practice Principles for Global Health Partnership Activities at Country Level*. Paris 14–15 November 2005. http://www.hlfhealthmdgs.org/Documents/GlobalHealthPartnerships.pdf (accessed November 2007).

Bennett S and Fairbank A (2006) *The System-wide Effects of the Global Fund to Fight AIDS, Tuberculosis and Malaria: A Conceptual Framework*. Abt Associates Inc: Bethesda, MD Partners for Health Reformplus. http://www.phrplus.org/Pubs/Tech031_fin.pdf (accessed February 2008).

Brugha R, Donoghue M, Starling M, et al. (2004) The Global Fund: managing great expectations. *Lancet* 364: 95–100.

Brugha R, Walt G, and Starling M (2002) GAVI, the first steps: lessons for the Global Fund. *Lancet* 359: 435–438.

Brundtland GH (1999) WHO – *The Way Ahead*. Statement by the Director-General to the 103rd Session of the Executive Board. Geneva, Switzerland: World Health Organization.

Buse K and Harmer A (2007) Seven habits of highly effective global public-private health partnerships: Practice and potential. *Social Science and Medicine* 64(2): 259–271.

Buse K and Walt G (1997) An unruly melange? Coordinating external resources to the health sector: A review. *Social Science and Medicine* 45(3): 449–463.

Buse K and Walt G (2000a) Global public-private partnerships: Part I – A new development in health? *Bulletin of the World Health Organization* 78(4): 549–561.

Buse K and Walt G (2000b) Global public-private partnerships: Part II – What are the health issues for global governance? *Bulletin of the World Health Organization* 78(5): 699–709.

Buse K, Mays N, and Walt G (2005) *Making Health Policy*. Maidenhead, UK: Open University Press.

Caines K (2005) *Background Paper: Key Evidence from Major Studies of Selected Global Health Partnerships*. Geneva, Switzerland: High Level Forum, Working Group on GHPs.

Caines K and Lush L (2004) *Impact of Public-Private Partnerships Addressing Access to Pharmaceuticals in Low and Middle Income Countries: A Synthesis Report from Studies in Botswana, Sri Lanka, Uganda and Zambia*. Geneva, Switzerland: Initiative on Public Private Partnerships for Health.
Caines K, Buse K, Carlson C, et al. (2004) *Assessing the Impact of Global Health Partnerships*. London: DfID Resource Centre.
Cassels A and Janovsky K (1998) Better health in developing countries: Are sector-wide approaches the way of the future. *Lancet* 352: 1777–1779.
Global Task Team (2005) *Global Task Team on Improving AIDS Coordination Among Multilateral Institutions and International Donors. Final Report*. 14 June 2005.
Lee K, Buse K, and Fustukian S (2002) An introduction to global health policy. In: Lee K, Buse K and Fustukian S (eds.) *Health Policy in a Globalising World*. Cambridge, UK: Cambridge University Press.
Lele U, Ridker R, and Upadhyay J (2005) *Health System Capacities in Developing Countries and Global Health Initiatives On Communicable Diseases*. Background paper prepared for the International Task Force on Global Public Goods. April 22 2005. http://www.umalele.org/publications/health_system_capacities.pdf (accessed November 2007).
McKinsey & Company (2005) *Global Health Partnerships: Assessing Country Consequences*. http://www.hlfhealthmdgs.org/Documents/GatesGHPNov2005.pdf (accessed November 2007).
Organisation for Economic Cooperation and Development (2003) *DAC Guidelines and Reference Series, 'Harmonising Donor Practices for Effective Aid Delivery'*. Paris, France: Organisation for Economic Cooperation and Development. http://www.oecd.org/dateoecd/o/48/20896122.pdf (accessed February 2008).
Organisation for Economic Cooperation and Development (2005) *Paris Declaration on Aid Effectiveness. Ownership, Harmonization, Alignment, Results and Mutual Accountability*. High Level Forum, Paris, February 28 – March 2 2005. Organisation for Economic Cooperation and Development. http://www.oecd.org/dataoecd/11/41/34428351.pdf (accessed November 2007).
Shakow A (2006) *Global Fund – World Bank HIV/AIDS Programs*. Comparative advantage study. January 19, 2006. http://www.hlfhealthmdgs.org/ReportGHPWorkingGroup28SepOS.doc.
Starling M, Brugha R, and Walt G (2005) *Global Fund Tracking Study, Tanzania Country Report*. London School of Hygiene and Tropical Medicine (LSHTM).
Stillman K and Bennett S (2005) *Systemwide Effects of the Global Fund: Interim Findings from Three Country Studies*. September 2005. Bethesda, MD: PHRPlus, Abt Associates. http://www.phrplus.org/Pubs/Tech080_fin.pdf (accessed November 2007).
Wilkinson D, Brugha R, Hewitt S, et al. (2006) *Assessment of the Proposal Development and Review Process of the Global Fund to Fight AIDS, Tuberculosis and Malaria: Assessment Report*. February 2006. Euro Health Group. http://www.theglobalfund.org/en/files/links_resources/library/studies/integrated_evaluations/EHG_Final_Report_Executive_Summary.pdf (accessed November 2007).
World Bank (2004) *Addressing the Challenges of Globalization. An Independent Evaluation of the World Bank's Approach to Global Programs*. Washington, DC: The World Bank.

Further Reading

Reich M (ed.) (2002) *Public-Private Partnerships for Public Health*. Cambridge, MA: Harvard Center for Population and Development Studies.

Relevant Websites

http://www.theglobalfund.org/en/links_resources/library/integrated_evaluations/ – Global Fund to Fight AIDS, Tuberculosis and Malaria. GFATM's resource library contains copies of internal and independent evaluations.
http://www.hlfhealthmdgs.org/Documents – Global HIV/AIDS Initiatives Network. High Level Forums (HLF) for the Millennium Development Goals (MDGs), with guidelines for Global Health Partnerships.
http://www.ghin.lshtm.ac.uk – Global HIV/AIDS Initiatives Research Network.
http://www.oecd.org/dataoecd/11/41/34428351.pdf – Organisation for Economic Cooperation and Development, Paris Declaration on Aid Effectiveness: Ownership, Harmonization, Alignment, Results and Mutual Accountability.
http://www.phrplus.org/swef.php – System-Wide Effects of the Fund.
http://www.worldbank.org/oed – The World Bank, with overviews of global health partnerships and information on its Multi-country AIDS Program (MAP).

Corruption and the Consequences for Public Health

T Vian, Boston University School of Public Health, Boston, MA, USA

© 2008 Elsevier Inc. All rights reserved.

Corruption is a huge challenge to achieving health goals. When public officials do not act in the public interest but instead use their positions to benefit themselves and their families, friends, or associates, we lose not only financial resources but hope and trust as well. It is a social, political, and economic problem that threatens international development, human rights, and peaceful social existence.

Corruption is a crime of calculation, relying on opportunity as well as inclination. Weak government institutions, lack of citizen involvement in public decisions, too much discretion in the hands of government officials, as well as eroding public values and moral standards, social and personal pressures, poverty, and inequality, all help create an environment where corruption can take hold and grow. These factors also show how corruption can be prevented: by increasing transparency and accountability in government performance, empowering citizens and giving them effective choices, altering economic incentives, promoting ethical standards, and changing attitudes to bring new hope.

In the health sector, corruption can take many forms depending on the structure of the health system and government. This article discusses types of corruption and their effects on health systems and outcomes. Prevention strategies are also discussed, giving examples from countries that have begun to tackle this important problem.

What Is Corruption?

Corruption has been defined as "abuse of public roles or resources, or use of illegitimate forms of political influence by public or private parties" (Johnston, 1997). In more simple terms, corruption is the misuse of office for personal gain (Klitgaard *et al.*, 2000). Corruption occurs when a government agent given authority to carry out the goals of a public institution instead uses his or her power and position to further personal interests. **Table 1** provides a summary of some of the common types of corruption that can be found in the health sector, while **Table 2** provides categories that are useful to distinguish the seriousness of the problem and to suggest the level at which interventions are needed.

Another way to look at corruption is from the viewpoint of the decision maker or stakeholder. Major stakeholders in health-care systems include patients and their families, providers, payers, government regulators, and suppliers. **Figure 1** shows the different types of abuses that can occur in the production and delivery of health-care services as these different stakeholders interact.

Corruption can be carried out alone, as with a government official who steals medical equipment or embezzles user fee revenues from a drug revolving fund. Or it may involve other parties, either private (a distributor offering a bribe to get a drug added to the government reimbursement list) or governmental (higher-level officials who require kickbacks from medical personnel to retain their jobs). Corruption can even be entirely private, as when company officials who are entrusted with the power to make decisions in the best interest of stockholders and staff instead drain the assets of the company to line their own pockets.

While most people would say corruption is 'wrong,' it is not always illegal. For example, to ensure that doctors do not put financial profit ahead of patient well-being, some countries tightly regulate physician conflict of interest in ownership of ancillary services such as laboratories and medical device companies, whereas other countries do not.

Even within a given country, not everyone will agree on the nature of corruption. In the United States, members of Food and Drug Administration advisory committees for drug approval routinely have financial ties to pharmaceutical companies: According to an analysis of committee records from 2000, in 55% of meetings, half or more of the advisors had conflicts of interest (Angell, 2004). This is not considered corruption, even though such ties have been shown to influence government decision making.

Another example is the practice of informal payments, which are unofficial payments given to government medical personnel for services that are supposed to be provided free of charge at point of delivery. These workers are already paid by the government to provide services, and citizens are entitled by law to free care in government facilities: thus, it seems clear that any additional 'unofficial' payments in exchange for services are bribes. But what if the amount given is intended as a gift, to express gratitude to a doctor who saved a patient's life or delivered a healthy new baby? Or what if the government neglects to pay its medical workers a living wage, forcing them to rely on the informal payments as a coping mechanism? What if a health worker has purchased drugs herself, from a private pharmacy, because the public supply system isn't working, and is asking patients to reimburse her for this service? In these cases, the intention of informal payments doesn't seem to fit our definition of corruption as abuse of public power for private gain. Economists note that informal payments may even serve a positive function, encouraging personnel not to abandon their public sector jobs for more lucrative employment. At the same time, such an unregulated, informal system operating within the public health structure cannot ensure that very poor and vulnerable populations will be protected, and may lead to inequality of access and quality of care.

The line between gifts and bribes, and the use of contacts or exchange of favors, are two other issues that make it hard to define corruption across cultures. Researchers have noted the cultural and historical importance of gift and favor exchanges to create webs of mutual obligation. In Albania, use of personal connections can sometimes help a person avoid having to make an informal payment to get medical services (Vian and Burak, 2005). Relationships are seen as an important resource in Africa as well.

Effects of Corruption on Health

Corruption has financial, economic, and social costs in all countries, but it is especially damaging in low-income countries because of its effects on development. On a macroeconomic level, corruption limits economic growth, since private firms see corruption as adding uncertainty and risk to their investment decisions. Although a particular multinational corporation might stand to gain by bribing an official to win a contract or tax break, Paulo Mauro's analysis of economic data from 68 countries suggests, that corruption creates an environment that reduces

Table 1 Types of corruption in the health sector

Area or process	Types of corruption and problems	Results
Construction and rehabilitation of health facilities	• Bribes, kickbacks, and political considerations influencing the contracting process • Contractors fail to perform and are not held accountable	• High-cost, low-quality facilities and construction work. Construction investments influenced by bribes may also lead to further waste if recurrent costs to operate facilities are not budgeted or inadequately financed • Location of facilities that does not correspond to need, resulting in inequities in access • Biased distribution of infrastructure favoring urban- and elite-focused services, high technology
Purchase of equipment and supplies, including drugs	• Bribes, kickbacks, and political considerations influence specifications and winners of bids • Collusion or bid rigging during procurement • Lack of incentives to choose low-cost and high-quality suppliers • Unethical drug promotion • Suppliers fail to deliver and are not held accountable	• High-cost, inappropriate, or duplicative drugs and equipment • Irrational prescribing • Inappropriate equipment located without consideration of true need • Substandard equipment and drugs • Inequities due to inadequate funds left to provide for all needs
Distribution and use of drugs and supplies in service delivery	• Theft (for personal use) or diversion (for private sector resale) of drugs and supplies at storage and distribution points • Sale of drugs or supplies that were supposed to be free	• Lower utilization • Patients do not get proper treatment • Patients must make informal payments to obtain drugs • Interruption of treatment or incomplete treatment, leading to development of antimicrobial resistance
Regulation of quality in products, services, facilities, and professionals	• Bribes to speed process or gain approval for drug registration, drug quality inspection, or certification of good manufacturing practices • Bribes or political considerations influence results of inspections or suppress findings • Biased application of sanitary regulations for restaurants, food production, and cosmetics • Biased application of accreditation, certification, or licensing procedures and standards	• Subtherapeutic or fake drugs allowed on market • Marginal suppliers are allowed to continue participating in bids, getting government work • Increased incidence of food poisoning • Spread of infectious and communicable diseases • Poor-quality facilities continue to function • Incompetent or fake professionals continue to practice
Human resources management	• Bribes to gain place in medical school or other preservice training • Bribes to obtain passing grades • Political influence, nepotism in selection of candidates for training opportunities or positions • Bribes or regular payoffs to obtain/maintain position in government health service or medical facilities	• Incompetent professionals practicing medicine or working in health professions • Loss of faith and freedom due to unfair system • Poor resource allocation decisions due to inaccurate health expenditure data (doesn't reflect payoffs to superiors, effectively a tax on salaries) • Increased informal payments, as health workers seek to finance required pay-offs to keep their job
Medical research	• Pseudo trials funded by drug companies that are really for marketing • Misunderstanding of informed consent and other issues of adequate standards in developing countries	• Violation of individual rights • Biases and inequities in research • Patients who receive unnecessary or harmful treatment
Financial management	• Embezzlement of budget allocation • Theft of user fee revenue • False recording of revenue to inflate or obscure financial position from stockholder or analysts (affects private health firms) • Billing or reimbursement fraud	• Reduced availability of public health programs and government medical services • Lower quality of care • Bankruptcy and loss of entrusted resources • Loss of state dollars to fraud
Service delivery	• Use of public facilities and equipment to see private patients • Diversion of patients to private practice or privately owned ancillary services	• Government loses value of investments without adequate compensation • Employees are not available to serve patients, leading to lower volume of services and unmet needs, and higher unit costs for health services actually delivered

Continued

Table 1 Continued

Area or process	Types of corruption and problems	Results
	• Utilization that is not medically indicated, in order to maximize income • Withholding of care that is medically indicated • Absenteeism • Informal payments required from patients for services that were supposed to be free of charge	• Reduced utilization of services by patients who cannot pay • Impoverishment as citizens use income, incur debt, and sell assets to pay for health care • Loss of citizen faith in government

Adapted from: Vian T (2005) The sectoral dimensions of corruption: Health care. In: Spector BI (ed.) *Fighting Corruption in Developing Countries*, pp. 45–46. Bloomfield, CT: Kumarian Press.

Table 2 Categories of corruption

- Grand corruption involves major embezzlement or exchange of resources such as bribes for advantages among elites at the highest levels of government and private industry. Considered serious due to scale of losses and because leaders are setting a bad example and eroding trust in government
- State capture happens when policies and laws meant to benefit the public good have instead been 'captured' (through bribes) and molded to favor private interests. Considered serious because it affects the rules of the game, creating systemic inequalities
- Vertical corruption indicates that multiple levels of government are colluding in corruption. Anticorruption strategies focused on hierarchical management tools (e.g., budgets or inventory systems) or limits on discretion may not be effective if corruption is vertical.
- Administrative corruption involves lower-level bureaucrats who demand bribes or speed money before performing their public duties. Sometimes called 'petty' corruption, this is considered less serious, but can be very visible and damaging to public morale

Sources: World Bank (2000) *Anticorruption in Transition: A Contribution to the Policy Debate*. Washington, DC: World Bank; USAID (2005) *USAID Anticorruption Strategy (PD-ACA-557)*. Washington, DC: USAID.

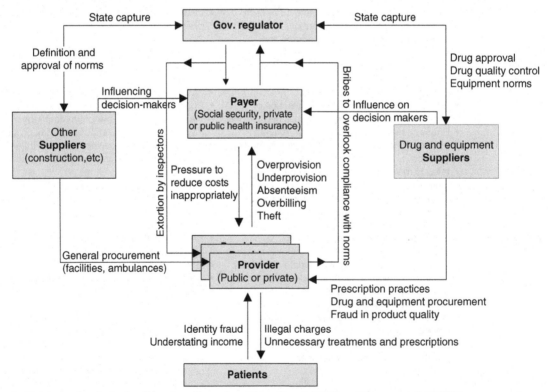

Figure 1 Five key actors in the health system. Reproduced from Savedoff WD and Hussmann K (2006) The causes of corruption in the health sector. In: Transparency International (ed.) *Global Corruption Report 2006*, p. 7. London: Pluto Press, with permission from Pluto Press.

overall magnitude of investment (Mauro, 1995). In turn, the lower economic growth results in less government revenue available for investment, including investment in the health sector.

Corruption also affects government choices in how to invest revenue, with corrupt governments more likely to invest in infrastructure-intensive sectors such as transport and military, where lucrative procurement contracts offer potential to extract bribes, rather than social sectors like health and education. Within the health sector, investments may also tend to favor construction of hospitals and purchase of expensive, high-tech equipment over primary health-care programs such as immunization and family planning, for the same reason.

Corruption in the health sector also has a direct negative effect on access and quality of patient care. As resources are drained from health budgets through embezzlement and procurement fraud, less funding is available to pay salaries and fund operations and maintenance, leading to demotivated staff, lower quality of care, and reduced service availability and use. Studies have shown that corruption has a significant, negative effect on health indicators such as infant and child mortality, even after adjusting for income, female education, health spending, and level of urbanization (Gupta et al., 2002). There is evidence that reducing corruption can improve health outcomes by increasing the effectiveness of public expenditures (Gupta et al., 2002).

A review of research in Eastern Europe and Central Asia found evidence that informal payments for care reduces access to services, especially for the poor, and causes delays in care-seeking behavior (Lewis, 2000). In Azerbaijan, studies have shown that about 35% of births in rural areas take place at home, mostly because of high charges for care in facilities where care was supposed to be free (World Bank, 2005). In Armenia, families are forced to sell livestock or assets, or borrow money from extended family and community members, in order to make the necessary informal payments to receive care.

Bribes to avoid government regulation of drugs and medicines clearly have adverse effects on health, as evidenced by incidents such as the dilution of vaccines in Uganda and the rising problem of counterfeit drugs in the world. Unregulated medicines that are of subtherapeutic value can contribute to the development of drug-resistant organisms and increase the threat of pandemic disease spread. In addition to fake drugs on the market, corruption can lead to shortages of drugs available in government facilities, due to theft and diversion to private pharmacies. This in turn leads to reduced utilization of public facilities. Procurement corruption can lead to inferior public infrastructure as well as increased prices paid for inputs, resulting in less money available for service provision.

Unethical drug promotion and physician conflict of interest can have negative effects on health outcomes as well. As estimated by Dr. Marcia Angell, former editor in chief of *The New England Journal of Medicine*, pharmaceutical companies spend about $54 billion each year on marketing to promote drugs (Angell, 2004), including industry-sponsored continuing education, drug information pamphlets and publications, and gifts and hospitality targeted to physicians. Companies also recruit doctors to serve as industry-paid consultants and speakers, sponsor clinical trials where physicians are paid to enroll patients, and provide 'unrestricted grants' to doctors, all of which help to align physicians' interests with those of the for-profit pharmaceutical companies and influence physician decision making. Interactions between physicians and the pharmaceutical industry can lead to nonrational prescribing (Wazana, 2000) and increased spending on medicines with little or no additional health benefit. Perverse incentives can endanger patients' health, as doctors enroll unqualified patients in trials or prescribe unnecessary and potentially harmful treatments in order to maximize profit.

Causes of Corruption

Strategies for prevention must address root causes. This requires some theoretical understanding about how corruption comes about. Two theories or models have been introduced to explain corruption. These include the rational choice model, which attempts to explain corruption from an economic systems point of view, and moral development theory, which examines how ethical value systems may contribute to corruption. Both models can help us to identify root causes of corruption and begin planning for prevention.

Rational Choice Model

As described by Klitgaard et al., (2000), the rational choice model assumes that people everywhere are motivated to pursue their own self-interest. Problems occur in government service, however, when the self-interest of the individual bureaucrat deviates from the public good that the institution is promoting. Where individual rewards of corruption are great, and the likelihood of being caught and punished is low, people are more likely to engage in corruption. Corruption prevention strategies therefore should try to change the equation by creating more advantages to act honestly and more disadvantages to acting corruptly. This might include higher salaries, more performance-based rewards, increased professionalism and codes of ethics, greater transparency, and penalties for corruption.

Moral Model

The moral model for explaining corruption assumes that people act corruptly because they don't understand what it means to be citizens or public servants or haven't been educated on professional values. Eroding public values and low moral consciousness create a vacuum in which corruption appears justified. Severe economic and political disruption, like what has occurred in post-communist Europe and Central Asia since 1991, can contribute to the problem by creating confusion over values: Capitalism suggests that 'everything has its price,' which seems to endorse aggressive pursuit of self-interest, even within government institutions (Miller *et al.*, 2001). Changing moral values such as increasing indifference toward the needs of others and a lack of personal sense of duty and social responsibility can make it more likely that public officials will misuse their power for personal gain. Under this model, strategies to prevent corruption might focus on citizenship education and development of shared ethical values, professional development, and promulgation of codes of ethical conduct.

Preventing Corruption

Experiences with anticorruption strategies are illustrated in **Table 3**. What are the common elements of these strategies, and why do they work? While the most effective anticorruption strategies are specifically adapted to the type of corruption and the context where it is occurring, we still can identify factors or 'mechanisms of action' that make an anticorruption strategy more effective. Five of these factors are discussed below, including transparency, accountability, discretion, management tools, and incentives.

Transparency

The first factor is transparency. Corruption is hard to measure because it is often illegal, and therefore hidden. Even in the case of actions that are widely practiced or commonly accepted, such as informal payments, there are few administrative records to measure the prevalence or scope of the problem. To combat corruption, therefore, we need to 'shine light in dark corners' and generate more information about what government is doing and what it is supposed to do. Transparency helps citizens to participate more in government by giving them needed information on which they can act or demand answers. Freedom of information acts have been adopted in many countries to help citizens gain access to information, and investigative journalism also plays a critical role in exposing areas vulnerable to corruption. But even more basic information strategies can work as well. Publishing price lists for services can help patients to understand the difference between official and unofficial services, while public dissemination of budget information can help prevent diversion of funds. Hospital 'report cards' measuring important statistics about patient care and access, and household expenditure surveys that document out-of-pocket expenditures (including informal payments), can reveal problems and create demand for solutions. Transparency also reduces the likelihood that officials can continue the corruption, by increasing the risk of shame, embarrassment, or potential punishment for revealed crimes.

Table 3 Anticorruption strategies in action

- The Ministry of Health in Argentina created a price monitoring system that tracked prices paid by public hospitals for common drugs, sharing these data with the reporting hospitals. Purchase prices for monitored items immediately fell by an average of 12%
- Chile's centralized health procurement agency, CENABAST, has prevented collusion and lowered prices by introducing a computerized, auction-style bidding system
- Due to diversion of funds, local allotments for health and education budgets under decentralization rarely reached the facility or school level in Uganda. The government used a newspaper campaign to inform parents about education budget transfers to districts and schools. This resulted in more funds flowing to schools, and higher school enrollment rates
- A study in Bolivia found that citizen health board activism was associated with lower rates of informal payments and lower prices paid by government procurement agents
- The Croatian Ministry of Health launched an initiative to require hospitals to publish open waiting lists. Combined with a hotline to monitor effectiveness, this initiative is designed to reduce favoritism and bribes used to allocate surgery
- Confronted with a problem of fee collection agents who were pocketing official hospital user fee revenue, a public hospital in Kenya implemented a system of networked electronic cash registers. Within three months, user fee revenue jumped 50% with no effect on utilization; within three years, annual user fee revenues were 400% higher
- A hospital in Cambodia has had success in reducing informal payments by formalizing user fees and promoting professionalism among staff. The hospital created individual contracts with personnel and increased pay scales while enforcing accountability and sanctioning poor performance
- The U.S. federal government gets a return of US$8 on every US$1 spent on fraud control. It recovered US$8 billion over 15 years through enforcement of the False Claims Act, about half of which was health-related

Sources: Vian T (2008) Review of corruption in the health sector theory, methods and interventions. *Health Policy and Planning* 23: 83–94. For more examples and country reports, see Transparency International's *Global Corruption Report 2006*, which focuses on corruption and health.

Accountability

A second way that anticorruption strategies work is by enhancing accountability. By making government more transparent, we increase the likelihood that officials can be held accountable for government performance. A health leader who wants to decrease corruption within her work unit can start by making sure everyone knows the goals, the objectives, and how performance will be measured. External accountability is also essential, especially to combat situations in which corruption entails collusion between different levels of government. Increasing citizen voice is an effective strategy, as shown in Bolivia, where citizen health board activism was associated with lower rates of informal payments and lower prices paid for goods procured.

Discretion

Effective anticorruption strategies try to clarify the discretion given to government officials to decide who gets how much of what services. Government officials or medical personnel who have too much discretion to allocate permits, decide on procurement contracts, or care for patients, may abuse that discretion by extorting bribes or allocating unfairly. We can control discretion by clearly defining objectives, rules, and procedures, making government processes more public and open to scrutiny, involving more people in the decision-making process by separating tasks, and creating teams or committees to provide additional oversight or review (Klitgaard *et al.*, 2000).

Somewhat counterintuitively, research in Colombia suggests that it may also be possible to reduce corruption by increasing a manager's discretion. A study funded by the Inter-American Development Bank found that increased hospital autonomy, especially in personnel management and budgeting, was associated with less corruption. The researchers hypothesized that the greater autonomy allowed hospital managers to enforce employee performance standards, thereby reducing corruption. However, in other studies, decentralizing management autonomy has led to greater corruption. For example, in Costa Rica, management reforms to give health-care facility managers new areas of authority and autonomy in human resources management led to higher rates of absenteeism (Garcia-Prado and Chawla, 2006). These different experiences highlight the need to adapt strategies to local context, and to evaluate the effectiveness of anticorruption interventions.

Controls on discretion work best in situations in which there is little evidence of collusion, or grand corruption. If the problem is that a particular 'agent' or government official is not being accountable, then a systems change to introduce checks and balances will probably improve the situation (as in the Argentina drug price monitoring scheme introduced by the Ministry of Health, described in **Table 3**). But if there is collusion or grand corruption, for example, if the hospital director and the head of the procurement office are both corrupt, or if corruption is vertical and spread throughout the highest offices in a ministry, then a new management system alone won't solve the problem. Systems reforms must be combined with efforts to address the grand corruption, perhaps through election reform or external transparency, in order to curb this type of corruption.

Management Tools

A fourth characteristic of many anticorruption activities is that they focus on management tools. Computerized accounting and billing systems coupled with internal and external audit procedures can help detect and deter embezzlement or misuse of funds. In Bogotá, Colombia, a revised hospital supply purchase system and other information systems changes produced substantial cost savings linked to reductions in theft, improper billing, and diversion of funds (Savedoff, 2005). Inventory control and asset management systems can help prevent theft of supplies and equipment, while management information systems report on inputs used to produce outputs, knowledge that can permit government officials to be held accountable for performance. Some management tools, such as internal and external financial audits, forensic accounting, and fraud control programs, may be specifically targeted to identifying corruption and abuse and prosecuting wrongdoers. Financial audits can detect diversion of funds and raise flags about spending that is not in line with approved plans or procedures, while system audits can be designed to detect other abuses such as inflated enrollment on insurance rosters, recording of 'ghost' patients, and overuse of health services by health workers who falsely declare themselves sick in order to collect and resell medications.

Incentives

Finally, effective anticorruption strategies alter the incentives of government agents in ways that reduce the net benefits of corruption. For example, increasing salaries of health personnel can reduce the need for corruption income, while increasing the probability that corruption will be detected and punished can make expected benefits lower. Another way to alter incentives is to increase the moral and legal cost of corruption by creating laws, and reinforcing moral values and professional ethics. As Swiss theologian Hans Küng, president of the Global Ethics Foundation, has said, "Laws without morality cannot endure, and no legal provisions against corruption can be implemented without moral consciousness based on elementary ethical standards." Qualitative research has highlighted the erosion of professional norms in the health sector as a cause for rising levels of corruption and other inappropriate behavior (Vian *et al.*, 2006). Health laws can help combat this undermining of professionalism and integrity by clarifying patient rights and regulating behaviors such as physician conflict of interest in ownership of facilities, use of public facilities in private practice, prescribing authority, and professional liability. Moral education and codes of ethics can instill positive values and promote an active role of civil society in combating corruption. Values education programs to increase social responsibility and citizen participation in anticorruption have been implemented in Italy, Argentina, Kazakhstan, and other countries.

Anticorruption and Health Reform

Health reforms being designed to address problems of efficiency, quality, and access to services should also incorporate strategies to reduce corruption and increase transparency. To do this, health reform efforts can incorporate strategies such as creating community oversight boards or restructuring payment systems to link pay or nonmonetary rewards to performance and minimize incentives to withhold care or to provide care that is not medically necessary. Reforms promoting competition or decentralization, if properly regulated, can increase citizen voice and choice, thereby creating additional pressure to reduce corruption. For example, in Bolivia, competition from private sector hospitals was associated with lower rates of informal payments in public hospitals nearby.

Health reforms can also help deal with corruption that happens at the nexus between the public and private sectors. For example, low worker satisfaction and lack of controls can result in elevated rates of absenteeism in public facilities, as workers shift more of their time to private sector activities. One World Bank study of absenteeism in Bangladesh found rates as high as 74% in rural health facilities, which severely reduced the public provision of health care in these areas (Chaudhury and Hammer, 2004). In addition, employees may use public sector supplies and equipment to treat private patients without compensating the public health facility. Changes in economic incentives through official recognition and regulation of the private sector can create more accountability and increase ethical conduct.

From the start of the health reform process, efforts to improve public health-care services through contracting, financing reform, or changes in provider payment systems should be reviewed from an anticorruption perspective. One project in Cambodia specifically evaluated the effect of such comprehensive health reforms on the level of corruption and informal activities of health workers. Working in eight districts, the project used a contracting approach coupled with performance-based staff incentives, official user fees, and new management controls and fee collection/exemption policies. After three years, the system successfully reduced total household health-care expenditures and increased utilization, despite increases in official user fees (Soeters and Griffiths, 2003). Monitoring systems specifically looked for evidence of overcharging, informal payment, ghost patients, and inflation of statistics, and used this information to address specific problems and make systematic changes. This type of integration of anticorruption tools and approaches into the traditional health reform process is perhaps the best strategy for preventing corruption.

Steps for the Future

Fighting corruption is a complex undertaking, but there are things policy makers and citizens can do to prevent corruption. Applied research is needed in several areas: policy research to evaluate which types of health reforms are most likely to reduce corruption; studies of the effectiveness of alternative roles for civil society in promoting transparency and accountability in health governance; and refinement of tools and methods to diagnose vulnerability to corruption in health systems and to reduce risk.

By closing opportunities for corruption while building ethical standards so that people are less inclined to abuse public power for personal gain, we can begin to curb corruption in the health sector. As David Nussbaum, the Chief Executive of Transparency International, wrote in his preface to the Global Corruption Report 2006:

> Corruption is a powerful force, but it is not inevitable or unavoidable. Diminishing its impact restores diverted resources to their intended purpose, bringing better health, nutrition, and education to victims of corruption around the world, and with them, opportunity and hope.
> (Transparency International, 2006).

See also: Economic Models of Hospital Behaviour; Governance Issues in Health Financing; Interest Groups and Civil Society, in Public Health Policy; Patient Empowerment in Health Care; Politics, and Public Health Policy Reform; The State in Public Health, The Role of.

Citations

Angell M (2004) *The Truth About the Drug Companies: How They Deceive Us and What to Do About It*. New York: Random House.

Chaudhury N and Hammer J (2004) Ghost doctors: Absenteeism in Bangladeshi rural health facilities. *World Bank Economic Review* 18(3): 423–441.

Garcia-Prado A and Chawla M (2006) The impact of hospital management reforms on absenteeism in Costa Rica. *Health Policy and Planning* 21(2): 91–100.

Gupta S, Davoodi HR, and Tiongson E (2002) Corruption and the provision of health care and education services. *Governance, Corruption and Economic Performance*, pp. 245–249. Washington, D.C: International Monetary Fund.

Johnston M (1997) Public officials, private interests, and sustainable democracy: When politics and corruption meet. In: Elliott KA (ed.) *Corruption in the Global Economy*, pp. 61–82. Washington, D.C: Institute for International Economics.

Kassirer J (2005) *On the Take: How Medicine's Complicity with Big Business Can Endanger Your Health*. New York: Oxford University Press.

Klitgaard R, Maclean-Abaroa R, and Lindsey Parris H (2000) *Corrupt Cities: A Practical Guide to Cure and Prevention*. Washington, D.C: World Bank Institute.

Lewis M (2000) *Who is Paying for Health Care in Eastern Europe Central Asia? Human Development Sector Unit, Europe and Central Asia Region*. Washington, DC: World Bank.

Mauro P (1995) Corruption and growth. *Quarterly Journal of Economics* 110(3): 631–712.

Miller WL, Grodeland AB, and Koshechkina TY (2001) *A Culture of Corruption? Coping with Government in Post-Communist Europe*. Hungary and New York: Central European University Press.

Savedoff WD (2005) *Transparency and Corruption in the Health Sector of Latin America and the Caribbean: A Conceptual Framework and Ideas for Action*. Washington, DC: Inter-American Development Bank.

Soeters R and Griffiths F (2003) Improving government health services through contract management: a case from Cambodia. *Health Policy Planning* 19: 22–32.

Transparency International (2006) *Global Corruption Report 2006: Special Focus on Corruption and Health*. London: Pluto Press.

USAID (2005) *USAID Anticorruption Strategy* (PD-ACA-557). Washington, DC: USAID.

Vian T and Burak L (2006) Beliefs about informal payments in Albania. *Health Policy and Planning* 21(5): 392–401.

Vian T, Gryboski K, Hall R, and Sinoimeri Z (2006) Informal payments in government health facilities in Albania: Results of a qualitative study. *Social Science and Medicine* 62: 877–887.

Vian T (2008) Review of corruption in the health sector theory, methods and interventions. *Health Policy and Planning* 23: 83–94.

Wazana A (2000) Physicians and the pharmaceutical industry: is a gift ever just a gift? *Journal of the American Medical Association* 283: 373–380.

World Bank (2000) *Anticorruption in Transition: a Contribution to the Policy Debate*. Washington, D.C: World Bank.

World Bank (2005) *Azerbaijan Health Sector Note, Volumes I and II*. Washington, DC: World Bank.

Relevant Websites

http://www.transparency.org/ – Transparency International.
http://www.globalcorruptionreport.org – Transparency International, Global Corruption Report.

HEALTH FINANCING

Health Care Financing and the Health System

C Normand and S Thomas, University of Dublin Trinity College, Dublin, Ireland

© 2008 Elsevier Inc. All rights reserved.

Introduction

Well-functioning health systems are of critical importance to the achievement of both national policy objectives and international policy commitments (such as the Millennium Development Goals [MDGs] of the United Nations). Financing systems should be the servants of policy – the choice of financing mechanisms should be informed by the type of health system that will meet overall policy objectives. This article analyzes the main types of health systems and financing systems across the world, exploring the policy objectives, the compatibility of financing mechanisms, and the overall objectives and the extent to which systems operate as they were intended. The article also emphasizes the importance of culture and history to the development of health systems and identifies factors that cause or constrain change. It is shown that systems are constantly undergoing change, that they frequently do not operate as originally envisaged, and that they are constantly subjected to pressures from both inside and outside.

Health Policy Objectives

It is common for governments to have stated (if sometimes somewhat vague) health policy objectives, and in some cases these are written into the constitution of a country. These normally cover protection against infectious diseases and other public health hazards, and access to important treatment and care when this is needed. There are several reasons why people may have difficulty in paying for care. First, because needs are very uncertain it may be important to insure the risks, and insurance is not always available to those who would need it. Second, since some services are very expensive there is a need to have funds available at the time of need. Third, some services may be considered important and cost-effective, but may be too expensive for some parts of the population to afford.

If a government has an objective of securing access for its citizens to some or all effective treatments, the chosen system of financing will have three main objectives – mobilizing funds for when they are needed, sharing risks, and subsidizing access, where needed, for those with low income. In the following section, the degree of risk sharing, or social solidarity, is an important defining feature for systems of health financing.

Financing of Current Health Systems

For the reasons given above, almost all governments accept that health systems cannot be left entirely to market forces to produce outcomes that are socially acceptable. There are two main reasons for this: First, in various technical ways there is market failure. For example, for some services (such as vaccination) the benefits of treatment are not exclusive to the individual who receives the intervention. Such externalities in consumption mean individuals will undervalue services from a societal viewpoint. Second, conditions for perfect markets, and their associated efficiency, are rarely found in health care. For instance, there is often an imbalance of information between supplier and consumer that can lead to induced demand. Further, there may be high costs in entering the market, so in many cases there is little effective competition. The most profitable services to provide are often not those that have the greatest impact on health.

The response of governments to this market failure includes regulation of the financing and provision of care, subsidies to individuals or providers of services, or in some cases direct provision by government agencies. Indeed, the state together with social security organizations are the largest funders of health services in many countries. According to the World Health Organization (WHO, 2007) general government funding accounted globally in 2004 for 56% of total health-care expenditure, increasing to an average of over 70% of funding in Europe. Further, over a third of all countries have 70% or more of their health-care funding coming from government sources (WHO, 2007). Nevertheless, markets do not have a monopoly on failure, and governments may also fail to achieve the best outcomes in their use of health system resources. (Criteria for evaluating system performance are reviewed later in this article.) As will be shown, there is no consensus on the ideal model for financing a health system. In most countries, several systems operate to provide access to different services or for different sectors of the population. The key archetypal financing models are now presented.

Archetypal Systems

As already outlined, systems of health financing aim to ensure resources are available when needed, and may also aim to share risk or subsidize the poor. Systems that remove barriers to access for the poor are often classified as being 'solidarity based,' in contrast to those that allow access to depend on being able to afford insurance or to pay for services directly.

Solidarity-based financing systems

Three solidarity-based financial systems merit attention: taxation, social health insurance, and community prepayment schemes.

Taxation

This method of financing the health system uses funds raised from general government taxation of the population. This can be either from direct taxes on income or wealth or from indirect (e.g., sales) taxes. Monies raised from taxation go into general government revenues to be used for a wide range of purposes, such as repaying debt and sectoral spending (defense, education, and policing). In government budget negotiations, health is allocated a proportion of general funds. In the stereotypical system, these funds are used for public providers such as hospitals, health centers, and public health programs and fund all line items such as staff, medicines, and other consumables. In this model, all health-care staff are employed by government. Services are then free (or available at low prices) at the point of contact for patients (i.e., there is no price mechanism to determine how the supply of goods and services matches the needs and wants of the population).

Under tax-based financing, risks are shared. Depending on the design of the tax system, it is also normal for tax systems to provide significant subsidies from richer to poorer people. Countries that use taxation as a major source of funds include the United Kingdom, Ireland, the Nordic countries, many countries in sub-Saharan Africa, and Canada.

Social Health Insurance (SHI)

The underlying principles of social health insurance (SHI) are: access to care is provided on the basis of need, and payment for insurance is based on income or the ability to pay. The basic characteristics of SHI are the following:

- Insured persons pay a regular contribution based on income or wealth, not on the cost of the services they are likely to use.
- Access to treatment and care is determined by clinical need and not ability to pay.
- Contributions to the social health insurance fund are kept separate from other government-mandated taxes and charges.
- The social health insurance fund finances care on behalf of the insured persons, and care is delivered by public and private health-care providers.

SHI funds are formally separate from general taxation funds, and may be organized and managed by autonomous organizations. Since SHI is separate from taxation and other publicly mandated systems, the income from contributions must cover the fees paid for the services to which members are entitled. However, it is common for SHI to be subsidized in two ways – from direct payments by government directly to providers of care (such as grants for capital developments) and through government payment of subscriptions for people unable to pay for themselves.

In terms of contributions and entitlement to services, the basic model has much in common with tax finance, although – despite the similarities – SHI has retained much of the tradition and rhetoric of insurance. In practice, the differences between SHI and tax-financed systems are more significant – for several reasons. First, the separate structures for collecting and managing funds tend to give the system greater transparency. Second, the fact that members are insured, and access to care is dependent on contributions to the fund, can give the patient the status of a customer. Third, to keep the system in balance, it is necessary to be more explicit about the range of services to which the contributor is entitled.

Under social health insurance, risks are shared. Depending on the rules for contributions, social health insurance systems usually provide significant subsidies from richer to poorer people, although some systems have a ceiling on such subsidies. Countries that use social health insurance as a major source of funds include Germany, many other countries in Central and Eastern Europe, Japan, and South Korea.

For many health services under taxation and social health insurance systems, access is either free or a modest user fee or copayment is charged. This removes financial barriers to access but also can lead to a tendency for people to want more than is available. In the case of SHI, this can be paid for by increasing the contribution (although there are limits to the acceptability of higher contributions), but in both cases there is some tendency for shortages to appear and rationing to be needed. Criteria for prioritizing what should be available and who should get the services include clinical need and cost-effectiveness of specific services.

There are interesting examples of approaches to rationing and equity in taxation and social health insurance systems. In some cases, a formula is used to distribute the resources to different regions based on some measures of need or disease burden. The aim of such a mechanism is to ensure that access to care is even across different areas. Many countries have explicit mechanisms, based on cost-effectiveness as a key criterion, for approving treatments and drugs to be included in the available packages. A more visible, and in many ways inefficient, mechanism for rationing access to care is the waiting list. Once the need for investigation or treatment has been determined, the person has to wait his or her turn. It is also common to have systems of triage and referral, in which access to specialist care is allowed only after assessment in primary care and referral by a primary care professional.

Community Prepayment Schemes

In countries where financial and government institutions are relatively weak, it can be difficult to develop access to high-quality care through government or social health insurance mechanisms. In such cases, there have been attempts to mobilize and manage resources locally, where there may be more trust from the population. This can be done through insurance at the community level or through firms or cooperatives. There are various versions of this idea, and different terminology is used, but in general the community-based schemes provide members with the opportunity to give a flat payment in advance in return for free or reduced-cost health care if they get sick. It can be useful in protecting communities against catastrophic costs of care and cash constraints due to seasonal income (Abel-Smith, 1994; Lambo, 1998). Nevertheless, it often requires high local motivation of communities, and there are few examples of schemes that have been replicated countrywide (Carrin and Vereecke, 1992; Abel-Smith, 1994; Witter, 2000). In some countries, there is a vision that community insurance or prepayment schemes can be the precursor of more formal social health insurance, but there are difficulties in achieving this development (Poletti *et al.*, 2007).

Community insurance systems have typically been developed in poor areas in poor countries, and an inevitable drawback is the overall lack of local resources. A second problem is that in many cases the risks facing individuals are not independent, because some health risks will occur at the same time for the whole local population (e.g., a flood or outbreak of an infectious disease). This makes community insurance schemes very vulnerable because they are not efficient in sharing risk. A possible solution is reinsurance (Dror, 2001). A problem with reinsurance generally is moral hazard. If, in effect, schemes are rewarded for failure, they will choose to fail. Reinsurance reduces the incentive to manage resources carefully, as those that run out of money are given more money.

Non-solidarity financing systems

The non-solidarity financial systems are: private risk-based health insurance, medical savings accounts, out-of-pocket prepayment, and informal fees.

Private risk-based health insurance

In a health system that relies on private risk-based insurance (private commercial health insurance), consumers choose insurance products covering a range of benefits and conditions, according to their willingness and ability to pay. Insurance only works if some people pay more in contributions than they take out in services. The ideal conditions for insurance to work well are when there is a small chance of a need for high-cost treatment, but neither the insurance company nor the insuree knows who will need the treatment. What both should know is the probability, so that an actuarially fair contribution can be set, but it should be difficult or expensive to identify the risks for individuals, according to McPake and Normand (2007). Typically, private insurance schemes set contributions on the basis of risk (Abel-Smith, 1994; Ensor and Jowett, 2000).

In the case of health care, the young are usually healthier than the old, and in many cases people who are at high risk have existing symptoms or signs. This means that the contribution charged to an old person with, for example, diabetes, will be high to reflect both that older people use more care and that people with diabetes are at high risk of related diseases and the need for some high-cost treatments. Other population groups, such as those who are unemployed or in dangerous jobs, may also find it difficult to afford private insurance and must fall back on publicly provided services (Normand and Weber, 1994; Thomas *et al.*, 2006).

Although people are good risks, they will seek the lower contributions available from private insurance or just pay their own way. Typically, this is when they are young and do not have dependants. When they get older and become worse risks, they are likely to be unable or unwilling to pay the contribution offered, and, in most countries that use private insurance, there are subsidized services for such groups. Risk-based insurance tends to fail when there is asymmetry in the knowledge of insurers and insurees. Individuals who know they are at high risk will want insurance. Individuals who know they are a low risk will consider the contribution too high, so those actually applying for insurance are likely to be the more risky cases. This further increases the contributions, since contributions must reflect this higher-than-average risk. In the end, contributions may become unaffordable for many, and the insurance breaks down as a financial protection mechanism. This is also associated with the concept of adverse selection (McPake and Normand, 2007).

Some countries make it illegal to use certain information on risk. For example, it may be illegal to require people to undergo HIV tests, but experience shows that it can be easy to get around such restrictions. There are typical strategies to avoid the problem of the fact that all those who want insurance are also those at high risk. These include the following, though none of these steps entirely resolves the problems:

- Qualifying conditions for membership: For example, pensioners can only participate if they have been members for 50% of their working life.
- Waiting periods: Voluntary members must have a waiting period before they can claim.
- Limited voluntary access: Each person has the chance only once in his or her life.

Another feature of health insurance is the presence of moral hazard. If health services are free or modestly priced at the point of contact, there is no incentive to limit demand because it is the insurance firm that pays. Requiring people to make co-payments and excluding specific services can reduce this moral hazard. The form of reimbursement for the supplier will also be critical to dissuading providers from inflating the quantity of services provided.

While private health insurance is often criticized as being highly inequitable, some authors argue that government regulation to ban risk-rating practices can improve welfare and the equity of financing of private health insurance for those within the risk pool (Feldman et al., 1998), if not for the system as a whole.

Private health insurance schemes are an important feature of financing in the Americas and in Southern Africa (WHO, 2007). Private health insurance rarely forms the main financing mechanism, although supplementary private health insurance is a growing phenomenon in high-income countries. The private funds flowing to health insurance in countries where they are a major financing mechanism are shown in **Figure 1**. The United States is the most frequently cited example of such a system, but South Africa and several Latin American countries also have relatively high enrollment in, and resources consumed by, private insurance. Private risk-based insurance helps to mobilize resources for when they are needed and provides some sharing of risks, but it is not designed to redistribute resources from richer to poorer people.

Medical savings accounts

As argued above, one function of financing systems is to ensure that resources are mobilized for use when needed. This has led to the development of some financing systems that do not specifically aim to share risk or provide solidarity, but which ensure that funds are saved and protected so as to be available when needed. Compulsory savings systems do this, of which the most popular version is the medical savings accounts system, used in Singapore (von Eiff et al., 2002) and increasingly being tried in other countries, including China (Dong, 2006).

The principle of medical savings accounts is simple – individuals or families must set aside funds into a special account until the funds reach a certain level. They can spend this money only on approved forms of medical costs, and when money is spent they must save again until the reserves are replenished. There are variants on the system – the funds can cover extended families so as to provide an element of intergenerational solidarity, and in some cases the remaining funds can be inherited in the event of a death. The main point is to ensure that people who have sufficient income to save for their medical expenses do so.

The two main limitations of systems of compulsory saving are the lack of explicit risk sharing and the inevitable need for other mechanisms to cover the very high costs of serious illness (Dixon, 2002). In Singapore, where there is the most extensive experience of compulsory savings, there are schemes to ensure good access to care for such circumstances, and there are some other

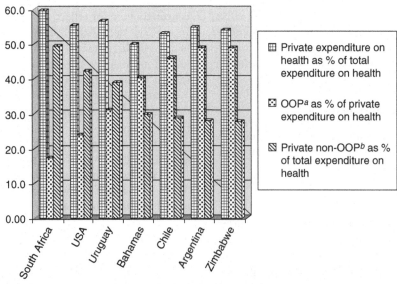

Figure 1 Private insurance financing in countries where it is a major financing mechanism, 2004 data. [a]OOP, out-of-pocket expenditure. [b]Private non-OOP includes both spending on private insurance and on prepayment mechanisms. Reproduced from WHO (2007) National Health Accounts statistics. http://www.who.int/nha/country/Annex1&2,%20March%205,%202007.xls.

government subsidies to providers of care, such as help with capital costs and some running cost subsidies. Hence, given limited experience with medical savings accounts, it is difficult to evaluate their performance in isolation from country contexts and parallel financing mechanisms (Hanvoravongchai, 2002).

Out-of-pocket payments

These are fees paid by the patient on use of health services. They include both user fees for public-sector services and payments to private providers at the point of contact. Proponents of public-sector user fees argue that they can both improve financial sustainability and referral patterns and dissuade consumers from unnecessary use of services (Akin et al., 1987; Shepard and Benjamin, 1993; Kutzin, 1995). Such arguments have been challenged by others who maintain that, in practice, the cost recovery potential of user fees is limited, particularly without retention of fees at the point of collection. Further, equity often suffers, especially through the failure of adequate exemption policies (Abel-Smith, 1994; Gilson et al., 1995; Nolan and Turbat, 1995; Russell and Gilson, 1995). Out-of-pocket payments are generally recognized as an extremely inequitable source of financing (Wagstaff and Van Doorslaer, 1993).

Out-of-pocket payments form the chief financing mechanism for health care in several countries in South and South-East Asia, Africa, the countries of Central and Eastern Europe, and the former Soviet Union. They are frequently the mainstay in conflict or postconflict situations and also in circumstances of regime upheaval where formal public systems have broken down (see the section 'Concluding remarks'). **Table 1** notes the 21 countries that are over 70% reliant on private household funding of health care and where the vast majority of this private funding is out-of-pocket. **Figure 2** highlights the six most reliant countries.

Informal fees

Informal or unofficial fees are payments – monetary or nonmonetary – made by an individual to a state healthcare worker during official hours of work that do not form part of the worker's official salary. These payments may be expected or unexpected and may be given for services that are routinely carried out or for an augmented or additional service (Killingsworth and Thomas, 2003). There has historically been very little systematic evidence on the extent of such payments, though there is now a growing body of research documenting and evaluating the practice (Gaal and McKee, 2004). There are several forms

Table 1 Countries in which out-of-pocket expenditure is the major financing source, 2004 data

	Private expenditure on health as a % of total expenditure on health	OOP as a % of private expenditure on health	OOP as a % of total expenditure on health
Afghanistan	83.1	97.7	81.2
Armenia	73.8	89.2	65.8
Azerbaijan	75.0	93.6	70.2
Bangladesh	71.9	88.3	63.5
Burundi	73.8	100.0	73.8
Cambodia	74.2	85.4	63.4
Cameroon	72.0	94.5	68.0
Cote d'Ivoire	76.2	88.7	67.6
Democratic Republic of Congo	71.9	100.0	71.9
Georgia	72.6	87.2	63.3
Guinea	86.8	99.5	86.4
Guinea-Bissau	72.7	90.0	65.4
India	82.7	93.8	77.6
Lao PDR	79.5	90.3	71.8
Lebanon	72.6	82.2	59.7
Myanmar	87.1	99.4	86.6
Nepal	73.7	88.1	64.9
Pakistan	80.4	98.0	78.8
Tajikistan	78.4	97.3	76.3
Togo	79.3	84.9	67.3
Vietnam	72.9	88.0	64.2

Reproduced from WHO (2007) National Health Accounts statistics. http://www.who.int/nha/country/Annex1&2,%20March%205,%202007.xls (accessed November 2007).

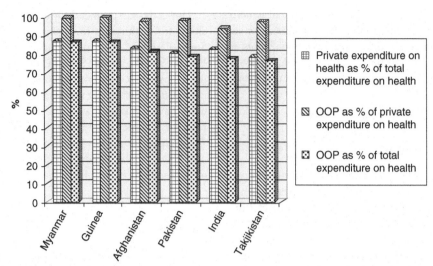

Figure 2 Private financing by type in countries most dependent on households' out-of-pocket payments for health care, 2004 data. Reproduced from WHO (2007) National Health Accounts statistics. http://www.who.int/nha/country/Annex1&2,%20March%205,%202007.xls.

of informal fees and a range of explanations for why they exist. Explanations include:

- 'legitimate' payments for doctors when state finances have collapsed, such as in some countries in the former Soviet bloc;
- the prevalence of a culture of rent-seeking and entitlement, such as in Bangladesh;
- the importance of gift-giving as a sign of respect in a transaction, such as with the practice of giving 'red packets' in China.

Informal fees tend to be supported by prevailing cultural values and conventions as well as the underfunding of the public sector. They also tend to worsen inequity (e.g., Szende and Culyer, 2006).

Funding by NGO and development aid partners

Donor funding

Many high-income countries have pledged to achieve the target of giving 0.7% of their gross national product (GNP) in aid, and this was reiterated with the Monterrey Consensus of 2002. Indeed, the MDGs have created a fresh impetus in generating funding for the world's poorest and most vulnerable groups. Given the importance of health and health-related targets in the MDGs, increasing funding for health systems in low-income countries is a priority for many donors. It is estimated that in 2004, 55 countries were reliant on external aid for over 10% of their total health-care funding. Of this number, 19 countries were heavily reliant on external support, which accounted for over 30% of their aggregate health-care spending (WHO, 2007). Regionally, Africa had the greatest dependence on external funding sources (9% and 21% of total and general government health-care funding, respectively) and this amounts to approximately $101 per person across the continent (expenditure on health at the international dollar rate during 2004). Many African countries are highly dependent on aid in the health sector. Further reliance on loans perpetuates the problem of debt where those loans are interest-bearing. Indeed, the extra resources provided by donors, to alleviate domestic resource shortages and address the mountain of health problems, come at a price. Berer (2002) notes:

> Although it is half a century since most developing countries became independent politically, all but a few have been kept economically dependent ... international institutions and donors are taking a larger and larger role in determining the health sector policies and priorities of middle- and low-income countries and have not always reached consensus with national governments on how best to do it.

Donor policy conditionalities have been a key driving force for the reform programs implemented across Africa, and donors will continue to be important players in any future changes in reform design. Many African governments have been able neither to withstand the pressure for reform nor to influence its design to a significant extent (see the section 'Concluding remarks'). A key factor in this is their resource dependence. In 2005, the Paris Declaration, signed by 91 countries, went some way toward agreeing to improve the local ownership of aid, remove conditionalities, and harmonize donor activity and funding while helping to build the capacity to absorb aid within recipient countries (Paris High Level Forum, 2005). The aid architecture for health care is also changing substantially with the growing number of Global Health Partnerships (GHPs). These are broad collaborations of governments, from both low- and high-income states, multilateral organizations, and private sector representatives, both for-profit and not-for-profit. Donors are channeling increasing proportions of their aid through these organizations (Pinet, 2003). The World Bank and IMF are also moving away from sector-specific strategies and toward Poverty Reduction Strategy Papers (PRSPs) for each country "as the basis of concessional assistance from the[se] two institutions" (World Bank, 2004). The effects of these changes on health system financing and performance are not yet well understood.

Funding by nongovernmental organizations and foundations

There has been a long tradition in many countries of health-care provision and some financing by charitable organizations. In some African countries, a significant part of the health system in rural areas is provided and managed by missions, and these are to some extent subsidized from donations from outside the countries as well as by governments. Over recent years, there has been an increasing role for charitable foundations, such as the Bill and Melinda Gates Foundation, in providing resources for certain services in developing countries. This, along with the other changes in aid architecture discussed above, has led to more complex patterns of funding.

Evaluating Health Financing and Health System Performance: Concepts, Criteria, and Measurement

In this section, we explore the evaluation of both health-care financing systems and health system performance as a whole. The two are clearly interlinked, and it is important not just to reflect on how the financing of health care can impact on overall performance, which it does, but how overall system performance affects health-care financing and helps to ground evaluation to further achieve policy goals. Indeed, we argue here that the choice of mechanisms for health-care delivery and finance should reflect policy objectives and the capacity of the chosen mechanisms to achieve these.

Attempts at global comparisons of health-care financing and health system performance (as carried out by the WHO in 2000) require that the objectives be specified, and must be assumed to be the same for all countries. Interestingly, the WHO stated that "the purpose of health financing is to make funding available, as well as to set the right financial incentives for providers, to ensure that all individuals have access to effective public health and personal health care" (as quoted in Carrin and James, 2005).

While such statements are a useful benchmark for international comparison of health-care financing systems, it may well be more just to analyze performance against the objectives chosen by individual countries. These are typically, but not universally, some combination of sufficient and sustainable resource generation, optimal resource use, and financial accessibility of health services to all (Carrin and James, 2005). Further, the weight accorded each component may well differ substantially from country to country according to local values and contexts.

Nevertheless, given scarce resources, it is important to review how resources are deployed, who is entitled to what, and how services are financed and organized. The key challenges in evaluating health-care financing and health system performance relate to:

- *The selection of policy goals against which performance must be measured.* There will often be trade-offs between different policy objectives, one of which is that between financial sustainability and equity. Different countries will favor different policy goals, depending on key challenges faced, and hence will choose different criteria and place different emphases on any standard criteria used to measure performance (Arah *et al.*, 2003). Therefore, any 'objective' measures of performance may well be artificial in their not taking into account the prevailing values of any particular country.
- *The selection (and interpretation) of indicators used to monitor and evaluate performance.* In order to be able to gauge progress, it is important to select indicators that can act as proxies for the goals/objectives of the health system. More than one indicator may be required for any particular objective to allow for triangulation. Hence, care needs to be taken that the right indicators have been chosen, often among several, or more ideally, indicators that are used for any particular objective to allow for triangulation. Analysts need to be aware that the relationship between indicators, context, and goals shifts over time and that which is the best measure today may not be the best measure tomorrow or in a different context. Hence, cross-country comparisons need always to be interpreted with care.
- *The calculation of indicators.* The old adage of 'rubbish in, rubbish out' applies here. The values and movement of indicators are only as good as the data available. Hence, in considering the most appropriate indicators when measuring performance, policy makers need to understand local constraints in data collection systems, what is collated regularly and to good standard, and what will require additional data collection efforts, whether one-off or continual. Arah *et al.* (2003: 392) note "the difficulty of building a conceptually sound framework around existing data and initiatives, while measuring performance gaps and maintaining international comparability."

Criteria for Evaluation

Since there are multiple (and sometimes competing) policy objectives that differ between countries, and because no indicator fully reflects these objectives, it is useful to base any judgments on a range of measures. The relative importance of each indicator needs to be weighted to reflect priorities. Such an approach is taken by the much-debated WHO report (WHO, 2000), which reviews the strengths and weaknesses of its methodology after considering specific criteria.

In setting health policy goals and in designing systems of health-care finance, system objectives are usually to ensure access to effective and appropriate care. This requires that resources are available for those who need them, when they need them, and that mobilizing such resources is possible without serious damage to the individual or the family. Risk sharing and solidarity can therefore be seen as mechanisms to ensure that people can gain access to appropriate care. It is therefore not surprising that attempts to evaluate the success of health systems tend to focus on the broader questions of whether they achieve fair and equal access and whether this access is for effective and appropriate services. They also focus on the burden that is placed on individuals and their families in the event of illness and the need for treatment or care. Specific criteria are explored next.

Equity

While there is often confusion over the precise definition of equity, most definitions relate to fairness of distribution (Mooney, 1983; Donaldson and Gerard, 1993). There are two general approaches to equity that can be applied both to the provision and to the financing of health care:

- Horizontal equity, implying the need for the equal treatment of equals;
- Vertical equity, implying the unequal but equitable treatment of unequals.

The translation of these approaches into working definitions of equity may take several forms relating to the equity of inputs, access, utilization, and outcomes (Mooney, 1983; Whitehead, 1992; Kutzin, 1995). Wagstaff and Van Doorslaer (1993) and Kutzin (1995) argue that equity in health-care financing relates to payment according to ability and treatment according to need, though the operationalization of this is open to significant interpretation (Culyer and Wagstaff, 1993). Mooney (1996) notes that while horizontal equity is more popular with policy makers, it may fail to narrow the gaps that exist between different groups in society. Certainly, vertical equity creates more upheaval to the distribution of resources, challenging vested interests, and as such may attract more opposition (see the section 'Concluding remarks').

One interesting application of equity to health-care financing is the assessment of the progressivity of different financing methods in 10 OECD (Organisation for Economic Co-operation and Development) countries by van Doorslaer and Wagstaff (1993). A financing method is said to be progressive when higher-income groups spend a larger proportion of their income for health care than lower-income groups. This fits in with the notion of paying for health care in accordance with ability to pay, that is, vertical equity. The results are summarized as follows:

- Direct taxes (personal income tax) were progressive in all 10 countries.
- Indirect taxes (such as VAT in the UK) tended to be regressive. Even when the tax rate is constant, richer people tend to spend less of their income on such taxes and so spend a smaller proportion of income on tax.
- Social health insurance schemes were regressive in those countries where they were the major financing source (e.g., the Netherlands) largely because of specific design features such as a ceiling on one's own contributions, which placed a limit on how much those who are well off pay. Where it was a supplementary financing mechanism, the results were mixed.
- Private health insurance was highly regressive when it formed the main financing source (United States). Nevertheless, it was found to be progressive when it was supplementary to other sources, as it allowed those who were well off to pay disproportionately more for their health care. There are problems of interpreting this result because access to care varies between different population groups.
- Out-of-pocket payments tended to be a highly regressive means of financing health care. In some respects this result understates the effects as it does not take into account differences in entitlements to services.

In a more recent study, Wagstaff *et al.* (1999) refined their methodology and revisited the same countries as well as three other high-income countries. Their results were similar to the earlier study, but social health insurance appeared to be more progressive (perhaps reflecting refinement of the designs of social health insurance in many countries), while private insurance appeared more regressive. It is interesting to note that most forms of health-care financing, apart from direct taxation, and possibly social health insurance, tend to be regressive.

Efficiency

There are two central approaches to efficiency in health economics. Allocative efficiency is concerned with maximizing the impact of health-promoting interventions across a broad range of activities (McGuire *et al.*, 1994; Witter, 2000). The idea of allocative efficiency focuses on asking whether we are doing the 'right' things. It relates to prioritizing some activities over others in relation to how they will meet set objectives, such as aggregate health status improvement. Many commentators believe that improving allocative efficiency was the primary objective of health reforms in the 1990s (Hammer and Berman, 1995; Murray, 1995; Gilson, 1998). Indeed, the movement to introduce essential packages of health services in many developing countries was an example of the pursuit of allocative efficiency (World Bank, 1993; Bobadilla et al., 1994). This controversial approach deployed a macro cost-effectiveness analysis to the prioritization of health-sector activities to meet the prevailing disease burden in each country.

Technical efficiency, in contrast, looks at the optimal combination of resources in any one activity to produce maximum output at minimum cost (Abel-Smith, 1994; McGuire et al., 1994; Witter, 2000). It is closer to the wider use of the concept of efficiency – asking whether we are doing things in the right way and if we are avoiding waste. While allocative efficiency focuses on which activity to pursue, technical efficiency is concerned with getting the right mix of inputs into a specific activity (Brown and Jackson, 1987; Smithson, 1996). Nevertheless, both are needed to improve overall efficiency in the use of resources in the health sector. Concern for technical efficiency, by definition, is associated with a more microeconomic perspective on reform, often concentrating at the facility level or on specific activities.

Financial sustainability and cost-containment

Another objective for evaluating system performance is financial sustainability. There are two prevailing definitions. The first discusses the financing of the health sector in relation to its dependency on external resources (LaFond, 1995). Of major concern here is the flow of foreign donor funds into the health system. The second definition is concerned with the sufficiency, predictability, and regularity of sources of finances in the health sector (McPake and Kutzin, 1997). Such an interpretation of financial sustainability is less concerned with the source of funds for financing a health sector and more interested in a steady future flow of finances and the affordability of future health-care services. The search for alternative financing mechanisms within the health-care reform movement was an endeavor by low-income countries to raise sufficient revenue to finance their desired health-care provision (Gilson and Mills, 1995).

Acceptability and satisfaction

Acceptability of a health system and satisfaction of its users can be seen as judgments on its performance in terms of equity and efficiency. However, consumer satisfaction may depend not only on how effective or fair is the use of resources, but also on features of the processes of delivery. For example, consumers may value politeness in staff and quality of facilities even when these have little impact on improving health status. In considering the views of users, it is important to understand their focus on process as well as outcome.

Ultimately, health-care services are consumed and financed by households. It is therefore appropriate for citizens of a country to have a role in evaluating the health services that they pay for and use. It is sometimes argued that health systems are too complex for the general public to make any meaningful judgment on their performance, or alternatively, that the expectations of the public reveal little about actual service delivery or that equivalent satisfaction scores mean different things in different contexts (see the fascinating exchange between Blendon et al., 2001 and Murray et al., 2001). It is, however, reasonable to give consumers a say in evaluating performance given their experience as end users. Indeed, the transparency of a system may be a good in itself in that people can see how their resources are being used. The Alma Ata Declaration on Health Services and Community Participation (International Conference on Primary Health Care, 1978) goes one step further and asserts that health-care services should not only be responsive to the needs of communities but actually should be defined by individual demands and preferences. It states in Article 1 that

> primary health care requires and promotes maximum community and individual self-reliance and participation in the planning, organization, operation and control of PHC, making fullest use of local, national and other available resources; and to this end develops through appropriate education the ability of the communities to participate.

As well, Article IV states that "the people have the right and duty to participate individually and collectively in the planning and implementation of their health care" "(International Conference on Primary Health Care, 1978:1)."

Evaluation Frameworks

As indicated, country governments can establish their own priorities given prevailing values and the features of the health system that they inherit. These will often be a mix of priorities. A useful guide to analysts wishing to evaluate their health-care financing system is to adapt the approach set out by Carrin and James (2005) to all health-care financing mechanisms in a particular country, taking into account the local settings and policy objectives.

The performance of health financing systems should be evaluated against key targets that relate to:

- resource generation (sufficient and sustainable);
- optimal resource use;
- financial accessibility of health services for all.

Performance in relation to these targets is analyzed by assessing the main functions of health financing against specified targets and indicators. Critical functions of health financing are:

- Revenue collection – the process by which the health system receives money from different sources, relating to generation of resources and accessibility of health services for the population;
  Key performance issues: population coverage and method of finance;
- Revenue pooling – the accumulation and management of revenues from individuals to share risk;
  Key performance issues: composition, fragmentation, and management of the risk pool;
- Purchasing – the process by which pooled contributions are used to pay providers to deliver specific health services;
  Key performance issues: package of services to be provided, provider payment mechanisms, and administrative efficiency.

For evaluating broader health system performance, the WHO in its World Health Report (2000) developed a groundbreaking, but controversial, health system performance evaluation framework, which it then applied to its 192 member states. They produced league tables of their performance, overall and in five key priority areas. Health system functions relate to stewardship, financing, resource generation, and service provision. There are five key components of health systems performance:

- Overall level of population health (25%);
- The distribution of health across the population (25%);
- The overall responsiveness of the health system (12.5%);
- The distribution of responsiveness of the health systems across the population (12.5%);
- The fairness of financing of the health system (25%).

The efficiency of the system, or its 'overall system performance,' is indicated by a single index that measures the actual achievement of these five goals compared to a maximum score it could have achieved given available resources. The weightings of each component in the index are indicated by the value in parentheses in the above list. The weights were derived from an internet-based survey of over 1000 public health practitioners.

Further, **Table 2** highlights the ten best performers overall, using the WHO (2000) data, and their scores against different performance criteria. The rankings have produced much criticism in relation to the selection of criteria of performance, the indicators used, the interpretation of the indicators, and the sources and reliability of data collected. At one level, it can be argued that an exercise such as this is inevitably flawed, since the judgment is against a somewhat arbitrary set of indicators with an arbitrary set of weights. Countries have different policy objectives and different weights for different features. It is interesting that some of the top performers are rated poorly by their own citizens, and conversely, according to Blendon et al. (2001), the two industrialized countries with the highest satisfaction scores rank at the bottom of the WHO ratings.

Nevertheless, this exercise has probably had some useful effects, both in making more explicit the potential policy objectives and in making countries more circumspect in making claims for the superiority of their systems. One effect of the exercise has been to develop a debate about what should be the criteria, how they should be measured, and how the analysis should be carried out (Gravelle et al., 2003; Richardson et al., 2003). While it is clear that the current frameworks and data limit the usefulness of the findings, it is likely that exercises of this sort will continue, and that techniques and data will improve. Skeptics will always be able to argue that if systems have different objectives, they cannot be fairly compared using a single set of objectives.

Two key issues that emerge from **Table 2** are not that certain systems of financing or service configuration are better for overall performance but rather, that matters of geography and lifestyle influence standing. The excellent performance of small states (3–7) suggests that health service delivery and access to services is easier in a small country. The excellent performance of southwest European countries (1–5 and 7) may indicate that lifestyle factors, such as red wine, sunshine, and a Mediterranean diet, are also important. If there are important nonhealth-system factors, these should be included in any assessment of system performance.

Performance of Archetypal Financing Systems

McPake and Normand (2007) suggest there are key features of performance of the archetypal systems. Public systems focus on social valuation but must ration services and are dependent on the tax base. SHI systems are often more popular to consumers but experience problems with cost control, and there are question marks about how well the poor and those in informal sectors are covered and their services financed. Private health insurance systems battle to control costs and will put profit above efficiency and equity. Systems in those countries that rely on private insurance as a chief financing mechanism tend to be more expensive than those in countries with mainly tax-based or SHI-based systems. To explore this, we review recent spending in high-income countries with different health systems.

The results shown in **Table 3** generally conform to expectations, with taxation-based countries spending less

Table 2 Ranking of states by attainment of goals, spending and systems performance: Highest system performance ranked states (1997 data)

	Attainment of goals					Fairness in financial contribution	Overall goal attainment	Health expenditure per capita in international dollars	Performance		
	Health		Responsiveness								
	Level (DALE)[a]	Distribution	Level	Distribution					On level of health		Overall health system
France	3	12	16–17	3–38		26–29	6	4	4		1
Italy	6	14	22–23	3–38		45–47	11	11	3		2
San Marino	11	9	32	3–38		30–32	21	21	5		3
Andorra	10	25	28	39–42		33–34	17	23	7		4
Malta	21	38	43–44	3–38		42–44	31	37	2		5
Singapore	30	29	20–21	3–38		101–102	27	38	14		6
Spain	5	11	34	3–38		26–29	19	24	6		7
Oman	72	59	83	49		56–57	59	62	1		8
Austria	17	8	12–13	3–38		12–15	10	6	15		9
Japan	1	3	6	3–38		8–11	1	13	9		10

Reproduced from World Health Organization (2000) *World Health Report, 2000. Health Systems: Improving Performance.* Geneva: World Health Organization.
[a]DALE, disability-adjusted life expectancy.

Table 3 Spending on health in selected high-income countries with different financing systems

	Total expenditure on health as % of GDP (2004)	Per capita total expenditure on health (international dollar rate) (2004)	Government expenditure on health as a % of total health exp (2004)	Average real annual growth in per capita total expenditure ($) on health 1997–2004
Dominated by tax-based funding				
UK	8.1	2560	86.3	12%
Denmark	8.6	2780	82.3	5%
Ireland	7.2	2618	79.5	12%
Sweden	9.1	2828	84.9	6%
Dominated by social health insurance				
France	10.5	3040	78.4	5%
Germany	10.6	3171	76.9	4%
The Netherlands	9.2	3092	62.4	7%
Private health insurance as a major funding source				
USA	15.4	6096	44.7	7%

Reproduced from WHO (2007) National Health Accounts statistics. http://www.who.int/nha/country/Annex1&2,%20March%205,%202007.xls (accessed November 2007).

per capita, and, as a proportion of GNP, than the other systems. Health systems with an important private health insurance component such as that in the United States are also the most expensive. Nevertheless, within this result it is interesting to see the high growth in spending in two tax-based countries: Ireland and the UK. In Ireland, there has historically been low spending on the health-care system. The period of analysis in **Table 3** saw a massive economic boom in Ireland during which the government also tried to boost its funding to the health sector to make up for historical underinvestment and meet consumer demands. There was also a large growth in the coverage of supplemental private insurance. In the UK, the Labour government was committed to expanding the funding of the National Health Service (NHS) and hence there were large increases in public-sector investment. Consequently, the data appear to indicate that there is a narrowing in the differential between systems, at least between the tax-based system and the SHI systems. This might be a result of two factors: SHI systems working better at controlling costs and tax-based systems responding to higher consumer expectations and higher income levels.

Out-of-pocket and free market systems

Unsurprisingly, those states that tend to have health-care financing composed largely of out-of-pocket payments by households tend to have worse-than-average equity of financing using the WHO (2000) fairness-of-financing index. The standard measures for equity of financing make no reference to access to services, however. Whereas individual payments for health affect access to services, measures of equity relating to financing will not adequately reflect the overall degree of inequity in the health system. Further, as noted before, the prevailing culture, values, history, and geography may be just as important in determining performance and therefore also need to be taken into account.

Mixed Financing Systems

No system conforms precisely to the archetypes. Even in the freest market with least organization of financing or regulation of service delivery there is some public spending on health care. Even in the most socialist of countries, such as Cuba, where government spending dominates, there is always some room for private spending on health-care services. Indeed, most health systems are a blend of different financing mechanisms. Some states, and in particular many in South America, have an equal balance between taxation-based financing, social health insurance, and out-of-pocket spending. Others are evolving from one system to another and do not conform clearly to the archetypes (see the section 'Archetypal systems').

Thus, care needs to be taken that the archetypal models do not hinder our understanding of the complexity of health systems. Consider Kierkegaard's maxim: 'Once you categorize me you negate me.' It is important not to limit analysis to the archetypal models but to build on them if we are to understand the performance of health systems and how systems are likely to evolve. This takes us beyond any individual financing mechanism and truly into an analysis of health systems, hence:

> A system is a set of elements connected together that form a whole, thereby possessing properties of the whole rather than of its component parts. Activity within a system is the result of the influence of one element over another. This influence is called feedback and can be positive (amplifying) or negative (balancing) in nature.

Systems are not chains of linear cause and effect relationships but complex networks of interrelationships.
(quoted in Iles and Sutherland, 2001)

A health system is made up of users, payers, providers, and regulators and can be defined by the relations between them. (McPake and Normand, 2008)

While it is useful to know the dominant financing mechanism, this does not give us a complete picture about the incentives in the health system and how different mechanisms combine to influence household, provider, and state behavior. Understanding the incentive structures and how they combine with culture is essential if we are to determine why health systems perform as they do. An interesting example is the case of the Republic of Ireland, which we look at next. It highlights the importance of understanding how different elements of the health system interact and understanding, specifically, how financing links with access and entitlement as well as how the values and culture of consumers determine health system structures.

The Tail That Wags the Dog – Private Financing and Public Resources in Ireland

A cursory examination of health system financing would indicate that Ireland should be classified as a taxation-based health-care system, with approximately 80% of all funds being provided by the state. However, a closer look reveals that private spending, although small, is extremely important because it unlocks access to many services. Over two-thirds of the Irish population must pay full charges for accessing their general practitioner (GP) and receiving the required drugs. Further, over half the population has supplementary private health insurance, which helps people jump the public-sector waiting lists for hospital services to see a consultant. Thus, how financing confers entitlements and access is key to performance. Further, in the Irish case, the private sector receives substantial subsidies from the state. Hence, what might appear to be a typical taxation-based system can be better understood as a system dominated by private insurance, as seen by the rapid cost escalation and problems with access for those in employment and on low incomes.

It is also no accident that the system is this way. The pay-your-own-way philosophy has deep roots in traditional Irish Catholic culture (Wren, 2003). This highlights why it is vital that we understand how values interact with health systems and how the public perceives the performance of health-care financing systems. This is the case not merely because the public is the key user and payer, as noted earlier, but also because such understanding will reveal how people interact with the system and intend to do so in the future. Understanding the public's values allows policy makers to evaluate not only current performance but also how the system can feasibly be improved to meet key goals.

Linkages between the Public and Private Sectors

There is much debate in the international literature about the value of private-sector activities to health service performance through their impact on the public sector. Arguments for and against a private health sector are presented in **Figure 3** and are frequently, and understandably, ideological. The extent to which these arguments hold in any particular setting is now a question for empirical research. Nevertheless, what is clear from this and the case study regarding Ireland is that even a small private

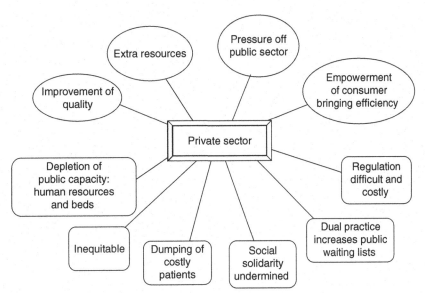

Figure 3 Arguments for and against private sector activity alongside the public sector.

sector can make a large impact on health system performance. (This is an important point and demonstrates one reason why a superficial analysis of financial flows of countries' health systems will often fail to reveal why systems perform as they do.)

Key issues to consider in evaluating the benefit of a parallel private sector relate to whether the private sector will assist overall performance by, for example, adding fresh resources and capacity to the system that allows government services to focus subsidies on the poor. Alternatively, the private sector may absorb scarce resources, dump costly patients on the public sector, and create a two-tier structure that helps undermine social solidarity and access to quality care for the poor and marginalized.

Public Values, History, and Culture

An important factor in the performance of any health system is the set of values and traditions within which it is set. This is very clear in the operation of the German sickness funds, in which unwritten rules were of particular importance; it may also explain the success of some more recent innovations (Krajewski-Siuda et al., 2007). As well, the relatively successful processes of reforms in the Nordic countries (Magnussen et al., 2007) may be explained partly by the strong consensus on objectives. Conversely, measures that undermine the old consensus may remove important mechanisms that provide quality and sustainability. The experience of the new financing mechanisms in Central and Eastern Europe illustrate the difficulty in implementing a system in the absence of supportive traditions (Voncina et al., 2007).

Concluding Remarks

This article has reviewed financing mechanisms and their likely impact on health system performance. It has emphasized the importance of making financing the servant of policy and of evaluating financing with reference to local goals and contexts. It has also explored the problems with superficially labeling health systems according to financial flows without exploring the incentives in the system and the values that are prevalent in the society.

Also, because health systems are subject to many and various stresses that can cause change, any evaluation of health-care financing or health system performance is only a snapshot of an evolving picture. Change factors are many and various but key ones relate to:

- vested interests in society that make pro-poor change very difficult;
- international trends and fashions, such as neoliberalism, which mean that policies can be transferred, sometimes coercively, from one context to another;
- deterioration of public taxation-based systems in certain resource-constrained contexts (e.g., sub-Saharan Africa or the former Soviet bloc).

An interesting feature of health system change and reforms is that there are only a limited number of options available for policy makers to choose from. Indeed, ideas often reemerge long after they have been tried and found wanting. Saltman and Figueras (1998: 86) comment, perhaps rather generously, that "health policy debates around the world comprise a complicated cocktail of validated evidence intermixed with presumption and ideology."

See also: Competiton in Health Care; The Demand for Health Care; Health Finance, Equity in; Insurance Plans and Programs - An Overview; The Private Sector in Health Care Provision, The Role of.

Citations

Abel-Smith B (1994) *An Introduction to Health Policy, Planning and Financing.* Harlow, Essex, UK: Longman Group Ltd.

Akin J, Birdsall N, and de Ferranti D (1987) *Financing Health Services in Developing Countries: An Agenda for Reform. A World Bank Policy Study.* Washington, DC: World Bank.

Arah OA, Klazinga NS, Delnoij DM, ten Asbroek AH, and Custers T (2003) Conceptual frameworks for health systems performance: A quest for effectiveness, quality and improvement. *International Journal for Quality in Health Care* 15(5): 377–398.

Berer M (2002) Health sector reforms: Implications for sexual and reproductive health services. *Reproductive Health Matters* 10(20): 6–15.

Blendon RJ, Kim M, and Benson JM (2001) The public versus the World Health Organization on health system performance. *Health Affairs* 20(3): 10–20.

Bobadilla JL, Cowley P, Musgrove P, and Saxenian H (1994) Design, content and financing of an essential national package of health services. *Bulletin of the World Health Organization* 72(4): 653–662.

Brown CV and Jackson PM (1987) *Public Sector Economics.* 3rd edn. Oxford, UK: Basil Blackwell.

Carrin G and James C (2005) Key performance indicators for the implementation of social health insurance. *Applied Health Economics and Health Policy* 4(1): 15–22.

Carrin G and Vereecke M (eds.) (1992) *Strategies for Health Care Finance in Developing Countries with a Focus on Community Financing in Sub-Saharan Africa.* Basingstoke, UK: Macmillan.

Culyer A and Wagstaff A (1993) Equity and equality in health and health care. *Journal of Health Economics* 12: 431–457.

Dixon A (2002) Are medical savings accounts a viable option for funding health care? *Croatian Medical Journal* 43(4): 408–416.

Donaldson C and Gerard K (1993) *Economics of Health Care Financing: The Visible Hand.* London: Macmillan.

Dong W (2006) Can health care financing policy be emulated? The Singaporean medical savings accounts model and its Shanghai replica. *Journal of Public Health (Oxf)* 28(3): 209–214.

Dror DM (2001) Reinsurance of health insurance for the informal sector. *Bulletin of the World Health Organization* 79(7): 672–678.

Ensor T and Jowett M (2000) Financing health services. In: Witter S, Ensor T, Jowett M, and Thompson R (eds.) *Health Economics for Developing Countries: A Practical Guide.* London and Oxford: Macmillan Education Ltd.

Feldman R, Escribano C, and Pellisé L (1998) The role of government in health insurance markets with adverse selection. *Health Economics* 7(8): 659–670.

Gaal P and McKee M (2004) Informal payment for health care and the theory of 'INXIT' *International Journal of Health Planning and Management* 19(2): 163–178.

Gilson L (1998) In defence and pursuit of equity. *Social Science and Medicine* 47(12): 1891–1896.

Gilson L and Mills A (1995) Health sector reforms in Sub-Saharan Africa: Lessons of the last 10 years. In: Berman P (ed.) *Health Sector Reform in Developing Countries: Making Health Development Sustainable, Harvard Series on Population and International Health*, pp. 277–316. Boston, MA: Harvard School of Public Health.

Gilson L, Russell S, and Buse K (1995) The political economy of user fees with targeting: developing equitable health financing policy. *Special Issue: Health Policies in Developing Countries. Journal of International Development* 7(3): 369–402.

Gravelle H, Jacobs R, Jones AM, and Street A (2003) Comparing the efficiency of national health systems: A sensitivity analysis of the WHO approach. *Applied Health Economics and Health Policy* 2(3): 141–147.

Hammer J and Berman P (1995) *Ends and Means in Public Sector Planning*. Boston, MA: Harvard School of Public Health.

Hanvoravongchai P (2002) *Medical Savings Accounts: Lessons Learned from International Experience*. EIP/HFS/PHF Discussion Paper No. 52. Geneva, Switzerland: World Health Organization.

High Level Forum (2005) *Paris Declaration on Aid Effectiveness: Ownership, Harmonisation, Alignment, Results and Mutual Acountability.* Paris, France. http://www1.worldbank.org/harmonization/paris/FINAL PARISDECLARATION.pdf (accessed 15 May 2007).

International Conference on Primary Health Care (1978) Declaration of Alma-Ata. Alma Ata, Russia. http://www.who.int/hpr/NPH/docs/declaration_almaata.pdf (accessed November 2007).

Iles V and Sutherland K (2001) *Organisational Change. A Review for Health Care Managers, Professionals and Researchers*. London: National Coordinating Centre for the NHA Service Delivery and Organization R & D.

Killingsworth J and Thomas S (2003) *Institutional aspects of health reforms and implications for informal fee practices in China and Bangladesh*. Conference paper: 4th International Health Economics Association (iHEA) World Congress: Global Health Economics–Bridging Research and Reforms. San Francisco, CA.

Krajewski-Siuda K, Romaniuk P, and Kaczmarek K (2006) The case of the Silesian regional sickness fund—did "social capital" determine the success of health reform in the Silesian Voivodeship, Poland? *Central European Journal of Public Health* 14(4): 200–207.

Kutzin J (1995) *Health Financing Reform: A Framework for Evaluation. National Health Systems and Policies Unit*. Geneva, Switzerland: World Health Organization.

LaFond A (1995) *Sustaining Primary Health Care. The Save the Children Fund*. London: Earthscan Publications Ltd.

Lambo E (1998) Aims and performance of pre-payment schemes. In: Beattie A, Doherty J, Gilson L, Lambo E, and Shaw P (eds.) *Sustainable Health Care Financing in Southern Africa*. Papers from an EDI Health Policy Seminar, Johannesburg, South Africa. Washington, DC: World Bank.

Magnussen J, Hagen TP, and Kaarboe OM (2007) Centralized or decentralized? A case study of Norwegian hospital reform. *Social Science and Medicine* 64(10): 2129–2137.

McGuire A, Henderson J, and Mooney G (1994) *The Economics of Health Care: An Introductory Text*. London and New York: Routledge.

McPake B and Kutzin J (1997) *Methods for Evaluation of Health System Performance and the Effects of Reforms*. Geneva, Switzerland: Department for International Development.

McPake B and Normand C (2008) *Health Economics: An International Perspective*. 2nd edn. London: Routledge.

Mooney GH (1983) Equity in health care: Confronting the confusion. *Effective Health Care* 1(4): 179–184.

Mooney GH (1996) And now for vertical equity? Some concerns arising from Aboriginal health in Australia. *Health Economics* 5: 99–103.

Murray CJL (1995) Towards an analytical approach to health sector reform. In: Berman P (ed.), *Health Sector Reform in Developing Countries. Making Health Development Sustainable*, pp. 121–142. Cambridge, MA: Harvard University Press.

Murray CJL, Kwawabata K, and Valentine N (2001) People's experience versus people's expectations. *Health Affairs* 20(3): 21–24.

Nolan B and Turbat V (1995) *Cost Recovery in Public Health Services in Sub-Saharan Africa. EDI Technical Materials*. Washington, DC: The World Bank.

Normand C and Weber A (1994) *Social Health Insurance: A Guidebook for Planning*. Geneva, Switzerland: World Health Organization and International Labour Office.

Pinet G (2003) Global partnerships: A key challenge and opportunity for implementation of international health law. *Medicine and Law* 22(4): 561–577.

Poletti T, Balabanova D, Ghazaryan O, et al. (2007) The desirability and feasibility of scaling up community health insurance in low-income settings –lessons from Armenia. *Social Science and Medicine* 64(3): 509–520.

Richardson J, Wildman J, and Robertson IK (2003) A critique of the World Health Organisation's evaluation of health system performance. *Health Economics* 12(5): 355–366.

Russell S and Gilson L (1995) User fees at government health services: Is equity being considered? Departmental Publication No. 15. Department of Public Health and Policy. London: London School of Hygiene and Tropical Medicine.

Saltman RB and Figueras J (1998) Analysing the evidence on European health care reforms. *Health Affairs* 17(2): 85–108.

Shepard DS and Benjamin ER (1993) User fees and health financing in developing countries: Mobilizing financial resources for health. In: Bell D and Reich M (eds.) *Health, Nutrition and Economic Crises: Approaches to Policy in the Third World*. Boston, MA: Harvard School of Public Health.

Smithson P (1996) Health financing and sustainability: A review and analysis of five country case studies. Save the Children Fund. Working Paper No. 10, London: Save the Children Fund (UK).

Szende A and Culyer AJ (2006) The inequity of informal payments for health care: the case of Hungary. *Health Policy* 75(3): 262–271.

Thomas S, Normand C, and Smith C (2006) *Social Health Insurance: Options for Ireland*. Dublin, Ireland: The Adelaide Hospital Society.

Von Eiff W, Massoro T, Voo YO, and Ziegenbein R (2002) Medical savings accounts: A core feature of Singapore's health care system. *European Journal of Health Economics* 3(3): 188–195.

Voncina L, Dzakula A, and Mastilica M (2007) Health care funding reforms in Croatia: A case of mistaken priorities. *Health Policy* 80(1): 144–157.

Wagstaff A and van Doorslaaer E (1993) Equity in the finance and delivery of health care: concepts and definitions. In: van Doorslaaer E, Wagstaff A, and Rutten F (eds.) *Equity in the Financing and Delivery of Health Care: An International Perspective*. Oxford, UK: Oxford University Press.

Wagstaff A and van Doorslaer E (1998) Equity in health care finance and delivery. In: Culyer AJ and Newhouse JP (eds.) *North Holland Handbook of Health Economics*, pp. 1803–1862. North Holland.

Wagstaff A, van Doorslaer E, van der Burg H, et al. (1999) Equity in the finance of health care: some further international comparisons. *Journal of Health Economics* 18: 263–290.

Whitehead M (1992) The concepts and principles of equity and health. *International Journal of Health Services* 22(3): 429–445.

Witter S (2000) Introduction to health economics. In: Witter S, Ensor T, Jowett M, and Thompson R (eds.) *Health Economics for Developing Countries: A Practical Guide*. London and Oxford: Macmillan Education Ltd.

World Bank (1993) *World Development Report: Investing in health*. Oxford, UK: Oxford University Press for The World Bank.

World Health Organization (2000) *World Health Report, 2000. Health Sysems: Improving Performance*. Geneva, Switzerland: World Health Organization.

WHO (2007) National Health Accounts statistics. http://www.who.int/nha/country/Annex1&2,%20March%205,%202007.xls (accessed November 2007).

Wren M-A (2003) *Unhealthy State: Anatomy of a Sick Society*. Dublin, Ireland: New Island.

Health Care Costs, Structures and Trends

T Tan-Torres Edejer, C Garg, P Hernandez, N Van de Maele, and C Indikadahena, World Health Organization, Geneva, Switzerland

© 2008 WHO. Published by Elsevier Inc. All rights reserved.

Definition of Health Expenditures and Their Accounting Frameworks

What Is a Health Expenditure?

A health expenditure is a consumption of a resource with the primary objective of promoting, restoring, and maintaining health. National or total health expenditure is the monetary representation of the totality of resources being consumed within the health system for a given year. The information on resources consumed is best reported within a formal accounting framework.

What Is Counted as a Health Expenditure Under a Health Accounting Framework?

From the above, it is clear that to be counted as a health expenditure, two criteria must be fulfilled: First, there must be a final consumption of a resource, and second, the primary objective of consumption of the resource is to promote, restore, and maintain health.

A consumption of a resource is clearly recognizable if there is a financial transaction. There is a producer of a good or a service on one side and there is a consumer on the other side. Their transaction can be translated into its monetary value. For example, hospitalizations, outpatient visits, including all the attendant diagnostic tests, medicines, and surgical procedures are clearly health expenditures. Alternative or complementary medicine and public health services would also be included. Many of these can be billed or costed. Informal payments for health goods and services, or in addition to formal payments, are also considered as financial transactions, though they may be more difficult to capture.

On the other hand, resources consumed in the course of production of health professionals would not be considered a final consumption. In the same way, the classification of capital expenditures in health such as investments in clinics and hospitals and medical equipment is tricky because consumption is ongoing throughout the life span of the resource.

The application of the second criterion of primary intent to promote, restore, or maintain health is clear in many situations. However, in some situations, the distinction between health and non-health or primary versus secondary intent is ambiguous. This lack of clarity arises particularly in case of vulnerable or dependent individuals, e.g., long-term care of the elderly or those with disability, or hospice care for terminally ill patients or care of HIV-positive orphans. In these cases, the distinction between health and non-health is facilitated by unbundling of the service and identification of the components as being health- or social welfare-related.

Intent is not necessarily defined by who delivers the care or where care is delivered. For example, school systems implement classes on safe sex or on basic sanitation and hygiene. Occupational health programs are delivered within business premises. The ministry of defense might run its own health subsystem and provide health services exclusively to its active duty personnel, veterans, and their families.

From the above, it is clear that the consumption of health resources occurs in different settings and through different mechanisms. To capture the universe of health spending entails a comprehensive and discerning approach. At the same time, to be able to use information on health expenditures in policy, it is necessary that the tracking of health expenditures be standardized and reported within a formal accounting framework. Every framework needs to address two main objectives:

1. To provide guidance on how to consistently estimate and report health expenditures that enable the documentation of trends across time and space. When there is ambiguity with regard to whether a substantial amount of resources represents final consumption or whether the primary intent to promote, restore, or maintain health, arbitrary decisions will need to be taken and codified into an accounting framework. In this way, the designation of the resource as health or non-health, even if arbitrary, can still inform policy. Everyone will have a common expectation of whether consumption of a particular resource will be routinely counted as a health expenditure or not, and can then make the necessary adjustments depending on the nature of their policy concerns.
2. To facilitate interpretation of health expenditures within the general economic accounting framework in the country. The health sector comprises a significant part of the economy. A health accounting system that is consistent with an accounting system that tracks the whole economy contributes to a greater understanding of the role of health within the economic life of the country.

Health Care Costs, Structures and Trends

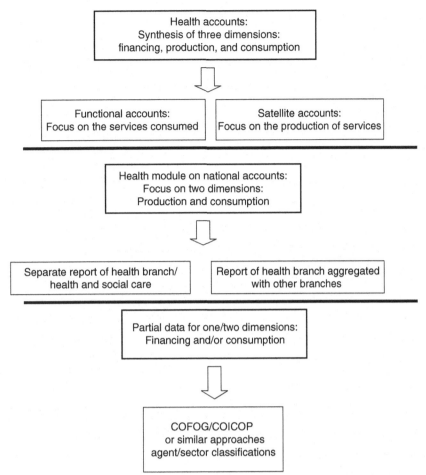

Figure 1 Descriptive summary of health accounting frameworks. COFOG, the classification of the functions of government (a classification used to identify the socioeconomic objectives of current transactions, capital outlays, and acquisition of financial assets by general government and its subsectors); COICOP, classification of individual consumption by purpose (a classification used to identify the objectives of both individual consumption expenditure and actual individual consumption). From System of National Accounts 93.

Figure 1 describes the three major health accounting systems that currently exist. In a few years, it is anticipated that a global health standard for health accounting will be developed that will both serve national needs and facilitate international comparisons.

How Are Health Expenditures Estimated and Reported?

Picturing the flow of funds and construction of national health account matrices

The unit of analysis in tracking health expenditure flows is the final consumption of a resource. For every resource consumed, there is a financier, a provider, and a consumer, illustrating the three analytical dimensions of accounting frameworks. The financing dimension covers both the funders (financing sources, or FS) and the purchasers who decide where the funds will be spent (financing agents or FA). The production dimension includes the providers (HP) and inputs to production (also called resource costs or RC and includes human resources, pharmaceuticals, capital). The consumption dimension is reflected in the use of the resource (health functions or HC) and consumer/beneficiary analysis by specific characteristics (age, sex, socioeconomic characteristics, health status, place of residence). The tracking of funds as they flow from financing, production to consumption (see **Figure 2**) is called national health accounting. National health accounts (NHA) cover both public and private sector spending.

Figure 2 could also be converted into a series of matrices illustrating several stages in the flow of expenditures, including:

- financing source by financing agent;
- financing agent by provider;
- provider by function.

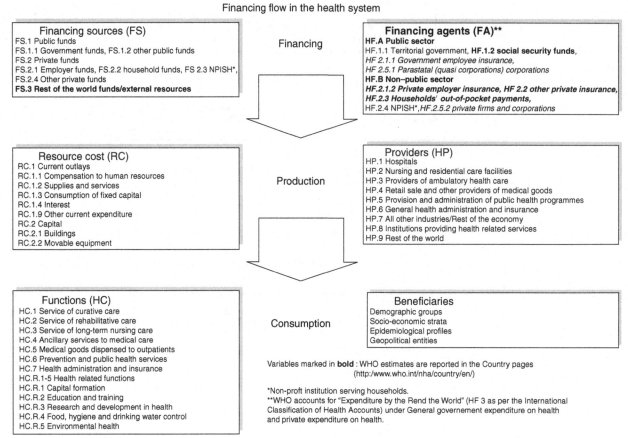

Figure 2 Financing flow in the health system.

More matrices could be constructed, depending on the policy need. The matrix approach ensures that at every level of transaction, there is a supplier and a recipient and that the expenditure, viewed from either perspective, does not change in quantity. This self-correcting characteristic of matrices is helpful for either estimation or validation purposes. More detailed information on estimation and validation techniques including data sources is available from the Guide to Producing National Health Accounts with special applications for low-income and middle-income countries or the System of Health Accounts.

Reporting conventions for time and place, including indicators

In capturing health spending, certain reporting conventions are observed. Expenditures are reported annually, based on calendar year and sometimes fiscal year. When there are missing data for some years, they are usually filled in by interpolation, on the assumption that it is business as usual. Recording in national currency units is on an accrual basis or at the time of consumption of the resource, rather than the time of payment.

Consistent with the definition of a health expenditure, expenditures are attributed to the country of residence of the consumer/beneficiary, rather than to the place where the service or good is provided. Medical tourism or cross-border care is treated in a similar way.

There are minimum indicators that are to be recommended to be reported annually. These indicators and their definitions are seen in **Table 1**.

The Global Picture of Health Spending

Data in this section are obtained from the latest year available from the WHO database on health expenditures of 193 Member States. More detailed information including a 10-year series for each Member State and methodology notes are available from the WHO NHA website.

Gross Domestic Product and Health Spending

In 2004, the world spent a total of US$4.1 trillion on health at exchange rates or I$4.9 trillion (International

Table 1 List of health spending indicators

Indicator	Definition
Total expenditure on health	Sum of general government and of private expenditure on health
General government expenditure on health	The sum of outlays for health maintenance, restoration or enhancement paid for in cash or in kind by government entities, such as the Ministry of Health, other ministries, parastatal organizations, social security agencies, (without double-counting the government transfers to social security and to extrabudgetary funds). Includes transfer payments to households to offset medical care costs and extrabudgetary funds to finance health. The revenue base of these entities may comprise multiple sources, including external funds
Social security and extra-budgetary funds on health	Expenditure by social security schemes and public social health insurance schemes to purchase health goods and services. These schemes refer to all compulsory schemes for a sizeable segment of the population. Extrabudgetary funds made up of publicly funded schemes that operate autonomously, such as university hospitals, foundations dealing with specific health risks, etc.
Private expenditure on health	Comprises the outlays of insurers and third-party payers other than social security, mandated and voluntary employer health services and other enterprises provided health services, nonprofit institutions and nongovernmental organizations (such as the International Committee of the Red Cross) financed health care, private investments in medical care facilities and household out-of-pocket spending
Prepaid private risk-pooling plans	The outlays of private and private social (with no government control over payment rates and participating providers but with only a broad outline from the government) insurance schemes, commercial and nonprofit (mutual) insurance schemes, health maintenance organizations, and other agents managing prepaid medical and paramedical benefits, including the operating costs of these schemes
Nongovernmental organizations' expenditure on health	Resources used to purchase health goods and services by enterprises that are not allowed to be a source of income, profit, or other financial gain for the units that establish, control, or finance them
Out-of-pocket spending on health	The direct outlays of households, including gratuities and payments in kind made to health practitioners and suppliers of pharmaceuticals, therapeutic appliances, and other goods and services, whose primary intent is to contribute to the restoration or to the enhancement of the health status of individuals or population groups. Includes household payments to public services, nonprofit institutions, or nongovernmental organizations. Includes nonreimbursable cost-sharing, deductibles, co-payments, and fee-for service. Excludes payments made by enterprises that deliver medical and paramedical benefits, mandated by law or not, to their employees. Excludes payments for overseas treatment
Tax-funded expenditure on health	All public outlays by territorial governments (Central/Federal, Provincial/Regional/State/District, Municipal/Local) on health, net of intergovernmental transfers, including subsidies to producers of medical goods and services, investment in medical facilities, transfer payments to households to offset medical care costs and extrabudgetary funds
External resources for health	Grants and loans for medical care and medical goods channelled through the Ministry of Health, other public agencies and nonprofit institutions. Grants in-kind (capital equipment, pharmaceutical supplies and vaccines, technical assistance such as experts) should be estimated at their monetary value. Grants to nongovernmental organizations should be accounted for under Nongovernmental Organizations' Expenditure on Health (NGOH) outlays in financing agent table. External resources are a financing source not shown explicitly under financing agents to prevent double counting as they are included under general government expenditure on health (GGHE) or NGOH

dollars taking into account the purchasing power of different national currencies). This constitutes approximately 10% of the global economy, measured in US dollars. Health spending by country as a share of gross domestic product (GDP) can be seen in **Figure 3** and ranges from 1.6 to 16.5%.

Per capita spending on health in 2004 was US$645 (I$777). Disaggregation by country income grouping shows that the average health spending per capita increases with increasing GDP per capita, as can be seen in **Table 2** and this trend is more clearly demonstrated in **Figure 4**.

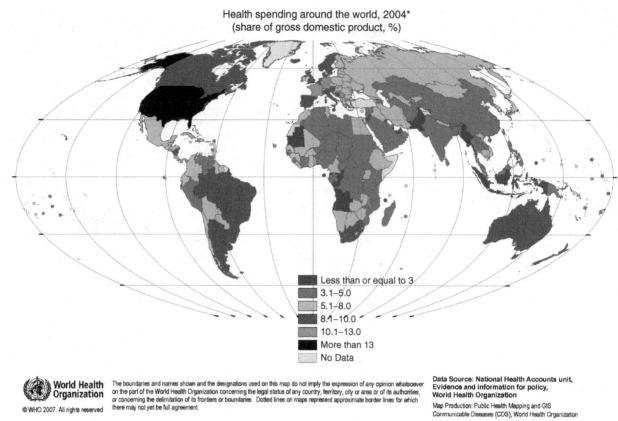

Figure 3 Total health expenditure as a share of gross domestic product.

Table 2 Average total health expenditure by capita according to country income groupings, 2004

Income level	Average[a] gross domestic product (per capita US$)	Average[a] total health expenditure (per capita US$)
High	33 496	3725
Upper middle	5229	348
Lower middle	1713	93
Low	516	24
World	6439	645

[a]Estimated as weighted average.

Distribution of Health Expenditure by Financing Agent

Of the total of US$4.1 trillion, 59% were general government health expenditures of which 25% were from social health insurance, while 19% were from private health insurance, and 18% were out-of-pocket expenditures. Again, the average global picture masks disparities. In **Figure 5**, one can see that low-income countries relied most heavily on out-of-pocket payments to finance health care. In these countries, the share of out-of-pocket payments in total health expenditures was 70% compared to only 15% in high-income countries. Health expenses in most high-income countries are raised largely through public prepayment mechanisms such as tax-based funding or social health insurance, with potential for cross-subsidizing and protecting households from financial catastrophe. These funds are channelled through private insurance, social security, and government agencies that purchase or provide health services.

Health Expenditures and Health Outcomes

Linking health expenditures to epidemiology, **Figure 6** shows that the poorer WHO regions like AFR and SEAR account for the largest share of the global burden of disease (over 50% of global disability-adjusted life years lost) and 37% of the world's population. However, they spend only about 2% of global health resources. Thirty OECD countries make up less than 20% of the world's population but spend 90% of the world's resources on health. Richer countries with smaller populations and lower disease burden use more health resources than poorer countries with larger populations and higher disease burden.

How can one judge whether spending is too much or too little? **Figure 7** shows that increasing health expenditure results in better health outcomes with steep

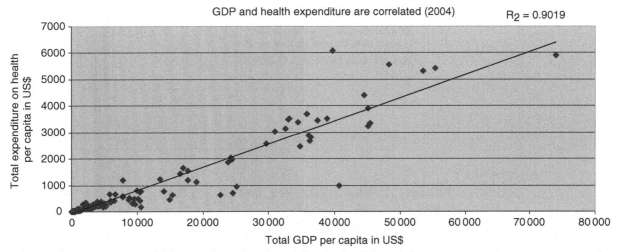

Figure 4 Correlation between GDP per capita and total expenditure on health per capita.

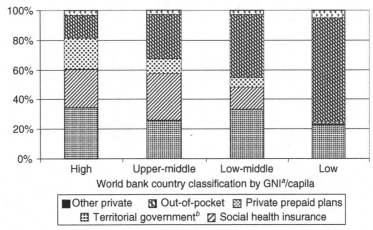

Figure 5 Components of health expenditure measured in US$, 2004. World Bank country classification by GNI/capita. High income, US$10 726 or more; upper middle income, US$3466–10 725; low middle income, US$ 876–3465; low income, US$ 875 or less.
[a]GNI is the sum of value added by all resident producers plus any product taxes (less subsidies) not included in the valuation of output plus net receipts of primary income (compensation of employees and property income) from abroad. GDP is sum of gross value added, at purchaser prices converted at market exchange rates to current U.S. dollars, by all resident producers in the economy plus any product taxes (less subsidies) not included in the valuation of output.
[b]Territorial government: the sum of central, regional and local government outlays on health, net of intra-government transfers.

returns in investment at low levels of per capita spending, gradually tapering until one reaches a plateau where increasing investments in health achieves only very marginal returns.

How Does Information on Health Expenditure Influence Policy at the Global and National Levels?

The standardization of estimation and reporting of health expenditure data allows us to describe and compare health expenditures by country at a global level. Clearly, many inequitable disparities exist. Tracking health expenditures at a global level allows one to clearly make the case for global solidarity in health financing. Low-income countries do not spend enough on health, the financial burden is borne directly by the population, and their health needs are overwhelming. Health expenditures in high-income countries are now increasingly getting a bigger share of the economy and raise questions of efficiency.

At the national level, describing the distribution of health expenditures can show striking results that lead to changes in health financing, whether it shows inadequate investments in health, inequities in expenditure by geographic area or by disease, high financial burden in accessing services because of user fees, or substantial dependence on donor funds. The value of the information provided by health expenditure estimates is also tremendously increased when it is interpreted in the

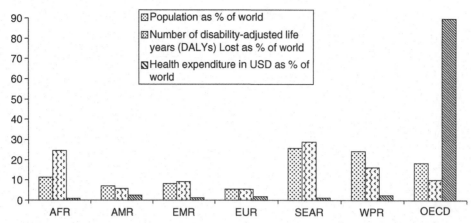

Figure 6 Percentage distribution of population, disability-adjusted life years[a], and total health expenditures[b] by WHO Regions and OECD[c], 2004.
[a]Disability-adjusted life years (DALYs) data are for 2002.
[b]Shares are calculated using total expenditure on health in exchange rate $.
[c]AFR, AMR, EMR, EUR, SEAR, WPR are World Health Organization Regions of Africa, Americas, Eastern Mediterranean, Europe, South-East Asia and Western Pacific, respectively. Totals for AMR, EUR and WPR regions have been calculated after subtracting out the 30 OECD countries from these groups.
OECD, Organization for Economic Co-operation and Development.

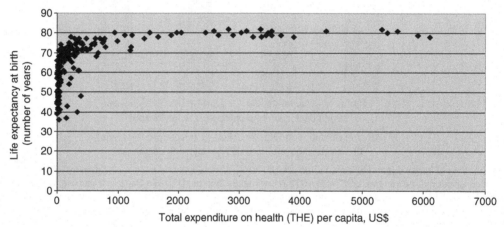

Figure 7 Correlation between expenditure on health and health outcomes.

context of other data such as health outcomes or coverage of interventions. Finally, trends in health expenditures can also be used to project expenditures into the future.

See also: Determinants of National Health Expenditure.

Further Reading

De S, Dmytraczenko T, Brinkerhoff D, and Tien M (2003) *Has Improved Availability of Health Expenditure Data Contributed to Evidence-Based Policymaking? Country Experiences with National Health Accounts*. Technical Report No. 022.Bethesda, MD: The Partners for Health Reform*plus* Project Abt Associates Inc.

Glassman A and Rasciborska D (2004) *Working Paper: Institutionalization of Health Resource Tracking in Low- and Middle-Income Countries: Approaches and Alternatives*. Washington, DC: Center for Global Development.

Institute of Policy Studies and Ministry of Health Sri Lanka (2003) Sri Lanka's National Health Accounts: National Health Expenditures 1990–1999. In: Yazbeck AS and Peters DH (eds.) *Health Policy Research in Asia: Guiding Reforms and Building Capacity*, pp. 163–194. Washington, DC: World Bank.

Musgrove P, Zeramdini R, and Carrin G (2002) Basic patterns in national health expenditure. *Bulletin of the World Health Organization* 80: 134–146.

Nandakumar AK, Bhawalkar M, Tien M, Ramos R, and Susna De (2004) *Synthesis of Findings from NHA Studies in Twenty-Six Countries*. Bethesda, MD: The Partners for Health Reform*plus* Project Abt Associates Inc.

OECD Health Policy Unit (2000) *A System of Health Accounts*. Paris, France: OECD.

Savedoff W (2003) *How Much Should Be Spent on Health?* Discussion Paper No. 2 EIP/FER/DP0.3.2.Geneva, Switzerland: World Health Organization. http://www.who.int/health_financing/documents/en/ (accessed October 2007).

World Health Organization (2003) *Guide to Producing National Health Accounts for Low and Middle Income Countries with Special Applications for Low Income and Middle Income Countries*. Geneva, Switzerland: World Health Organization.

Relevant Websites

http://www.oecd.org/health/sha – Organisation for Economic Co-operation and Development, A System of Health Accounts.

http://www.phrplus.org/nha.html – Third CIS NHA workshop: Progress to Date and Future Steps.

http://www.who.int/topics/global_burden_of_disease/en/ – World Health Organization, Global burden of disease.

www.who.int/nha/en/ – World Health Organization, National Health Accounts.

Determinants of National Health Expenditure

A K Nandakumar and M E Farag, Brandeis University, Waltham, MA, USA

© 2008 Elsevier Inc. All rights reserved.

How Much Does the World Spend on Health?

In 1998, the world spent nearly 7.9% of global income on health care, which amounted to 3.1 trillion international dollars or 523 international dollars per capita (Poullier *et al.*, 2002). The world not only spends a significant share of its resources on health care but countries at all levels of economic development are concerned about how resources are mobilized, allocated, and the value proposition of investing in health.

There are large variations in health spending across countries. For example, 2004 data obtained from the World Health Organization (WHO) indicate that total health expenditures as a percentage of gross domestic product (GDP) ranged from a low of 1.6% in Equatorial Guinea to a high of 16.6% in Tuvalu followed by 15.4% in the United States; on a per capita basis health expenditures ranged from 15.3 international dollars in Democratic Republic of the Congo to 6096.2 international dollars in the United States. These differentials are not restricted to low- and high-income countries but exist within and across countries at the same level of economic development. For example, if one were to consider countries of the Organization for Economic Co-operation and Development (OECD), the Republic of Korea spends 5.5% of its GDP on health as compared with the United States, which spends 15.4% of its GDP on health (WHO, 2007). Over the decades growth in health expenditures has tended to outstrip general inflation rates in most countries, although Sweden did report a negative growth in health spending in 1999–2000.

In its simplest form total health expenditure is a product of the quantities of different health services consumed and their unit prices. In this article, we analyze and identify factors that determine health expenditures. Where data are available we try to analyze how these determinants vary across countries at different levels of economic development. We rely mainly on secondary sources of information in addition to conducting analysis of the available published data.

Determinants of National Health Expenditures

In **Figure 1** we provide a framework within which to analyze determinants of national health expenditures. The main factors affecting health expenditures are the following:

- How the health system is organized and managed
- The health needs of the population
- The level of economic development, per capita income, and income distribution
- The supply of health services
- Technology.

Governance and Organization of the Health System

How a health-care system in a country is managed and organized influences how much that country spends on health care. Management of the health system is an important function that governments perform and involves policy formulation, defining the roles of the public and private sectors in the financing and provision of health services, setting priorities on allocating scarce health resources, monitoring the performance of the health system, and regulating and protecting consumers against the adverse effects of market failures in health care. At the most

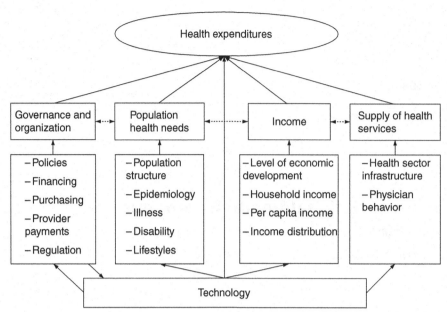

Figure 1 A framework for analyzing the determinants of health expenditures.

fundamental level the policies that governments enact and the role they play in managing the health system influences all inputs into the health system, the mix of services produced, access to health care, prices in the market place for health-care goods, and eventually health outcomes and expenditures. For example, in the United States, where the government has much less direct control over health spending, the result has been higher rates of increase of health expenditures as compared with other OECD countries (Altman and Rodwin, 1988; Reinhardt, 1993). The U.S. government's relatively lower degree of control over expenditures stems from the fact that it has little direct influence over expenditures in the private sector, whereas in Canada and European countries, for example, the government can use tools such as negotiations with medical unions, budget caps, and claw-back mechanisms to control expenditures.

Health-care financing consists of mobilizing health funds, pooling these funds, and using them to purchase health-care services. Governments can use a mix of financing methods to mobilize health funds. These include general tax revenues, earmarked taxes, social health insurance, private health insurance, medical savings accounts, out-of-pocket expenditures, and external assistance. The mix of resource mobilization methods used reflects social values, the level of socioeconomic development, and the particular aspects of market failure that the government would like to address. For example, social health insurance schemes such as those in Europe reflect an explicit contract between the government and its citizens, assure universal coverage, and are reasonably effective in dealing with adverse selection. The use of insurance mechanisms – either social or private – is facilitated by the existence of a large formal sector and effective collection, pooling, and disbursements systems. Insurance systems take time to design and implement and involve large investments. National Health Accounts studies have shown that low- and middle-income countries use a multiplicity of financing methods and have underdeveloped insurance markets and high out-of-pocket expenditures.

Purchasing of health services refers to what services are purchased, how they are purchased, from whom they are purchased, who and how many perform the purchasing function, and how the purchasing pools are funded. There exists significant variation across countries in how the purchasing function is organized. For example, Germany, on the one hand, has a mix of social insurance health funds and private insurance schemes that can provide services to those outside the social health insurance scheme. Finland, on the other hand, has devolved responsibility of purchasing health services to local municipal councils that receive funds from the government on a prospective, needs-based budget. The organization of the purchasing function influences services produced, prices paid to providers, and access to care. All these factors, in turn, affect overall health expenditures. An important distinction to keep in mind is that under social insurance the total amount spent on health can be decided by government, whereas in a private insurance system this decision is a result of the market and the power of the various stakeholders.

Provider payment refers to the mechanism by which health providers are reimbursed at the point of service. The main aim of provider payment is to create incentives that influence the behavior of providers to achieve policy objectives of the government such as equity, efficiency, and increased access to care. There are three principal methods of provider payment. In the first the purchaser pays salaries and makes available facilities and medical supplies; the second is contracting for services; the third is allocating an annual budget that could be set on the basis of expected services or enrolled population. More recently, the term 'pay for performance' or 'P4P' has made its way into the vocabulary of policy analysts and researchers. One definition refers to P4P as the "transfer of money or material goods conditional on taking a measurable action or achieving a predetermined performance target" (Eichler, 2006). Pay for performance refers to incentives to address both demand and supply-side issues. On the demand side, examples include cash transfer programs or vouchers; on the supply side examples encompass the entire range of incentive payments designed to affect provider behavior.

Once again, how providers are reimbursed influences health-care costs. For example, until the 1970s in the United States hospitals were paid retrospectively. In other words, hospitals first spent then billed for their services. Since the revenues of a hospital are a function of the costs of services provided there was little incentive to balance the cost of care against the patient benefits. The result was double-digit increases in health expenditures, rising private insurance premiums, rapid increase in the expenditure of the public programs Medicare and Medicaid, and an increased share of GDP allocated to health. In response to escalating costs, the government changed its payment method to a prospective payment system and Health Maintenance Organizations were established. Both these developments were designed to provide incentives to the provider to be more cost conscious and share in the risk of health-care costs. Subsequent to these changes the rate of growth of medical expenditures slowed, at least in the short-term.

Decisions about how health care will be financed, purchased, and paid for all have a direct impact on the demand for health-care services, investments that will be made by the private sector in creating health infrastructure and R&D, the type, quantity, and intensity of health services provided, and the price of health services in the marketplace, and these in turn affect health expenditures.

Health Needs of the Population

Demographic transition posits that with improvements in health, mortality rates start to drop faster than fertility rates. This results in a short-lived increase in family size. Due to the lag between mortality and fertility, population will increase. The sheer increase in the number of individuals in a country increases health needs. However, over time as fertility rates decline the proportion of elderly tends to increase as a percentage of the total population, and this change in population structure affects the need and demand of health-care services. Another factor affecting health needs is the epidemiological transition that countries go through. 'Epidemiological transition' refers to the fact that with economic development and declines in fertility rates the disease profile of countries changes from a preponderance of communicable diseases, maternal and perinatal conditions, and nutritional deficiencies to one in which noncommunicable conditions account for a large part of the disease burden. Thus both the demographic and epidemiological transitions affect the health needs and subsequently the health demands of populations, and this in turn has an impact on health expenditures.

In the next 50 years, the share of world population aged 60 or more will double from 10% to 22%, tripling to 30% by 2100. The root causes for this are advances in medical care, improved nutrition, changes in lifestyle, and decreased fertility.

How will this change in demographics affect health expenditures? An article by Alistair Gray of the University of Oxford analyzed data from 13 OECD countries where data were available and concluded that population aging would increase age-related expenditures from under 19% of GDP in 2000 to almost 26% of GDP by 2050 with expenditures on health accounting for half of these increases (Gray, 2005). Other studies conducted with developed country data also support the hypothesis that the demographic structure of a population is a significant variable in explaining health expenditures (Anderson et al., 2003). In a recent study published in *Health Affairs* the authors project that health spending in the United States is expected to account for 20% of GDP by 2015 and that population aging will account for a "small but rising" share of total health expenditures between 2004 and 2015 (Borger et al., 2006).

In recent years there have been a few studies that have tried to estimate the impact of aging on health expenditures in low- and middle-income countries. Two studies conducted under the Partners for Health Reform Plus (PHRplus) project funded by USAID analyzed this issue in the context of Jordan and the Philippines. The Jordan study modeled expenditures on the elderly under different scenarios of macro-economic growth. The study concluded that whereas the elderly as a percentage of the population were projected to increase from 7% in 2000 to 9% in 2015, their share of total health expenditures was projected to increase from 20.2% in 2000 to 23.2% under the high-growth scenario, to 32.7% under the medium-growth scenario, and to 38% under low-growth assumptions. The study done in the Philippines concluded that the share of health expenditures going to services for the elderly will rise from 19.5% in the year 2000 to 29.5% in the year 2020. In the Philippines most of this increase was due to the aging of the population, but this would not affect the share of health spending going to the young. However, the study concluded that this is likely to change beyond 2020 when significant aging in the Philippines will begin to take place (Mason *et al.*, 2004).

Lifestyles also affect health expenditures. Healthy lifestyles tend to improve health and reduce health expenditures, and unhealthy lifestyles result in poor health and increased health expenditures. A good example of this is to look at how obesity affects health expenditures in the United States. It is estimated that in 1998 overweight and obesity attributable medical expenditures accounted for 9.1% of total health expenditures amounting to $78.5 billion dollars. Medicare and Medicaid financed roughly half these costs (Finkelstein *et al.*, 2003).

The Effect of Income on Health Expenditures

Evidence exists for a strong and positive correlation between income and health expenditures at the level of countries and households. What lies behind the relationship between income and health expenditures?

Our own analysis of 2004 data for 190 countries obtained from the World Health Organization (WHO, 2007) shows the following three facts:

1. There exists a positive correlation between GDP per capita and share of total health expenditures as a percentage of GDP, as shown in **Figure 2a**; an Ordinary Least Squares (OLS) regression line shows the positive correlation between percentage of GDP spent on health in a country and the country's GDP per capita.
2. There exists a positive correlation between GDP per capita and per capita health expenditures. **Figure 2b** shows that the higher the GDP per capita measured in international dollars/PPPs, the higher the per capita health expenditures in international dollars/PPPs. The simple OLS regression line can only indicate the correlation between GDP per capita and health spending per capita. However, it cannot establish causality, since it does not consider all the other possible factors that could have an influence on health spending.
3. There exists a positive correlation between GDP per capita and the government share of total health expenditures as shown in **Figure 2c** using simple OLS regression.

The patterns observed above are consistent with the findings of Musgrove *et al.* (2002), who found that total health spending rises from around 2–3% of gross domestic product (GDP) at low incomes (<US$1000 per capita) to about 8–9% at high incomes (>US$7000). They also found that public financing constitutes a larger share of GDP as income increases, and converges at high incomes. Their research also shows that the health share of total public expenditures increases as income rises from 5–6% to 10% (Musgrove *et al.*, 2002).

However, a synthesis of National Health Accounts from 26 low- and middle-income countries published by the PHRplus project appears to indicate that with regard to countries in Latin America and the Caribbean there actually was a negative correlation between the percentage of GDP a country spends on health and that country's per capita income. The second hypothesis tested in the study was whether there was a positive correlation between per capita incomes and the share of public expenditures to total health expenditures. Once again the study found that for middle-income countries from Latin America and the Caribbean and those in the Middle East and North Africa the hypothesis did not hold. A number of factors might have accounted for these findings, including the number of countries included in the sample, classification and validity of data, and how the underlying health systems are organized. However, the study does highlight two important facts: first, that relationships observed in high-income countries might not hold in low- and middle-income countries and, second, that more research is needed to understand these relationships in low- and middle-income countries.

The report of the Commission on Macroeconomics (2001) and health argues very strongly for the link between health and economic development. The commission report shows that health status is important in explaining the differences in economic growth rates across countries even when one controls for macro-economic variables. Given that ill health and its consequences disproportionately affect the poor, the commission argues that increased investments for combating health conditions affecting the poor will stimulate economic development and help alleviate poverty. A World Bank report authored by Lance Pritchett and Laurence H. Summers using cross-country longitudinal data showed that the relationship between incomes and health is "not only associative but causal and structural" (Pritchett and Summers, 1993).

Grossman pioneered the use of the theory of human capital to study the demand for health care (Grossman, 1972). According to Grossman, individuals aim at increasing their income and in order to do so will invest in themselves. Thus investments that individuals make in health are a means to an end and not an end in itself. The "health of an individual" is a commodity that is used up over multiple time periods and hence can be viewed as a capital good. Individuals increase their capital of health by both purchasing and producing health. Subsequent applications of the Grossman approach have shown that the demand for health goes up with income and education.

Families facing high infant mortality tend to overcompensate by having more children than needed to adjust for mortality and thus have fewer resources to invest per child. This is sometimes referred to as the "quality/quantity" trade-off. As the probability of child survival increases, families start having fewer children and invest more in

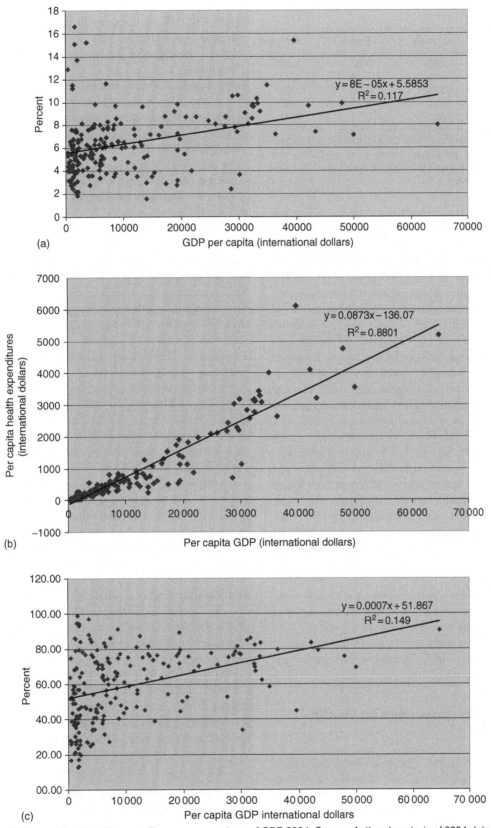

Figure 2 (a) Share of total health expenditures as percentage of GDP 2004. Source: Authors' analysis of 2004 data from WHO. (b) Per capita GDP by per capita health expenditures. (c) Per capita GDP and government share of total health expenditures.

Table 1 Per capita utilization of health outpatient services by income quintiles

Income quintile	Jordan	Egypt	Kenya
Lowest	3.63	2.32	1.72
Second	4.03	2.91	1.75
Third	3.78	3.40	1.93
Fourth	3.40	3.79	2.07
Highest	2.91	5.11	2.27

Source: Jordan Household Health Care Utilization and Expenditure Survey, Egypt Household Health Care Utilization and Expenditure Survey, Kenya Household Health Care Utilization and Expenditure Survey.

these children and hence family size starts declining; this cycle results in a change in the population structure that is referred to as the demographic transition (Barro and Becker, 1998). Studies conducted in both developed and developing countries bear out the positive relationship between household income and the health status of children.

Household income also is a strong predictor of the demand for health-care services and expenditures (**Table 1**). A study of the inequality of health-care use and expenditures from eight developing countries and countries in transition found that individuals in higher-income groups had a higher probability of using care when sick, were more likely to be seen by a doctor, and also spent more in absolute terms on health care as compared with individuals in lower-income groups (Makinen et al., 2000). We analyzed data from three nationally representative household health-care utilization and expenditure survey reports and found that in both Kenya and Egypt those in the higher-income quintiles used more outpatient visits per capita as compared with those in the lower-income quintiles. Jordan is an exception to the rule in the case of low- and middle-income countries: in Jordan the use of outpatient care actually declines with increasing income. This fact reflects in part the strong commitment to health of the population by the country, the extensive and well-financed health infrastructure, and the availability of physicians and drugs at the facilities.

In conclusion, income is an important determinant of health expenditures at both the level of the country and households.

Effect of Health Insurance on Health Expenditures

Economic theory suggests that risk-averse individuals would prefer to protect against unpredictable costs through the purchase of insurance. In a seminal paper titled "Uncertainty and the Welfare Economics of Medical Care," Kenneth Arrow identifies situations in which markets for health insurance might fail and argues that because of welfare gains associated with insurance, "governments should undertake insurance where the market, for whatever reason, has failed to emerge" (Arrow, 1963). What insurance does is lower the marginal cost faced by individuals and, as a consequence, it can increase utilization of services by the individual. This phenomenon is also known as 'moral hazard.' Mark Pauly showed that moral hazard was a rational economic response to the presence of insurance and that "even if all individuals are risk averters, some uncertain medical care expenses will not and should not be insured in an optimal situation" (Pauly, 1968).

In the United States, the Rand Corporation undertook the first randomized study to examine the impact of insurance on demand and expenditures. The key findings from this study are reported in "Health Insurance and the Demand for Medical Care: Evidence from a Randomized Experiment" (Manning et al., 1987). The Rand study showed that "demand elasticities for medical care are non zero and indeed the response to cost sharing is nontrivial." Rand researchers also examined the effect of insurance on the increase in health expenditures in the United States since World War II. They concluded that insurance accounted for only 10% of the total increase in health expenditures. This means that the expansion in health insurance coverage would account for only 70% of the 700% increase in health expenditures in the United States.

Analysis of Household Health Care Expenditures and Utilization Surveys in middle-income countries do not always support the hypothesis that the presence of insurance increases demand and expenditures on health care. For example, in Egypt it was found that insurance was not a significant variable in determining demand for health-care services (Nandakumar et al., 2000). In Jordan it was observed that holding other factors constant, age, income, and insurance were not significant in explaining the demand for health-care services. The reasons for these findings vary by country. In Egypt the reasons probably revolved around the design and management of the social health insurance scheme, whereas in Jordan it had more to do with a well-functioning health system that spends over 9% of its GDP on health, has an extensive network of primary health-care facilities within easy reach of the population, and has a very strong commitment to public health and primary health care. These studies indicate that the significant association observed in the United States and other developed countries between insurance and demand, as well as expenditures on health care, might not hold in the case of low- and middle-income countries.

The Effect of Physician Behavior on Health Expenditures

The presence of asymmetries in information and their effect on the physician–patient relationship have been the focus of extensive research. Robert Evans was probably the first economist to postulate the hypothesis that physicians have the ability to "shift out" demand for their services through "inducing activities" (Evans, 1974). David Dranove, in an important paper published in 1985, used a game theory approach to present a model in which physician inducement can be better understood (Dranove, 1985). In this model the game is played between the physician and the patient. The physician's income is based on payments received for services provided to the patient. The physician has the ability to induce demand and this will positively affect the physician's income. However, the physician runs the risk of losing the patient's business if the latter comes to the conclusion that the physician overprescribes services. According to Dranove the physician will choose the optimal level of inducement that "balances the gains from recommending and performing expensive treatments and the losses from possessing a bad reputation." The level of inducement will depend on various factors, including the reimbursement rate for the treatment, the level of knowledge of the patient, and the value placed on the treatment by the patient. Various studies appear to validate Dranove's hypothesis. For example, a study on ordering of laboratory tests showed that roughly 50% of these tests were unwarranted (Kaplan *et al.*, 1985). Another study conducted with data from the 1977 National Medical Care Expenditure Survey in the United States showed that a decrease of 1% in the out-of-pocket price of physician visits increased physician-initiated visits by 0.17% and that physician-initiated visits decreased with the education level of the patient (Wilenky and Rossiter, 1983).

Giuffrida and Gravelle (2001) analyzed the demand and supply of night visits in primary care in the UK by using panel data. They found that the introduction of differential fees for general practitioner (GP) and deputy visits in 1990 led GPs to increase their own visits and to reduce the number made by deputies. Xirasagar and Lin (2006) examined the earnings of 8106 office-based (FTE) physicians in 2002 in Taiwan and found evidence of a steady earnings increase with increasing total physician density, thus confirming their hypothesis about the presence of physician-induced demand in an office setting.

It is important to point out that there are others who argue that it is neither the profit-maximizing nor income-maximizing behavior of physicians that results in excess care being prescribed but rather the uncertainty of medical diagnosis and the desire of physicians to optimize health outcomes for their patients that can lead to excess care being prescribed. Some economists have argued that as physician supply increases physicians induce demand in order to protect their incomes. Yet others argue that in countries where the fear of medical malpractice suits is high physicians tend to practice defensive medicine: "the use of diagnostic and end-treatment measures explicitly for the purposes of averting malpractice suits" (Tancredi and Barondess, 1978), which in turn leads to unnecessary health services (Rodriguez *et al.*, 2007) and increased costs.

The United States is one country where the issue of the effect of defensive medicine on health expenditures has been studied quite extensively; most studies show that it accounts for less than 1% of total health expenditures.

Whatever one's views might be on the ability of physicians to induce demand, thereby affecting health expenditures, it cannot be denied that treatment decisions taken by physicians whether in an inpatient or outpatient setting are critical in deciding the type, intensity, and duration of care that is provided, and hence their role in determining health expenditures should not be underestimated.

The Role of Technology in Determining Health Expenditures

There is an emerging consensus among researchers that the development, diffusion, and adoption of technologies are an important determinant of health expenditures. Technology, by its very nature, is a complex commodity that takes time to develop and requires large investments in Research and Development (R&D). Burton Weisbrod (1991), in an important paper entitled "The Health Care Quadrilemma: An Essay on Technological Change, Insurance, Quality of Care, and Cost Containment," examined the relationship between the expansion of insurance and the development of "cost increasing technologies" in the United States. Weisbrod argues that there is a reciprocal relationship between health insurance and technology.

New interventions are usually expensive and companies spending on R&D factor into their investment decisions either existing financing mechanisms or those that will be in place when these technologies enter the market. This is best illustrated by considering the effect of a technology such as kidney or liver transplant. With these technologies it is now possible to treat conditions that were previously untreatable but at a cost that most individuals cannot afford to pay out-of-pocket. The catastrophic nature of these expenditures means that the demand will grow to pay for such treatment either from government funds or through insurance. According to Weisbrod, "the long run growth of health care expenditures is a by product of the interaction of the R&D process with the health insurance system." Some technologies, such as the polio vaccine, can be viewed as a public good. In this instance the financing comes largely from public sources or donor assistance. Therefore it is not necessary that all technologies will stimulate a demand for insurance.

In the United States health insurance has largely paid for facility-based treatment, with coverage for preventive care being limited. Hence the R&D sector has little incentive to focus on prevention rather than on treatment. Thus, the type of health insurance and how providers and manufacturers are reimbursed for the use of technology will determine the direction of R&D but also the balance between cure and prevention.

An article published in *Health Affairs* examines the relationship between technology availability and health-care spending in the United States (Baker *et al.*, 2003). The authors found that, for those with private insurance, an increase in one non-hospital-based magnetic resonance imaging (MRI) machine led to a 0.93% increase in per beneficiary spending on outpatient MRI. Similarly, increases in free-standing computer tomography (CT) units were significantly associated with increased use and spending by Medicare and private insurance beneficiaries. The authors conclude that "the general pattern in our results is that more availability is associated with higher use and expenditures." Joseph Newhouse in his analysis of the determinants of increases in health expenditures in the United States concluded that aging, increased insurance, increased income, and supplier-induced demand accounted for perhaps a quarter of the increases in medical expenditures over a 50-year span. He goes on to say the bulk of "the residual increase is attributable to technological change, or what might loosely be called the march of science and the increased capabilities of medicine" (Newhouse, 1992).

Not many studies exist on the development, diffusion, and adoption of technology and its impact on health expenditures in low- and middle-income countries. However, information contained in the National Health Accounts study for Lebanon provides a useful insight into this issue (Ammar *et al.*, 2000). Lebanon spends over 14% of its GDP on health care. It has a highly pluralistic health financing system made up of government spending; social health insurance; private health insurance, and out-of-pocket expenditures. The public and private financing agents purchase services from the private sector, which is growing rapidly and is largely unregulated. The National Health Accounts study showed that in 1998, pharmaceutical expenditures accounted for over 25% of total health expenditures. Ninety-eight percent of pharmaceuticals sold in the country are brand-name drugs and 94% of drugs consumed in the country are imported. The growth in expenditures on pharmaceuticals has been accompanied by a rapid increase in the number of pharmacies. In the 1990s the government decided to pay for open heart surgery, kidney transplantation, and the treatment of burns. By 1998, these three procedures accounted for 20% of total government expenditures on health. Between 1992 and 1998 the number of open heart surgery centers grew from two to eight, the number of open heart surgeries from 600 to 1600, and expenditures from roughly 10 billion Lebanese pounds to 25 billion Lebanese pounds.

The endogenous and reciprocal relationship between insurance (health financing) and technology observed in the United States need not hold for other developed countries. For many of the OECD countries, R&D and development of new technology appears to be exogenous to the mode of health financing.

Expenditures on Pharmaceuticals

In both developed and developing countries considerable attention has focused on the impact of prescription drugs on total health expenditures. In the past decade, spending on outpatient prescription drugs in the United States has grown at an annual rate of 15–20%, with total expenditures increasing from $40 billion annually to over $160 billion (Thomas *et al.*, 2002).

Figure 3 compares expenditures on pharmaceuticals as percentage of GDP for select OECD countries for which data were available for the year 2000. We find that spending on pharmaceuticals ranges from a low of 0.6% of GDP in Ireland to a high of 1.9% in France.

Figure 4 examines the share of pharmaceuticals to total health expenditures. We observe that this ranges from a low of 9% in Ireland to 22.2% in France.

A synthesis of National Health Accounts findings from 26 low- and middle-income countries showed that expenditures on pharmaceuticals accounted for a significant proportion of total health expenditures. For example, for countries in eastern and southern Africa, excluding two countries whose data were unreliable, the share of pharmaceuticals to total health expenditures ranged from a

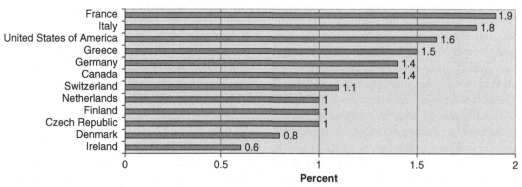

Figure 3 Expenditure on pharmaceuticals as percentage of GDP, 2000, from OECD data, 2002.

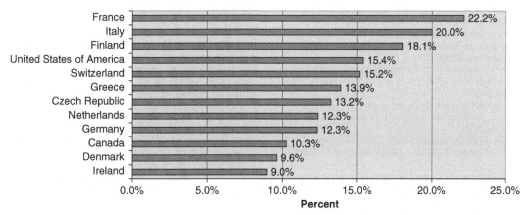

Figure 4 Pharmaceuticals as share of total health expenditures 2000 (of countries for which 2000 data are available).

low of 14% in South Africa to a high of 53% in Ethiopia. For countries in the Middle East and north Africa, spending by Iran and Djibouti on pharmaceuticals was 15% of their total health expenditures; Lebanon and Jordan spent over 25% of total health expenditures on pharmaceuticals; and Egypt, Morocco, and Yemen all spent over 35% of total health expenditures on pharmaceuticals. For countries in Latin America and the Caribbean, expenditures on pharmaceuticals as a share of total health expenditures ranged from 4% in the Dominican Republic to 33% in Nicaragua. Ecuador, El Salvador, Nicaragua, and Peru all spent over 20% of total health expenditures on pharmaceuticals (Nandakumar et al., 2004).

Our analysis shows that in countries at all levels of economic development, expenditures on pharmaceuticals represent a fairly significant proportion of total health expenditures, and the current consensus is that this will increase over time.

We would like to end the discussion on technology and its impact on health systems by pointing out that the Commission on Health Research and Development in its 1990 report observed that 10% of global R&D spending is directed at health problems of 90% of the global population (Commission on Health Research for Development, 1990). We do not believe this imbalance has been reduced in the past decade. The Commission on Macroeconomics and Health observes that for diseases that are incident in both rich and poor countries, R&D exists in rich countries, products are available, and the issue for poor countries is access to technology; for diseases that are incident in both rich and poor countries but the majority is in poor countries, R&D spending is not commensurate with the needs of poor countries; and finally for those diseases which are incident primarily in poor countries, little or no R&D investment takes place.

Conclusion

Many countries consider health care to be a basic human right because of its ability to extend and improve the quality of life of individuals. This in turn means that society expects governments to intervene proactively in the health sector to increase access to health care, protect consumers against the adverse effects of market failures, and provide safety nets for the poor. Our analysis of the determinants of health expenditures shows that how health systems are organized and managed; the health needs of the population; the level of economic development and per capita income; the presence of health insurance; the behavior of health providers, and, last but not least, technology all impact upon health expenditures. The magnitude and share of these determinants in health expenditures varies across countries. Most of the research to date has focused on high-income or developed countries. There is a need to more systematically study this issue in the context of low- and middle-income countries.

Acknowledgments

The views expressed in this article reflect those of the authors, and any omissions or errors are theirs.

See also: Demand and Supply of Human Resources for Health; The Demand for Health Care; Governance Issues in Health Financing; Insurance Plans and Programs - An Overview.

Citations

Altman SH and Rodwin M (1988) Halfway competitive markets and ineffective regulation: The American health care system. In: Greenberg W (ed.) *Competition in the Health Care Sector: Ten Years Later.* Durham, NC: Duke University Press.

Ammar W, Fakha H, Azzam O, et al. (2000) *Lebanon National Health Accounts, December.* Ministry of Health, WHO, and WB. http://www.who.int/nha/docs/en/Lebanon_NHA_report_english.pdf.

Anderson G, Reinhardt U, Hussey P, and Petrosyan V (2003) It's the price, stupid: Why the United States is so different from other countries? *Health Affairs* 22(3).

Arrow KJ (1963) Uncertainty and the welfare economics of medical care. *The American Economic Review* L111(5, 53): 941–973.

Baker L, Birnbaum H, Geppert J, Mishol D, and Moyneur E (2003) The relationship between technology availability and health care spending. *Health Affairs* (web exclusive) W3–537.

Barro R and Becker G (1998) Fertility choice in a model of economic growth. *Econometrica* 57: 481–501.

Borger C, Smith S, Truffer C, et al. (2006) Health spending projections through 2015: Changes on the horizon. *Health Affairs* 10.1377/htlhaff.25.w61.

Commission on Health Research for Development (1990) Report. *Health Research: Essential Link to Equity in Development*. Geneva, Switzerland: COHRED.

Commission on Macroeconomics and Health (2001) *Investing in Health for Economic Development*. Geneva, Switzerland: World Health Organization.

Dranove D (1988) Demand inducement and the physician/patient relationship. *Economic Inquiry* 26: 281–298.

Eichler R (2006) *Can "Pay for Performance" Increase Utilization by the Poor and Improve The Quality of Health Services?* Washington, D.C: Center for Global Development.

Evans R (1974) Supplier-induced demand: Some empirical evidence and implications. In: Perlman M (ed.) *The Economics of Medical Car*. New York: Wiley.

Finkelstein E, Fiebelkorn I, and Wang G (2003) National medical spending attributable to overweight and obesity: How much, and who's paying? *Health Affairs*, Web exclusive W3–219.

Giuffrida A and Gravelle H (2001) Inducing or restraining demand: the market for night visits in primary care. *Journal of Health Economics* 20 (2001): 755–779.

Gray A (2005) Population ageing and health care expenditure. *Oxford Institute of Ageing, Ageing Horizons* Issue No. 2, 15–20.

Grossman M (1972) On the concept of health capital and the demand for health. *Journal of Political Economy*, Vol. 80 (2): 223–255.

Kaplan S, Sheiner L, Boeckmann A, et al. (1985) The usefulness of preoperative laboratory screening. *Journal of Medical Associations* 3576–3581.

Makinen M, Waters H, Rauch M, et al. (2000) Inequalities in health care use and expenditures: Empirical data from eight developing countries and countries in transition. *Bulletin of the World Health Organization* 78: 55–65.

Manning WG, Newhouse JP, Duan N, Keeler EB, Leibowitz A, and Marquis SM (1987) Health insurance and the demand for medical care: Evidence from a randomized experiment. *The American Economic Review* Vol. 77: No. 3: 251–277.

Mason A, Racelis R, Russo G, and Wongkaren T (2004) *Technical Report on Projections and Their Implications: Philippines 1994–2020*. PHRplus July 2004.

Musgrove P, Zeramdini R, and Carrin G (2002) Basic patterns in national health expenditures. *Bulletin of the World Health Organization 2002* 80(2).

Nandakumar AK, Chawla M, and Khan M (2000) Demand for outpatient health care in Egypt: Perception and reality. *World Development* 28(1): 187–196.

Nandakumar AK, Bhawalkar M, Tien M, Ramos R, and Susna D (2004) *Synthesis of findings from NHA studies in twenty six countries. PhRplus project*. Bethesda, MD: Abt Associates.

Newhouse JP (1992) Medical care costs: How much welfare loss? *Journal of Economic Perspectives* 6(3): 3–21.

Pauly MV (1968) The economics of moral hazard: Comment. *American Economic Review* 58: 531–537.

Poullier JP, Hernandez P, Kawabata K, and D Savedoff W (2002) *Patterns of Global Health Expenditures: Results for 191 Countries*. EIP/HFS/FAR Discussion Paper No. 51. Geneva, Switzerland: World Health Organization.

Pritchett L and Summers L (1993) *Wealthier Is Healthier. Policy Research Working Paper for World Development Report 1993*. WPS 1150. Washington D.C: World Bank.

Reinhardt UE (1993) Reforming the health care system: The universal dilemma. *American Journal of Law and Medicine* 19(1, 2).

Rodriguez RM, Anglin D, Hankin A MD, et al. (2007) *Longitudinal Study of Emergency Medicine Residents' Malpractice Fear and Defensive Medicine*. Lansing, MI: Society for Academic Emergency Medicine.

Tancredi LR and Barondess JA (1978) The problem of defensive medicine. *Science, New Series* 200(4344): 879–882.

Thomas CP, Wallack SS, Lee S, and Ritter GA (2002) Impact of health plan design on retirees' prescription drug use and spending in 2001. *Health Tracking* W 408.

Weisbrod BA (1991) The health care quadrilemma: An essay on technological change, quality of care and cost containment. *Journal of Economic Literature* 29: 523–552.

Wilenky G and Rossiter L (1983) The relative importance of physician induced demand on the demand for medical care. *Milbank Memorial Fund Quarterly* 252–277.

World Health Organization (2007) http://www.who.int/whosis/en/ (accessed January 2008).

Xirasagar S and Lin H-C (2006) Physician supply, supplier-induced demand and competition: empirical evidence from a single-payer system. *International Journal of Health Planning and Management* 21: 117–131.

Further Reading

Bilgel F (2003) *The Determinants of Health Care Expenditure in Turkey, 1927–1996: An Econometric Analysis*. Istanbul, Turkey: Department of Business-Economics, Istanbul Bilgi University.

Hansen P and King K (1996) The determinants of health care expenditure: A co-integration approach. *Journal of Health Economics* 15: 127–137.

Matteo L di (2005) The macro determinants of health expenditure in the United States and Canada: Assessing the impact of income, age distribution and time. *Health Policy* 71(1): 23–42.

International Perspectives on Resource Allocation

D K Martin, University of Toronto, Toronto, Ontario, Canada
S R Benatar, University of Cape Town, Cape Town, South Africa

© 2008 Elsevier Inc. All rights reserved.

Introduction

Resource allocation, or priority setting, is arguably the most significant and challenging health policy issue of the twenty-first century. It may be defined as the distribution of goods and services (e.g., funds, professional time, beds, drugs, etc.) among competing programs or people (e.g., prevention, acute care, clinical programs, groups, individuals, etc.). No health system, whether public, private, or mixed, can afford to provide everything that may be demanded of it. Therefore, resource allocation choices are inevitable and those choices are complex, difficult, and morally problematic.

Justice, the primary moral concern of health systems, requires that the benefits and burdens of health-related services be distributed according to morally relevant criteria. Knowing what resource allocation decisions to make would be quite simple if we could agree on the criteria to guide allocations. However, examination of international experience has provided two key observations: there is no consensus about what allocation decisions should be made, and the politics of 'rationing' favors the evasion of responsibility (Ham and Coulter, 2001).

Traditional disciplinary approaches are only partially helpful. Philosophical theories of justice such as utilitarianism, egalitarianism, and communitarianism lead to different outcomes and there is no agreement about which theory is correct. Economic approaches such as cost-effectiveness analysis are helpful, but are practically limited and emphasize values (e.g., efficiency) about which there is no consensus. Legal approaches tell us what is unacceptable (e.g., discrimination), not what is right.

Different people emphasize different morally relevant criteria – for example, need, benefit, cost, cost-effectiveness, equity, equality, rule-of-rescue, and more. These criteria often conflict and there is no overarching moral theory that can resolve the conflicts. For example, when should large benefits to a few people outweigh smaller benefits to many?

In this article, we examine the current state of knowledge about resource allocation at mega (global), macro (health system), meso (institutional), and micro (clinical) levels, and suggest guidance to help decision makers address these thorny problems.

Mega-Level Resource Allocation: Global

Despite unprecedented growth of the global economy (sevenfold in the latter half of the twentieth century) and impressive progress in knowledge and technology, the world at the beginning of the twenty-first century is characterized by enormous and widening disparities in wealth and health. A century ago, the wealthiest 20% of the world's population were 9 times richer than the poorest 20%. This ratio has grown progressively to 30 times by 1960 and to over 86 times by 2000. Such economic disparities are associated with similar wide disparities in health and longevity that have been described as a form of global apartheid. Life expectancy is well over 70 years and rising in highly industrialized countries, but below 40 years and dropping in some African countries – largely due to the HIV/AIDS pandemic. Disparities in health and life expectancy are also observed between rich and poor within rich countries.

In 2002, 88% of the US$3.2 trillion spent on health care (about 10% of global GDP) was spent on about 16% of the world's population (who bear less than 10% of the global burden of diseases) (Zaracostas, 2006). Per capita expenditure on health now ranges from over $3000 annually in most advanced modern societies down to less than $15 in countries containing half the world's population. For the poorest 1 billion people in the world, most of the medical progress made in the last 100 years is almost irrelevant.

Similarly, 90% of annual global expenditure on medical research (about US$106 billion in 2001) is spent on those diseases that account for 10% of the global burden of disease (Global Forum, 2006). These ongoing and seemingly intractable imbalances in expenditure of resources on health research and health care are augmented by the degree to which they have been driven increasingly by commercial interests (**Table 1**) (Relman and Angell, 2002). For example, of 1393 new chemical entities marketed between 1975 and 1999 only 16 were for tropical diseases and tuberculosis, even though these latter diseases account for enormous mortality and morbidity (Troullier *et al.*, 2002).

A few decades ago there was hope that the major infectious diseases affecting the vast majority of humankind could be eliminated. The World Health Organization's (WHO) unprecedented success with smallpox was a remarkable model. However, the recrudescence of tuberculosis and malaria in multiresistant forms, and the appearance of HIV infection and other new infectious diseases such as SARS, have dashed such hopes and have illustrated the limitations of a narrowly focused scientific approach to public health. Communicable diseases continue to be leading causes of loss of human life and potential, as illustrated by the threat of the next pandemic of avian influenza.

The historical, political, and economic factors that sustain poverty and contribute to the ecological niches conducive to the rise and spread of these diseases cannot be

Table 1 The unique place of the paramaceutical industry

The pharmaceutical industry enjoys an almost unique place as a business. Its marketing and administrative costs amount to 30% of revenue, while research and development costs amount to only 12% of revenue. Profits, at 19% of revenue, exceed profits of commercial banks (15.8%) and those of other industries (0.5–12.1%). Moreover, the tax rate for the pharmaceutical industry (16.2% for 1993–1996) is much lower than for major American industries (27.3%). As 60% of global pharmaceutical industry profits are made in the USA, and Federal Drug and Administration links to industry are growing (with funding and staffing conflicts of interest implications, and with neither the FDA nor the U.S. patent office taking action against abuses of the patent system) it is not surprising that American interests in market-based individual health care dominate globally, and that public health is neglected

Source: Relman AS and Angell M (2002) How the drug industry distorts medicine and politics: America's other drug problem. *The New Republic* 227(25): 27–41.

ignored. Moreover, infections have no respect for geographic boundaries, particularly in an era of extensive and rapid transportation. The control of infectious diseases is not merely a problem for individual nations but for the whole world. In addition, chronic diseases are also becoming more prevalent in developing countries, producing a double burden of disease. Violence associated with the trade in small arms, illicit drugs, and commercial sex are additional factors adversely affecting health.

Negligible progress in improving global health has many sources:

1. The pursuit of economic growth has progressively superseded all other values.
2. Doing research appears to take precedence over using knowledge, unless it is commercially profitable.
3. Global health interventions tend to focus narrowly on 'vertical programs,' which constrains the way in which needy nations can address their own systemic problems.
4. There is insufficient attention to the social determinants of health.
5. Action by charitable organizations can only achieve limited results.
6. There is political reluctance to address the complex global system forces that underlie poverty and the many concomitant fatal diseases (Benatar, 2005).

Because we seem to be more interested in economic growth and in advancing knowledge than in using such knowledge to improve lives and ameliorate inequities, unless it is commercially profitable, we encourage and support the pursuit of scientific progress over social progress. This mind set has allowed global economic processes to extract material and human resources from many poor countries, erode the value of their currencies, and place their economies at the mercy of global organizations such as the International Monetary Fund and the World Bank.

Within Western societies, civil and political rights are generally ranked above socioeconomic rights and civic duties. The Universal Declaration of Human Rights defines all rights, including socioeconomic rights, as inalienable and interdependent. Failure to achieve socioeconomic rights is to a considerable extent the result of powerful upstream forces that control the global economy (Benatar, 1998). By emphasizing the rights and freedoms of capital, or capital owners, reflected in such international agreements as the North America Free Trade Alliance (NAFTA) and the World Trade Organization (WTO), the rights and freedoms of millions of individuals are sacrificed for the benefit of the wealthy.

Alternatively, the Global Fund, the Bill and Melinda Gates Foundation, and the generosity of many others present an innovative strategy to voluntarily address many pressing health issues in the developing world. However, such attitudes result in a linear, vertical approach to health problems rather than an integrated horizontal approach to the complex systems within which health is embedded. Moreover, the limited success in raising the required resources illustrates the lack of meaningful support by wealthy nations for this ambitious endeavor.

Another example of political rights ranking over socioeconomic ones is that more people die every day from malnutrition and preventable childhood diseases than they do from AIDS. Yet, we see concerted efforts to provide widespread access to antiretroviral drugs with minimal attention to the provision of food and to the prevention of avoidable deaths from easily treatable conditions in children.

Poverty and the sad state of global health can only be effectively addressed by recognizing that poor health, poverty, and human rights abuses are related to the structural forces built into modes of living that favor some over others. It is essential to modify the upstream forces, including trade rules, that sustain poverty and disadvantage poor nations.

Arguably, the key resource allocation problem is that reasonable people will undoubtedly disagree about how to proceed. Health 'maximizers' will wish to intervene to improve overall aggregate health, often by targeting those who are in some way already advantaged and ignoring the worst off, thereby exacerbating inequities. So, for example, the three health-related Millennium Development Goals (MDGs) focus on health aggregates (e.g., mortality of children). Moreover, as already noted, geopolitical structures and monetary incentives favor the maximizers. Health 'egalitarians,' on the other hand, will wish to intervene on behalf of the worst off first, which may help ameliorate inequities but will not maximize global health gains in aggregate. The problem is this: There is no consensus about which perspective is correct and no overarching moral principle to resolve the differences. Consequently, we propose that a framework for fair deliberation about competing visions regarding improving global health be applied within institutions of the international community to, at the very minimum, bring into the open the values that lie at the heart of this debate.

A global agenda must extend beyond the rhetoric of universal human rights to include greater attention to duties, social justice, and interdependence. While it may be unrealistic to expect that it is possible to find commonality in our approaches to such issues in a highly diverse world, ethics provide a framework within which such an agenda could be developed and promoted across borders and cultures (Benatar *et al.*, 2003).

Ultimately, at the global or mega-level, the paucity of resources and lack of moral imagination devoted to such activities belies any serious major commitment to human well-being at a population level – a vivid indication that some lives are valued much more than others. Moreover, a reluctance to engage in fair, open deliberation about improving global population health suggests reluctance on the part of the powerful to recognize their interdependence with the powerless.

Macro-Level Resource Allocation: Health Systems

At the macro level, politicians, who hold responsibility for allocating resources in the health sector, seek to avoid blame for complex and controversial decisions, and delegate the responsibility to bureaucrats and 'technical' experts who make recommendations based on the analysis of scientific evidence and economic evaluations. Consequently, the difficult value conflicts that lie at the heart of allocation decisions are avoided, and patients (for whom the system exists) and members of the public (who fund the system) have very little input into these difficult decisions.

Several large-scale initiatives to guide resource allocation in health systems have focused on developing information and tools. Two examples are: The WHO's Choosing Health Interventions that are Cost-Effective (CHOICE) project and Disease Control Priorities in Developing Countries (Jamison et al., 2006). The common objectives of these initiatives are to develop and disseminate information and tools for priority setting that emphasize and rely upon evidence-based medicine and cost-effectiveness analysis. However, international experience with this approach has shown limited acceptance because, within their health systems, different countries emphasize different sets of values that go beyond evidence-based medicine and cost-effectiveness analysis (Martin and Singer, 2000; Kapiriri et al., 2004).

The greatest driver of skyrocketing costs in health systems is drug costs (Burns et al., 2003). Technocratic bodies that make recommendations about drug funding – for example, the National Institute for Health and Clinical Excellence (UK) or the Canadian Expert Drug Advisory Committee (Canada) – focus almost exclusively on information derived from scientific literature and pharmacoeconomics. Thus, the decisions that generate the most controversy are avoided. These controversial decisions include: When should we fund a drug that provides a small benefit to many people or those that provide a large benefit to a few? When should we fund expensive drugs that provide only a small benefit? When should we fund drugs for children rather than those for seniors?

In addition, macro-level decision makers must allocate resources to address other vital systemic questions, such as: Should we build and staff primary care clinics in rural areas where people cannot access care, or in urban areas where there are many people? How should we allocate resources between public health/preventive measures and care for acute and chronic medical problems?

The key issue at stake for macro-level decision makers is the sustainability of their health systems. In our current era of rising costs and limited budgets, those systems that will be sustainable are those that will have the capacity to limit spending, and that capacity can only function properly within an environment where the public determines that it is acceptable to say 'No' – that is, an environment of fairness.

While individual decision makers in parts of the system (e.g., hospitals) have tried to develop a priority-setting environment that meets the conditions of fairness, no macro-level leaders have done so for an entire health system.

Arguably, the main barrier to improving resource allocation practices in health systems is the disjointed nature of decision making both within and between systems. Every policy maker in every system, even those with very different structures, faces the same resource allocation problems. But, there is no systematic mechanism for capturing and sharing lessons between contexts. Leaders in every country are seeking better ways of making these difficult decisions and would benefit from the identification of good practices and strategies for improvement.

'Accountability for reasonableness' (see section 'Meso-level resource allocation: Institutions') provides a standard of fairness toward which health systems may aspire, an evaluation framework for capturing and sharing lessons between contexts, and a common language to facilitate public learning about reasonable limit-setting that connects allocation decisions to broader theoretical issues involving fundamental democratic deliberative processes. A way forward would include cultivating an environment of fair decision making in which limit-setting decisions will be perceived to be acceptable, developing mechanisms for capturing and sharing lessons of good practice, and developing strategies for improvement between decision-making contexts.

Meso-Level Resource Allocation: Institutions

Many crucial resource allocation decisions in a health system have been 'downloaded' by macro-level policy makers to the so-called meso level, which includes Regional and District Health Authorities (RHAs, DHAs), private health insurers, and hospitals – all of which struggle to meet growing demands, affordably, without compromising delivery of services (Daniels and Sabin, 1997; Gibson et al., 2005). Hospitals are a particular focal point of controversy for allocation decisions, as they account for a large portion of health-related spending – up to one-third in Canada. Moreover, hospitals everywhere remain stressed from severe financial constraints, mergers and closures, increasing demands for beds and operating room time, overcrowded emergency rooms, and an inadequate supply of resources for discharged patients.

Recently, several scholars have advocated principles or criteria that priority-setting decision makers in meso-level institutions should apply (Cookson and Dolan, 2000; Mooney, 2000). Other studies have described the criteria that meso-level decision makers actually do apply (Martin *et al.*, 2000; Kapiriri *et al.*, 2003). The range of criteria identified in this literature illuminates the competing interests (e.g., clinical vs. budgetary, local vs. systemic, strategic vs. operational) and multiple stakeholder relationships that must be considered in the meso-level context. This is consistent with previous findings that simple technical solutions have only limited influence on priority setting and are insufficient to guide decision making (Holm, 2000).

In response to these challenges, Daniels and Sabin have developed a framework to help meso-level institutions to allocate their limited resources in a way that is morally defensible. Accountability for reasonableness is a conceptual framework for legitimate and fair priority setting. It is theoretically grounded in justice theories emphasizing democratic deliberation, and was developed in the context of real-world allocation processes. It has emerged as the preferred ethical framework for developing best priority-setting practices in meso-level institutions (Coulter and Ham, 2000; Daniels and Sabin, 2002).

According to accountability for reasonableness, a fair allocation process meets four conditions: relevance, publicity, revisions/appeals, and enforcement (**Table 2**).

Table 2 The four conditions of 'accountability for reasonableness'

Relevance	Relationship for priority-setting decisions must rest on reasons (evidence and principles) that 'fair-minded' people can agree are relevant in the context. 'Fair-minded' people seek to cooperate according to terms they can justify to each other – this narrows, though does not eliminate, the scope of controversy, which is further narrowed by specifying that reasons must be relevant to the specific context
Publicity	Priority-setting decisions and their rationales must be publicly accessible – justice requires openness where people's well being is concerned
Revisions/ appeals	There must be a mechanism for challenge, including the opportunity for revising decisions in light of considerations that stakeholders may raise
Enforcement	There must be either voluntary or public regulation of the process to ensure that the first three conditions are met

Reproduced from Martin D and Singer P (2003) A Strategy to Improve Priority Setting in Health Care Institutions. Health Care Analysis. 11(1): 59–68, with kind permission of Springer Science and Business Media.

Micro-Level Resource Allocation: Bedside

Health-care professionals decide which individuals are cared for first, which patients receive which diagnostic tests and which drugs, which patients are admitted to a hospital bed, and which patients are taken to the operating theater. In emergencies, triage conventions require that life-threatening situations be addressed first. But, in non-emergency situations, the allocation conventions are unclear and variable.

Critical care studies (Mielke *et al.*, 2000; Cooper *et al.*, 2005) have shown that ICU admission decisions varied from clinician to clinician – some prioritized need, others the potential for benefit; some prioritized the young, others the elderly. Often, referring physicians who pushed the hardest and loudest found a bed for their patient. Even in contexts where admission policies exist, they were seldom well known.

A study of elective cardiac surgery revealed that a complex and unstandardized mélange of clinical reasons (e.g., pathology and anatomy) and nonclinical reasons (e.g., social supports, clinician-specific experiences, and remuneration schemes) were used by surgeons making allocation decisions (Walton *et al.*, 2006). Where standardized Urgency Rating Scores had been developed to help cardiac surgeons prioritize patients on waiting lists, the scores were used for record-keeping purposes only, not for allocation decisions.

At the micro-level, clinicians are thus forced to act as gatekeepers for the health system – a task for which they are neither trained nor inclined. They are often abandoned by policy makers to struggle with these complex allocation decisions without support or guidance. Consequently, clinicians often rely on clinical guidelines that are typically based on the narrow range of values inherent in evidence-based medicine, and not the entire range of values relevant to these difficult allocation decisions (Norheim, 1999). Institutional leaders have an obligation to support their frontline clinicians with policies that are legitimately developed and practically applicable.

Conclusions

Health systems are caring institutions that share timeless and universal aspirations for improving human health and well-being. The practice of medicine not only involves individuals, but also their families, whole cultures, societies, social institutions, and indeed whole populations globally. In the modern world, the universal humanitarian and caring goals of medicine, as well as the motives of health professionals and policy makers, are being eroded by progressive commercialization of health care, commodification of the human body, and judgments about whose lives are and are not valuable. Trust in physicians and policy makers has been undermined because their work is seen to be self-serving and directed by market and managerial forces rather than directed to meeting the needs of individuals and whole populations. Among many different activities needed to promote and preserve professionalism and ensure equity in access to health care, is a more rational, ethical, and publicly accountable process of allocating resources within and between health systems.

See also: Agenda Setting in Public Health Policy; Evidence-Based Public Health Policy; Global Health Initiatives and Public Health Policy; Governance Issues in Health Financing; Health Care Costs, Structures and Trends; Health Care Financing and the Health System; Health Finance, Equity in; Health Inequalities; Health Policy: Overview; Human Rights, Approach to Public Health Policy; Politics, and Public Health Policy Reform; The Demand for Health Care.

Citations

Benatar SR (1998) Global disparities in health and human rights. *American Journal of Public Health* 88: 295–300.

Benatar SR (2005) Moral imagination: The missing component in global health. *Public Library of Science Medicine* 2(12): e400.

Benatar SR, Daar A, and Singer PA (2003) Global health ethics: The rationale for mutual caring. *International Affairs* 79: 107–138.

Burns H, Beever C, and Hutchens R (2003) *What's Driving Prescription Drug Costs?* http://www.strategy-business.com/enewsarticle/enews092903.

Cookson R and Dolan P (2000) Principles of justice in health care rationing. *Journal of Medical Ethics* 26: 323–329.

Cooper AB, Joglekar AS, Gibson JL, Swota AH, and Martin DK (2005) Communication of bed allocation decisions in a critical care unit and accountability for reasonableness. *BioMed Central Health Services Research* 5: 67.

Coulter A and Ham C (2000) *The Global Challenge of Health Care Rationing*. Buckingham, UK: Open University Press.

Daniels N and Sabin JE (1997) Limits to health care: Fair procedures, democratic deliberation and the legitimacy problem for insurers. *Philosophy and Public Affairs* 26(4): 303–502.

Daniels N and Sabin JE (2002) *Setting Limits Fairly: Can We Learn to Share Medical Resources?* Oxford, UK: Oxford University Press.

Gibson JL, Martin DK, and Singer PA (2005) Evidence, economics and ethics: Resource allocation in health services organizations. *Health Care Quarterly* 8: 50–59.

Global Forum for Health Research (2006) Monitoring flows for health research. http://www.globalforumhealth.org (accessed December 2007).

Ham C and Coulter A (2001) Explicit and implicit rationing: Taking responsibility and avoiding blame for health care choices. *Journal of Health Services Research and Policy* 6: 163–169.

Holm S (2000) Developments in Nordic countries – goodbye to the simple solutions. In: Coulter A and Ham C (eds.) *The Global Challenge of Health Care Rationing*, pp. 29–37. Buckingham, UK: Open University Press

Jamison DT, Breman JG, Measham AR, et al. (eds.) (2006) *Disease Control Priorities in Developing Countries,* 2nd edn. Washington, DC: World Bank.

Kapiriri L, Norheim OF, and Heggenhougen K (2003) Using burden of disease information for health planning in developing countries: The experience from Uganda. *Social Science and Medicine* 56: 2433–2441.

Kapiriri L, Arnesen T, and Norheim OF (2004) Is cost-effectiveness analysis preferred to severity of disease as the main guiding principle in priority setting in resource poor settings? The case of Uganda. *Cost-Effectiveness and Resource Allocation* 2: 1–11.

Martin DK, Bernstein M, and Singer PA (2003) Neurosurgery patients' access to ICU beds: Priority setting in the ICU – a qualitative case study and evaluation. *Journal of Neurology, Neurosurgery and Psychiatry* 74: 1299–1303.

Martin DK and Singer PA (2000) Priority setting and health technology assessment: Beyond evidence based medicine and cost-effectiveness analysis. In: Coulter A and Ham C (eds.) *The Global Challenge of Health Care Rationing*, pp. 135–145. Buckingham, UK: Open University Press

Martin DK, Pater JL, and Singer PA (2001) Priority setting decisions for new cancer drugs: A qualitative study. *Lancet* 358: 1676–1681.

Mielke J, Martin DK, and Singer PA (2003) Priority setting in critical care: A qualitative case study. *Critical Care Medicine* 31: 2764–2768.

Mooney G (2000) Vertical equity in health care resource allocation. *Health Care Analysis* 8: 203–215.

Norheim OF (1999) Health care rationing – are additional criteria needed for assessing evidence based clinical practise guidelines? *British Medical Journal* 319: 1426–1429.

Relman AS and Angell M (2002) How the drug industry distorts medicine and politics: America's other drug problem. *The New Republic* 227(25): 27–41.

Troullier P, Oliaro P, Torreele E, Orbinski J, Laing R, and Ford N (2002) Drug development for neglected diseases: A deficient market and a public health failure. *The Lancet* 359: 2188–2194.

Walton N, Martin DK, Peter E, Pringle D, and Singer PA (2006) Priority setting in cardiac surgery: A qualitative study. *Health Policy* 80(3): 444–458.

Zaracostas J (2006) World Bank warns of financial crises in healthcare systems. *British Medical Journal* 332: 1293.

Further Reading

Action Aid International USA (2005) *Changing Course: Alternative Approaches to Achieve the Millennium Development Goals and Fight HIV/AIDS*. Washington DC: Action Aid International USA. http://www.actionaidusa.org/pdf/Changing%20Course%20Report.pdf (accessed December 2007).

Alexander T (1996) *Unraveling Global Apartheid: An Overview of World Politics*. Cambridge, MA: Polity Press.

Bakker I and Gill S (2003) *Power, Production and Social Reproduction*. New York: Palgrave Press.

Daniels N (2008) *Just Health: Meeting Health Needs Fairly*. Cambridge, UK: Cambridge University Press.

Farmer P (2005) Never again: Reflections on human values and human rights. The Tanner Lectures on Human Values and Human Rights. http://www.tannerlectures.utah.edu/lectures.documents/Farmer_2006.pdf.

Friman HR and Andreas P (eds.) (1999) *Illicit Global Economy and State Power*. New York: Rowman and Littlefield.

Kassalow JS (2001) *Why Health Is Important to U.S. Foreign Policy*. New York: Council on Foreign Relations and Milbank Memorial Fund.

The Global Fund (2003) *The Global Fund Annual Report 2002/2003*. Geneva, Switzerland: The Global Fund. http://www.theglobalfund.org (accessed December 2007).

Pogge T (2002) *World Poverty and Human Rights*. Cambridge, MA: Polity Press.

Sreenivasan G and Benatar SR (2006) Challenges for global health in the 21st century: Some upstream considerations. *Theoretical Medicine and Bioethics* 27(1): 1–114.

United Nations Development Report (UNDP) (2000) *Human Development Report 2000: Human Rights and Human Development*. New York: Oxford University Press.

Wilkinson RG (1996) *Unhealthy Societies: The Afflictions of Inequality*. London: Routledge.

Cost-Influenced Treatment Decisions and Cost Effectiveness Analysis

D B Evans, World Health Organization, Geneva, Switzerland

© 2008 WHO. Published by Elsevier Inc. All rights reserved.

Introduction

Health financing systems are a means to an end, designed to support the overall health system in its fundamental goal of maintaining and improving health. All systems face three fundamental challenges, linked to the key functions of a health system, which is to raise revenues, pool them to spread risks, and use them to purchase or provide services (Savedoff et al., 2003; Xu et al., 2007). The challenges are:

- how to raise sufficient funds for health;
- how to raise them in a way that allows people to use services when needed, but protects them from suffering financial hardship;
- how to ensure that the resources that are raised are used efficiently and effectively.

Cost-effectiveness analysis is concerned with the third challenge, providing valuable information to policy makers on how available or new resources could be used most efficiently. The bulk of the applied studies have focused on maximizing health outcomes for the resources devoted to a particular health problem such as maternal mortality, often termed technical efficiency studies by health economists. More recently, sectoral cost-effectiveness has examined which sets of interventions would maximize population health for different levels of resource availability, requiring comparisons of interventions targeting prevention, promotion, treatment, and rehabilitation, as well as interventions dealing with all possible health problems. This type of study is sometimes said to address questions of allocative efficiency, how best to choose the most appropriate mix of inputs (here, interventions) after taking into account their impact and prices (see Tan-Torres Edejer et al., 2003).

In poorer countries, between US$35 and US$50 per capita would be required each year to ensure universal access to a minimum set of critical health interventions (World Health Organization, 2007b). This assumes that all interventions are delivered relatively efficiently and only the most critical interventions are funded, so the real needs would be substantially higher. Yet the World Health Organization reports that in 2004, 59 of its 193 member countries spent less than US$50 per capita, a figure that includes the funds provided by external sources such as bilateral donors and foundations. Per capita spending did not reach US$25 in 39 countries, and was less than US$10 in 11 (World Health Organization, 2007b). This is despite recent rapid increases in external assistance for health and is one of the fundamental reasons that a minority of countries are on track to achieve the health-related Millennium Development Goals (Sahn and Stifel, 2002). It is not surprising that the major focus of attention in low-income countries has been on ways of increasing the funds available for health.

In richer countries, policy makers have also been vitally interested in the extent of funding available for health, but more from the perspective of restraining the growth of health spending. The fact that health expenditure increases as a percent of gross domestic product as incomes rise has surprisingly been seen as undesirable, even though we know that people are willing to devote increasingly higher proportions of their incomes to protect or improve their own health as their incomes rise (Hall and Jones, 2007).

A number of factors explain the desire to constrain health spending. The first is linked to the fact that governments generally contribute a higher proportion to overall health expenditures as incomes rise, and all governments face many competing demands on their available resources. Restricting expenditures in one area releases funds for another. They also face considerable pressure to either reduce taxation or at least not increase it substantially. The second contributing factor is the continual development of new health technologies, many of which are relatively expensive but offer at best small improvements in health or wellbeing. The third is a concern that at least some of the increase in observed health expenditure is unnecessary, induced largely by suppliers of services (e.g., health workers, pharmaceutical companies, hospitals, etc.) rather than because of need. This is possible because of the well-known information asymmetry in health where patients or consumers do not have the necessary information to judge if the services offered to them are truly warranted (Retchin, 2007).

With this background, it is not surprising that the question of economic efficiency has become increasingly important in richer countries. The literature on the economic evaluation (including cost-effectiveness analysis) of health interventions has grown substantially in recent years, and a vast majority of the published papers have focused on developed countries. Moreover, the instances in which economic evaluation has been introduced into routine decision making are found in OECD countries, mostly to aid decision making about public subsidies for pharmaceuticals.

While this focus is understandable, there is also increasing acceptance that efficiency considerations need to be considered in low-income countries as well. While it is true that the gains from introducing greater efficiency in systems spending less than $10 per capita on health will be outweighed by the potential gains from doubling or tripling overall expenditures, population health could still be higher than it currently is – in the most basic terms, more lives could be saved – if current and new resources are used more efficiently. In response, the literature applying cost-effectiveness techniques to the health problems faced by developing countries is also expanding.

The impact of this literature on policy is, however, not clear (Chisholm and Evans, 2007). This article does not seek to review the literature but focuses on a number of common problems that restrict the value of many cost-effectiveness studies to practical decision making.

Efficiency of New Versus Existing Resources

Cost-effectiveness analysis is dominated by concerns about small changes at the margin, most often focusing on the relative costs and effects of a new intervention compared to existing practice. This poses a major problem for policy. There is ample evidence from different settings that many interventions of relatively poor cost-effectiveness are undertaken while those that are more efficient are not, or not implemented fully (e.g., Tengs *et al.*, 1995; Jamison *et al.*, 2006).

Incremental analysis could be used to assess whether the current activity should have been undertaken in the first place, or more broadly, whether the current mix of interventions is the most efficient, but this would require assessment of the resource savings and the associated reductions in health outcomes associated with a contraction of all current activities. The results would then have to be compared with the costs and effectiveness of expanding all activities as well as introducing new ones. This is computationally intense and has not been done, one of the reasons why generalized cost-effectiveness analysis was developed, a method that has been described elsewhere (Tan-Torres Edejer *et al.*, 2003; Evans *et al.*, 2006).

The undoubted difficulties involved in reallocating resources from inefficient to efficient interventions should not prevent analysts seeking to shed light on where there are current inefficiencies and the possibilities for redressing them. To date, little attention has been paid to understanding the sources of current inefficiencies.

The Appropriate Scale

Substantial increases in external funding for health have been made available to low-income countries in recent years, and in some domestically sourced expenditure has also increased. More is still required, but already activities are being expanded well beyond the scale assessed in traditional incremental cost-effectiveness analyses. This raises the question of whether unit costs increase or decrease as the scale of the intervention increases (referred to in economics as diseconomies and economies of scale, respectively), as well as possible changes in the overall impact in health or each unit of additional coverage. This may lead to nonlinear rather than linear cost and effectiveness curves.

Unit costs can fall with increasing coverage where there is excess capacity (Adam *et al.*, 2005), but they can also rise substantially if new health facilities need to be constructed, new health workers trained or where particular groups in the community do not recognize the value of an intervention. The gains in effectiveness from each unit of expansion can also vary; as screening moves beyond high-risk people to the general population the gains in population health per person screened are reduced. On the other hand, if coverage expands from relatively affluent to poorer geographical areas where disease prevalence is higher, the benefits from each unit of expansion in coverage might increase.

The combination of nonlinear cost and effectiveness curves means that it is rarely possible to claim that an intervention is cost-effective *per se*, although many studies imply this finding. Expanding coverage of childhood immunization from 30% to 40% might be very cost-effective, but expanding from 85% to 95% might not be, yet rarely do cost-effectiveness studies give policy makers an indication of the desirable scale of the activity for the resources available in their settings.

Interactions Between Interventions

In practice, health interventions are never undertaken in isolation, but with very few exceptions, they are evaluated assuming their costs and effects are independent. The population impact – and therefore the cost-effectiveness – of a program to screen and treat people with hypertension will depend on whether active smoking reduction interventions exist or are likely to be introduced. The costs of expanding coverage of case finding and treatment for tuberculosis will depend on whether there are programs for the prevention and treatment of HIV. The economics literature calls the reduction in unit costs associated with interactions between programs undertaken concurrently economies of scope, and both economies and diseconomies are possible.

Incremental analysis undertaken in a specific setting implicitly takes into account, at least in theory, what other interventions are currently being undertaken in that they assess costs and effectiveness in that setting. In reality, many borrow effectiveness data from other settings without assessing whether the mix of interventions undertaken in the setting where the effectiveness data were produced is, or will be, undertaken in the study area. Moreover, most studies do not examine the impact on their estimated cost-effectiveness that would result from the introduction of other interventions at the same time or in the future, even if those interventions are already in the pipe line (Drummond et al., 1992).

It is admittedly difficult to undertake studies that account for all the possible interactions between interventions, partly because efficacy or efficiency studies generally consider one intervention in isolation from others. However, this is the type of information that is required for informed decision making.

Ex Ante Versus *Ex Post* Cost-Effectiveness Analysis

Most cost-effectiveness studies are undertaken from an *ex ante* perspective, seeking to determine what would happen if the intervention were to be undertaken. However, when the interventions are new, or new to a country, assumptions must be made about the costs and effectiveness in that situation. Experience in other settings or from trials or experiments can be used to guide assumptions on effectiveness, but questions of costs are often guided by the advice of experts that provide information on what inputs would be required to implement a program locally.

The advice of experts could introduce a number of possible biases. For example, it is possible that experts might underappreciate the complexities of introducing and running a new activity either because of a lack of knowledge or because they are advocates for its introduction. They may well overestimate their own abilities to implement an intervention at low cost, or to achieve high levels of effectiveness. On the other hand, experts who oppose the introduction of a new intervention may well have the opposite biases.

There is not a large literature comparing the results of *ex ante* analyses with *ex post* attainments, but at this stage there is no conclusive evidence that *ex ante* costs are consistently underestimated and *ex ante* effects consistently overestimated. For example, Hammitt (2001) reports that the *ex ante* costs of introducing environmental control in the US were actually overestimated; Townsend and others (2003) found that *ex post* effectiveness was about equivalent to *ex ante* estimates for two studies in the UK. More work in this area, however, is required before generalizable conclusions can be reached.

If all interventions were evaluated with the same biases, the relative preference ordering would be the same. However, this is unlikely. For example, it would not be the case when evaluating new technologies with current practice, where actual costs and effectiveness of current practice would be compared with estimates of what would happen with the new technology. While waiting for a more comprehensive empirical analysis of the biases in *ex ante* analysis, it is suggested that the bounds of the uncertainty or sensitivity analyses should be widened to allow for possible biases, particularly where expert advice has been used.

The problems are compounded with sectoral cost-effectiveness analyses, which attempt to provide guidance to policy makers on an efficient set of interventions for the health sector as a whole, across a range of diseases and conditions (e.g. Jamison et al., 2006; World Health Organization, 2007a). Because of the need to compare many different interventions, it has been necessary to borrow information on effectiveness and costs from different studies and settings to present an overall picture of the mix of interventions that would add most to population health for the available resources. This has been done most commonly for subregions of the world, sometimes in ways that can be adapted by country analysts (World Health Organization, 2007a).

This poses particular difficulties because the technical efficiency with which each intervention is implemented could well vary across countries according to factors such as the degree of excess capacity in health facilities or the way providers are paid (Robinson, 2001; Adam et al., 2005). The WHO-CHOICE project addressed this issue by presenting results for 14 subregions of the world, assuming that all interventions would be undertaken at 80% capacity utilization. This reveals the mix of interventions that would be optimal if all the interventions were implemented relatively efficiently and country analysts could adapt the technical efficiency assumptions to their local settings.

The logic for a consistent assumption about technical efficiency across interventions is clear; it is not very useful telling decision makers that a particular set of interventions would be optimal if they were all done very badly, or if half were done badly and half well. However, the data necessary to address the varying levels of capacity utilization across facilities in a given country, for example, are rarely available, so adaptation of the results to each country is complex.

This issue remains a vexing problem for cost-effectiveness analysis. In the short run, understanding more about whether there are consistent biases in *ex ante* analysis is important. A second implication is that comparisons of new technologies with current practice should also take into account the possibility that the technical efficiency of current practice could be improved. This can be done by comparing not only the cost-effectiveness of current practice with the cost-effectiveness of new technologies, but by adding a third arm: the cost-effectiveness of improving the efficiency of current practice.

Concluding Remarks

One of the fundamental questions facing any financing system is to provide incentives for the efficient use of resources, new and existing. But before incentives can be designed, there must be an understanding of the nature of the changes that are desirable. Although there is not universal acceptance among economists that cost-effectiveness analysis is the preferred form of economic evaluation, by revealing the relative efficiency of different ways of using scarce resources, it can provide valuable guidance on how health could be improved for the available resources.

There are still, however, some issues that prevent cost-effectiveness analysis from being of more practical use to decision makers, the main focus of this article. Until they are addressed, it is unlikely that the number of countries in which the technique has been institutionalized as a guide to policy making will increase substantially.

See also: Governance Issues in Health Financing; Determinants of National Health Expenditure; Innovative Financing of Health Promotion.

Citations

Adam DB, Amorim DB, Edwards DB, Amaral DB, and Evans DB (2005) Capacity constraints to the adoption of new interventions: Consultation time and the integrated management of childhood illness in Brazil. *Health Policy and Planning* 20: i49–i57.

Chisholm D and Evans DB (2007) Economic evaluation in health: Saving money or improving care? *Journal of Medical Economics* 10: 325–327.

Drummond MF, Bloom BS, Carrin G, et al. (1992) Issues in the cross-national assessment of health technology. *International Journal of Technology Assessment in Health Care* 8: 671–682.

Evans DB, Chisholm D, and Tan-Torres Edejer T (2006) Generalized cost-effectiveness analysis. In: Jones A (ed.) *The Elgar Companion to Health Economics.* Cheltenham, UK: Edward Elgar Press.

Hall RE and Jones CI (2007) The value of life and the rise in health spending. *Quarterly Journal of Economics* 122: 39–72.

Hammitt JK (2001) Are the costs of proposed environmental regulations overestimated? Evidence from the CFC phaseout. *Environmental and Resource Economics* 16: 281–301.

Jamison D, Breman J, Measham A, et al. (eds.) (2006) *Disease Control Priorities in Developing Countries*, 2nd edn. New York: Oxford University Press.

Retchin SM (2007) Overcoming information asymmetry in consumer-directed health plans. *American Journal of Managed Care* 13: 173–176.

Robinson JC (2001) Theory and practice in the design of physician payment incentives. *Milbank Quarterly* 79: 149–177.

Sahn DE and Stifel DC (2003) Progress toward the millennium development goals in Africa. *World Development* 31: 23–52.

Savedoff WD, Carrin GK, Kawabata K, and Mechbal A (2003) Monitoring the health financing function. In: Murray CJ and Evans DB (eds.) *Health System Performance Assessment. Debates, Methods and Empiricism*, pp. 205–210. Geneva, Switzerland: World Health Organization.

Tan-Torres Edejer T, Baltussen R, Adam T, et al. (2003) *Making Choices in Health: WHO Guide to Cost-effectiveness Analysis.* Geneva, Switzerland: World Health Organization.

Tengs TO, Adams ME, Pliskin JS, et al. (1995) Five-hundred life-saving interventions and their cost-effectiveness. *Risk Analysis* 15: 369–390.

Townsend J, Buxton M, and Harper G (2003) Prioritisation of health technology assessment. The PATHS model: Methods and case studies. *Health Technology Assessment* 7: 1–94.

World Health Organization (2007a) CHOosing Interventions that are Cost Effective (WHO-CHOICE). www.who.int/choice (accessed October 2007).

World Health Organization (2007b) National Health Accounts. www.who.int/nha (accessed October 2007).

Xu K, Evans DB, Carrin G, et al. (2007) Protecting households from catastrophic health expenditures. *Health Affairs* 26: 972–983.

Further Reading

Dayton J (1998) *World Bank HIV/AIDS Interventions: Ex-ante and Ex-post Evaluation.* Washington, DC: World Bank.

Drummond M, Jonsson B, and Rutten F (1997) The role of economic evaluation in the pricing and reimbursement of medicines. *Health Policy* 40: 199–215.

Evans DB, Lim SS, Adam T, and Tan-Torres Edejer T the WHO-CHOICE MDG Team (2005) Achieving the Millennium Development Goals for health: Methods to assess the costs and health effects of interventions for improving health in developing countries. *British Medical Journal* 331: 1137–1140.

Gonzalez-Pier E, Gutierrez-Delgado C, Stevens G, et al. (2006) Priority setting for health interventions in Mexico's system of social protection in health. *Lancet* 368: 1608–1618.

Hoffmann C, Stoykova BA, Nixon J, et al. (2002) Do health-care decision makers find economic evaluations useful? The findings of focus group research in UK health authorities. *Value Health* 5: 71–78.

Hutubessy R, Chisholm D, and Tan-Torres Edejer T (2003) Generalized cost-effectiveness analysis for national-level priority-setting in the health sector. *Cost Effectiveness and Resource Allocation* 1: 8.

Iglesias CP, Drummond MF, and Rovira J NEVALAT Project Group (2005) Health-care decision-making processes in Latin America: Problems and prospects for the use of economic evaluation. *International Journal of Technology Assessment in Health Care* 21: 1–14.

Kanavos P, Trueman P, and Bosilevac A (2000) Can economic evaluation guidelines improve efficiency in resource allocation? The cases of Portugal, The Netherlands, Finland, and the United Kingdom. *International Journal of Technology Assessment in Health Care* 16: 1179–1192.

Murray CJ, Evans DB, Acharya A, and Baltussen RM (2000) Development of WHO guidelines on generalized cost-effectiveness analysis. *Health Economics* 9: 235–251.

World Health Organization (2001) *Macroeconomics and Health: Investing in Health for Economic Development.* Report of the Commission on Macroeconomics and Health. Geneva, Switzerland: World Health Organization.

Decision Analytic Modeling

P Muennig, Columbia University, New York, NY, USA

© 2008 Elsevier Inc. All rights reserved.

Introduction

Life is full of uncertainties. You could invest in a mutual fund or a certificate of deposit account. You could buy a home or rent. You could go to public health school or write a novel.

If you knew the risks and benefits of each alternative, the decision would be a lot easier. Decision analysis provides a mathematical framework for making decisions under conditions of uncertainty. Let's see how this works by using an example.

Imagine that you have $100 000 to invest. You've always wanted to study public health, but you've also dreamed about writing a novel ever since you were in college. If you write a novel, you reason, you can simply invest the money in a mutual fund and earn interest, making small withdrawals as needed. Since you are undecided between the two options, you decide to examine which will be the better option financially.

Decision analysis is based on a concept called expected value, in which the value of an uncertain event (such as making $10 000 in the stock market) is weighed against the chances that the event will occur. For example, if you know that the historical average increase in a particular mutual fund is 10% per year, then the expected value of the return on your $100 000 investment is $0.1 \times \$100\,000 = \$10\,000$ over one year.

You set your sights five years down the road and assume that if you go to public health school, all of the $100 000 would be spent on your education after living expenses are taken into account, but you would be able to earn about $50 000 per year working in public health. After taxes and living expenses, you estimate that you would save about $10 000 over the 3 years after graduation.

If you decide to write a novel, you will have spent your $100 000, along with the interest on the mutual fund, on living expenses over the 5-year period. But if you publish the novel, you could earn an additional $30 000. Your college English professor advises you that there is about a 1% chance that you will be published. Therefore, the 'invest and write' option will produce a probabilistically weighted return of $\$30\,000 \times 0.01 = \$300$.

Since $10 000 is more than $300, you might go for the career in public health. However, you might not be satisfied with your calculations; there is a chance that the mutual fund could do very well, but there is also a chance that you could lose money. If it does well, you could end up with leftover money from your mutual fund investment at the end of 5 years. So if you write the book, you might make money even if you don't publish (perhaps better than spending it on tuition). But if the mutual fund loses money, you might not be able to finish your novel, which would be quite depressing.

There is also a chance that you will not find a job right out of public health school, which would also be discouraging. Ideally, you would want to have a rough idea not only of the difference in earnings associated with each decision, but also the difference in utility, or happiness. This way, you'll not only have a better idea of which decision is riskiest, but you'll also know the chances of your relative satisfaction with each choice.

The various options that one is deciding between are called 'competing alternatives.' Decision analysis can thus be described as the process of making an optimal choice among competing alternatives under conditions of uncertainty (Gold *et al.*, 1996).

In public health or medicine, decision analysis is most commonly employed in cost-effectiveness analyses. Here, the competing alternatives are the different health interventions under study. Therefore, rather than net improvement in cash flow and personal utility, cost-effectiveness analysis provides the user with information on incremental costs and health gains.

In the past, researchers performing a cost-effectiveness analysis had to write a computer program that would calculate the cost and effectiveness of different medical interventions, or attempt to do so by using a spreadsheet program. Today, most cost-effectiveness analyses can be easily assembled with decision analysis software.

Decision analysis software provides a graphical framework for estimating the costs and effectiveness values (usually represented as quality-adjusted life years, or QALYs) associated with a given medical or public health strategy. Let's take a look at a concrete example of how this works in public health.

Decision Analysis Models

In **Figure 1**, we wish to compare two strategies for dealing with influenza virus during the flu season. The first is to provide supportive care to people who become ill (Muennig and Khan, 2001). The second is to attempt to prevent infection with an influenza vaccination.

In this figure, the two alternatives are represented in branches separated by a square called a decision node.

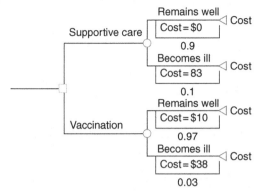

Figure 1 Decision analysis tree comparing supportive care to vaccination.

The decision node is like a referee holding the competing alternatives apart as they set out to do battle. Following this square, you'll see a circle. The circle is called a chance node. A chance node is followed by two or more possible outcomes. In **Figure 1**, the outcomes are 'remains well' and 'becomes ill.'

Notice that each 'remains well' and 'becomes ill' branch in the decision analysis tree is associated with a cost and a probability. In the supportive care option, the cost associated with remaining well is $0. But in the vaccinate option, everyone gets a $10 influenza vaccine at the start of influenza season. Thus, whether or not folks receiving the vaccine would have gotten sick, they must pay for the vaccination.

However, vaccination greatly reduces the chances of becoming ill during influenza season. If, during the average season, there is a 10% chance of developing the flu among unvaccinated persons, there is only a 3% chance of developing the flu among vaccinated persons. Moreover, among those who get sick despite vaccination, the infection will be much less severe. Therefore, the costs will be lower. (In **Figure 1**, those becoming ill incur a cost of $83 if unvaccinated and $38 if vaccinated.)

So, how does this work? The model merely provides a framework for calculating probabilistically weighted costs. Thus, we see that there is a $0.97 \times \$10 + 0.03 \times \$38 = \$11$ average cost among those receiving vaccination, and a $0.1 \times \$84 + 0.9 \times \$0 = \$8$ average cost among those receiving supportive care alone.

Note that **Figure 1** only deals with costs for simplicity. Moreover, it is a bit simplistic in other ways; there is a lot more uncertainty associated with these two competing alternatives than simply remaining well or becoming ill.

Figure 2 presents a more complete representation of the decision between supportive care and vaccination. Here, we see that someone who becomes ill has a chance of seeing a doctor or being hospitalized. As before, the risk of each is much lower among vaccinated persons.

There are a few things to note about **Figure 2**. First, the costs are represented as running totals. It is not necessary to set up a decision analysis model this way, but it helps to illustrate a key point; each event is associated with a cost, and that cost is added to the events that preceded it. Thus, the cost at the end of each branch in the tree represents the probabilistically weighted cost of a given pathway of events. Thus, the initial cost of becoming ill along the top branch is $12 (the cost of over-the-counter medications). Since there is only a 10% chance of incurring this cost, the average cost will be $0.1 \times \$12 = \$1.20$. But if the person sees a doctor, the cost will be $\$110 \times 0.2 = \$22$, and this gets added to the $1.20, for a running total of $23.20 at the 'sees doctor' event in the pathway.

The second thing to note about **Figure 2** is that all costs are incurred at one point in time. In other words, we calculate the average cost of each of the events in the pathway as if they happened in one day. This is fine for a disease like influenza, which tends to make someone ill for a short time. However, it might not work so well for cancer, which, depending on the type of cancer a person has, can drag on for many years. We return to this problem in the next section.

The above example provides an illustration of how decision analysis modeling works. As you can see, decision analysis provides probabilistically weighted values of a series of outcomes of interest. The average value of any competing option is called its 'expected value.' Although all trees provide a probabilistically weighted expected value, different models arrive at this value in very different ways.

Types of Decision Analysis Models

There are different types of decision analysis models (Gold et al., 1996). The type of model that analysts choose depends on the problem under evaluation.

Simple decision trees

The most basic is a simple decision tree, such as the one presented in the above example. Simple decision trees are usually employed to examine events that will occur in the near future. They are therefore best suited to evaluate interventions to prevent or treat illnesses of a short duration, such as acute infectious diseases (Muennig et al., 1999). They may also be used to evaluate chronic diseases that may be cured (for example, by surgical intervention). When these trees are used to evaluate diseases that change over time, they sometimes become too unruly to be useful.

Markov modeling

For chronic or complex diseases, it is best to use a state transition model, also known as a Markov model (Sonnenberg and Beck, 1993). This type of model allows the researcher to incorporate changes in health states over time into the analysis. For example, if a person has cancer,

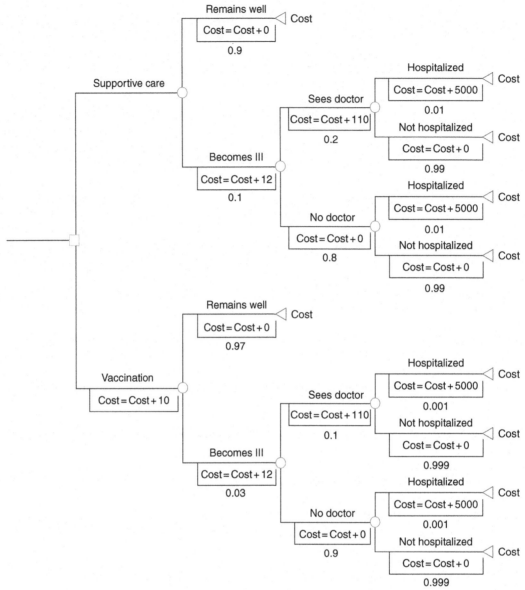

Figure 2 A more complete decision analysis tree comparing supportive care to vaccination.

there is a chance that the person will recover within a year and then relapse. There is also a chance that the person will remain sick for some time or will die soon.

With every passing year, the cost of treatment changes. More importantly, the chances of survival, recovery, or deterioration change. Markov models allow researchers to track changes in the quality of life, the quantity of life, and the cost of a disease over time when different health interventions are applied (Sonnenberg and Beck, 1993).

Most interventions in public health or medicine that target diseases have some component of time to them. To model screening mammography, for instance, it is necessary to have some way to measure the progression of breast cancer over time. This way, differences in the progression of disease can be compared when treated and when left untreated.

Using a Markov model, we can incorporate a temporal element into our decision analysis model (Sonnenberg and Beck, 1993). Markov models count the years that accrue as the model completes cycles and the medical costs, living costs, and changes in health-related quality of life scores over these years. Of course, days, months, or decades can be modeled, too.

For instance, suppose we are interested in calculating the lifelong cost associated with breast cancer in patients who have been diagnosed via a screening mammogram. We would start the model by using the average age of onset of breast cancer. The number of survivors would be determined by using the probability of death specific to women who have been diagnosed with breast cancer via screening mammography. Each patient who is still living at the end of the year gains 1 year of additional life

(1 person-year). But she can also be assigned medical costs, home health-care costs, transportation costs, and so forth. Women who die do not accrue such costs, so these women gain neither a year of life nor any costs.

Thus, if the average annual cost of living with breast cancer were $10 000, a group of 10 women would incur a cost of 10 × $10 000 = $100 000 in year 1. Now imagine that by year 2, one woman died. Thus, year 2 costs would be 9 × $10 000 = $90 000. If we continued this process until the last subject died, we would not only have the average number of life years lived, but we would also have the total cost incurred by these women over that period (See **Table 1**).

In this example, we are measuring various relevant health outcomes over a discrete interval of time. We know that the average woman lived 48 years of life/10 women = 4.8 years over the 6-year interval. The average cost of this treatment was $450 000/10 women = $45 000.

In a Markov model, **Table 1** is represented graphically as a chain of events rather than a table. This makes sense given that, for most diseases, subjects do not merely progress slowly toward death due to the disease under study. Rather, they can become better, die from other causes, or develop other diseases.

Thus, to model events that unfold over time realistically, we will want some sort of recursive component in our model. A recursive event is one that repeats over and over (see **Figure 3**). Thus, at the end of each year of a subject's life, he or she is assigned a cost value and a QALY value, and then reenters the next year of life (or dies). This process is repeated until all subjects are dead or the evaluation period ends.

As in the examples evaluating influenza infection via simple decision analysis trees discussed previously, each arrow in **Figure 3** is assigned a probability value. For instance, the likelihood of remaining well over any given year might be 0.98 in the typical cohort of healthy persons.

Markov models can also be used to simulate the life experience of the average individual with a particular disease before and after treatment, the health effects of a particular medical intervention, or even the benefits of having health insurance over a lifetime (Mandelblatt *et al.*, 2004; Muennig *et al.*, 2004, 2005).

For instance, we might wish to compare the advantages of folate supplementation to no intervention. Since folate prevents birth defects, one branch of the model might record the health-related quality of life and health costs of the average infant with a spinal cord defect as time progressed. In the other branch, we might simulate the health-related quality of life and health costs of the typical baby without a spinal cord defect as time progressed. As in the table above, each would account for differences in mortality rates, and thus calculate the average life expectancy of each group. The model would then tell us the differences in QALYs and costs over the entire lifetime of babies who did and did not have a spinal cord defect.

Worked examples of Markov models can be found at http://www.pceo.org/. This site provides free self-instruction manuals and links to government websites that provide data free of charge.

Sensitivity Analysis

The value of decision analysis model inputs can be very difficult to establish with absolute certainty. For instance, health-related quality of life scores – a key ingredient in the calculation of QALYs – can be obtained from various instruments, each producing a slightly different number (Gold and Muennig, 2002). Because these differences arise due to differences in the way the studies are designed, they represent a form of nonrandom error.

Table 1 Progression of a cohort of 10 women with breast cancer over a 6-year period

Year	Women surviving	Years lived in interval[a]	Cost of treating breast cancer
1	10	10	$100 000
2	9	9.5	$90 000
3	8	8.5	$80 000
4	7	7.5	$70 000
5	6	6.5	$60 000
6	5	5.5	$50 000
Total		48	$450 000

[a]Those dying were assumed to die, on average, in June of the reference year. They are therefore given 0.5 years of life in that year.

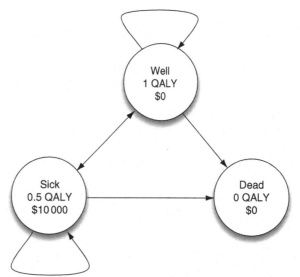

Figure 3 Conceptual representation of a Markov model. Subjects who are well can remain well, become sick (e.g., from breast cancer), or can die (e.g., from an accident) over the course of a year. Likewise, subjects who are sick can remain sick, become well, or die. This process is repeated, accruing a mean cost and QALY value. (Each arrow represents a transition probability over the course of 1 year.)

Most model inputs will be derived from a sample, and therefore also contain random error.

We can usually guess the range of plausible values within which the true value might lie. For instance, looking through the literature, we might see that the health-related quality of life score for the disease we are studying varies by roughly 20% when using different instruments. We might also know the standard error in datasets or published values.

The inputs we are least likely to be certain about are the assumptions we have made. In the earlier influenza example, we might have made an assumption about the amount of time it takes for a nurse to administer the influenza vaccine. There are other values that we might be fairly confident about, such as the cost of the influenza vaccine itself. (The average wholesale price is usually easy to get.)

The parameters the researcher is least certain about should be tested over the widest range of values (because it is plausible that the values are much higher or much lower than our baseline estimate). Parameters that the researcher is somewhat more confident about can be tested over a narrower range of values. When a particular strategy remains dominant over the range of plausible values for the inputs that we are uncertain about, the model is said to be robust.

There are many different ways of testing variables in a sensitivity analysis. These include a one-way (univariate) sensitivity analysis, in which a single variable is tested over its range of plausible values while all other variables are held at a constant value; a two-way (bivariate) sensitivity analysis, in which two variables are simultaneously tested over their range of plausible values while all others are held constant; a multi-way sensitivity analysis, in which more than two variables are tested; and a tornado analysis (or influence diagram), in which each variable is sequentially tested in a one-way sensitivity analysis. The tornado analysis is used to rank order the different variables in order of their overall influence on the magnitude of the model outputs.

Figure 4 presents a typical one-way sensitivity analysis. Returning to the influenza example above, let's assume that we wish to know how changes in the estimated value of the vaccine cost will influence the overall expected value of each strategy.

In this instance, we'll add a treatment arm (there are anti-influenza drugs that can be used to treat the infection in early stages). Because the cost of the vaccine does not influence other arms of the analysis, we see that their expected value is not influenced by changes in the cost of the influenza vaccine.

Ideally, we would want to generate some estimate of the impact of all sources of error in the study on the cost and effectiveness values generated by the decision analysis model. One way to generate such an estimate is via Monte Carlo simulation (Halpern *et al.*, 2000). Named after the famous gambling enclave, this type of analysis

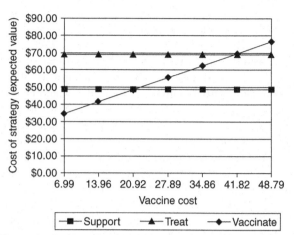

Figure 4 One-way sensitivity analysis examining how the cost of providing the influenza vaccine influences a vaccination, supportive care, and treatment intervention.

allows for the generation of a single confidence interval around multiple variables.

In a Monte Carlo simulation, a hypothetical cohort of subjects enters into the decision analysis model. As subjects pass through the model, they encounter a number of different probabilities such as the chance of developing influenza-like illness, the chance of seeing a doctor, the chance of being hospitalized, and so on. Each time a subject encounters one of these variables, the value that the variable assumes is determined by its probability distribution.

The net result is a weighted mean value for each sampled distribution of each subject randomly entered into the model. (Although this isn't exactly the way that the models are always calculated, it is the easiest way to think about it.) The final standard error associated with all subjects who pass through the model is the overall standard error of all of the distributions sampled.

The basic theory of cost-effectiveness analysis, decision analysis modeling, health-related quality of life scores, and data collection can be found in a number of books and textbooks (Drummond *et al.*, 2005; Muennig, 2007). The methods for standardizing cost-effectiveness analysis are also available in book form (Gold *et al.*, 1996).

Summary

Decision analysis is a formalized approach to making optimal choices under conditions of uncertainty. It allows the user to enter costs, probabilities, and health-related quality of life values among other inputs of interest, and then calculates probabilistically weighted means of these outcome measures. In public health, these outcome measures usually include costs and QALYs. Typically, therefore, decision analysis is the heart of cost-effectiveness analyses in public health and medicine (Gold *et al.*, 1998).

However, just about any outcome measure can be modeled, including vaccine-preventable illnesses averted, deaths avoided, and so forth. Therefore, local health departments, pharmaceutical companies, or other agencies can use decision analysis for internal decision-making processes. Decision analysis is often used by non-health businesses interested in deciding whether they should release a product, perform internal restructuring, and so forth.

One great strength of decision analysis modeling is that it allows for the calculation of a range of possible values around a given mean. This approach, called 'sensitivity analysis,' allows the user to better understand the chances that he or she will make a bad decision if a given strategy is taken.

Decision analysis, like cost-effectiveness analysis, is highly dependent on the accuracy and completeness of model inputs, as well as the assumptions that the analysts make. Drugs can have unforeseen side effects, or interventions can have long-term costs that may not be apparent to the analysts. Any of these effects can lead to suboptimal outcomes.

For instance, the optimal treatment strategy for tuberculosis in most instances is a low-cost combination of medications that can be effectively delivered in developing countries. By using the most cost-effective medications, it is possible to maximize the number of lives saved within a given budget. However, as Farmer points out, these medications will be wasted if delivered to populations with a high percentage of drug-resistant tuberculosis (Farmer, 2004). Therefore, decision analysis and cost-effectiveness analysis must be viewed as an adjunct to optimal decision making rather than the final word in health policy.

Citations

Drummond MF, O'Brien BO, Stoddart GL, and Torrance GW (2005) *Methods for the Economic Evaluation of Health Care Programmes*, 3rd edn. London: Oxford University Press.
Farmer P (2004) *Pathologies of Power: Health, Human Rights, and the New War on the Poor*. Berkeley, CA: University of California Press.
Gold M, Siegel J, Russell L, and Weinstein M (1996) *Cost-Effectiveness in Health and Medicine*. New York: Oxford University Press.

Gold MR, Franks P, McCoy KI, and Fryback DG (1998) Toward consistency in cost-utility analyses: Using national measures to create condition-specific values. *Medical Care* 36(6): 778–792.
Gold MR and Muennig P (2002) Measure-dependent variation in burden of disease estimates: Implications for policy. *Medical Care* 40(3): 260–266.
Halpern EF, Weinstein MC, Hunink MG, and Gazelle GS (2000) Representing both first- and second-order uncertainties by Monte Carlo simulation for groups of patients. *Medical Decision Making* 20(3): 314–322.
Mandelblatt JS, Schechter CB, Yabroff KR, et al. (2004) Benefits and costs of interventions to improve breast cancer outcomes in African American women. *Journal of Clinical Oncology* 22(13): 2554–2566.
Muennig P (2007) *Cost-Effectiveness Analysis in Health, a Practical Approach*. San Francisco, CA: Jossey-Bass.
Muennig P, Pallin D, Sell RL, and Chan MS (1999) The cost effectiveness of strategies for the treatment of intestinal parasites in immigrants. *New England Journal of Medicine* 340(10): 773–779.
Muennig P, Pallin D, Challah C, and Khan K (2004) The cost-effectiveness of ivermectin vs. albendazole in the presumptive treatment of strongyloidiasis in immigrants to the United States. *Epidemiology and Infection* 132(6): 1055–1063.
Muennig P, Franks P, and Gold M (2005) The cost effectiveness of health insurance. *American Journal of Preventive Medicine* 28(1): 59–64.
Muennig PA and Khan K (2001) Cost-effectiveness of vaccination versus treatment of influenza in healthy adolescents and adults. *Clinical and Infectious Disease* 33(11): 1879–1885.
Sonnenberg FA and Beck JR (1993) Markov models in medical decision making: A practical guide. *Medical Decision Making* 13(4): 322–338.

Further Reading

Drummond MF, O'Brien BO, Stoddart GL, and Torrance GW (2005) *Methods for the Economic Evaluation of Health Care Programmes*, 3rd edn. London: Oxford University Press.
Gold MR, Siegel JE, Russell LB and Weinstein MC (eds.) (1996) *Cost-Effectiveness in Health and Medicine*. New York: Oxford University Press.
Hunink M, Glasziou P, Siegel JE, et al. (2001) *Decision Making in Health and Medicine*. Cambridge, UK: Cambridge University Press.
Muennig P (2002) *Designing and Conducting Cost-Effectiveness Analysis in Health and Medicine*. San Francisco, CA: Jossey-Bass.
Muennig P (2007) *Cost-Effectiveness Analysis in Health, a Practical Approach*. San Francisco, CA: Jossey-Bass.
Sonnenberg FA and Beck JR (1993) Markov models in medical decision making: A practical guide. *Medical Decision Making* 13(4): 322.
Weinstein MC, Fineberg HV, Elstein AS, et al. (1980) *Clinical Decision Analysis*. Philadelphia, PA: W. B. Saunders.

Health Finance, Equity in

D De Graeve, University of Antwerp, Antwerp, Belgium
K Xu, World Health Organization, Geneva, Switzerland

© 2008 Elsevier Inc. All rights reserved.

Concept of Equity in Health Financing

What Is Equity in Health Financing?

The question of what constitutes equity is a normative one; it has to do with what a person ought to have, as of right. Philosophers and also economists have reflected on the issue and have formulated various theories of distributional justice in general. Equity in health financing is about fairness in the distribution of health-care payments across the population. Who pays how much for health care is the central question in any discussion of equity in health financing. During the past decade, the equity issue has been of growing importance to policy makers, health workers, and researchers. Since the beginning of the 1990s, the European Union (EU) has financed cross-EU country comparative research measuring equity in the finance of health care (Van Doorslaer et al., 1993). In the 2000 World Health Report, the World Health Organization (WHO) suggested a framework for evaluation of health system performance in which fairness is one of the three goals of the health system along with health and responsiveness (World Health Organization, 2000).

Work has been done to specify what could constitute equity in the finance of medical care. There seems to be broad consensus on the normative assumption that health-care payments should be linked to ability to pay with use related to need, and that all households should be protected against catastrophic financial losses related to ill health (Van Doorslaer et al., 1993; Murray et al., 2003). This implies a disconnection between the payment and the use of services. Given equal access to needed care, people with high capacity to pay should contribute more to a health system than those with lower capacity to pay. Furthermore, people with the same capacity contribute the same amount. The former is vertical equity or progressivity and the latter is horizontal equity. The contribution to a health system includes all payments made by a household through general taxation (direct tax and indirect tax), social health insurance premiums (payroll tax), voluntary prepayment schemes, and out-of-pocket payments.

What Do We Care?

Following the principle that payment for health care should correspond to capacity to pay, the equity concern nevertheless is perceived differently in societies with different economic, political, cultural, and historical contexts. For example, most OECD countries have reached universal coverage of essential health care through a tax-based system, social health insurance, or mixed mechanisms. Few households face severe financial hardship or impoverishment by paying for health care. These societies focus more on whether health payments worsen the overall equity of income (Wagstaff, 2002).

In middle- and low-income countries, health-care financing relies heavily on out-of-pocket payments. As a result, some portions of the population, particularly the poor, are unable to access needed care because they can not afford it. For those who do get needed care, catastrophic expenditure and impoverishment are a frequent result. In this context, the reduction of financial burden and prevention of impoverishment are the primary equity concerns.

Methodologies in Measuring Equity in Health Financing

In short, to measure equity in health financing is to assess the variation in health payments across the population. However, not all variations are regarded as inequitable. Equity implies some social judgments. Many indicators are applicable to measuring equity in health financing, among which two main approaches are widely used, namely, the income approach and the financial burden approach. Both of them require micro-level (household) data.

The income approach is derived from the equity measure of public finance where progressivity is the main concern. This approach has been used mostly for OECD countries. The financial burden approach argues that the burden of paying for health care should be equally distributed across all households. It puts more emphasis on catastrophic health spending and is more applicable to developing countries. Both approaches are in fact complementary and accept the fundamental principle that funds for health care should be collected according to capacity to pay.

Household's Capacity to Pay

Defining capacity to pay is essential in measuring equity in health-care financing. Theoretically, a household's capacity to pay is equal to the total resources that a household can mobilize for purchasing health services, including savings, selling assets, and borrowing from financial institutions, relatives, and friends. Practically, different variables have been used as a proxy for household capacity to pay because the information required is not always available from a cross-section household survey.

Gross Income or Net Income?

In the taxation literature, pre-tax gross equivalent income is used as a proxy for capacity to pay and one is essentially interested in the move from the pre-tax to the post-tax income distribution. Taxes (and social security contributions) are regressive (the poor pay a higher percentage of their income than the rich), neutral (proportional to income) or progressive (the poor pay a lower percentage of income than the rich) if they deteriorate equity in income, leave it unchanged, or improve it. In most European countries, gross income has been used to examine the progressivity of health-care payments. Health-care payments, however, include public (taxes and compulsory insurance) as well as private sources (voluntary prepayment and out-of-pocket payments). Van Ourti argues for using disposable income instead of gross income for the private payments since it is a more adequate indicator of a household's ability to pay and redistribution is not a purpose of these payments (Van Ourti, 2004).

Household Income or Expenditure?

The choice between income and expenditure often depends on the accuracy of available data. In most OECD countries, income data often are linked to the registration system and they are more reliable than reported expenditure from a household survey. By contrast, in most developing countries where registered income data are not available, reported expenditures in household surveys are considered more reliable than reported income. But also for developed countries there is an argument to use expenditures instead of current income because expenditures are less liable to short-term fluctuations, and therefore better approximate ability to pay.

Household Non-food Expenditure or Non-subsistence Spending?

In the WHO World Health Report 2000, household non-food expenditure was used as a proxy for capacity to pay, and this variable has been adopted in various subsequent studies. The argument for using non-food expenditure is that a household should first meet its basic food requirement (although other basic needs such as shelter and clothing also need to be fulfilled) before considering its potential contribution to a health system.

Although food is considered as a household's basic need, empirical data show that a rich household spends much more money on food than a poor household.

So the same subsistence spending for all households with adjustment for household size should be defined. The one-dollar-a-day poverty line and a national poverty line have been used as subsistence spending. In order to reduce unnecessary bias and improve the comparability across countries, WHO has proposed using the food expenditure of the household whose food share of total household expenditure is at the middle of all households in the country (Xu *et al.*, 2005a).

Summary Indices

Income approach

The commonly used indexes are the concentration index (CI), the Kakwani index (KI), and the redistributive effect (RE) (van Doorslaer *et al.*, 1999) (**Figure 1**). The horizontal axis of the figure represents the cumulative percentage of the population ranked according to gross income (poorest first). The vertical axis measures the cumulative share of health care payments (X) and gross income (Y). The curve $L_{X,Y}(p)$ is the concentration curve of health-care payments. When all individuals have exactly the same amount of health-care payments, $L_{X,Y}(p)$ will coincide with the diagonal. When the surface of the rectangle is standardized to 1, the CI is defined as twice the area below $L_{X,Y}(p) - 1$ and thus is a measure of inequality in health-care payments. The CI ranges from -1 to 1. The distribution of health payments is progressive when the CI is positive, regressive when CI is negative, and neutral when CI is zero. Analogously, the Lorenz curve $L_Y(p)$ and the Gini coefficient measure inequality in gross income. By comparing

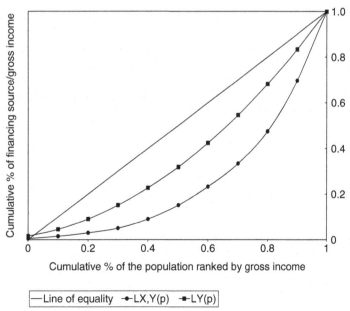

Figure 1 Graphical representation of inequality indexes.

$L_{X,Y}(p)$ with $L_Y(p)$, we can see whether health-care payments increase income inequity. This will be the case when $L_{X,Y}(p)$ lies below $L_Y(p)$. The Kakwani index is defined as the difference between the concentration index and the Gini coefficient; it coincides with twice the area between the two curves. The KI ranges from -2 to 1. A positive value indicates that health payments reduce income inequality, a negative value indicates that health payments increase income inequality and zero indicates that health payments do not change equity in income. The RE is defined as the difference between two income Gini coefficients: income before health payments and income after health payments. The RE takes into consideration both vertical and horizontal equity and is dependent on the share of health-care payments in income. It ranges from -1 to 1 with the same interpretation as the Kakwani index.

All three indexes have the property of scale invariance, which means that when every household doubles its payments, the indexes do not change (Jenkins, 1991). Also, these indexes are more sensitive to changes in payments for households that are in the middle of the distribution.

Financial burden approach

The financial burden approach argues that although progressivity is desirable for a health financing system, most societies do not seek to redistribute income through financing health care but do expect health payments to be arranged in a fair way (World Health Organization, 2000). At any given level of total revenue from health-care services, each individual should carry the same burden. The burden is measured as a share of total household spending on health to a household capacity to pay (nonsubsistence spending). The fairness in financial contribution (FFC) index is used to summarize the distribution of the burden across the population. The FFC index is between 0 and 1, with 1 indicating the perfect situation that the share of the total health spending of household capacity to pay is identical for all households. The index will be less than 1 if shares differ. All deviations are treated alike; no distinction is made between inequities due to pro- or regressivity of payments. Zero represents the maximum unfairness. The FFC index has the property of constant invariance, which means that by adding or subtracting the same amount of burden from all households the index remains the same. The FFC index is more sensitive to health payments made by households at the tail of the distribution (Xu et al., 2003b).

According to the financial burden approach, a fairly financed health system collects its revenue in a progressive manner since payment of an equal share of nonsubsistence spending by all households implies that a high-income household pays a higher share of its total expenditure than a low-income household. It also implies that no household should face financial catastrophe.

The most commonly used measure in the financial burden approach is the percentage of households facing catastrophic health expenditure. The percentage of households with catastrophic expenditure also gives the flexibility in setting different thresholds according to different country situations. The WHO has used 40% of the out-of-pocket payment in a household's nonsubsistence spending as a threshold for its cross-country studies.

Other indexes

A wide range of equity measures can also be used to analyze the distribution of households' health payments such as entropy measures, Atkinson's index, and variance. The entropy measures, including Theil and mean logarithmic deviation (MLD), are derived from the notion of entropy in information theory. The Theil and MLD give more weight to the individuals at the tail of the distribution. Atkinson's index has its origins in the social welfare literature. Through changing levels of inequality aversion, Atkinson's index allows one to explore the consequence of different weighting systems. A higher inequality aversion implies higher weights on the households at the tail of the distribution.

The Limitation of the Indexes

Equity or fairness in health financing is defined under the condition that every person can access services when needed. None of the measures take into consideration the actual use of health services. It has been argued that equity in health payments and equity in access to care imply separate policies. While it may not be necessary or desirable to combine the two into one index, a further analysis of the distribution of access to health care should provide a more comprehensive picture of equity. Related to this discussion is the issue of the origin of health-care payments. Health-care payments can be the result of characteristics for which the individual can be held responsible or not. Think about the health expenditure following a skiing accident versus that resulting from a genetic defect. High payments may also be associated with the individual's choice of a very expensive, but not more effective, physician. Furthermore, each equity index has its own focus. The choice among the indexes depends on the purpose of the study. For example, the income approach gives more of an overall picture, while the burden approach focuses on vulnerable groups.

Apart from the methodological concern, the characteristics of data used in measuring equity or fairness are critical. Most measures use sampled household survey data. The quality of data, the recall period of total household expenditures and expenditures for health care, and the questions phrased in the survey may all have an impact on the results.

Empirical Results on Equity in Health Financing

Global Inequity

Despite continuous efforts made at the global and national levels, equity in health-care financing is still far below expectation. Statistics in the World Health Report (World Health Organization, 2005b) show that in the year 2002 approximately 85% of the global population spent only 20% of total health expenditure (**Figure 2**). The per capita total health spending is less than $10 in 13 countries, between $10 and $20 in 25 countries, and between $20 and $50 in another 28 countries.

Furthermore, every year approximately 44 million households, or more than 150 million individuals, throughout the world face catastrophic expenditure, about 25 million households or more than 100 million individuals are pushed into poverty by the need to pay for services and 1.3 billion people do not have access to effective and affordable health care (Preker et al., 2002; Xu et al., 2005b).

Cross-Country Comparison

There is a rich literature on equity of health financing, among which two groups of studies have made a great effort to undertake cross-country comparisons. The first group was started in the late 1980s in the OECD countries by Wagstaff and van Doorslaer, who used income approach indexes to examine the progressivity of different means of health financing (Wagstaff et al., 1999; De Graeve and Van Ourti, 2003; Murray et al., 2003). Later on in the early 2000s, the same methodology was applied to a group of countries in the Asia Pacific region (Wagstaff and Van Doorslaer, 2003; Donnell et al., 2005, 2006).

The overall progressivity of a health financing system depends on the progressivity of health payments from various sources (general government tax revenue, social health insurance, etc.) and their share in total health payments. The study by Wagstaff and van Doorslaer in OECD countries (Wagstaff et al., 1999; De Graeve and Van Ourti, 2003) found that the overall health payments were regressive in seven out of the 14 countries (**Table 1**). The United States and Switzerland were the worst in terms of equity, while the United Kingdom was the best. The variability across countries in the Kakwani index of total payments is small, however (range, −0.045 to 0.051), with the US and Switzerland being outliers. Payments made through direct taxes such as income tax and property tax were progressive in all countries, while payments made through indirect taxes, such as value added tax, sales tax, and excise duties were regressive. Social health insurance contributions through payroll tax were progressive except in Germany and the Netherlands, where until recent reforms high-income earners could opt out or are excluded from social insurance. Private health insurance varied across countries, due to the variety of roles and market shares. The out-of-pocket payments were the most regressive financing source in all countries included in this study (except for Italy and the Netherlands). Out-of-pocket payments are related to demand for health-care consumption, which is higher in low-income groups who incur more illnesses.

The Asia Pacific region study included ten countries, most of which belong to the developing world. Compared to OECD countries, the results from the Asia Pacific region were somewhat surprising except for health payments financed via direct taxes. Among the ten countries included in the study, only Taiwan had a regressive health financing system (**Table 1**). Health payments financed via direct taxes were generally progressive, as with the OECD countries. Unlike the OECD countries, the health payments financed via indirect taxes in the Asia Pacific region were all progressive except in Sri Lanka. Out-of-pocket payments were progressive except in mainland China, Kyrgyzstan, and Taiwan. Social health insurance was prevalent in eight countries in this study, but most on a small scale except in Taiwan, Japan, and the Republic of Korea, where it covered nearly the entire population. Surprisingly, social health insurance contributions were progressive in all countries except the three that nearly reached universal coverage.

The second group of comparative studies were conducted within the framework of health system performance assessment proposed by WHO. The studies focused on fairness and catastrophic health expenditure and used the burden approach measures. Data for 59 countries have so far been analyzed (World Health Organization, 2000).

Results from the second group of studies found significant variations in the FFC index across countries. It ranged from 0.74 in Brazil to 0.94 in Slovakia (**Table 2**). The percentage of households with catastrophic expenditure ranged from less than 0.1% in Belgium, Canada, Czech Republic, France, Germany, Romania, Slovakia, Slovenia, South Africa, and UK to over 10% in Brazil and Vietnam. In general, the high-income OECD countries scored high

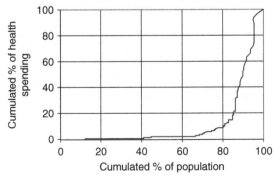

Figure 2 Distribution of total heath spending globally.

Table 1 Progressivity of health-care financing by components (Kakwani index)

	Direct taxes	Indirect taxes	Social insurance	Private insurance	Out-of-pocket payments	Total financing
Early study in OECD countries						
Belgium (1997)	0.180	−0.180	0.102	−0.0210	−0.260	−0.000
Denmark (1987)	0.0624	−0.1126		0.0313	−0.2654	−0.0047
Finland (1990)	0.1272	−0.0969	0.0937	0.000	−0.2419	0.0181
France (1989)			0.1112	−0.1956	−0.3396	0.0012
Germany (1989)	0.2488	−0.0922	−0.0977	0.1219	−0.0963	−0.0452
Ireland (1987)	0.2666		0.1263	−0.0210	−0.1472	
Italy (1991)	0.1554	−0.1135	0.1072	0.1705	−0.0807	0.0413
Netherlands (1992)	0.2003	−0.0885	−0.1286	0.0833	−0.0377	−0.0703
Portugal (1990)	0.2180	−0.0347	0.1845	0.1371	−0.2424	−0.0445
Spain (1990)	0.2125	−0.1533	0.0615	−0.0224	−0.1801	0.0004
Sweden (1990)	0.0529	−0.0827	0.0100		−0.2402	−0.0158
Switzerland (1992)	0.2055	−0.0722	0.0551	−0.2548	−0.3619	−0.1402
United Kingdom (1993)	0.2843	−0.1522	0.1867	0.0766	−0.2229	0.051
United States (1987)	0.2104	−0.0674	0.0181	−0.2374	−0.3874	−0.1303
Asia Pacific region						
Bangladesh (1999–2000)	0.5523	0.1110			0.2192	0.2142
China mainland (2000)	0.1521	0.0398	0.2348		−0.0168	0.0404
Hong Kong (1999–2000)	0.3940	0.1102		0.0403	0.0113	0.1663
Indonesia (2001)	0.1962	0.0741	0.3057		0.1761	0.1737
Japan (1998)	0.0950	−0.2232	−0.0415		−0.2691	−0.0688
Republic of Korea (2000)	0.2683	0.0379	−0.1634		0.0124	−0.0239
Kyrgyzstan (2000)	0.2395	0.0508	0.1422		−0.0520	0.0087
Nepal (1995–96)	0.1436	0.1143			0.0533	0.0625
Philippines (1999)	0.3809	0.0024	0.2048	0.1199	0.1391	0.1631
Sri Lanka (1996–7)	0.5693	−0.0100			0.0687	0.0850
Taiwan (2000)	0.2438	0.0404	−0.0749	0.2053	−0.0780	−0.0292
Thailand (2002)	0.5101	0.1819	0.1803	0.0039	0.0907	0.1972

From De Graeve D and Van Ourti (2003) The distributional impact of health financing in Europe: A review. *The World Economy* 26(10): 1459–1479; Donnell O, Van Doorslaer E, Rannan-Eliya R, and Somanathan A (2005) *Who Pays for Health Care in Asia.* EQUITAP project: working paper.

in FFC and a low percentage of households were facing catastrophic expenditure, but there was considerable variation even among OECD countries. For example, the United States and Switzerland were far behind most of the other OECD countries. Catastrophic expenditure was highest in some countries in transition and in certain Latin American countries.

A further study has explored the link between catastrophic expenditure and health system indicators (Xu et al., 2003a). The study identified three key preconditions for catastrophic payments: The availability of health services requiring out-of-pocket payment, low capacity to pay, and the lack of a prepayment mechanism. The results showed that the higher the percentage of out-of-pocket payment in total health-care spending and the larger the population below the poverty line, the higher the percentage of households with catastrophic expenditure. Holding these two factors constant, a higher ratio of total health spending to gross domestic product (GDP) led to a higher percentage of catastrophic expenditure; GDP is a proxy for availability of services. Out-of-pocket payments were specifically highlighted in causing catastrophic expenditure. **Figure 3** shows the relationship between the percentage of catastrophic expenditure and the percentage of out-of-pocket payments in total health spending.

Within-Country Differences

There are also country case studies exploring the differences in health payments across socioeconomic groups and their impact on households' financial situation. Many studies related to developing countries find that the poor carry a larger burden than the rest of the population. The poor also use fewer services. Furthermore, households with senior members and those living in rural areas are more likely to face financial catastrophe. Using public facilities does not protect households against financial loss because of user charges. Health insurance schemes frequently play a limited role in financial risk protection because of their insufficient population coverage and the inappropriate benefit package (Fabricant et al., 1999; Falkingham, 2004; Gotsadze et al., 2005; Su et al., 2006; Xu et al., 2006). The information from these studies is useful for identifying and targeting disadvantaged population groups.

Table 2 Fairness in financial contribution and catastrophic payments

Country	FFC index	% Of households[a]	Country	FFC index	% Of households[a]
Argentina	0.785	5.77	Lebanon	0.844	5.17
Azerbaijan	0.748	7.15	Lithuania	0.875	1.34
Bangladesh	0.868	1.21	Mauritius	0.861	1.28
Belgium	0.903	0.09	Mexico	0.857	1.54
Brazil	0.740	10.27	Morocco	0.913	0.17
Bulgaria	0.862	2.00	Namibia	0.877	0.11
Cambodia	0.805	5.02	Nicaragua	0.829	2.05
Canada	0.913	0.09	Norway	0.888	0.28
Colombia	0.809	6.26	Panama	0.801	2.35
Costa Rica	0.861	0.12	Paraguay	0.815	3.51
Croatia	0.865	0.20	Peru	0.813	3.21
Czech	0.904	0.00	Philippines	0.886	0.78
Denmark	0.920	0.07	Portugal	0.845	2.71
Djibouti	0.853	0.32	Romania	0.901	0.09
Egypt	0.835	2.80	Senegal	0.892	0.55
Estonia	0.872	0.31	Slovakia	0.941	0.00
Finland	0.901	0.44	Slovenia	0.890	0.06
France	0.889	0.01	South Africa	0.894	0.03
Germany	0.913	0.03	Spain	0.899	0.48
Ghana	0.862	1.30	Sri Lanka	0.865	1.25
Greece	0.858	2.17	Sweden	0.920	0.18
Guyana	0.887	0.60	Switzerland	0.875	0.57
Hungary	0.905	0.20	Thailand	0.888	0.80
Iceland	0.891	0.30	UK	0.921	0.04
Indonesia	0.859	1.26	Ukraine	0.788	3.87
Israel	0.897	0.35	United States	0.860	0.55
Jamaica	0.787	1.86	Vietnam	0.762	10.45
Korea	0.847	1.73	Yemen	0.853	1.66
Kyrgyzstan	0.875	0.62	Zambia	0.816	2.29
Latvia	0.828	2.75			

[a]Only out-of-pocket payments are included.
From Murray C, Xu K, Klavus J, et al. (2003) Assessing the distribution of household financial contributions to the health system: Concepts and empirical application. In: Murray CJL and Evans DB (eds.) *Health Systems Performance Assessment: Debates, Methods and Empiricism*, pp. 513–531. Geneva, Switzerland: World Health Organization.

Policy Implications in Improving Equity in Health Financing

Different Policy Focuses in Different Settings

Equity in health financing is a common concern of many countries. Diverse socioeconomic and political settings have produced different perspectives on how to address the equity issue. For example, in Africa user fees, the official fees charged by public facilities, have been a central focus during the past 15 years. Some studies found that user fees reduced the level of equity not only in health-care financing but also in access to basic care, such as in Burkina Faso, Burundi, Ghana, and Tanzania (Hussein and Mujinja, 1997; Nyonator and Kutzin, 1999; Bate and Witter, 2003; Riddle, 2003). Other studies, for example in Cameroon, Mauritania, Benin, and Guinea, found that the quality of services had improved after introducing user fees, and that with an effective exemption mechanism the poor can also benefit from high-quality services (Litvack and Bodart, 1993; Soucat and Gandaho, 1997; Audibert and Mathonnat, 2000).

Obviously, there is no final conclusion on the impact of user fees. Through debate, people realize that user fees do not constitute the sole cause of inequity in health-care financing and access to services. Alternative financing mechanisms aiming to reduce the overall out-of-pocket payments are key in improving equity.

Equity in health financing has been on the agenda of recent reforms in many Latin American countries where social health insurance has a long history. The challenge for those countries is to reduce the gap between the insured and the uninsured. Countries such as Colombia, Mexico, Chile, and Argentina are making efforts to include the poor or other vulnerable groups in the overall social protection program by either subsidizing social health insurance premiums or providing nearly free basic health services through public facilities (Bitran et al., 2000; Frenk et al., 2003; Lloyd-Sherlock, 2005).

Countries previously under a centralized planned economic regime had enjoyed nearly free health-care service from public facilities financed by the government. Following market-oriented economic reform, these health

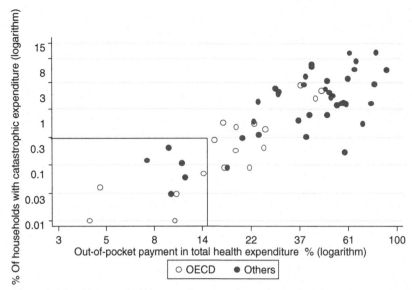

Figure 3 Proportion of households with catastrophic expenditures vs share of out-of-pocket payment in total health expenditure. From Xu K, Evans D, Carrin G, and Aguilar A (2005b) *Designing Health Financing Systems to Reduce Catastrophic Health Expenditure.* World Health Organization Technical Briefs for Policy-Makers.

systems solely funded by the government could not be maintained, however. In order to make up for the shortage in government funding, user charges became a common practice in public facilities and equity decreased (Ensor and Savelyeva, 1998; Makinen et al., 2000; Gao et al., 2002). In these circumstances, many countries have considered social health insurance as an attractive alternative financing mechanism (Saltman et al., 2004). However, the risk is that social health insurance would start with formal sector employees leaving behind the self-employed and the poor. Furthermore, the lack of experience in organizing social health insurance adds more challenges to current reform efforts.

Finally the most developed OECD countries face the challenge of maintaining their relatively equitable public health financing systems. Most of these countries have reached nearly universal coverage, but now need to cope with tight government budgets having to finance increasing health-care costs. Therefore, some have decreased the public financing share in total health expenditure and shifted financing to out-of-pocket payments and private insurance. Differential user charges, exemptions, and deductibles are also being explored to avoid catastrophic expenditures of some (unfortunate) households.

Is One Method Better than Another in Revenue Collection?

Funds used for health care are mainly from government general taxation, payroll taxes, private insurance premiums, out-of-pocket payments, and external resources (especially for low-income countries). There is strong evidence that out-of-pocket payment is the most inequitable way to finance health care, although some modest level of out-of-pocket payments can be maintained to stimulate the rational use of health services. However, out-of-pocket payment should remain affordable, which is not the case for a large proportion of the population in developing countries. Reducing out-of-pocket payment and increasing the role of prepayment schemes in overall revenue collection is still the main task for most developing countries.

There are two broad types of public prepayment schemes: The tax-based financing system and the social health insurance system. In the former, funds collected are used to provide basic health services to the general population through public health facilities. Whether a tax-based system is the most equitable way to collect funds depends on the equity of the overall taxation system. Income taxes are usually more progressive than indirect taxes such as value added taxes (VAT), sale taxes, and excise duties. In many developing countries, government taxation mainly relies on indirect taxes so that progressivity is not guaranteed.

In a social health insurance system, funds are collected from payroll taxes that are generally proportional to income. In most cases a ceiling is applied, reducing the potential contribution of the high-wage population. On the other hand, there can be exemptions for the lower-wage population. In recent health financing reforms, many countries have been struggling to choose between tax-based and social health insurance mechanisms (William, 2004). In practice, we also see mixes of the two systems. For example, governments may subsidize social health insurance by paying the premiums for the poor or unemployed or by providing services through public facilities at a low cost for the uninsured population. The choice between a tax-based system, social health insurance, or some mixed system depends on a country's specific situation.

Private health insurance, which is important in the United States, is problematic from an equity point of view. While more limited in the rest of the world, its market share is growing in some highly developed countries. These increased resources for health care can make health care more responsive to the insured, but vulnerable groups can be refused cover or priced out the market by risk-rated premiums. Policy makers should be aware of this and regulate the role of private health insurance (e.g., specify rules of access). Community-based schemes or mutual fund programs have found favor in some African countries, such as Rwanda and Senegal (Scheider and Hanson, 2006). External resources are very important in financing health care for some low-income countries. For example, in Rwanda 55% of total health expenditure is from external funding sources. In Zambia, external funding accounts for 45% and in Mozambique and Comoros 41%. External resources accounted for more than 20% of total health expenditure in 14 out of 46 African countries in 2003 (World Health Organization, 2006). External funding can both offset shortages of public resources and also improve equity if they are used properly in these countries.

How to Improve Equity in Health Financing?

In 2005, the World Health Assembly adopted a resolution, Sustainable Health Financing, Universal Coverage, and Social Health Insurance (World Health Organization, 2005a). This resolution encourages countries to increase the extent of prepayment and reduce the reliance on out-of-pocket payments in order to improve equity in health financing. Such reforms on revenue collection should run parallel with modifications to the other two functions of health financing, namely pooling and purchasing (World Health Organization, 2000). An appropriate pooling system allows for cross subsidies from the healthy to the ill and from the rich to the poor (Kawabata et al., 2002). The more people that are covered by a prepayment scheme, the more efficient the pooling function is. The purchasing function contributes to equity through carefully choosing a benefit package and setting a cost-sharing scale. A benefit package that is too small or has a sharing rate that is too high will not be able to improve equity, while an overly generous benefit package or a sharing rate that is too low can make the program unsustainable and compromise equity in the long run.

The ideal situation of universal coverage cannot be reached within a short period of time. In most developed countries, the transitional period has lasted several decades, and this is likely also to be the case for developing countries. During the transition, various kinds of prepayment schemes should be encouraged, not only taxation and social health insurance, but also community-, cooperative- and enterprise-based health insurance and other forms of private health insurance. There is no golden standard or universal path that can be applied to all countries. The choices have to be made within the social, economic, historical, and cultural context of each country. Above all, governments' political will and good leadership are critical to ensure that the equity component is taken into consideration in any reform process. Once reached, there should be a continuing concern to keep the system equitable and to guarantee access to the basic benefit package to all income groups, including the poor.

See also: Determinants of National Health Expenditure; Managed Care; The Private Sector in Health Care Provision, The Role of; Universal Coverage in Developing Countries, Transition to.

Citations

Audibert M and Mathonnat J (2000) Cost recovery in Mauritania: Initial lessons. *Health Policy and Planning* 15(1): 66–75.
Bate A and Witter S (2003) *Coping with Community Health Financing: Illness Cost and Their Implementations for Poor Households' Abilities to Pay for Health Care and Children's Access to Health Services.* London: Save the Children UK.
Bitran R, Munoz J, Aguad P, Navarrete M, and Ubilla G (2000) Equity in the financing of social security for health in Chile. *Health Policy* 50(3): 171–196.
De Graeve D and Van Ourti T (2003) The distributional impact of health financing in Europe: A review. *The World Economy* 26(10): 1459–1479.
Ensor T and Savelyeva L (1998) Informal payments for health care in the former Soviet Union: Some evidence from Kazakstan. *Health Policy and Planning* 13(1): 41–49.
Fabricant SJ, Kamara CW, and Mills A (1999) Why the poor pay more: Household curative expenditures in rural Sierra Leone. *International Journal of Health Planning and Management* 14(3): 179–199.
Falkingham J (2004) Poverty, out-of-pocket payments and access to health care: Evidence from Tajikistan. *Social Science and Medicine* 58(2): 247–258.
Frenk J, Sepulveda J, Gomez-Dantes O, and Knaul F (2003) Evidence-based health policy: Three generations of reform in Mexico. *The Lancet* 362: 1667–1671.
Gao J, Qian JC, Tang SL, Eriksson B, and Blas E (2002) Health equity in transition from planned to market economy in China. *Health Policy and Planning* 17: 20–29.
Gotsadze G, Bennett S, Ranson K, and Gzirishvili D (2005) Health care-seeking behaviour and out-of-pocket payments in Tbilisi, Georgia. *Health Policy and Planning* 20(4): 232–242.
Hussein A and Mujinja P (1997) Impact of user charges on government health facilities in Tanzania. *Journal of East African Medicine* 74(12): 310–321.
Jenkins S (1991) The measurement of income inequality. In: Osberg L (ed.) *Economic Inequality and Poverty International Perspectives*, pp. 3–38. London: Sharpe ME.
Kawabata K, Xu K, and Carrin G (2002) Preventing impoverishment through protection against catastrophic health expenditure. *Bulletin of the World Health Organization* 80(8): 612.
Litvack JI and Bodart C (1993) User fees plus quality equals improved access to health-care – Results of a field experiment in Cameroon. *Social Science and Medicine* 37(3): 369–383.
Lloyd-Sherlock P (2005) Health sector reform in Argentina: A cautionary tale. *Social Science and Medicine* 60: 1893–1903.
Makinen M, Waters H, Rauch M, et al. (2000) Inequalities in health care use and expenditures: Empirical data from eight developing countries and countries in transition. *Bulletin of the World Health Organization* 78(1): 55–65.

Murray C, Xu K, Klavus J, et al. (2003) Assessing the distribution of household financial contributions to the health system: Concepts and empirical application. In: Murray CJL and Evans DB (eds.) *Health Systems Performance Assessment: Debates, Methods and Empiricism*, pp. 513–531. Geneva, Switzerland: World Health Organization.

Nyonator F and Kutzin J (1999) Health for some? The effects of user fees in the Volta Region of Ghana. *Health Policy and Planning* 14(4): 329–341.

O'Donnell O, Van Doorslaer E, Rannan-Eliya R, and Somanathan A (2005) *Who Pays for Health Care in Asia*. EQUITAP project: working paper.

O'Donnell O, Van Doorslaer E, Rannan-Eliya R, and Somanathan P (2006) *Explaining the Incidence of Catastrophic Expenditures on Health Care: Comparative Evidence from Asia*. EQUITAP Project: Working Paper #5.

Preker A, Langenbrunner J, and Jakab M (2002) Rich-poor differences in health care financing. In: Dror D and Preker A (eds.) *Social Re-insurance – A New Approach to Sustainable Community Health Care Financing*, pp. 21–36. Washington DC: the World Bank.

Ridde V (2003) Fees-for-services, cost recovery, and equity in a district of Burkina Faso operating the Bamako Initiative. *Bulletin of the World Health Organization* 81(7): 532–538.

Saltman R, Busse R, and Figueras J (2004) *Social Health Insurance Systems in Western Europe*. New York: Open University Press.

Schneider P and Hanson K (2006) Horizontal equity in utilisation of care and fairness of health financing: A comparison of micro-health insurance and user fees in Rwanda. *Health Economics* 15(1): 19–31.

Soucat A and Gandaho T (1997) Health seeking behavior and household health expenditures in Benin and Guinea: The equity implementation of Bamako Initiative. *International Journal of Health Planning and Management* 12(supplement 1): s137–s163.

Su T, Kouyaté B, and Flessa S (2006) Catastrophic household expenditure for heath care in a low income society: A study from Nouna District, Burkina Faso. *Bulletin of the World Health Organization* 84(1): 21–27.

Van Doorslaer E, Wagstaff A, and Rutten F (1993) *Equity in the Finance and Delivery of Health Care: An International Perspective*. Oxford, UK: Oxford Medical Publications.

Van Doorslaer E, Wagstaff A, van der Burg H, et al. (1999) The redistributive effect of health care finance in twelve OECD countries. *Journal of Health Economics* 18(3): 291–313.

Van Ourti T (2004) *Essays on Inequality Measurement in Health, Health Care and Finance of Health Care*. PhD Thesis. University of Antwerp.

Wagstaff A (2002) Poverty and health sector inequalities. *Bulletin of the World Health Organization* 80(2): 97–105.

Wagstaff A and Van Doorslaer E (2003) Catastrophe and impoverishment in paying for health care with applications to Vietnam 1993–1998. *Health Economics* 12(11): 921–934.

Wagstaff A, van Doorslaer E, van der Burg H, et al. (1999) Equity in the finance of health care: Some further international comparisons. *Journal of Health Economics* 18(3): 263–290.

William S (2004) Is there a case for social insurance? *Health Policy and Planning* 19(3): 183–184.

World Health Organization (2000) *The World Health Report 2000: Health Systems: Improving Performance*. Geneva, Switzerland: World Health Organization.

World Health Organization (2005a) *Sustainable Health Financing, Universal Coverage and Social Health Insurance*. A58/20. Geneva, Switzerland: World Health Organization.

World Health Organization (2005b) *The World Health Report 2005*. Geneva, Switzerland: World Health Organization.

World Health Organization (2006) *World Health Report 2006*. Geneva, Switzerland: World Health Organization.

Xu K, Evans D, Kawabata K, Zeramdini R, Klavus J, and Murray C (2003a) Household catastrophic health expenditure: A multicountry analysis. *The Lancet* 362: 111–117.

Xu K, Klavus J, Aguilar-Rivera A, Carrin G, Zeramdini R, and Murray C (2003b) Summary measures of the distribution of household financial contributions to health. In: Murray CJL and Evans DB (eds.) *Health Systems Performance Assessment: Debates, Methods and Empiricism*. Geneva, Switzerland: World Health Organization.

Xu K, Aguilar A, Carrin G, and Evans D (2005a) *Distribution of Health Payments and Catastrophic Expenditures: Methodology*. WHO Health Financing Policydiscussion paper.

Xu K, Evans D, Carrin G, and Aguilar A (2005b) *Designing Health Financing Systems to Reduce Catastrophic Health Expenditure*. World Health OrganizationTechnical Briefs for Policy-Makers.

Xu K, Evans D, Kadama P, et al. (2006) Understanding the impact of eliminating user fees: Utilization and catastrophic health expenditures in Uganda. *Social Science and Medicine* 62: 866–876.

Further Reading

Wagstaff A and Van Doorslaer E (1993) *Equity in the Finance and Delivery of Health Care: An International Perspective*. Oxford, UK: Oxford Medical Publications.

Governance Issues in Health Financing

M Lewis, World Bank, Washington, DC, USA
P Musgrove, Health Affairs, Bethesda, MD, USA

© 2008 Elsevier Inc. All rights reserved.

Paying for Health Care and the Functions of a Health System

Financing is one of the four basic functions of a health system, as classified by the World Health Organization (WHO, 2000), and is what pays for two others, investment in people, buildings, and equipment and the delivery of health services. The fourth function, stewardship (often referred to as regulation or oversight), corresponds closely to governance since it prevents irregular behavior or outright corruption. While the other functions can be carried out by many different actors, public and private, stewardship is an inalienable responsibility of government, to be exercised over all the other functions. Good governance ensures that government is ultimately accountable to its citizens. This can take the form of physicians responding to patient requests, local government ensuring that clinics are opened and staffed, or that physician performance meets basic standards set by the government or a private oversight body. The extreme of poor governance is corruption, where individuals use public positions for private gain and are not called to account for such behavior. The concept of accountability – answering for actions taken in the name of the government – implies oversight or regulation to ensure compliance. In finance it applies to collection of revenues, spending, and procurement and flow of funds, and follows the sequence of tasks that constitute health-care financing.

Poor governance and corruption stem from inadequate oversight of finance, investment, and delivery. These are all abstract, high-level functions; to identify specific issues for the governance of financing, they must be broken down and related to the instruments at governments' command. The latter can be classified in various partially overlapping ways, two of which are (Musgrove, 2004a; Roberts et al., 2004): Regulations specifying how something is to be done, or who is licensed to do it (which may or may not be distinguished from mandates requiring that something be done), imply rules for behavior and some mechanism to enforce those rules through penalties.

Funding, Pooling, and Buying Goods and Services

Financing is best thought of in three stages: Revenue raising (also called funding); pooling, for all forms of funding except out-of-pocket payments; and purchasing, or buying services and the inputs to them. Payment refers to how purchases are made, the payment system, the way providers are remunerated, for example by salary, capitation, fee-for-service, or other forms. Each of these stages presents particular challenges for good governance.

For funding and pooling, good practice means distributing the financial burden fairly, while minimizing the deadweight loss to the economy from taxes (see Musgrave and Musgrave, 1989); good governance specifically implies minimizing the theft or diversion of funds through corruption. Governments can directly determine and collect taxes, including those for social insurance, but they can affect what people spend out of pocket only indirectly, by regulating private insurance, setting fees or allowing facilities to set fees, and by financing services through public prepayment (see **Figure 1**). Informal or under-the-table payments, in contrast, are a sign of poor governance. Choices about taxes and insurance will affect how much of health spending is pooled so as to share risks, how many pools there are, which people are included in them, and from which financial risks they are protected.

In most poor countries, there is very little private insurance, and if social insurance exists, it covers only a few percent of the population. In middle-income countries, both kinds of insurance are more common, but with great variety in how they are defined and regulated. In Chile, people can direct their payroll tax to the public National Health Fund or to a private insurer; in the Netherlands until recent reforms, the rich were excluded from the public pool and required to insure privately through regulated insurance funds. Social insurance agencies sometimes provide services to those not insured, but more often do not. The most important indicator of how

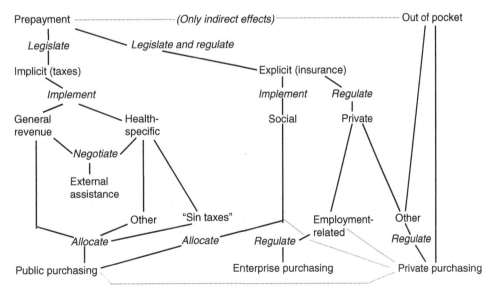

Figure 1 Sources of funding for health and governance relations. Adapted from Musgrove P (2004b) Introduction. In: Musgrove P (ed.) *Health Economics in Development*. Washington, DC: World Bank.

well people are protected financially is the share of total health spending that is out of pocket, which is quite high on average (and also quite variable) in poor countries (Musgrove et al., 2002). However, while that share is associated with great inequity, it cannot be interpreted as an indicator of bad governance, since it is the result of pricing and the decisions on financing levels by government, not inefficiency or ineptitude in public service delivery. While funding and pooling arrangements can be judged according to the equity of the tax burden, and its drag on the economy and the probability of catastrophic expense for a household, no measures of governance specific to health financing have yet been devised.

The buying or purchasing stage of financing presents more complicated challenges for governance, for two reasons: There are many more choices to make among inputs, people, diseases, and services; and the opportunities for corruption, incompetence, and fraud are multiplied. Whereas poorly controlled funding and pooling may lead to theft of funds, the purchase of services or the payment of suppliers and providers allows for the theft of supplies, especially drugs; of time; and of the use of public equipment and facilities for private gain. While much discussion has emphasized outright corruption, including theft and bribes, other problems such as unauthorized absenteeism by staff also represent poor governance and a clear lack of accountability of public sector employees.

It may be reasonable to allow staff on the public payroll to operate private practices; indeed, that may be necessary for recruiting staff at salaries the government can afford. Abuse of such arrangements by absenteeism, recruiting patients for private care and diversion or abuse of public supplies and equipment implies underperformance of public duties, requiring oversight by hospital directors or chief physicians empowered to ensure compliance. Accountability implies that those who underperform or engage in irregular behavior will be disciplined in some manner. Without a means of reward and discipline, oversight becomes meaningless and public employees cannot be held accountable for their actions. At this level, stewardship or oversight cannot be exercised from on high; it requires supervision and accountability at the level of individual providers, suppliers, and procedures.

Once money has been spent or allocated, financing shades into investment and service delivery and out of the scope of this article. Unfortunately, good governance is just as crucial or more so beyond that point, since resources will still be wasted if providers do not know what to do or do not do what is required to meet patients' needs. Such incompetence, the failure to follow protocols, and medical errors are alarmingly common in both public and private facilities, and not only in poor countries, as studies have shown in the United States (Asch *et al.*, 2006), Mexico, Paraguay, India, Indonesia, and Tanzania (Das and Gertler, 2005). Good governance in financing can only prevent such failings upstream from the point where patients and providers meet.

Peculiarities of Health and Consequences for Governance

The differences between health care and other sectors of the economy are rooted in biology, specifically in the fact that the asset one wants to protect cannot – in contrast to nonhuman assets such as a dwelling or a vehicle – be alienated or replaced. This fact has consequences for the difference between health insurance and insurance for other goods, which create problems for health finance and for its governance (see **Table 1**). In particular, health expenditure has to cover both predictable events, which are technically uninsurable because they are too predictable – but which must be paid out of pocket if not insured, causing risks for (poor) people – and catastrophic events that may have almost no upper limit on cost. It is either impossible, or regarded as unjust, to rely on the market and on individual healthful behavior to limit risks or to pay for

Table 1 Differences between health insurance and insurance for nonhuman assets

Characteristics of insurance	Type of asset			Consequences
	House	Car	Body	
Is the asset itself insured?	Yes	Yes	No	No market price/no upper limit on cost
Can the asset be replaced?	Yes	Yes	No	Expense determined by cost of repairs/treatment
Covers catastrophic costs?	Yes	Yes	Yes	Very skewed distribution of expenses
Covers ordinary wear and tear?	No	No	Yes	Costs of predictable high-frequency (uninsurable) events included
Owner responsible for protecting the asset?	Yes	Yes	Only partly	Cannot always hold patient responsible: children, elderly, victims of bad luck, including genetic
Risk and cost related to behavior?	No	Yes	Only partly	Requires efforts to change behavior; not easy, and too little known about behavior/health links
Third-party payment of premium?	No	No	Yes	Moral hazard and adverse selection

Adapted from Musgrove P (2004b) Introduction. In: Musgrove P (ed.) *Health Economics in Development*. Washington, DC: World Bank.

all needed care, even for the nonpoor. The complexities of paying for health drive the importance of regulation and the use of information and persuasion to change behavior, just as it does to ensure that financing is fair, transparent, and reaches its intended spending objectives.

Specific Challenges for Governance in Health Finance: Measurement

Good governance can be difficult to measure. More straightforward is the lack of governance, that is, corruption. The extent and nature of corruption in any given setting can be assessed by compiling perceptions of corruption from government officials, the business community, and citizens (Kauffman et al., 2005). The health sector is sometimes included in such surveys, but less often than more generic measures. Nonetheless, it can be helpful in determining relative governance across countries, and tracking changes in perceptions of corruption in the sector. In some countries, health is identified as among the most corrupt of sectors, so this is not a trivial concern. **Figure 2** shows the share of respondents who perceive corruption in the health sector in 19 countries, ranging from less than 10% in only two countries to 60% or more in eight countries (Lewis, 2006).

The view that the health sector is corrupt may be strongly influenced by absenteeism among public sector health workers; **Figure 3** shows estimated rates of absence among such workers in nine countries. Rural staff invariably are absent from their jobs more often than their urban counterparts, and physicians are more likely to neglect their duties than other levels of staff, often because they are less accountable and therefore harder to supervise and discipline (Lewis, 2006).

Reforms in how health care in a country is financed may be due as much to such governance failings as to misguided policies, but consistent, effective, and comprehensive measurement of governance in health-care financing does not yet exist.

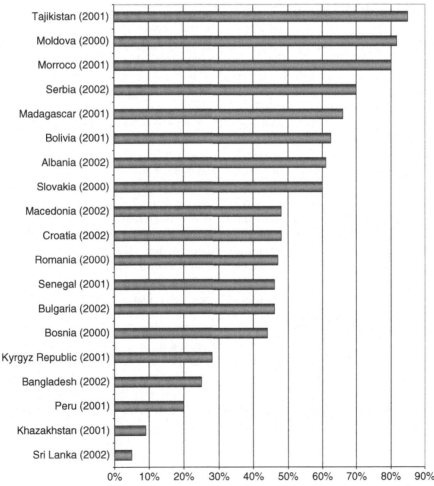

Figure 2 Percent perceiving corruption in the health sector. From Lewis M (2006) *Governance and Corruption in Public Health Care Systems*. Working paper No. 78. Washington, DC: Center for Global Development (www.cgdev.org).

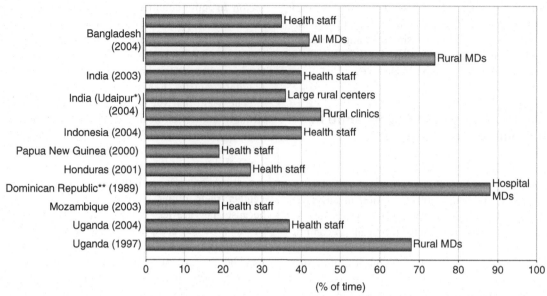

Figure 3 Absence rates among health workers in selected countries. From Lewis M (2006) *Governance and Corruption in Public Health Care Systems*. Working paper No. 78. Washington, DC: Center for Global Development (www.cgdev.org).

Governance and Health Outcomes

Governance in health care, or the lack of it, extends far beyond what is usually defined as financing. It is also true that health outcomes respond to so many factors that attributing them to particular policies or how those policies are respected or subverted is very difficult. Aggregate measures of governance are correlated with some outcome measures, and that is the case even when controlling for other factors. **Figure 4** shows the relationship between governance indicators using three measures of perception of governance specifically – government effectiveness, control of corruption, and voice and accountability – and two health outcomes, immunization rates for measles and child mortality (deaths before age 5 per 1000 births). The governance measures are expressed in standard deviations from the mean for all countries, while the health indicators are expressed as rates or percentages (Lewis, 2006). Each graph includes a regression line relating the governance measure alone to the health outcome, which explains the relatively poor fit to the data.

More complete regression analyses, including income and other variables expected to affect health outcomes, including indicators of female education, are given in **Tables 2** and **3**. Even when these other explanatory variables are included, the governance measures remain statistically significant in all but two of the specifications, both for child mortality. Gross domestic product (GDP), interestingly, affects only child mortality, perhaps reflecting the fact that child mortality is an even better predictor of economic direction than of health service effectiveness (Lewis, 2006).

All the graphs have two features in common. First, and not surprisingly, as governance improves, so does the health indicator, immunization climbing toward 100% and child mortality falling, indicating that good governance and the absence of corruption improves the effectiveness of health interventions. Second, as governance improves, the variation among countries narrows dramatically. Well-governed countries, with few exceptions, have quite similar outcomes on these two health measures; countries with less effective governments, or poor governance overall, vary much more among themselves in health results. A very similar pattern occurs when health measures are related to the degree to which corruption is believed to be controlled, although it is not clear how much corruption specifically interferes with efforts to save children's lives or immunize them. It is also striking that the pattern of narrowing variance in **Figure 4** resembles that for out-of-pocket spending, mentioned above: As countries are richer, such spending becomes much less important on average as a source of health funding, and the share converges from large differences among countries to very little variation. To the extent that out-of-pocket spending impoverishes families or makes it difficult to provide their children with adequate nutrition or health care, these different relations may be displaying aspects of the same phenomenon: Good governance – and probably more competent government – by limiting waste and corruption and protecting households from financial risk, also makes it easier for them to protect their children's health.

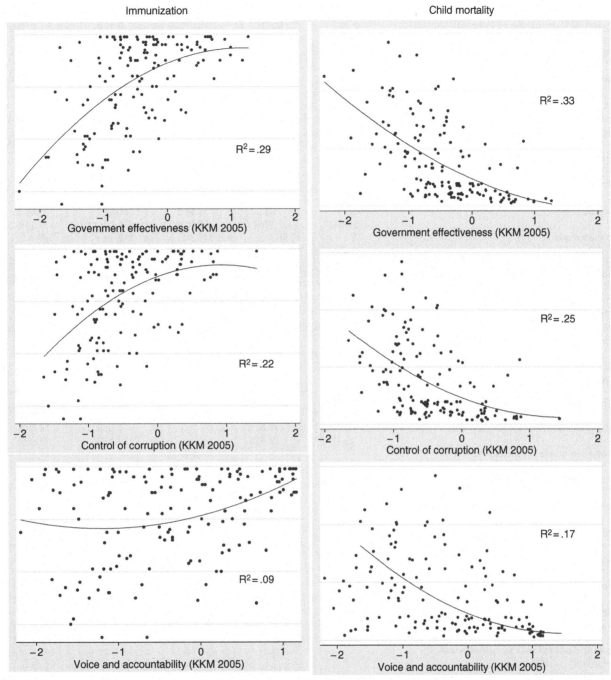

Figure 4 Relationship between corruption and health outcome indicators. From Lewis M (2006) *Governance and Corruption in Public Health Care Systems*. Working paper No. 78. Washington, DC: Center for Global Development (www.cgdev.org).

Governance as an International Issue

Governance is usually thought of as a national phenomenon since that is where government responsibility can be located. But the concept can be applied internationally as well. Donor organizations can be as guilty of bad governance as the governments they wish to help, to the extent that donors support corrupt governments or unsuccessful programs (Easterly, 2006). Even when donors provide substantially increased revenue, pooling of funds can be a problem if donors either impede it or insist on pooling their funds in ways that make it harder to use them well, such as limiting purchases to their own countries' exports. Poor governance with aid financing shows up most readily in purchasing, where corruption is more likely than at earlier stages of financing.

Table 2 OLS results for measles immunization coverage (% of children ages 12–23 months)

Log of GDP per capita, PPP (const. 2000 int'l $)	2.351	0.808	0.487	0.136	−1.378
	−3.489	−3.561	−2.451	−2.609	−4.212
Aggregate governance		6.152		5.201	
		(3.124)*		(2.442)**	
Government effectiveness	7.026		6.812		8.221
	(3.218)**		(2.345)***		(3.607)**
Ethnolinguistic fractionalization		−6.021		−4.059	−6.671
		(2.271)**		(2.263)*	(2.284)***
Average years of schooling, adult females (15+)	1.888	1.763			2.337
	(0.981)*	(1.008)*			(1.071)**
Primary completion rate, female			0.293	0.309	
			(0.067)***	(0.073)***	
Road density					−0.037
					(0.015)**
Constant	56.18	77.12	57.689	66.128	94.809
	(25.664)**	(27.959)***	(17.318)***	(19.704)***	(33.118)***
Observations	71	68	119	112	68
R-squared	0.434	0.473	0.444	0.47	0.497

Robust standard errors in parentheses.
*significant at 10%;
**significant at 5%;
***significant at 1%.
From Lewis M (2006) Governance and corruption in public health care systems. Working paper No. 78. Washington, DC: Center for Global Development (www.cgdev.org).

Table 3 OLS results for under-5 mortality rate

Log of GDP per capita, PPP (constant 2000 int'l $)	−66.447	−55.263	−29.148	−24.932	−55.649
	(7.853)***	(9.847)***	(8.403)***	(8.390)***	(9.856)***
Aggregate governance	18.747	16.828		−3.069	18.644
	(9.167)**	(9.426)*		−7.588	(9.866)*
Government effectiveness (KKZ 2005)			−4.773		
			−8.576		
Ethnolinguistic fractionalization		19.222		20.169	
		(8.220)**		(5.525)***	
Average years of schooling, adult females (15+)	−3.819	−3.893			−3.563
	−2.483	−2.551			−2.504
Primary completion rate, female			−1.261	−1.197	18.934
			(0.194)***	(0.213)***	(8.155)**
Road density					−0.054
					−0.073
Constant	639.747	521.888	408.635	342.705	526.372
	(60.938)***	(85.021)***	(60.448)***	(62.343)***	(85.128)***
Observations	71	68	119	112	68
R-squared	0.748	0.764	0.745	0.769	0.766

Robust standard errors in parentheses.
*significant at 10%;
**significant at 5%;
***significant at 1%.
From Lewis M (2006) Governance and corruption in public health care systems. Working paper No. 78. Washington, DC: Center for Global Development (www.cgdev.org).

Assistance to health may sometimes be less susceptible to such failings than aid in other sectors, as shown by the several large-scale successes in health even in very poor countries that have benefited from external funds and expert technical assistance, including the global eradication of smallpox or the control of onchocerciasis in Africa (Levine et al., 2004). Such success requires good governance and little or no corruption in the disease control programs and is therefore hard to replicate throughout a public system.

Comparably good governance would be required to implement a recent proposal for a subsidy for combination drug therapy against malaria (Laxminarayan et al., 2006). Every country using the therapy would have to assure that the subsidy actually went to make the combination of drugs as cheap as existing but increasingly ineffective monotherapies, or resistance would develop and the subsidy would be wasted.

As WHO expresses it metaphorically, failure of stewardship can be identified with three kinds of visual limitations. Turning a blind eye to corruption is a clear example of bad governance, whereas myopia and tunnel vision, the other two failings, are not. Good governance requires oversight, clear standards, and the ability to hold providers and payers accountable. Where these do not exist, it is unlikely that health systems will work, services will be delivered, and health status will improve. Poor governance undermines the quality of services and the acquisition and spending of public funds. Corruption eats away at the foundation of health-care finance, diverting funds during collection of premiums, undermining procurement rules in the purchase of inputs and allowing funds to disappear between the point of collection and points of delivery. Absent physicians effectively steal from the public sector; petty theft of drugs, light bulbs, or food is just as much robbery. Even absent such corruption, underperformance by health-care providers leads to spending that has no impact. Addressing these problems entails clear rules, oversight, and enforceable discipline for those who violate public trust.

See also: Corruption and the Consequences for Public Health; Cost-influenced Treatment Decisions and Cost Effectiveness Analysis; The Private Sector in Health Care Provision, The Role of; The State in Public Health, The Role of.

Citations

Asch SM, Kerr EA, Keesey J, et al. (2006) Who is at greatest risk for receiving poor-quality health care? *New England Journal of Medicine* 354: 1147–1156.
Das J and Gertler PJ (2005) Practice-quality variation in five low-income countries: A conceptual overview. *Health Affairs* 26: w296–w309.
Easterly W (2006) *The White Man's Burden: Why the West's Efforts to Aid the Rest Have Done So Much Ill and So Little Good*. New York: Penguin Press.
Kaufmann D, Kraay A, and Mastruzzi M (2005) Measuring governance using cross-country perceptions data. In: Rose-Ackerman S (ed.) *The Handbook of Economic Corruption*. Camberley, UK: Edward Elgar Publishing.
Laxminarayan R, Over M, and Smith D (2006) Will subsidies for antimalarials save lives? *Health Affairs* 25: 325–336.
Levine R and the What Works Working Group, with Kinder M (2004) *Millions Saved: Proven Successes in Global Health*. Washington, DC: Center for Global Development.
Lewis M (2006) *Governance and Corruption in Public Health Care Systems*. Working paper No. 78. Washington, DC: Center for Global Development.
Musgrave R and Musgrave P (1989) *Public Finance in Theory and Practice*. New York: McGraw Hill.
Musgrove P (2004a) Public and private roles in health. In: Musgrove P (ed.) *Health Economics in Development*, pp. 1–22. Washington, DC: World Bank.
Musgrove P (2004b) Introduction. In: Musgrove P (ed.) *Health Economics in Development*, pp. 35–76. Washington, DC: World Bank.
Musgrove P, Carrin G, and Zeramdini R (2002) Basic patterns in national health expenditure. *Bulletin of the World Health Organization* 80(2): 134–142.
Roberts MJ, Hsiao W, Berman P, and Reich MR (2004) *Getting Health Reform Right: A Guide to Improving Performance and Equity*. Oxford, UK: Oxford University Press.
World Health Organization (2000) *World Health Report. Health Systems: Improving Performance*. Geneva, Switzerland: World Health Organization.

Further Reading

Goddard M, Hauck K, Preker A, and Smith PC (2006) Priority setting in health – A political economy perspective. *Health Economics Policy and Law* 1: 79–90.
Schieber G and Gottret P (2006) *Health Financing Revisited: a Practitioner's Guide*. Washington, DC: World Bank.

Universal Coverage in Developing Countries, Transition to

T Ensor, Oxford Policy Management, York, UK

© 2008 Elsevier Inc. All rights reserved.

Glossary

Benefits package The range of benefits financed by a given insurance contribution.
Community insurance System of voluntary risk-pooling aimed at those working outside the formal sector usually based on community rate contributions paid into not-for-profit funds. Community insurance is a common term for voluntary health insurance schemes, organized at the level of the community. These may be alternatively labeled as mutual health organizations, medical aid schemes, medical aid societies, or micro-insurance schemes (see Carrin et al., 2005).
Community rating Procedure for setting equal insurance contributions for all contributors within a particular group. The premium is the sum of total costs, administration, profit, and contingency divided by the number enrolled.

> **Health insurance** Mechanism by which the costs of illness are pooled across a population. Protection is based on a contract, implicit or explicit, that secures members against financial loss arising from ill health in return for a regular payment.
> **Risk rating** Procedure for setting insurance contributions that are based on the likelihood of using services based on information on past utilization and other risk factors.
> **Social health insurance** This is often part of a wider framework of social insurance embracing pensions, sickness, unemployment, as well as health benefits. System of compulsory risk pooling provided to those making wage-related contributions and to their dependants. Government may pay for nonworking groups and the poor to be enrolled.
> **Solidarity-based system** insurance system based on income-related contributions and incorporating both rich and poor members.

Paying for Health Care and Pooling Risk

Paying for Health Care

Individuals pay for medical care in two ways: Directly in return for service or, indirectly, through payment in return for an entitlement to treatment if sick. Direct payments include user charges paid around the time of illness; savings-based schemes, where users pay ahead of time; and loan schemes, where payment is deferred until after treatment. Savings schemes include provident funds that are often offered to civil servants in developing countries and medical savings accounts, used in Singapore, China, and some states in the United States. Prepayment systems have the advantage over user fees that people do not face large bills when they are sick but can spread the cost of care over their lifetime. They may be viewed as an interim stage in the progress towards inter-personal risk pooling.

Indirect payments, or insurance entitlement, cover a much larger potential cost of treatment than is reflected in the contribution but is only effective in the event of illness. Contributions from members reflect the costs of the scheme including administration, contingency, and cost of treatment. The serious and financially catastrophic nature of some illnesses means that risk pooling is preferred, particularly for payments for major illness. A latent demand for insurance is indicated in the observation that individuals tend to be risk averse. This means that if offered the choice between a certain income and an uncertain, but mathematically equivalent, expected income, they prefer the certain option.

Indirect payment systems can be provided through explicit insurance, where members knowingly pay contributions in return for coverage, or through implicit insurance, where coverage is financed by taxation for part or all of a population (see WHO, 2000: Chapter 5). With implicit systems of insurance coverage, citizens or residents or a particular community are covered regardless of whether they make a contribution. These are mainly financed out of general taxation. Universal funding is closely linked with the ability to administer a system of taxation. While most OECD countries collect more than 30% of GDP in taxes, in low-income countries the figure is usually less than 20% and sometimes as low as 5%.

Explicit systems tend to limit coverage to those that have made a contribution or to those where the contribution is explicitly financed from another source. A variety of explicit systems exist. One type is voluntary commercial insurance organized by the private sector, on a profit or non-profit-making basis, as a service for paying contributors. In order to maximize profits and minimize the problem of adverse risk selection (see below), contributors are charged a premium related to their risk status (risk rating).

Another type of financing is social health insurance, which differs from private insurance in that it is generally offered on a noncommercial basis and financed from compulsory deductions from employee wages. Employers and government may also make a matching contribution. Social health insurance is usually instituted by government but can be managed by nongovernment bodies such as employment-based organizations, unions, or locally based mutualities. Government may finance the elderly and poor, while insured members often cover dependants. Even though contributions are related to income or wages, the adverse selection problem is avoided by making the scheme compulsory for a well-defined group of the population.

Social insurance is based on the existence of an identifiable payroll and on a relatively stable workforce. Yet the context in many middle- and low-income countries is that the workforce is transient, employment is casual, and no formal payroll exists. In addition, there is often a distrust of the state and considerable avoidance of taxation. Community insurance offers a slightly different way of developing risk coverage. Although there are many types of community schemes, most provide a limited package of benefits, often restricted to local facilities and limited referral, and based on voluntary enrollment on payment of a flat rate premium. The schemes have much in common with those offered by friendly societies and mutualities in Europe during the nineteenth and twentieth centuries. Adverse selection is an important issue since the scheme is voluntary.

Organized health financing mechanisms also have other important functions that can be achieved only by pooling contributions for health care. One function is to finance the cost of public health interventions or treatments that have significant externalities. Positive externalities are where treatments benefit people in addition to those actually using the service; an example is the additional protection afforded to members of the community as a result of a vaccination against a disease.

A further role of organized state funding is as a mechanism for income redistribution by transferring resources from the healthy who are often also relatively wealthy to the sick and impoverished. This is achieved in systems that base contributions on income such as social insurance and universal systems based on progressive or proportional taxation regimes. There is less scope for redistribution in voluntary community schemes where contributions are generally flat rate. Income redistribution plays no part in commercial systems of insurance.

Another important function of organized risk pools is to provide a stimulus for active purchasing. This term describes a range of tools used to induce improvements in the effectiveness and efficiency of provision such as selective contracting, quality assurance, treatment protocols and provider payment incentives. These tools may be used both by social and private insurers in order to extract better value for resources used. Closely related are means to control consumer demand in order to improve the distribution of services toward those most able to benefit or in most need. Tools include access rules such as primary care gatekeepers, prioritization of services, and waiting lists.

Technical Concerns in Extending Coverage

Extending health insurance cover to a population – however financed – raises a number of practical issues. The first, adverse risk-selection, relates to the method of assessing contributions. This problem arises because people often know more about their risk status than does the potential insurer: Individuals know if they have a chronic condition, have been ill in the past or have a lifestyle habit, such as smoking, that predisposes them to more illness. As a consequence, a voluntary system with income or flat-rated contributions tends to attract high-risk individuals and to deter those who are at low risk from joining the scheme. This disturbs the central objective of insurance, which is to pool risk between risk types, and can lead to a substantial increase in premium for those that are still willing to join.

The private sector solution to adverse risk selection is to base premiums on risk rather than income. This increases the cost of insurance to those more likely to get sick who are also often in lower income groups. Since many people cannot afford risk-rated insurance, commercial insurance is not a good way of extending universal coverage.

The problem of adverse risk selection means that the most reliable way of extending coverage to a population is by making insurance compulsory. Contributions can then be based on ability to pay.

Further technical issues concern the practical difficulties of identifying potential members, assessing contributions, and collecting premiums. These difficulties are particularly acute where communities are not based on well-defined static groups such as formal employment. Where coverage is compulsory, all three issues are pertinent in developing a solidarity-based system. Where coverage is voluntary, identification is mainly a matter of marketing the scheme and selling policies to those that require cover.

Sustaining the finance for a scheme is important for the long-term development of coverage. Contributions must be based on an accurate assessment of the risk of those insured. To cover unexpectedly large costs, calculations must build in the accumulation of a reserve. Since the probability of incurring greater than average costs diminishes with the number of contributors, large insurance groups are much less at risk than smaller groups. This is a particularly important issue for smaller community funds, which are highly exposed to such uncertainty. Some state systems operate on a cash limited pay-as-you-go basis, which rations the level of care according to the amount of funds available.

Another issue that affects the sustainability of extending coverage is the excess use associated with care that is free to patients at point-of-delivery. This problem, known as moral hazard, has been particularly important in OECD countries that have invested substantial technical resources in minimizing its effects. The problem is exacerbated where providers are paid in direct proportion to levels of activity since neither consumer nor provider has an incentive to contain demand. In recent years both the Czech and Korean systems have suffered from rampant increase in costs resulting from this problem.

What is Universal Coverage?

Universal coverage can be described as the attainment of complete insurance coverage of a population for the costs of a specified package of priority health care. The target has two dimensions described by Kutzin as breadth and depth (Kutzin, 1998). Breadth refers to the proportion of a population group covered by the insurance scheme; the target is 100% of all citizens or permanent residents of a country. Depth relates to the types of service included in the benefits package. There is no absolute benchmark, although a guide is provided by the ILO's 1952 Social

Security Convention, which specifies the minimum coverage to be provided under a social security scheme. This includes:

- general practitioner care, including home visits;
- specialist care in hospitals and similar institutions for inpatients and outpatients and such specialist care as may be available outside hospitals;
- essential pharmaceutical supplies;
- prenatal, confinement, and postnatal care by medical practitioners or qualified midwives;
- hospitalization where necessary.

The definition emphasizes levels of care whereas other approaches place greater emphasis on the types of illness for which treatment should be offered and the treatment technologies themselves. A further refinement is to restrict coverage to those technologies that are proven to be effective or cost-effective. Faced with the rapidly increasing availability of new drugs and technologies, such evaluation is increasingly being carried out in countries including Australia, Canada, and the United Kingdom.

In most cases, the transition to universal coverage cannot be accomplished quickly. A number of factors are important. Given that total spending on health care is mainly determined by the macro-economy, the most important question is whether total resources available are sufficient to match the needs of universal coverage. A second factor is whether a sufficient proportion of total spending on health care can be channeled to finance a core package. Both questions are of importance in low- and middle-income countries. While average health spending in the OECD is around US$2500 per capita (unweighted average in 2004 at purchasing power parity; see OECD website), in low-income countries spending is less than US$15. In addition, most low-income countries pool a much smaller proportion of total health-care spending. A rich country such as the United Kingdom, for example, pools more than $2400 per capita, whereas a low-income country such as Bangladesh pools around $5 per capita (see **Table 1**).

Countries that are not able to afford an ILO-style package sometimes specify a lower level of coverage that can be financed on a universal basis from public funds. This is the central concept behind the package of essential services described in the 1993 World Development Report (World Bank, 1993). This report suggests concentrating public funding on a small number of highly cost-effective services. It is important to realize that many of these services are of a public health or primary care nature and high-cost curative hospital services are mostly not included. Additional services are then financed by individuals using voluntary insurance or in the gradual addition of groups covered by more extensive, social or voluntary, insurance.

The high-breadth, low-depth issue is particularly acute in those low- and middle-income countries that claim to offer universal coverage on the basis that all citizens can walk into public health facilities and obtain consultation and treatment without official payment. Shortage of resources often means that people must wait long periods or make additional unofficial payments before treatment is forthcoming. This has been common in many postcolonial countries of Africa and South Asia that have attempted to extend systems inherited from their colonizers but without the resources to make the claim to comprehensive cover truly effective.

Paths to Universal Coverage: OECD Countries

The extent to which countries have achieved universal coverage varies enormously across the world. Those countries that have the most well-established and stable risk-pooling systems are predominantly concentrated in the OECD. (Much of this discussion focuses on the original members of the OECD: Western Europe, North America, Australia, and New Zealand. Later members only partly fit this profile.) A characteristic of the transition in these countries has been the gradual development of coverage. While it is tempting to focus on key events – the 1883 Insurance Act in Germany or the 1946 National Health Service Act in the United Kingdom, for example – these events might be seen more as milestones in a much longer process of transition.

Table 1 Degree of pooling in four representative countries

		Spending			Amount pooled	
		US$	% GDP	% Pooled	US$	% GDP
Bangladesh	2003	$14	3.4%	35.0%	5	1.2%
Chile	2003	$282	6.1%	76.0%	214	4.6%
Egypt	2003	$55	5.8%	47.0%	26	2.7%
United Kingdom	2003	$2428	8.1%	90.0%	2185	7.3%

Data from World Health Organization (2006) *The World Health Report 2006: Working Together for Health.* Geneva: World Health Organization and OECD, online statistics.
GDP, gross domestic product.

Most established market economies extended risk coverage through compulsory insurance for employees and later their dependants. Beyond this there is a dichotomy. First, there are countries that base coverage on the gradual filling of gaps in existing coverage based on explicit insurance. Second, some countries have chosen, at some point, to legislate for 100% coverage financed from general taxation (implicit insurance). Those taking the latter route have generally first reached a significant level of explicit coverage of the population. It is important to recognize that while the explicit approach is less dramatic than the implicit, universal approach, it still requires committed and sustained policy effort.

Germany

The foremost example of the explicit insurance approach is the German system. Often known as the Bismarck model after the nineteenth-century German Chancellor (Count Otto von Bismarck, 1815–1898), it is based on coverage through compulsory membership of employment-related risk pools financed by wage-based contributions. This is referred to by Mesa Lago as the social insurance approach, with separate programs for different risks such as unemployment, old age pensions, and sickness (Mesa-Lago, 1991).

The impetus to universal coverage was the 1883 Insurance Act, which made social insurance compulsory for certain categories of workers. Much of the social legislation of Bismarck, including this act, was part of an orchestrated attempt to undermine the allure of socialism by providing workers with a broad welfare safety net. The main focal group was industrial workers who, together with the trade unions they joined, were most influenced by the wave of social democratic sentiment. An added benefit was that it was easier to collect contributions from this relatively well-paid group in steady employment.

The 1883 act prepared the ground for the extension of coverage but built on a variety of existing organizations and legal obligations. Trade guilds traditionally offered assistance to vulnerable members to finance funeral, food, and housing expenses. Employers were legally responsible for the cost of accidents to employees, although this often placed an unsustainable burden on smaller enterprises. Employees also found that the requirement to prove liability meant that obligations were often not met. Furthermore, poor relief, which was the responsibility of manorial estates, often put a considerable strain on these rural communities. Thus while legislation was not uncontentious and its urgency arose from political expediency, it was undoubtedly assisted by the way in which it relieved burdens at the same time as imposing new obligations on employers, workers, and the state.

Initially the insurance act covered approximately 26% of blue-collar employees, roughly 10% of the population. Civil servants were covered in 1914, the unemployed in 1918, and self-employed agricultural workers in 1972. Students were not included until 1975, 92 years after the original act. Today less than 0.1% of the population is without cover. Reforms introduced in 2007 will mean that by 2009 coverage will be mandatory for all residents either through private or social insurance – 125 years since the original insurance act.

The system is financed from compulsory contributions for those in employment. Solidarity between rich and poor was assured by the compulsory nature of the system, although an opt-out for the better-off was permitted from 1914.

Following Germany, both Austria (1888) and Hungary (1891) enacted legislation on a similar basis. France also followed a social insurance model but retained an important role for top-up insurance provided by mutual insurers. Switzerland for a long time rejected similar legislation and it was not until 1996 that health insurance became universal.

United Kingdom

An alternative path to universal coverage is to legislate for 100% cover by including all groups based on citizenship or residency rather than contribution. This is sometimes known as the Beveridge model after the civil servant W.H. Beveridge, who designed the British system introduced after the Second World War. It is important to note, however, that several other universal systems, notably the system in New Zealand, actually predate legislation in the United Kingdom.

In the United Kingdom, the 1946 act was the culmination of more than a century of change in the approach to financing health care. The system in the UK could easily have followed the German model. Social policy during the nineteenth century focused on punitive welfare designed to encourage workers out of poverty. Ever since the Middle Ages, the parish had responsibility for providing poor relief, which was consolidated through revisions to the Poor Law in 1834. An enlightened policy toward the improvement of public health was largely pursued on the grounds that "labourers are suddenly thrown by infectious disease into a state of destitution" (Edwin Chadwick, public health reformer, 1800–1890). For the same reason, the Poor Law benefit was restricted to discourage indigence.

By the beginning of the twentieth century, while public health had largely been included in the duties of the state, coverage for personal health care was still extremely fragmented. For the rich, treatment was paid for by commercial insurance and out-of-pocket payments. For those on low incomes, there were free Poor Law (public) and charitable hospitals to which doctors gave some of their time without charge. For the aspiring working class, the friendly societies organized provident funds for health and funeral expenses. By the end of the nineteenth century, however, many of these were in financial trouble as members were living too long and payouts exceeded contributions.

A major departure from the Victorian emphasis on morality was articulated by Winston Churchill, then President of the Board of Trade, who advocated a principle of universality rather than attempting to distinguish between deserving and undeserving poor. Both Churchill and David Lloyd-George (Finance Minister, later Prime Minister) favored a broad social insurance package, similar to that adopted in Germany, which eventually became universal. The National Insurance Act of 1911 was more circumscribed, including sickness benefit, primary care contacts, and some specified services such as TB sanatoria but no general hospital benefit. One reason was the severe opposition from both professions and friendly societies. The latter were clearly threatened by this state intrusion on their virtual monopoly over prepayment for health care. Another reason was that a comprehensive benefit was simply not affordable at that time.

Interclass solidarity that built up during the Second World War provided the much needed impetus to the creation of a universal insurance system institutionalized in the National Health Service (NHS). The 1942 report on social insurance and allied services, known as the Beveridge report after its main author (William H. Beveridge, 1879–1963), sketched out the fundamentals of the modern welfare state. The central principles were comprehensiveness, contributions related to means, and benefits based on need. Importantly, and in contrast to Germany, the envisaged system integrated both financing and provision of care.

The universal, implicit insurance approach has also been adopted in New Zealand where coverage was extended first for inpatient care (1939) and subsequently outpatient and pharmaceuticals (1941). Sweden legislated for universal coverage in 1953 followed by other Scandinavian countries (Norway 1956; Finland, 1963; Denmark, 1971; Iceland, 1972). Canada (1966) and Australia (1974) followed with similar legislation. More recently, legislation has been introduced in the southern European countries of Portugal (1978), Spain (1978), and Italy (1980).

Russia

In Russia, parallels to the German experience were recognizable in the late nineteenth century. The state, as part of a general policy of liberalization, intervened in the funding and provision of services. Following the emancipation of the serfs, a medical system was integrated into the local government structure that provided polyclinic and inpatient services. The 1912 Insurance Act, introduced during the Fourth State Duma, placed an obligation on employers to bear the costs of accidents, sickness, and death of employees and dependants. As in Germany, these benefits were aimed to assuage the demands of an increasingly militant labor movement. But this was too little too late, and the revolution led to a much more fundamental transformation of medical care.

The Soviet system that developed following the second revolution of 1917 was greatly influenced by the physician A.N. Semaschko (1874–1949) who was head of the Central People's Commissariat of Health from 1918. The nationalized health service, as in other sectors, placed emphasis on the contribution of medicine to the process of industrialization. Party congresses continually laid great stress on the productivity losses arising from illness. As a result, the three separate subsystems of industrial medicine and public health, adult medicine, and pediatric care developed. Specialized polyclinic care provided the entry point and the system remained highly specialized and horizontally segregated when patients were referred. The rural health service, created during the late czarist regime, remained and was eventually integrated into the Semaschko system. Although the system evolved during the 1920s, it was not until 1935 that a centralized structure was finally agreed, creating the Ministry of Health as supreme administrative body. The head of the Ministry, always a doctor, was made a permanent member of the cabinet. The Semaschko system was used throughout the Soviet Union and, in modified form, in most of Eastern Europe.

General Trends in Establishing Universal Coverage in the OECD

A number of general features are evident in the transition to universal coverage across the OECD.

1. Developing universal coverage was a slow process. Building upon medieval structures, it took up to a century to extend coverage to much of the population of Western Europe.
2. Indigenous mechanisms for risk pooling existed in all countries and attempts to extend coverage built on these systems. This is exemplified in the integration of the friendly societies into the administration of national insurance after the First World War in Britain and incorporation of the *mutuelles* in France. The latter still have an important role today in providing supplementary insurance.
3. Historic obligations on local authorities to provide Poor-Law relief and on employers to provide accident and sickness assistance promoted the need to create more effective structures for risk pooling. It is also noticeable across Europe that while a number of institutions provided the basis for a developing system of

social protection, state intervention was required to unify, and sometimes pacify, disparate forces.
4. The administration of the provider network changed relatively little with the development of universal coverage. The major exception is the UK, which nationalized its system after the Beveridge reforms, and the Soviet Union where the entire system was taken into state hands.
5. In almost all OECD countries, near universal coverage required substantial state involvement. Intervention ranged from the regulation of funds and their redistribution in social insurance systems to the integrated systems common in Scandinavia, New Zealand, the UK, and southern Europe. The United States stands out as the only one of the original members of the OECD with substantially less than universal coverage.
6. Political factors were of considerable importance as a catalyst to the development in a number of countries. German social insurance was initially designed to reduce socialist opposition, while the social reforms of the Russian Fourth Duma were designed to do the same for communism. Social insurance in Italy between the wars was seen as a way of reinforcing the classlessness espoused by National Socialism. The Beveridge reforms partly came from a sense of solidarity generated by the Second World War.
7. Those systems legislating for universality had already achieved coverage of the overwhelming majority of their population. The cost of extending coverage, in addition to social and political factors, prevented some systems from establishing universal coverage even earlier.

Paths to Universal Coverage: Developing and Transitional Countries

Coverage of developing and transition countries is generally much lower than in the OECD, both in breadth and depth. There is considerable diversity across countries.

Latin America

Much of Latin America has adopted the social insurance model as a way of developing coverage between groups. The region, encouraged by the International Labour Organization (ILO), began to introduce social insurance soon after the First World War. Mesa-Lago identifies three waves of activity. In the first wave, the pioneer countries Argentina, Brazil, Chile, Uruguay, and Cuba introduced insurance on a piecemeal basis beginning with civil servants followed by formal blue and white collar workers in key large-scale industry: Transport, energy, banking, and communications. Schemes were later extended to other urban workers, agriculture, and the self-employed. The result was a series of schemes offering very different packages. Key industries and civil servants received more substantive coverage than other groups. Subsequently, this made unification of the schemes difficult: Leveling up to the best plan has proved too costly, while a reduction is resisted by those with more comprehensive cover.

In Argentina, social insurance was based, until recently, on compulsory contributions by workers and employers to union-administered funds (Obras Sociales). There are more than 300 funds, although the largest 30 account for more than 70% of members. Many of these originated in the nineteenth century. The schemes cover both workers and their dependants. In addition, there are funds in each of the 23 provinces to cover public workers. A separate organization covers retired workers.

A number of problems have been identified. One is the monopolistic nature of the funds since employees were often obligated to obtain insurance from sometimes inefficient schemes. Another is the substantial difference in level of remuneration offered with the result that members of poorer funds are forced to make significant out-of-pocket co-payments for treatment. New mechanisms to guarantee minimum funding, through a redistribution fund, were approved in 1994. Attempts are also underway to establish a minimum package of services to be guaranteed by each fund.

Chile was one of the first countries to introduce social insurance in the 1920s. Starting in a traditional way with insurance for workers in industry, by 1970 approximately 75% of the population were covered. As in the Argentinean system, there were substantial variations in benefits between groups. Nonmanual and, in particular, government workers generally had access to better quality services than manual workers.

Major changes were introduced by the Pinochet government, which attempted to widen the role of the private sector by allowing people to opt out of the social insurance system and purchase private coverage. This undermined the solidarity principle of risk pooling across income and risk groups. Those insuring privately are predominantly low-risk, wealthier employees. This group is able to obtain attractive coverage, choosing between a wide range of providers at relatively low premiums. The elderly, chronically ill, and very young are generally more expensive and less profitable and are mostly covered by the public insurance fund. Combined with general reductions in public funding for health, this has reduced the quality of the public service, creating a two-tier system. Drop-out from the public system in Chile has been much greater than in other countries that permit opt-outs. One reason is that whereas in the Netherlands and Germany opt-outs are only permitted above a certain income, the Chilean system permits opt-outs at any income.

Brazil is the only country in Latin America to legislate for universal coverage. This followed the development of employment-based social insurance coverage. The 1988 constitution introduced the Unified and Decentralized Health System (SUDS) and established a citizen's right to use any public health service in the country. Various factors have restricted the depth of coverage. Fundamental to this are the large geographic differences in economic status across the country. Central government provides funding to states based on size of population, which are then supplemented from local resources. Poorer states are unable to top-up to the same degree as wealthier states and the result is large differences in effective cover.

A second wave of social insurance adoption commenced in the 1940s heavily influenced by the International Labour Organization (ILO). The countries involved – Mexico, Colombia, Peru, Panama, Ecuador, Bolivia, Paraguay, and Venezuela – were relatively developed but still predominantly rural economies. Coverage has closely followed the industrialization of each economy. The Mexican social security system, for example, currently covers around 50% of the population, mostly formal employees and their families. The remainder have access to the state-run system or, for those able to pay, to the extensive network of private facilities. Unlike Brazil, where people now have access to a wide variety of facilities, the Mexican system remains vertically integrated, with social security facilities reserved for those who are covered under the scheme. Considerable discussion is now underway regarding ways to achieve near universal coverage through, for example, publicly subsidized access to an essential services package aimed at the uninsured, in particular the poor (Frenk *et al.*, 2007).

A final wave of insurance coverage expansion during the 1950s and 1960s is evident in poorer countries of the region. The group includes Dominican Republic, Guatemala, El Salvador, Nicaragua, and Honduras. Extension of coverage is hampered by the low levels of GDP, a relatively small industrial workforce, and a scattered rural population.

Former Soviet Union and Eastern Europe

Since the collapse of the Soviet Union, there has been widespread adoption of entitlement-based social insurance across the region. The trend is important because it represents a move away from the Semashko system that, in theory, already offered universal coverage. The transition is based on the growing reality that depth of cover has, in reality, never been comprehensive. Furthermore, it has been deteriorating in recent years. The system probably always offered a two- or even three-tier service. Party workers – the nomenclature – received the highest standard of service, followed by industrial workers in key sectors, with the remainder of the population receiving a varying quality of services often based on what they were able to trade in return.

A number of motives were apparent in the development of insurance legislation. Of paramount importance was the need to provide additional and earmarked funding for health care. Another reason was to improve the efficiency of provision through the selective contracting of services by nascent insurance funds. In theory this can motivate competition between providers for insurance fund contracts and so improve the efficiency of the system. It is possible, in principle, to create a split through a division in organizational responsibilities within a country's ministry of health. In countries where highly centralized control has been the norm, as in the Former Soviet Union (FSU), this separation can prove difficult. Establishing a fund creates a split between the purchaser of care (the insurance fund) and the providers, a change that may enable the system to respond to consumer needs rather than the concerns of providers.

A further development in some FSU countries has been to encourage the creation of a competitive market in which social insurers, like private insurers, compete for business. For competition to exist, employees must have a choice of a number of funds. The employee and employer contribution is then allocated to the chosen fund. This objective of competition was pursued most vigorously in the Russian Federation where the design of the new system allowed people to choose between competing funds. In practice, however, this competition often does not function effectively because employers make the decision regarding which fund to enroll workers into or because only one fund operates in a given geographic area.

A key problem with the imposition of social insurance in the FSU was that it imposed a burden in the form of a health tax on employers just at the time when many were already suffering from the impact of economic transition. Newly created insurance agencies expected to improve the quality of services. Yet the funds were often ill equipped to induce a fundamental change in the provider system. Some evidence in Russia, where regions have developed insurance at differential speeds, suggests that even in the most advanced regions the insurance funds have little changed the way in which they purchase services (Twigg, 1999).

A weakness of the development of insurance in FSU countries has been a failure to address the issue of declining risk pooling for health care. A characteristic of all the countries has been increasing out-of-pocket payments, official and unofficial, and a contracting formal workforce. Since dissolution of the Soviet Union, most economies have experienced a significant contraction in their economies in real terms – between 10% and 90% across the region – and a break-up of state industries. Yet the reforms offered were based on organizational mechanisms to cover the formal, largely state, sector based on a payroll tax. Particularly in the poorer states of the FSU – Central Asia and the Caucuses – formal insurance may not have addressed the economic realities of increasing unemployment and fragmentation of the labor market. Social insurance has appeared to take root relatively successfully in the wealthier and highly industrialized countries of Eastern Europe: Hungary, the Czech Republic, and the Baltic States. All have formal industrial sectors exceeding 70% of total employment.

Low-Income Countries

A key feature of most low-income countries (average GDP $410 per capita, 1999) is that funding for health care is dominated by direct payments for care. More than 59% of spending on health is estimated to be private, the majority out of pocket.

In most Sub-Saharan African and low-income Asian economies, the main source of pooled funding is direct taxation (supplemented by donor funding), which is used to finance a publicly managed health center and hospital system. These public systems tend to be underfinanced and access favors urban residents and higher income groups. Many governments now attempt to prioritize certain services that are particularly cost-effective, such as public health care. The strategy may have a considerable impact on population health, but it still leaves individuals exposed to the risk of high-cost catastrophic illness.

Extending risk pooling to populations in low-income countries has followed a number of routes. One is through traditional work-based social insurance. A variety of countries have extended payroll-based insurance to the public and private formal sector. The problem is that in most low-income countries these sectors are extremely small, perhaps constituting 6–10% of the population. Another issue is that even for formal employers the obligations to provide health care and protect employees from accidents may be absent or not enforced. As a consequence, there is little incentive for employers to seek to develop insurance coverage for their employees. Those that tend to benefit most are civil servants who, as a relatively privileged subgroup, have less exposure to catastrophic financial risk. They are also male-dominated since the majority of civil servants and formal sector employees are men, although coverage of families widens coverage somewhat.

In almost all sub-Saharan countries (excluding South Africa), formal sector insurance covers less than 5% of the population. The exceptions are Kenya, which has a formal sector scheme that includes dependants covering around 25% of the population, and Senegal and Burundi that cover public sector workers constituting perhaps 10–15%. A number of African countries are now attempting to extend social insurance to a wider population. In Kenya, action has begun to enlarge the existing base of formal sector workers and civil servants to include a larger number of small enterprises and self-employed workers. In Ghana, a system that ties together an existing social insurance scheme for formal workers with district-based mutual insurance for the rural population subsidized by taxation is now being introduced (Appiah-Denkyira and Preker, 2007).

A similar situation characterizes low-income South Asian countries. In Bangladesh and Pakistan, social insurance is limited to a variety of provident funds for civil servants, although the formal sector is increasingly turning to the private sector for health insurance coverage for employees. All these countries maintain an extensive but often decaying public system open to all on payment of unofficial payments, and a vibrant private sector offering almost anything on a fee-for-service and largely unregulated basis.

Patterns of Transition

In recent times, both Korea and more recently Thailand have taken the step of legislating for universal coverage. The problems arising offer interesting lessons for the extension of coverage in other low- and middle-income countries.

South Korea

One of the most dramatic extensions of coverage is recorded in South Korea. A voluntary insurance law was passed in 1963, but by 1977 less than 9% of the population was covered. From 1977 compulsory insurance was gradually extended, at first to large enterprises, through employment and area-based insurance societies. Later coverage was extended to civil servants (1978), smaller companies (from 1981), the self-employed (1981), and other rural workers. A separate scheme for the poor was also established based on strict eligibility criteria. By 1987, almost 60% of the population was covered by one of the schemes and in 1989 health insurance was made compulsory for all long-term residents of the country.

Korea is an example of a system that has achieved good breadth of cover in a short period. An important factor was rapid economic growth that averaged more than 10% from 1970 to 1990, while the proportion of the labor force working in agriculture fell from more than 49% to 18%. Some of the growth in breadth was at the expense of depth of coverage. Insurance funds include all the items mentioned in the ILO social security convention, although some expensive diagnostics such as MRI and PET are excluded (until 1996 CT was also excluded). Significant co-payments are, however, an important feature of the system. Users contribute between 30% and 55% of the cost of ambulatory care and 20% of the cost of inpatient care. A monetary limitation is also placed on the reimbursable cost of each 30-day period of illness. The substantial co-payments are partly the consequence of regional economic recession toward the end of the 1990s. They can also be traced back to the fee-for-service basis for remuneration, which has made cost containment difficult.

Thailand

In Thailand, from the 1970s, and more strongly from the early 1980s, voluntary insurance was extended to a largely rural population by marketing health cards. Later this movement lost ground when the initiators left office. More recently, the scheme has been revived and developed into a national scheme covering approximately 50% of the target group. Social insurance (Social Security Scheme, SSS) was introduced for the formal sector in 1991 and has been progressively extended to smaller companies. A separate scheme for civil servants, including teachers and medical staff, is financed fully by the government. Finally, a system of public assistance has been extended to those on low incomes.

In 2001, a new government was elected promising to combine the schemes and make coverage universal. Unification is difficult because of the varied contributions and benefits provided to members of the different schemes. By 2000, all schemes covered roughly 70% of the population, although offering uneven depth of coverage. The contributions for the scheme for civil servants, which are paid fully by government, for example, are ten times the contributions paid for the voluntary health card scheme. While both civil servants and SSS members have access to public and private facilities, health card and public assistance members were restricted to public facilities. Since 2001, while the schemes for civil servants and employees remain separate, a universal scheme has replaced health cards and the scheme for the poor to cover the remainder (74%) of the population. Recent studies indicate that this scheme is progressive in targeting benefits toward those with lower incomes, particularly at the lowest levels of the system and financed by those most able to pay (Tangcharoensathien et al., 2007). The study suggests that this is largely because of the heavy role played by general taxation in the financing of the scheme.

China

A reverse process of transition is evident in China. Three schemes were established during the 1950s: The Government Employees System (GIS), the Labor Insurance System (LIS), and Cooperative Medical Schemes (CMS). Until 1980, universal coverage in China in rural areas was ensured through the CMS, financed out of commune funds. Members were entitled to free outpatient and inpatient care as well as medicines. By 1979, more than 90% of the rural population were covered by CMS. In urban areas, the LIS and GIS provided protection for most industrial sector employees.

In the early 1980s, there was a rapid collapse in CMS. A number of factors have been suggested, including the market reforms of Deng Xiaoping (1904–1997), which introduced individual rather than collective responsibility for agriculture and an erosion in commune funds, increased income opportunities for medical workers, and the demand by farmers for more sophisticated and costly services. At the same time, medicine in both urban and rural areas has become increasingly market-oriented. This has led to rapid cost escalation and a deterioration in access to services by vulnerable parts of the population. Trends suggest a reverse process, with coverage of the population deteriorating, a decline in risk pooling, and greater reliance on direct payments for health care. While the catalyst to change has been economic, the process itself indicates the importance of retaining the support of society. The difficulty in recapturing a sense of community solidarity, through the reinvention of the CMS system, has proved difficult given the general distrust for state-run social schemes. There is now a new attempt to restore some government credibility through the establishment of a new CMS that will be run both with individual contributions and matching contributions from local and central government.

Risk Coverage for the Informal Sector

The speed toward universal coverage is likely to vary enormously according to country context. Studies examining the historic transition agree that there are a number of key facilitating factors, including a fast-growing economy, a high level of formalization and industrialization of the workforce, urbanization, good governance, and a high level of social solidarity (Ensor, 1999; Carrin and James, 2005). Yet in many low-income countries, these conditions will not exist for many years. Indeed, the difficulty involved in extending social insurance mechanisms to a wider population has led to alternative approaches. These are usually based on networks that exist outside the formal industrial sector: Specific communities, occupation, or social groupings. In principle, schemes can be voluntary or compulsory. A number of countries, including Korea and Taiwan, have now developed organizations and levels of economic development that permit them to make the schemes compulsory for the entire population.

Compulsory insurance for the informal sector in many low- and middle-income countries is made difficult because individuals can often evade contributions as they do other taxes. Many cannot afford premiums and the potential benefits, in terms of existing local health services, do not provide adequate compensation for their contribution. In response to this, a variety of voluntary systems, collectively known as community insurance, have developed. In general, these approaches are based on voluntary enrollment, usually, but not always, based on a fixed premium. These offer clearly identified benefits that are highly valued. Beyond this, there is remarkable diversity in approaches both in the services covered and in the way they are set up to attract enrollees. Some offer primary care only, while others include referral services.

A few voluntary schemes succeed in covering the majority of the population in a given area. The Bwamanda scheme in the Democratic Republic of Congo (former Zaire) covers more than 60% and Goalpara in India 90%. One study found, in a survey of 62 schemes, that most schemes cover no more than 30–40% of the target group (Bennett *et al.*, 1998).

Atim suggests that within the general category of insurance for the informal sector there exists a wide range of different types (Atim, 1999). These range from traditional social solidarity networks based on tribal or ethnic group through more inclusive mutual health associations. Both of these place considerable emphasis on participation in the governance of the schemes by members. This approach has been labeled micro-insurance (Dror and Jacquier, 1999). Individual micro-insurance schemes may be linked into networks to enable wider pooling of risks and shared training and management support structures. In essence, the approach attempts to get much closer to indigenous systems for developing risk pooling, with the aim that these are more likely to succeed than schemes that are imposed from the outside.

A separate approach has been for organizations running health-care facilities – government or nongovernment – to develop prepayment and insurance schemes to promote access to their facilities. A scheme may be established either by the facility management or the parent body, often an NGO. This is probably the dominant model in both Africa and Asia. Facilities may even make it compulsory for users to join the scheme before they can use facilities. The schemes tie the users to a particular type of care. Some provide for member involvement in running the scheme, although the majority do not.

In Bangladesh, widespread NGO-run micro-credit programs are being used to extend prepayment and risk pooling. A number of Civil Society Organizations (CSOs) now offer insurance to credit members providing low-cost access to their health facilities. Some organizations are investigating how these could be extended to coverage for treatment provided at referral level facilities. The nature of microcredit is that most members are women, although insurance coverage may also be offered to family members.

Schemes in both Thailand (in the 1980s) and Vietnam (in the 1990s) were initially launched by government at a national level, although they operated on different principles. In Vietnam, local pilot projects preceded countrywide implementation, but a national scheme was quickly introduced that allowed little local variation and provided unlimited benefits. In contrast, the Thai system permitted extensive local variation and involvement of communities. In many areas, it limited benefits to a maximum number of consultations in any year. The Vietnam scheme was launched simultaneously with a parallel scheme for the formal sector. While the formal scheme expanded quite rapidly, the voluntary scheme has achieved far less penetration.

Insurance for schoolchildren has been used by governments in several countries as a relatively low-cost way of enrolling children and their families into insurance schemes. Although sometimes thought of as a community approach, it is closer to formal-sector insurance in that the focus is on the semi-compulsory enrollment of all studying within a specified organization. School insurance is attractive since the population is easy to identify and contributions can be collected at a fixed time in each school. The group also tends to be quite low-risk since school children of ages 5–15 are some of the lightest users of medical care. In Vietnam, the mass enrollment of school children enabled the struggling insurance scheme to boost coverage at low cost in a short period (more than 3.4 million enrolled within 3 years). In Egypt, more than 70% of children are now covered by a similar scheme.

A number of design weaknesses have become evident in community insurance schemes. One is that the small scale of most schemes means that they cannot accumulate a sufficient reserve to pool unexpectedly large claims. Another is that the problem of adverse risk selection is endemic since flat-rate contributions mean that low-risk individuals tend not to join. In turn this leads to smaller, high-risk pools and greater costs. Finally, the administrative costs tend to be large. Bennett *et al.* found that administrative costs range from between 5% and 17%, although in some cases the amounts are much higher. They also point out that the costs usually cover only the basic administration of the scheme since the more sophisticated active purchasing function is generally absent.

In addition to technical issues, there are wider factors that relate to the extent which community insurance can stimulate change and promote universal coverage. One identified in the success of schemes has been the extent to which they take account of local institutions. This was the norm in Western Europe, where the development of social insurance often incorporated, at least initially, existing systems of risk pooling and took advantage of worker groups and employer obligations. This is not only a matter of involving some community members in governance but also involves taking account of context-specific factors that influence the desirability of particular forms of risk pooling. The success of one scheme in Cameroon, for example, has been attributed to the active participation of members in premium and benefit setting, a strong ethnic base, and the incorporation of other benefits valued by the community, including financial relief in the event of death. Conversely, imposing a scheme without taking account of indigenous social structures may lead to greater exclusion of people that, while part of the indigenous social network of mutual aid, are unable to pay for the imposed insurance system.

There is more scope for the insurer to promote system change if it is not strongly linked with a particular health facility but has the flexibility to negotiate with a range of facilities to secure low prices or higher quality. Most community schemes have not so far developed as strong purchasers of services. They tend to provide what consumers think they need – often medication – rather than attempting to rationalize service use. There are exceptions. Schemes such as those of the Sajida Foundation in Bangladesh and Bwamanda in former Zaire place an emphasis on preventive care, contracts with local facilities, and a strict referral system to higher levels.

Equity between and within community schemes is a major issue. While a network permits the creation of a large risk pool or enables a reinsurance function, the reallocation of funds from rich to poor schemes is hampered by the voluntary nature of association and membership. Even in China, where commune insurance was more or less compulsory until the early 1980s, evidence suggests large differences in the wealth of schemes. As a consequence, it is not usually feasible to expect large reallocations between schemes.

A further equity issue is the extent to which poor income groups are able to join the scheme. Some schemes, such as Gonoshastya Kendra in Bangladesh and MUGEF-CI in Côte d'Ivoire, have a sliding contribution scale according to income. The problem is that overcoming adverse risk selection tends to militate against sliding fees on the basis that those with high incomes tend to have less need of care and the scheme would risk losing the low risk from the pool. In the context of schemes based on indigenous institutions, it may be that members are more willing to cross-subsidize. This is less likely in schemes imposed by external agencies where social alliances are weaker. It is probably inescapable that, in order to enroll a large proportion of the very poor, some form of external subsidy is required. One way to do this is through the provision of government-purchased free cards, as occurred in Thailand and, to a lesser extent, Vietnam.

Conclusion

There are many ways in which a country can achieve universal coverage and each country's experience is in one sense unique. At the same time, there are some clear patterns that emerge from the experience, particularly in the decision of whether to rely on an explicit entitlement approach or the more implicit approach based on residency. From a policy perspective, the role of government in facilitating the transition is crucial. This includes providing a legislative framework for mandating employers to provide social security for workers or opting into established state-run schemes, ensuring that the poor are provided with a basic guarantee of access, not only to essential services, but also insurance coverage for catastrophic expenses, and also in helping small community schemes to expand to cover the informal sector.

Extending coverage may sometimes imply a contradiction between encouraging indigenous schemes based on local institutions and scaling up for universal coverage. The latter tends to require more uniformity and consistency in contracts, which in turn may erode the traditional forms of social solidarity. One way forward is to accept that scaling will lead to changes in structure and that such changes impose a cost on members, and to make that cost acceptable. The benefits from change must exceed the costs. Government roles in the extension of insurance are often ambiguous. While government management of the scheme may damage the local participation and attractiveness of the scheme, a clear role is seen in the provision of technical advice, developing networks of schemes for reinsurance and other purposes, ensuring smooth entry and exit from the market, and subsidizing low-income members.

See also: Community Health Insurance in Developing Countries; Competiton in Health Care; Determinants of National Health Expenditure; Health Finance, Equity in; Innovative Financing of Health Promotion; Insurance Plans and Programs - An Overview; Managed Care; Provider Payment Methods and Incentives; The Private Sector in Health Care Provision, The Role of.

Citations

Appiah-Denkyira E and Preker A (2007) *Reaching the Poor in Ghana with National Health Insurance – An Experience from the Districts of the Eastern Region of Ghana. Extending Social Protection in Health.* Berlin, Germany: GTZ/ILO/WHO.

Atim C (1999) Social movements and health insurance: A critical evaluation of voluntary, non-profit insurance schemes with case studies from Ghana and Cameroon. *Social Science and Medicine* 48(7): 881–896.

Bennett S, Creese A, and Monasch R (1998) *Health Insurance Schemes for People Outside Formal Sector Employment.* Geneva, Switzerland: WHO Analysis Research and Assessment Division.

Carrin G and James C (2005) Social health insurance: Key factors affecting the transition towards universal coverage. *International Social Security Review* 58: 45–64.

Carrin G, Waelkens MP, and Criel B (2005) Community-based health insurance in developing countries: A study of its contribution to the performance of health financing systems. *Tropical Medicine and International Health* 10(8): 799–811.

Dror D and Jacquier C (1999) Micro-insurance: Extending health insurance to the excluded. *International Social Security Review* 52(1): 71–97.
Ensor T (1999) Developing health insurance in transitional Asia. *Social Science and Medicine* 48(7): 871–879.
Frenk J, Knaul F, Gonzalez-Pier E, and Barraza-Llorens M (2007) *Poverty Health and Social Protection. Extending Social Protection in Health*. Berlin, Germany: GTZ/ILO/WHO.
Kutzin J (1998) Enhancing the insurance function of health systems: A proposed conceptual framework. In: Nitayarumphong S and Mills A (eds.) *Achieving Universal Coverage of Health Care*, pp. 27–101. Bangkok, Thailand: Nontaburi Ministry of Public Health Thailand.
Mesa-Lago C (1991) Social security in Latin America and the Caribbean: A comparative assessment. In: Ahmed E, Dreze J, Hills J, and Sen A (eds.) *Social Security in Developing Countries*, pp. 356–394. New York: Oxford University Press.
Tangcharoensathien V, Prakongsai P, Patcharanarumol W, and Jongudomsuk P (2007) *University Coverage in Thailand: The Respective Roles of Social Health Insurance and Tax-Based Financing. Extending Social Protection in Health*. Berlin, Germany: GTZ/ILO/WHO.
Twigg J (1999) Regional variation in Russian medical insurance: Lessons from Moscow and Nizhny Novgorod. *Health and Place* 5(3): 235–245.
World Bank (1993) *World Development Report 1993: Investing in Health Executive Summary*. Washington, DC: World Bank.
World Health Organization (2000) *The World Health Report 2000, Health Systems: Improving Performance*. Geneva, Switzerland: World Health Organization.
World Health Organization (2006) *The World Health Report 2006: Working Together for Health*. Geneva, Switzerland: World Health Organization.

Further Reading

Barnighausen T and Sauerborn R (2002) One hundred and eighteen years of the German health insurance system: Are there any lessons for middle- and low-income countries? *Social Science and Medicine* 54(10): 1559–1587.
Dror DM and Preker AS (eds.) (2002) *Social re-insurance: A new approach to sustainable community health financing*. Washington, DC: ILO and World Bank.
Gertler PJ (1998) On the road to social health insurance: The Asian experience. *World Development* 26(4): 717–732.
International Labour Organization (1999) Social Health Insurance. Geneva, Switzerland: International Labour Organisation/International Social Security Association.
Nitayarumphong S and Mills A (eds.) *Achieving Universal Coverage of Health Care*. Bangkok, Thailand: Nontaburi Ministry of Public Health Thailand.
Ron A and Scheil-Adlung X (2001) Recent Health Policy Innovations in Social Security. New Brunswick, NJ: New Jersey Transaction Publishers.

Relevant Websites

http://www.ilo.org – International Labour Organization (ILO).
http://www.OECD.org – Organisation for Economic Co-operation and Development (OECD).
http://www.worldbank.org – World Bank.
http://www.who.int/health_financing – World Health Organization, Health Financing Policy.

Insurance Plans and Programs: An Overview

S Greß, University of Applied Sciences, Fulda, Germany
J Wasem, University of Duisburg Essen, Essen, Germany

© 2008 Elsevier Inc. All rights reserved.

Introduction

The purpose of this article is to provide an overview on the principles of health insurance plans and programs. (On a system level, we use the term health insurance program. On the level of the individual health insurance entity, we use the term health plan. It is important to note that this article does not cover the tax-financed schemes that are predominant in some parts of Europe such as Scandinavia, the UK, and Italy and Canada.) In doing so, we endeavor to discuss the major theoretical issues that make the design of health insurance plans and programs difficult. The diversity of health insurance designs around the world is the consequence of these difficulties. One of these theoretical problems is adverse selection in competitive health insurance markets: As a consequence of market failures, comprehensive coverage by health insurance is difficult if not impossible to obtain. Another important problem is to ascertain the value of health insurance: While comprehensive coverage health insurance coverage is valued highly in many countries, the incomplete coverage in the United States can – among other reasons – be explained by the conviction that health insurance leads to wasteful overconsumption of health care because the price of health services for the consumer is too low.

This article is organized as follows. The section titled 'Design of health insurance programs' provides a summary and nontechnical discussion about the research that has been conducted on two of the most important theoretical problems of health insurance: The value of health insurance and adverse selection in competitive health insurance markets. This section also provides an analytical framework to classify real-world health insurance programs. The following sections analyze real-world health insurance programs in more detail. 'Private health insurance programs' discusses the design of private health insurance programs that typically calculate risk-related premiums. We find that even in the United States supposedly purely private health insurance is not dominant: Typically designers of health insurance programs prefer comprehensive coverage, which is difficult to obtain by using private health insurance with risk-related premiums. Therefore, the section titled 'Social health insurance programs' reviews the more predominant social health insurance programs. Social health insurance implies that extensive regulation – most importantly premium rate restrictions, standardization of benefits, and mandatory coverage – leads to comprehensive coverage. However, some important differences between social health insurance programs can be established, most importantly the difference between competitive multipayer programs and noncompetitive single-payer programs. Finally, 'Health insurance in low- and middle-income countries' reviews the evidence on the health outcomes of health insurance programs.

Design of Health Insurance Programs

This section discusses two of the most important theoretical problems of the design of health insurance programs: The trade-off between comprehensive coverage and wasteful overconsumption of health care and the trade-off between competition and selection. The section titled 'Calculation of premiums in health insurance programs' introduces an analytical framework to classify real-world health insurance programs.

The Value of Health Insurance

The value of health insurance is derived from the uncertainty and unpredictability of health spending. Of any given population, only a very small fraction of individuals incurs a very large fraction of health spending. For Germany, this fact is illustrated by **Figure 1**. The distribution of health spending at any given time (and over time as well) is highly skewed, in Germany as well as in other countries. Although individuals have some information about their health status and their needs for health spending, the exact amount is highly uncertain. As a consequence, health insurance is an important tool to spread risks and by this to enhance welfare.

Insurance is superior to borrowing and saving (Cutler and Zeckhauser, 2000). Individuals might borrow money when they are sick and repay their loans when they are healthy again. However, individuals might not be able to live long enough to pay back their loans. Moreover, savings might be able to cover everyday health expenses.

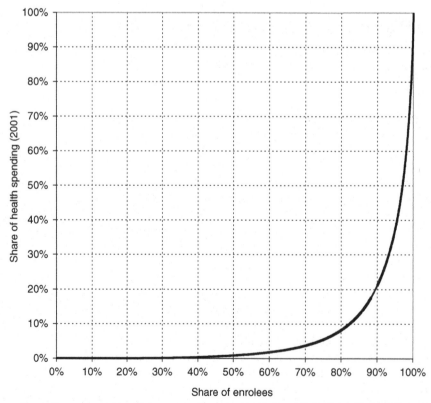

Figure 1 Health spending in German social health insurance. From Jacobs K, Reschke P, Cassel D, and Wasem J (2002) *Zur Wirkung des Risikostrukturausgleichs in der gesetzlichen Krankenversicherung.* Baden-Baden, Germany: Nomos.

However, medical episodes will possibly incur very substantial health expenses, which cannot be covered by savings. As a consequence, risk spreading of health insurance is highly valuable for individuals. Moreover, it is highly valuable from a societal perspective as well. In most developed industrial countries – with the notable exception of the United States – comprehensive coverage against the financial risk of health spending is highly valued by society. Moreover, comprehensive mandatory coverage avoids market failures such as adverse selection and free-rider behavior (see the section titled 'Adverse selection in competitive health insurance markets').

The value of health insurance, determined by spreading medical risks, is, however, diminished by incentive problems caused by health insurance. There is a substantial body of literature that presumes that the existence of health insurance leads to overspending (Pauly, 1968). Individuals with health insurance use more health services than they would if they were paying for these health services themselves. This behavior is called moral hazard. The term does not refer to some moral failure of individuals. Moral hazard simply implies that individuals adapt their behavior to incentives set by health insurance: "The response of seeking more health care with insurance than in its absence is a result not of moral perfidy, but of rational economic behaviour (Pauly, 1968: 535). The economic analysis of the welfare implications of moral hazard actually led to the conclusion that moral hazard substantially reduces the value of health insurance and consumers might even incur a negative value from health insurance if the coinsurance rate is very low (Manning and Marquis, 1996). This welfare loss occurs because with health insurance patients consume additional services that provide little benefit to them (Rice, 2002).

A rather famous natural experiment found that (higher) coverage of health insurance indeed leads to higher utilization rates of health services. The RAND Insurance Experiment randomized about 6000 individuals in six areas in the United States into different insurance programs. The insurance programs differed by coinsurance rates – between 0% and 95% (see **Table 1**). Without coinsurance, total health spending per capita was considerably higher than with some degree of coinsurance (Manning et al., 1987; Newhouse and Insurance Experiment Group, 1993). However, the RAND Insurance Experiment also found that individuals are unable to distinguish between highly effective and less effective treatments. In other words, more coinsurance may indeed lead to less utilization of health services – useful services as well as useless services – "... cost sharing did not seem to have a selective effect in prompting people to forgo care only or mainly in circumstances when such care probably would be of relatively little value" (Lohr et al., 1986: S36).

The design of health insurance programs involves a trade-off between risk spreading and appropriate incentives. More generous health insurance programs spread risk more broadly but also led to more overspending due to moral hazard. Several studies simulate optimal coinsurance rates, ranging between 25% and 58% (Cutler and Zeckhauser, 2000). From a societal point of view, these coinsurance rates are – at least outside the United States – difficult to accept. Still, modest coinsurance rates are part of most social health insurance programs. Therefore, most countries accept some degree of moral hazard in order to gain the benefits which are due to risk spreading: "Perhaps the most persuasive empirical evidence regarding the value of health insurance is the extent to which health insurance is purchased voluntarily, or provided to the citizens of democratic states. This evidence, represented by the high proportion of U.S. consumers who are insured and the high proportion of developed democracies that have some form of national health insurance, suggests that the value of health insurance is overwhelmingly positive" (Nyman, 2006: 102).

Adverse Selection in Competitive Health Insurance Markets

In the previous section we discussed the trade-off between risk spreading and appropriate incentives. In this section, we discuss another trade-off that is essential for the design of health insurance programs: The trade-off between competition and selection. Of course, this trade-off is not relevant for noncompetitive single-payer health insurance programs. However, designers of health insurance

Table 1 Results of the RAND health insurance experiment

Co-insurance rate	Outpatient expenses (1984$)	Inpatient expenses (1984$)	Total expenses (1984$)	Physician visits	Admissions
0 (Free)	340	409	749	4.55	0.128
25%	260	373	634	3.33	0.105
50%	224	450	674	3.03	0.092
95%	203	315	518	2.73	0.099

From Manning WG, Newhouse JP, Duan N, et al. (1987) Health insurance and the demand for medical care: Evidence from a randomized experiment. *American Economic Review* 77(3): 251–277, with permission from American Economic Association.

programs in many countries rely on competition as a means to stimulate innovation and – at least to some degree – to enhance consumer choice as a way to meet individual preferences. As a consequence, consumers who are shopping around for the lowest price and the best product at least theoretically stimulate price competition and the development of new products. The benefits of competing health insurers are similar to the benefits of competition in other markets (Cutler and Zeckhauser, 2000).

Unfortunately, health insurance is different. In contrast to other markets, some characteristics of the consumer of health insurance programs most probably affect the price of the product. If health insurance programs are charging risk-related premiums (see the section titled 'Calculation of premiums in health insurance programs') sick individuals pay more for an identical product than healthy individuals. Moreover, sick individuals prefer health plans with more generous benefits and low coinsurance rates. Since individuals also tend to have more information about their health status than the health plan, the latter is unable to calculate actuarially fair premiums. As a consequence, health plans charge some kind of average price. However, more generous health plans attract a high share of sick individuals and less generous health plans attract a high share of healthy individuals. As a result of this process of adverse selection, premiums of more generous health plans go up, which drives out the remaining healthy individuals, which in turn increase premiums even further. The empirical evidence for adverse selection is rather strong and unambiguous (Cutler and Zeckhauser, 2000; Geoffard, 2006).

Adverse selection makes it extremely difficult – if not impossible – to reach market equilibrium that ensures risk spreading for both groups, sick individuals as well as healthy individuals. Moreover, health plans have incentives to distort benefits in order to make themselves unattractive for sick individuals. What is more, they face disincentives to develop product innovations that are likely to attract sick individuals. This outcome is rather undesirable from a societal point of view.

As a consequence, designers of social health insurance programs in many countries strive to prevent the consequences of adverse selection. They do so by introducing mandatory coverage, standardizing benefits, and abolishing risk-related premiums. (Alternatively, health insurance programs could also charge risk-related premiums if bad risks (sick individuals) received premium subsidies, for example by the government: The sicker an individual, the higher the premium subsidy (see Zweifel and Breuer, 2006). However, this solution is not applied in practice.) However, the trade-off between competition and selection remains an important issue in highly regulated health insurance programs as well, because some kind of risk adjustment system needs to neutralize incentives for risk selection (see the sections titled 'Private health insurance programs' and 'Social health insurance programs').

Calculation of Premiums in Health Insurance Programs

We have seen in the previous section that adverse selection is an important reason why the design of health insurance plans is regulated quite heavily. One of the most important fields of regulation is the method of premium calculation in health insurance plans. In this section, we introduce some basic distinctions of premium calculation in health insurance programs and discuss the implications. **Table 2** displays the basic methods of premium calculation and some real world examples of health insurance programs.

Adverse selection is an important reason for the regulation of health insurance programs. Moreover – and maybe even more importantly – societies in many OECD countries place a high priority on fairness or solidarity as a policy objective in health-care financing (Wagstaff and van Doorslaer, 1992, 2000). Several dimensions of solidarity need to be distinguished (van de Ven and Ellis, 2000), the most important being risk solidarity and income solidarity. The most basic dimension of solidarity is risk solidarity. Looking in more detail, it can be distinguished in *ex ante* risk solidarity and *ex-post* risk solidarity between the healthy and the sick. *Ex-post* solidarity means that there is a limited redistribution of resources from the unexpectedly healthy toward the unexpectedly sick. *Ex-post* risk solidarity between the healthy and the sick can also be considered to be the basic (health) insurance function, which can even be

Table 2 Calculation of premium in health insurance programs

Method of premium calculation	Income-related contributions	Community rating	Risk-related premiums
Health insurance program	Germany (social)	Switzerland	United States (individual)
			Germany (private)
		United States (group)	
	France		
	Netherlands	Netherlands	

Based on Wasem J, Greß S, and Okma KGH (2004) The role of private health insurance in social health insurance countries. In: Saltman R, Busse R, and Figueras J (eds.) *Social Health Insurance in Western Europe*, pp. 227–247. London: Open University Press.

achieved in private health insurance programs that calculate risk-related premiums. For the sake of simplification we classify health insurance programs as private if they primarily rely on risk-related premiums. If health insurance programs are required to calculate community-rated premiums or income-dependent premiums, we classify them as social insurance programs. The private U.S. group health insurance programs are somewhere in between. Note that the classification 'private' does not refer to the legal status of insurance companies: In the Netherlands, the social health insurance program is now carried out by private health insurance companies.

Ex-ante risk solidarity implies a redistribution from those who are expected to be healthy to those who are expected to be sick. This cannot be achieved with risk-related premiums, as they charge those expected to be sick higher premiums. This is the natural result that can be observed on more or less unregulated health insurance markets. However, OECD countries do not want to restrict their health-care system to *ex post* risk solidarity. Therefore – with the notable exception of individual private health insurance markets in the United States and Germany (in both countries individual health insurance calculates risk-related premiums and has a market share of approximately 10%) – designers of social healthcare financing systems prefer to implement modes of financing, which provide an enhanced degree of solidarity and redistribution. The introduction of premium rate restrictions, for example community rating (community-rated premiums are the same for all enrollees in the same health plan) – and mandatory enrollment lead to *ex-ante* risk solidarity as well as *ex-post* risk solidarity between the healthy and the sick, because health insurance programs have to refrain from charging higher premiums for high health risks (see the section titled 'Social health insurance programs' for the implications this regulatory requirement has for the trade-off between competition and selection).

Moreover, income solidarity between the rich and the poor may be another fundamental feature of health insurance programs as well, but not necessarily so. If health insurance programs are required to calculate community-rated premiums, these premiums are independent of income. As a consequence, these health insurance programs do not redistribute resources from the rich to the poor. What is more, the consequences of community-rated premiums are regressive: The higher the income, the smaller the share which is spent for health insurance premiums. In those OECD countries that use social health insurance as the predominant mode of health-care financing, these consequences are not acceptable to designers of health insurance programs. Therefore, they either implement a system of community-rated premiums and tax-financed and needs-tested premium subsidies to the poor (Switzerland) or use income-dependent premiums as a mode of financing (the social health insurance market in Germany, France). In the Netherlands, both approaches are applied, as half of the contribution in social health insurance is income-dependent, half is community-rated. The income consequences of community-rated premiums with tax-financed and needs-tested premium subsidies on the one hand and income-dependent premiums on the other hand can be equivalent (Breyer, 2002).

Private Health Insurance Programs

Compared to other sources of health-care finance, private health insurance programs are of minor importance in most OECD countries. Within the OECD, it is only in the United States that private health insurance programs account for more than 30% of health spending. Still, adequately regulated private health insurance programs are attractive alternatives to so-called socialized medicine for proponents of market-oriented reforms not only in the United States (Pauly and Herring, 1999) but also in Western Europe (Henke, 1999). What are then the problems of adequate regulation of private health insurance programs? The next section briefly describes the various functions private health insurance programs can perform in health-care systems. The section titled 'Regulation of private health insurance programs' analyzes regulation of private health insurance programs. Finally, we will discuss the relationship of private health insurance programs with health-care providers ('Provision of health-care services').

Functions of Private Health Insurance Programs

Private health insurance programs (PHIs) cover a wide range of arrangements. Private health insurance programs are supplied by commercial insurance firms (both stockholder and mutual; among them also plans owned by the state) as well as not-for-profit agencies. Insurance business can be run by conventional indemnity plans, which only reimburse costs, as well as by more innovative plans, which provide some form of managed care. On the demand side of PHI markets, individuals as well as groups or corporate actors (e.g., employers, professional organizations) may ask for insurance. In general, contracts between insurer and enrollee are voluntary for both sides. However, mandatory contracts (for one or both sides) are realized in some countries (and discussed in others) as well. Risk spreading between the parties involved (insurer, insured, health-care providers, and employers) varies considerably.

Regulation of private health insurance programs in different countries results from specific historical national as well as international developments. In the past international developments have been of minor importance for

PHI regulation. However, in Europe European Union regulation is of increasing importance. The third EU directive on Non-Life Insurance has forced several member states to adapt their regulatory framework for private health insurance programs. However, they also reflect the particular function of private health insurance programs. Basically three functions of PHI in health-care systems can be observed in international comparisons.

Private health insurance programs may be the only system of coverage available for some part of the population, because these people are not included in public schemes. Private health insurance programs thus perform the function of an alternative to public arrangements. This is the case particularly in countries with means-tested public health benefit schemes (Medicaid in the United States) or if eligibility to social health insurance programs depends on income and/or employment status (Germany) or age (Medicare in the United States). The need for regulation of alternative private health insurance programs is particularly high, because an unregulated market does not guarantee that people who are not entitled to the public system will receive adequate insurance coverage (see the section titled 'Adverse selection in competitive health insurance markets').

The second function of private health insurance programs is to supplement public schemes. Supplementary private health insurance programs can offer coverage for services not covered in the public system (e.g., dental care for adults in the Netherlands as well as dental care and pharmaceuticals in Canada but also upgraded hospital services such as private or semi-private rooms in almost every country). Supplementary private health insurance programs also offer coverage for services not completely covered by public schemes and thus reduces co-payments and deductibles (e.g., Medigap insurance in the United States, coverage for co-payments in France, dental care in Germany). If benefit schemes of the public system are rather comprehensive and of good quality, supplementary private health insurance programs basically cover luxury goods (e.g., more comfortable board and lodging in hospitals in Belgium). As a consequence, a smaller degree of regulation for supplementary private health insurance programs than for alternative private health insurance programs is more justifiable in terms of social acceptability.

The third function of private health insurance programs is to complement public schemes. Thus private health insurance programs provide double cover: People who are entitled to benefits of the public system might buy private insurance that covers at least partly the same benefits as the public system. People purchase complementary private health insurance programs for a variety of reasons: They want to get services quicker than in the public system (queue jumping), they want to get better or more comfortable services, or they want to contact health-care providers who are excluded from delivering services within the public system. Complementary private health insurance programs seem to occur primarily in tax-financed health-care systems – for example, in the United Kingdom, Australia, and Canada (Flood *et al.*, 2005) – but play a role in systems with mandatory social health insurance programs as well, for example in the Netherlands (Brouwer *et al.*, 2003). Regulation of complementary private health insurance programs primarily concerns the question whether it may be supplied at all. In Canada, 100% of the population is covered by the public health insurance scheme, which is run by the provinces. Most provinces prohibit the supply of complementary private health insurance programs. However, this regulation was challenged by the Supreme Court in June 2005. In a narrow 4:3 decision, the Supreme Court of Canada struck down Quebec laws prohibiting the sale of complementary PHI on the basis that they violate Quebec's Charter of Human Rights and Freedoms. The result makes further Charter challenges to similar laws in other provinces inevitable, but the question of whether they will succeed remains unanswered for the time being (Flood *et al.*, 2005).

Regulation of Private Health Insurance Programs

We have shown that unregulated private health insurance markets would not lead to socially desirable outcomes (see the section titled 'Design of health insurance programs'). In this section, we review the regulation of (mostly alternative) private health insurance programs that aim to increase access for unfavorable risks. The term unfavorable risks is applied to individuals who are expected to have high health spending in the future.

To increase access to private health insurance programs for unfavorable risks, a variety of approaches is possible and many have been tried during the last few decades. Most of them have been implemented only for alternative private health insurance programs or (in the case of Ireland) for complementary private health insurance programs. Discrimination against unfavorable risks in supplementary private health insurance programs is widespread, which might become less acceptable the more benefits in public schemes are limited. The attempt of the French government to increase access for low-income persons to supplementary private health insurance programs by providing means-tested subsidies (Turquet, 2004) and the initiative of the European Parliament for the revision of European regulation for supplementary private health insurance programs (Rocard, 2000) are first indicators for more regulation in that particular area of private health insurance programs.

One possible way to safeguard access to health care for unfavorable risks is to offer access to a public scheme for those individuals. Deficiencies of the risk spreading capabilities of competitive private health insurance programs thus would be compensated for. This type of approach has been realized in parts of the United States. Premium income generally covers only parts of health spending for high risks in these schemes. The deficit is covered by the fiscal budgets (Achman and Chollet, 2001).

Instead of implementing a public scheme for unfavorable risks, private health insurance programs may be directly regulated in order to increase access: Mandatory open enrollment, prohibition of preexisting condition limitations and/or prohibiting or premium rate restrictions are instruments of direct regulation. Similar to the first approach, most of these measures imply a subsidization of unfavorable risks. Here, subsidies would be financed not through taxes but by favorable risks insured with private health insurance programs. A similar approach was applied in alternative private health insurance programs in the Netherlands before the 2006 health insurance reform and will be applied in alternative private health insurance programs in Germany in 2009. Even the United States has implemented federal legislation in order to increase access for unfavorable risks, especially for small group and individual contracts. Since 1996, the extent to which private health insurers may impose preexisting conditions limitation is limited. Furthermore, private health insurers in the United States are not allowed to discriminate against unfavorable risks in group contracts (Jost, 2001).

Mandatory open enrollment, prohibition of preexisting condition limitations, and premium rate restrictions are important tools to increase access in private health insurance programs. However, they also create new incentives for adverse selection. Favorable risks could seek very low coverage first and change to more comprehensive coverage when they happen to become unfavorable risks. It is difficult to neutralize these incentives for adverse selection. One way is to restrict access to private health insurance programs to a limited time period, for example after losing coverage in public schemes or in social health insurance programs.

Regulation to increased access for unfavorable risks in private health insurance programs does not only produce problems of adverse selection. It might also produce problems of unequal risk distribution and incentives for risk selection (cream skimming) between competing health insurers, which would not occur if insurers could exclude unfavorable risks or charge them an extra premium reflecting their unfavorable health status. As a consequence, some type of risk adjustment scheme needs to neutralize incentives for risk selection (van de Ven and Ellis, 2000; Glazer and McGuire, 2006).

Provision of Health-Care Services

Traditionally, private health insurance programs – in the United States and elsewhere – do not influence incentives on the supply side, for example, remuneration systems for physicians. One important exception is the development of managed care insurance in the United States (Glied, 2000). However, managed care has been developed because third-party payers (employers, government) put pressure on private health insurance programs to contain health spending. Managed care is virtually nonexistent in individual private health insurance programs in the United States. In general, private health insurance programs instead use instruments at the demand side to influence costs. Insurance contracts include mechanisms such as co-payments and deductibles to increase consumers' cost-consciousness. These mechanisms in turn are supposed to put indirect pressure on the behavior of providers.

Moreover, private health insurance programs usually are unable to influence the supply of health-care providers. The market power of private health insurance programs in most cases is too small to play an active role in determining the supply of health-care providers. Moreover, policy makers (at least in most of Europe and in Canada) are first of all interested in the viability of public schemes. Thus, they want to cut expenditures and growth rates of expenditures primarily within these systems. Cost containment in private health insurance programs is of secondary importance to them. Therefore, we often observe that the attempt to contain costs in the public sector leads to cost shifting toward private health insurance programs. It is very common that health-care providers compensate for budgets, spending cuts, and the like in the public sector by raising volume and/or prices for services in private health insurance programs. Governments may even purposefully shift costs from public schemes to private health insurance programs by allowing higher fee levels in private health insurance programs to compensate providers for cost-containment measures in the public sector.

Social Health Insurance Programs

Designers of competitive multipayer health insurance programs in many countries strive to prevent the consequences of adverse selection. This problem can be avoided by designing single-payer health insurance programs (such as in Korea) or noncompetitive multiple-payer health insurance programs (e.g., in France and Austria). As a consequence, potential benefits of competitive health insurance markets can also not be achieved (**Table 3**).

In competitive multi-payer social health insurance programs (e.g., Germany, Switzerland, and the Netherlands), adverse selection is prevented by introducing mandatory coverage, standardizing benefits, and abolishing risk-related premiums. However, the trade-off between competition and selection remains an important issue in these health insurance programs as well, because some kind of risk adjustment system needs to neutralize incentives

Table 3 Typology of social health insurance programs

	Single payer	Multiple payers
Competitive	–	Germany, Netherlands, Switzerland
Noncompetitive	Korea	France, Austria

for risk selection by health insurers. In this section, we analyze the relationship between risk adjustment and consumer choice in three social health insurance programs in Germany, the Netherlands, and Switzerland (Greß, 2006).

Risk Adjustment

The objectives guiding health-care reforms in Germany, Switzerland, and the Netherlands leading toward more competition in social health insurance programs in the middle of the 1990s have been quite similar. These objectives can be summarized as efficiency and consumer satisfaction in the provision of health-care services while maintaining solidarity of health-care financing and effective containment of health-care costs (van de Ven *et al.*, 2003). One of the most important prerequisites for competition in social health insurance programs to be successful is an effective mechanism for risk adjustment. Since premium rate restrictions prohibit risk-rated premiums in any of the three social health insurance programs, without risk adjustment health plans have ample incentives for the selection of risks. If risk adjustment is absent or incomplete, it is more profitable for health plans to select risks than to manage health services. This behavior may be rational from the viewpoint of health plans. However, it definitely contradicts the objectives of the health-care reforms mentioned above.

Systematically, three adverse effects of incentives to select risks can be separated (van de Ven *et al.*, 2004). First, health plans face a disincentive to react to the preferences of bad risks. It is rational for health plans to provide good service for profitable, i.e., favorable, risks. Moreover, it is also rational for health plans to provide bad service for unprofitable, i.e., unfavorable, risks since investments in preferred risk selection (cream skimming) have higher returns than investments in improving the efficiency of health services. From a public health point of view, these disincentives are fatal, since unfavorable risks are usually patients who are chronically ill and need services that are better than average. Neither health plans nor health-care providers have incentives to gain a reputation for treating the chronically ill efficiently and effectively (van de Ven and Ellis, 2000).

Second, if cream skimming is successful, it will eventually lead to market segmentation. Unfavorable risks (high-risk patients) will be members of sickness funds with high contributions. Conversely, favorable risks (low-risk patients) will be members of sickness funds with low contributions. This situation is not compatible with the idea of solidarity in social health insurance programs since in fact it paves the way for risk-related premiums.

Third, preferred risk selection strategies that are highly rational from an individual health plan point of view create welfare losses for society. Investments for the identification of favorable risks (e.g., information technology) and investments for the attraction of favorable risks and the deterrence of unfavorable risks (e.g., resources used for developing effective marketing strategies) do not create any societal gains. Therefore, resources spent on preferred risk selection represent a welfare loss (van de Ven and Ellis, 2000). Moreover, preferred risk selection strategies may create an unstable market if some sickness funds refrain from selecting risks. These funds may be forced to declare bankruptcy due to adverse selection of risks. This consequence also represents a welfare loss to society.

Research is unanimous in concluding that adjusters based on sex and age (demographic adjusters) predict actual health-care expenditures of individuals very poorly (van de Ven and Ellis, 2000). If the risk adjustment formula takes into account information of prior diagnosis and/or prior costs, the risk adjustment formula predicts actual health-care expenses of individuals more accurately. Thus, it neutralizes incentives of sickness funds to select risks more effectively. The difference between actuarially predicted expenses and revenue from contributions and the risk adjustment mechanism is much smaller.

In all three social health insurance programs – in Germany, the Netherlands, and Switzerland – some kind of risk adjustment system has been implemented. However, only in the Netherlands is risk adjustment health-based (van de Ven *et al.*, 2004). As a consequence, only in the Dutch social health insurance program are incentives for cream skimming of health plans neutralized quite effectively (Prinsze and van Vliet, 2005). The rather crude risk adjustment mechanisms in Germany and Switzerland leave ample incentives for health plans to make risk selection worthwhile (Beck *et al.*, 2003; Behrend *et al.*, 2004). Accordingly, risk selection for health plans in Germany and Switzerland is less profitable than it would be in a situation without risk adjustment at all. However, it is still profitable enough to make selection strategies worthwhile. This is not the case in the Netherlands. Even if health plans may have small financial incentives for the selection of favorable risks, they also have to consider the costs for pursuing these strategies. These costs consist not only of costs for identifying and attracting favorable risks but also consist of negative public relations effects if these strategies become public knowledge.

Consumer Choice

Another important prerequisite for competition to be successful is free consumer choice. Consumers – the insured – need to have an exit option in order to search successfully for more efficient sickness funds: "... the exit option is widely held to be uniquely powerful: by inflicting revenue losses on delinquent management, exit is expected to induce that 'wonderful concentration of the mind' akin to the one Samuel Johnson attributed to the prospect of being hanged" (Hirschmann, 1970: 21). Free choice of health plans – open enrollment – has been established in all three health insurance programs. Open enrollment implies that consumers are able to switch health plans and each health plan must accept all applicants. Usually there is an open enrollment period during which consumers can switch to another fund. Incentives for consumer choice are enhanced if the benefits of switching (lower premiums) are substantial enough to outweigh the costs of switching (information costs, search costs, administration costs). Moreover, incentives for consumer choice are enhanced if consumers can realize the full benefits of lower premiums after switching health plans. If this is not the case, consumers may refrain from switching, although they might do so if they were able to collect the full benefits of switching.

Free consumer choice of health plans has been established in Germany, the Netherlands, and Switzerland. However, incentives for consumer choice vary. Open enrollment has been established in all countries. Whether consumers can realize the full benefits of switching to a lower-priced health plan depends on the manner premiums are calculated (see the section titled 'Calculation of premiums in health insurance programs'). In Switzerland, contributions are community-rated and independent of income. Therefore, consumers can realize the full benefits of switching to another health plan. The same is true in the Netherlands, since health plans have different community-rated premiums. This is not the case in Germany where employer and employee pay 50% each of an income-dependent premium that differs between health plans. If consumers switch to a lower-priced health plan, they realize only 50% of the pecuniary benefits.

Price differences between health plans in Germany, Switzerland, and the Netherlands reflect differences in efficiency as well as differences in the risk structure on members. Since risk adjustment does not neutralize incentives for risk selection effectively in Germany and Switzerland, price differences are high and constitute powerful incentives for consumers to switch. Therefore, in both Germany and Switzerland price differences between sickness funds should be substantial enough to offset the costs of switching for consumers. In the Netherlands, this is less obvious. Price differences are smaller, since they do not reflect diverging risk structures of sickness funds as strongly as in Germany and Switzerland.

In contrast to Germany (Tamm *et al.*, 2007), it is quite surprising that consumers in Switzerland in fact are very reluctant to switch to lower-priced health plans, since incentives to switch are high. This might be partly explained by poor consumer information (Beck *et al.*, 2003). Moreover, the analysis of incentives for consumer mobility does not explain why healthy consumers switch more often than less-healthy consumers in all three countries, in Germany and Switzerland more so than in the Netherlands. Since sickness funds do not calculate risk-related premiums, price differences are the same for healthy and less-healthy consumers. Moreover, open enrollment applies to all consumers. Different switching behavior of different risk groups therefore points to risk selection of sickness funds (Laske-Aldershof *et al.*, 2004).

Provision of Health-Care Services

Even if there were few incentives for health plans to select risks in a competitive environment and incentives for consumer choice were high, health plans are only able to influence the efficiency of the provision of health service if they have sufficient instruments do so. Otherwise, "...under competition dissatisfaction takes the form of ineffective flitting back and forth of groups of consumers from one deteriorating firm to another without any firm getting a signal that something has gone awry" (Hirschmann, 1970: 26). In order to avoid this "ineffective flitting back and worth of consumers," health plans need to be able to develop innovative contractual arrangements with health-care providers that take into account consumers' preferences. Accordingly, health plans must be able to decide which providers to contract with and must be able to negotiate freely about the content of those contracts.

If health plans are not able to contract selectively with health-care providers they will not be able to gain competitive advantages. The potential for developing innovative arrangements for the provision of health care will instead be small when health plans are obliged to contract collectively, i.e., with every willing licensed health-care provider. Even if health plans are able to contract selectively, contractual freedom can be diminished by public regulation intended to contain costs. However, public regulation to contain costs (restrictions on prices, budgets, and other contract parameters) may severely restrict the contractual freedom of health plans and health-care providers.

There is some opportunity for health plans to contract selectively with health-care providers in all three social health insurance programs. However, these opportunities are limited (Greß, 2006). Only in the Netherlands are health plans legally allowed to choose health-care providers. However, a governmental agency determines maximum tariffs for prices in ambulatory care and hospital care. In contrast to the Netherlands, collective contracting is still the legal norm in Germany and in Switzerland. Yet there are exceptions from this norm in both countries. In Germany, sickness funds are allowed to contract selectively with general practitioners in order to offer gatekeeping models (Greß et al., 2004). Moreover, the legislator has earmarked 1% of overall budgets of ambulatory care and hospital care for integrated care projects. Sickness funds are free to determine their contractual partners for these projects (Greß et al., 2006). In Switzerland sickness funds are only allowed to contract selectively with health-care providers if their insured enroll in managed care plans.

Health Insurance in Low- and Middle-Income Countries

The trade-offs between risk spreading and appropriate incentives and between competition and selection that we focused on in this article are relevant for low- and middle-income countries as well as for high-income countries. For low- and middle-income countries, however, specific chances but also specific challenges exist, with regard to the implementation of health insurance. In the last few decades, quite a large number of low- and middle-income countries have started to implement mechanisms of health insurance as an approach to solve their often dramatic health funding problems. Implementing health insurance has been identified as a strategy to contribute to the solution of these problems for three reasons (Carrin and James, 2005a, 2005b; Carrin et al., 2007; Hsiao and Shaw, 2007; McIntyre, 2007):

- Revenue collection: It is well known that low- and middle-income countries spend even smaller portions of their GDP on health than high-income countries. Many low-income countries spend considerably less than the 5% of GDP. Often an underfinanced health sector with poor performance is financed by taxes, and private (formal but often as well informal) payments add some resources. Social health insurance has been seen by several countries as an instrument to increase available resources for health. Especially if people feel that they are getting value for money and draw additional benefit from health insurance, they often are willing to contribute.

  Mandatory social health insurance, however, is easier to implement in the formal sector of the economy. If most of the labor force is in the informal sector, small-scale, voluntary community health insurance may be a more appropriate approach; its main obstacle, however, is adverse selection (as described in more detail in the section titled 'Health insurance programs and health outcomes'), as the healthy might wait until they join.

- Pooling of funds: Often medium-size and large expenditures for medical treatment lead to impoverishment, debts, etc. in low- and middle-income countries. This is because, even if a tax-financed health system exists, its coverage for expensive surgery and drugs is often rather limited or available only in certain regions or for certain groups of the population. As we analyzed in more detail in the section titled 'The value of health insurance,' the value of health insurance is derived from the uncertainty and unpredictability of health spending. At the time of illness, health insurance is pooling funds from many contribution payers to cover the costs of treatment. It is sharing risks. Poor people pay small contributions to health insurance regularly and are entitled to receive services in case of illness. Health insurance is enabling medical treatment for parts of the population who would not be able to finance it without insurance. Pooling of resources might be accompanied by *ex ante* redistribution of resources, from the healthy to the sick, from higher income to the poor. Health insurance might therefore contribute to narrowing somewhat the often extreme gap between the large majority of rather poor and a small minority of rich in low- and middle-income countries.

- Purchasing of health-care services: Health insurance agencies buy health services for their insured on health-care markets. They therefore have some market power and can negotiate for quality and cost-effective services, whereas the individual, especially when in need of health services, cannot. As performance of the health sector in low- and middle-income countries often is low, implementing health insurance might be a strategy, therefore, to increase quality of services. Also, as the insured have paid contributions to health insurance, they can argue that they are entitled to services of a certain quality.

Although there are some strong arguments that implementing health insurance might contribute to quantity and quality of health services and a fair distribution of the burden of finance, health insurance is far from being a *deus ex machina*, which would solve all the health sector's problems easily. Whether implementing health insurance will be a success story in low- and middle-income countries depends on a variety of factors. In particular, there must be a political framework and a climate in society that allows success for health insurance (Carrin and James, 2005b).

Health Insurance Programs and Health Outcomes

The final section of this article reviews empirical research about the relationship between different health insurance programs and health outcomes. First of all, it is quite evident that the health consequences of not having insurance at all can be quite dramatic. Research on the consequences of being uninsured in the United States has shown consistently that individuals without health insurance "receive fewer preventive and diagnostic services, tend to be more severely ill when diagnosed, and receive less therapeutic care" (Hadley, 2003: 3S). More importantly, having health insurance would decrease mortality of the uninsured in the United States significantly.

One might expect that similar findings are available for differences between health insurance programs. For example, enrollment in more generous health insurance programs – such as high-coverage and low coinsurance plans – might result in superior health outcomes compared to enrollment in less generous health insurance programs, such as managed-care insurance and high coinsurance plans. However, there are also tendencies counteracting these assumptions. For example, fee-for-service plans might increase incentives for the overuse and misuse of services, which might be beneficial for the income of the health-care provider but may be harmful for the patient's health. What is more, the use of evidence-based guidelines in managed care might decrease the overuse and misuse of health services, which might be beneficial for health outcomes (Cutler and Zeckhauser, 2000).

Evidence on the health consequences of different health insurance programs is scarce and rather ambiguous. The RAND Health Insurance Experiment has found some relationship between the level of coinsurance and health outcomes, although the findings were less dramatic and less conclusive than the relationship between the level of coinsurance and health spending (see the section titled 'The value of health insurance'). Actually, health outcomes did not differ across plans for most individuals. However, it has to be noted that the RAND Health Insurance Experiment was limited to a short time period: "Increased primary and preventive care, even if strongly beneficial, might not be so important in such a short period of time" (Cutler and Zeckhauser, 2000: 629).

Moreover, maybe even more importantly,

"health among the sick poor – approximately the most disadvantaged 6 percent of the population – was adversely affected ... In particular, the poor who began the experiment with elevated blood pressure had their blood pressure lowered more on the free care plan than on the cost-sharing plans. The effect on predicted mortality rates – a fall of about 10 percent – was substantial for this group. In addition, free care marginally improved both near and far corrected vision ... and increased the likelihood that a decayed tooth would be filled" (Newhouse and Insurance Experiment Group, 1993: 339).

Evidence on the health outcome of managed care insurance is ambiguous as well. A review of the empirical literature comparing health outcomes of managed care insurance and fee-for-service indemnity insurance did not find clear differences. About half of the studies have found that managed care improves health outcome (quality of care), while the other half have found that managed care has a negative impact on health outcomes (Miller and Luft, 2002).

Moreover, there is no clear empirical evidence of health outcomes in private health insurance programs compared to health outcomes in social health insurance programs (e.g., comparing health outcomes in Germany social health insurance and in German alternative private health insurance).

Conclusions

The design of health insurance programs and plans is determined by important trade-offs. First, designers of health insurers need to consider the trade-off between risk spreading and appropriate incentives. More generous health insurance programs spread risk more broadly but may also lead to more overspending due to moral hazard. However, most countries – with the notable exception of the United States – accept some degree of moral hazard in order to gain the benefits stemming from risk spreading and comprehensive coverage. Even in the United States the fact that employers can deduct health insurance premiums for their employees from their tax sheet sets incentives for more generous health insurance policies (Pauly, 1986). Second, designers of health insurance programs need to consider the trade-off between competition and selection. Many countries rely on competitive health insurance programs as a means to stimulate innovation and – at least to some degree – to enhance consumer choice as a way to meet individual preferences. However, if health insurance programs are calculating risk-related premiums, adverse selection makes it extremely difficult – if not impossible – to reach market equilibrium, which ensures risk spreading for both groups: Sick individuals as well as healthy individuals. As a consequence, designers of health insurance programs in many countries strive to prevent the consequences of adverse selection.

Mandatory open enrollment, prohibition of preexisting condition limitations and premium rate restrictions are important tools to increase access to private health insurance programs. However, regulation also creates new incentives for adverse selection. Moreover, regulation might also produce problems of unequal risk distribution and incentives for risk selection (cream skimming) between competing health insurers. Moreover, regulation of private health insurance programs reflects the particular function of private health insurance programs. The need for regulation of alternative private health insurance programs is particularly high, because an unregulated market will not guarantee that individuals who are not entitled to the public system will receive adequate insurance coverage. In contrast, less-extensive regulation for supplementary health insurance is socially acceptable. Discrimination against unfavorable risks in supplementary private health insurance programs is widespread. However, it might become less acceptable the more benefits in public schemes are limited.

Adverse selection can be prevented by designing single-payer or noncompetitive multiple-payer social health insurance programs. Designers of competitive multiple-payer social health insurance programs prevent the consequences of adverse selection by introducing mandatory coverage, standardizing benefits, and abolishing risk-related premiums. However, the trade-off between competition and selection remains an important issue in these health insurance programs as well, because some kind of risk adjustment system needs to neutralize incentives for risk selection by health plans. Even if there were few incentives for health plans to select risks in a competitive environment and incentives for consumer choice were high, health plans are only able to influence the efficiency of the provision of health service if they have sufficient instruments do so.

Evidence on the health consequences of different health insurance programs is scarce and rather ambiguous. The health consequences of not having insurance at all can be quite dramatic. Having health insurance would decrease mortality of the uninsured in the United States significantly. The RAND Health Insurance Experiment has found some relationship between the level of coinsurance and health outcomes, although the findings were less dramatic and less conclusive than the relationship between the level of coinsurance and health spending. Evidence on the health outcome of managed-care insurance is ambiguous as well. Moreover, there is no clear empirical evidence of health outcomes in private health insurance programs compared to health outcomes in social health insurance programs.

Health insurance can contribute to the problems of health sector financing in low- and middle-income countries as well. In particular, it can make revenue collection easier and therefore allow for an increase in quantity and quality of services, it may support the pooling of risks and therefore avoid impoverishment because of illness, and it may be a vehicle for prudent purchasing of health care. Whether implementing health insurance in low- and middle-income countries will be a success story depends on many factors, however, political and societal support being the most important among them.

See also: Universal Coverage in Developing Countries, Transition to.

Citations

Achman L and Chollet D (2001) *High Risk Pools of Limited Help to the Uninsurable.* New York: The Commonwealth Fund.

Beck K, Spycher S, Holly A, and Gardiol L (2003) Risk adjustment in Switzerland. *Health Policy* 65(1): 63–74.

Behrend C, Greß S, Holle P, et al. (2004) Zur Erklärungskraft des heutigen soziodemografischen Risikostrukturausgleichsmodells. Ergebnisse empirischer Analysen an Prozessdaten einer ostdeutschen Regionalkasse. *Journal of Public Health* 12(1): 20–31.

Breyer F (2002) Einkommensbezogene versus pauschale GKV-Beiträge – eine Begriffsklärung. *Schmollers Jahrbuch* 122: 605–616.

Brouwer W, v. Exel J, Hermans B, and Stoop A (2003) Should I stay or should I go? Waiting lists and cross-border care in the Netherlands. *Health Policy* 63: 289–298.

Carrin G and James C (2005a) Key performance indicators for the implementation of social health insurance. *Applied Health Economics and Health Policy* 4(1): 15–22.

Carrin G and James C (2005b) Social health insurance: Key factors affecting the transition towards universal coverage. *International Social Security Review* 58(1): 46–63.

Carrin G, James C, Adelhardt M, et al. (2007) Health financing reform in Kenya – Assessing the social health insurance proposal. *South African Medical Journal* 97(2): 130–135.

Cutler DM and Zeckhauser RJ (2000) The Anatomy of Health Insurance. In: Culyer AJ and Newhouse J (eds.) *Handbook of Health Economics*, pp. 563–643. Amsterdam, the Netherlands: Elsevier.

Flood C, Sossin L, and Roach K (eds.) (2005) *Access to Care Access to Justice: The Legal Debate Over Private Health Insurance in Canada.* Toronto, Canada: University of Toronto Press.

Geoffard P-Y (2006) Incentives and selection effects in health insurance. In: Jones A (ed.) *The Elgar Companion to Health Economics*, pp. 104–113. Cheltenham/Northampton, UK: Edward Elgar.

Glazer J and McGuire T (2006) Optimal risk adjustment. In: Jones A (ed.) *The Elgar Companion to Health Economcis*, pp. 279–285. Cheltenham/Northampton, UK: Edward Elgar.

Glied S (2000) Managed care. Handbook of health economics. In: Culyer AJ and Newhouse J (eds.) *Handbook of Health Economics*, pp. 707–753. Amsterdam, the Netherlands: Elsevier.

Greß S (2006) Regulated Competition in Social Health Insurance: A Three-Country Comparison. *International Social Security Review* 59(3): 27–47.

Greß S, Hessel F, Schulze S, and Wasem J (2004) Prospects of gatekeeping in German social health insurance based on national and international experience. *Journal of Public Health* 12(4): 250–258.

Greß S, Focke A, Hessel F, and Wasem J (2006) Financial incentives for disease management programmes and integrated care in German social health insurance. *Health Policy* 78(2–3): 295–305.

Hadley J (2003) Sicker and poorer. The consequences of being uninsured: A review of the research on the relationship between health insurance, medical care use, health, work, and income. *Medical Care and Research Review* 60(supplement 2): 3S–75S; discussion 76S–112S.

Henke K-D (1999) Socially bounded competition in Germany. *Health Affairs* 18(4): 203–206.

Hirschmann A (1970) Exit, voice and loyalty. *Responses to Decline in Firms, Organizations and States*. Cambridge, MA: Harvard University Press.

Hsiao W and Shaw P (2007) *Social Health Insurance for Developing Nations*. Washington, DC: World Bank.

Jacobs K, Reschke P, Cassel D, and Wasem J (2002) *Zur Wirkung des Risikostrukturausgleichs in der gesetzlichen Krankenversicherung*. Baden-Baden: Nomos.

Jost TS (2001) Private or public approaches to insuring the uninsured: Lessons from international experience with private insurance. New York: University Law Review 76(2): 419–493.

Laske-Aldershof T, Schut FT, Beck K, et al. (2004) Consumer mobility in social health insurance markets: A five-country comparison. *Applied Health Economics and Health Policy* 3(4): 229–241.

Lohr K, Brook R, and Camberg C (1986) Effect of cost sharing on use of medically effective and less effective care. *Medical Care* 29(supplement 9): 31–38.

Manning W and Marquis S (1996) Health insurance: The trade-off between risk pooling and moral hazard. *Journal of Health Economics* 15(5): 609–640.

Manning WG, Newhouse JP, Duan N, et al. (1987) Health insurance and the demand for medical care: Evidence from a randomized experiment. *American Economic Review* 77(3): 251–277.

McIntyre D (2007) *Learning from Experience: Health care financing in low and middle-income countries*. Global Forum for Health Research. http://www.globalforumhealth.org (accessed October 2007).

Miller RH and Luft HS (2002) HMO plan performance update: An analysis of the literature, 1997–2001. *Health Affairs* 21(4): 63–86.

Newhouse JP Insurance Experiment Group (1993) *Free for All? Lessons from the RAND Health Insurance Experiment*. Cambridge, MA: Harvard University Press.

Nyman J (2006) The value of health insurance. In: Jones A (ed.) *The Elgar Companion to Health Economics*, pp. 95–103. Cheltenham/Northampton, UK: Edward Elgar.

Pauly M and Herring B (1999) *Pooling Health Insurance Risks*. Washington, DC: AEI Press.

Pauly MV (1968) The economics of moral hazard: Comment. *American Economic Review* 58(3): 531–536.

Pauly MV (1986) Taxation health insurance, and market failure in the medical economy. *Journal of Economic Literature* XXIV: 629–675.

Prinsze FJ and van Vliet RCJA (2005) *Health-Based Risk Adjustment: Improving the Pharmacy-Based Cost Group Model by Addition of Diagnostic Cost Groups*. Erasmus Medical Centre: Rotterdam Institute of Health Policy and Management.

Rice T (2002) *The Economics of Health Reconsidered*. Chicago, IL: Health Administration Press.

Rocard M (2000) *Report on Supplementary Health Insurance* (A5–0266/2000). Brussels, Belgium: European Parliament.

Tamm M, Tauchmann H, Wasem J, and Greß S (2007) Elasticities of market shares and social health insurance choice in Germany – A dynamic panel data approach. *Health Economics* 16(3): 243–256.

Turquet P (2004) A stronger role for the private sector in France's health insurance? *International Social Security Review* 57(4): 67–90.

van de Ven WPMM and Ellis R (2000) Risk adjustment in competitive health plan markets. Handbook of Health Economics. In: Culyer AJ and Newhouse J (eds.) *Handbook of Health Economics*, pp. 755–845. Amsterdam, the Netherlands: Elsevier.

van de Ven WPMM, Beck K, Buchner F, et al. (2003) Risk adjustment and risk selection on the sickness fund insurance market in five European countries. *Health Policy* 65(1): 75–98.

van de Ven WPMM, van Vliet RCJA, and Lamers LM (2004) Health-adjusted premium subsidies in the Netherlands. *Health Affairs* 23(3): 45–55.

Wagstaff A and van Doorslaer E (1992) Equity in the finance of health care: Some international comparisons. *Journal of Health Economics* 11: 361–387.

Wagstaff A and van Doorslaer E (2000) Equity in health care finance and delivery. Handbook of Health Economics. In: Culyer AJ and Newhouse J (eds.) *Handbook of Health Economics*, pp. 1803–1857. Amsterdam, the Netherlands: Elsevier.

Wasem J, Greß S, and Okma KGH (2004) The role of private health insurance in social health insurance countries. In: Saltman R, Busse R, and Figueras J (eds.) *Social Health Insurance in Western Europe*, pp. 227–247. London: Open University Press.

Zweifel P and Breuer M (2006) The case for risk-based premiums in public health insurance. *Health Economics Policy and Law* 1: 171–188.

Further Reading

Drechsler D and Jütting J (2007) Different countries, different needs: the role of private health insurance in developing countries. *Journal of Health Politics, Policy and Law* 32(3): 497–534.

Eanthoven A and Fuchs V (2006) Employment-based health insurance: Past, present, and future. *Health Affairs* 25(6): 1538–1547.

Gottret P and Schieber G (2006) *Health Financing Revisited. A Practitioner's Guide*. Washington, DC: The World Bank.

Goodmann J (2006) Employer-sponsored, personal and portable health insurance. *Health Affairs* 25(6): 1556–1566.

Hussey P and Anderson GF (2003) A comparison of single- and multi-payer health insurance systems and options for reform. *Health Policy* 66: 215–228.

Maarse H and Paulus A (2003) Has solidarity survived? A comparative analysis of the effect of social health insurance reform in four European countries. *Journal of Health Politics, Policy and Law* 28(4): 585–614.

Mossialos E and Thomson S (2004) *Voluntary Health Insurance in the European Union*. Copenhagen, Denmark: World Health Organization on behalf of the European Observatory on Health Systems and Policies.

The OECD Health Project (2004) *Private Health Insurance in OECD Countries*. Paris, France: OECD.

Sekhri N and Savedoff W (2004) Private Health Insurance: Implications for Developing Countries. *Bulletin of the World Health Organization* 83: 127–134.

van Doorslaer E and Wagstaff A (1999) The redistributive effect of health care finance in twelve OECD countries. *Journal of Health Economics* 18(3): 291–313.

Woolhandler S and Himmelstein D (2002) Paying for national health insurance – And not getting it. *Health Affairs* 21(4): 88–98.

Community Health Insurance in Developing Countries

B Criel, M-P Waelkens, and W Soors, Public Health Department Prince Leopold Institute of Tropical Medicine, Antwerp, Belgium
N Devadasan, Institute of Public Health, Bangalore, India
C Atim, PATH Malaria Vaccine Initiative, France

© 2008 Elsevier Inc. All rights reserved.

Scope and Origin of an Evolving Approach

Community Health Insurance (CHI) is an exciting yet elusive concept. Indeed, the term CHI covers a wide variety of health insurance schemes, each in its distinctive setting and each designed for different population groups. In theory, there are five characteristics that CHI schemes all share:

- solidarity, where risk sharing is as inclusive as possible and membership premiums are independent of individual health risks;
- community-based social dynamics, where the schemes are organized by and for individuals who share common characteristics (geographical, occupational, ethnic, religious, gender, etc.);
- participatory decision making and management;
- nonprofit character;
- voluntary participation.

In practice however, all CHI schemes apply all of these principles to a greater or lesser extent. Schemes set up by health-care providers, for example, might not permit the full development of participatory decision making and management. A trade union might decide to make subscription to a CHI scheme compulsory for its affiliates, thus not upholding the principle of voluntary participation.

In the English-language literature, the term CHI is the phrase used to describe all such schemes. Less common is the descriptor mutual health organization, although its French equivalent *Mutuelle de Santé* is widely employed in francophone Africa. In West Africa especially, the social and political dimensions of CHI come to the forefront and scheme management relies considerably on community participation. On the other hand in East Africa, where provider-driven schemes are encountered more frequently, the financial dimensions of CHI attract more attention. This latter approach to CHI is reflected in the use of the term health micro insurance, a phrase endorsed over recent years by the International Labour Organization (ILO). The ILO denomination is, however, less specific than CHI, as it does not refer to participatory decision making or to the independence of premium calculation from individual health risks. CHI is concentrated in, but not limited to, the informal labor sector. Resource-pooling initiatives taken by workers' organizations in the formal sector, in search of better access to health care, are also included. CHI is not necessarily an informal business either: The insurance may be purchased from an existing insurance company, as is often the case in India.

The wide variety of CHI models has led to various attempts at classification (Bennett *et al.*, 1998). Until now, CHI has been classified by ownership, management, membership, and risk coverage:

- Classification by ownership refers to the initiator of a CHI scheme rather than to strict legal ownership. Essentially, such a scheme can be initiated and run by a group of people with similar health-care needs (community-based) or by a health-care provider (provider-driven). By extension, a community-based scheme can also be owned by representative organizations within a community, for example, a nongovernmental organization (NGO) or a trade union. Provider-driven schemes can further be categorized according to the character of the provider. Common examples include faith-based providers wishing to improve access to their health-care facilities, other private providers wanting to improve income flow, or governmental institutions attempting to implement CHI at the district level.
- Classification by management differentiates between schemes on the basis of organization and control and is thus somewhat more specific. A CHI scheme can either be managed by elected representatives of the membership, by an NGO with existing connections to the scheme, or by a health-care provider, or the management may be contracted out to a third party such as a professional insurer.
- Classification by membership can provide useful additional information. Membership of a CHI scheme may be defined on a geographical basis (for example, people living in the same village or district, or using the same health facility), on the grounds of occupation, ethnicity, religion or gender, or on membership in another organization.
- Classification by risk coverage distinguishes between CHI schemes covering infrequent but costly events (such as hospital admissions) and those covering common low-cost events (e.g., first-line consultations). Such a distinction assumes a direct relation between high-cost events and high risk, whereas others have

reported that frequent low-cost events can also lead to catastrophic health expenditure (Segall *et al.*, 2000). In addition, classification by risk coverage is becoming obsolete since more and more CHI schemes set out to cover both high-cost and low-cost events, and – in some cases – even indirect costs.

It is essential to consider CHI within the framework of health insurance as a whole and to highlight both the common features and the distinctions that exist across commercial, community, and social health insurance schemes (see **Table 1**). All three types of schemes, being risk-sharing arrangements, accomplish risk reduction by pooling prepaid premiums in a fund earmarked for the health-care expenses of their affiliates. What differentiates them is a series of characteristics based on their different rationale, resulting in a narrower or broader insurance spectrum:

- Commercial health insurance generally operates in a private-for-profit environment. Premiums are a function of the expected cost of health care and set on the basis of individual risk assessment of the client. Clients with high health risks pay more, while those with low health risks pay less. Solidarity and cross-subsidy play no role. Subscription is usually voluntary.
- CHI – as already described in this section – thrives on community solidarity and has a social purpose in a private nonprofit environment. Premiums are generally fixed according to the risk faced by the average scheme member, i.e., a system of community rating, independent of individual income. Thus there is an element of cross-subsidy from the healthier to the less healthy but not from richer to poorer affiliates, except where the very poor are exempted from premium payments. Subscription is usually voluntary.
- Social health insurance (SHI) pursues nationwide risk sharing from a public rights-based perspective and in a nonprofit environment. Premiums are generally proportional to income, independent of the individual risk, and paid principally by employees and their employers through legislation and financial levies. SHI implies both cross-subsidy from the healthy to those with poor health, and from the rich to the poor, provided that affiliation is mandatory and universal.

In the European countries where it originated, social health insurance (the so-called Bismarck model, referring to the German chancellor Otto von Bismarck who introduced the first national compulsory health insurance scheme in 1884) delivers almost universal coverage, thus maximizing the benefits of solidarity. Non-European high-income countries such as Japan and the Republic of Korea followed a similar path. Other European countries attained the same goal by providing tax-financed health care (the so-called Beveridge model, referring to the British academician William Beveridge whose 1942 Report to the Parliament on Social Insurance and Allied Services was at the basis of the National Health Service's establishment in 1948). The financing models on which both systems are based are far from incompatible and blends of both models are the rule rather than the exception. The fact that Bismarck included state subsidies in the first SHI scheme is often overlooked. Recent history shows that SHI systems in the world increasingly rely on revenue from general taxation, partly in response to the explosion of health-care costs that occurred in the late twentieth century and the need to subsidize or pay for the contributions of vulnerable groups such as the unemployed and low-income pensioners. With health insurance defined as effective health-care risk protection, a national pool of tax contributions to pay individual health-care expenses can be seen as the consummate manifestation of the health insurance function. From this perspective, a British citizen is equally as well insured as his German counterpart, albeit without a formal insurance arrangement (Kutzin, 1998). Clearly, the successes of both the Bismarck and the Beveridge models are related to a particular context: Combinations of civic voice, political stability, government stewardship, and administrative competence that most developing countries can only covet (Criel and Van Dormael, 1999). Only a few low- and middle-income countries share these characteristics and were able to approximate universal coverage. Historic examples are Costa Rica (by and large following the SHI path) and

Table 1 Types of health insurance

Commercial health insurance	Community health insurance	Social health insurance
Private for-profit rationale	Private nonprofit rationale	Public nonprofit rationale
Premium is a function of individual risk	Premium is a function of average risk	Premium is a function of individual income
Limited cross-subsidy from the healthier to the less healthy	Cross-subsidy from the healthier to the less healthy	Cross-subsidy from the healthier to the less healthy
No cross-subsidy from the wealthier to the less wealthy	Limited cross-subsidy from the wealthier to the less wealthy	Cross-subsidy from the wealthier to the less wealthy
Individual or corporate client	Member of a community	Citizen of a state
Usually voluntary affiliation	Usually voluntary affiliation	Mandatory affiliation

Cuba (using state revenues). In most developing countries, neither of the two models succeeded. Most developing countries' social health insurance systems remained at best highly fragmented (of which core exemplars can be found in Latin America) or restricted to civil servants (typical of Africa). The case of Africa is illuminating: In the 1960s and 1970s, neither SHI nor free health care at the point of use brought the desired welfare state any closer. In fact, both SHI and the free care concept were inherited from colonial powers and lacked the underpinning of autonomous socio-political development (Criel, 1998). During the 1970s, the African public health systems deteriorated in parallel with the deepening economic crisis. From the 1980s on, the introduction of user fees further impeded access to care, in Africa as elsewhere. In many cases, it was the emergence of widespread problems with exclusion from effective health care that prompted the development of CHI in the late 1980s and early 1990s.

Community Health Insurance in Africa

CHI in Africa must be seen in the context of large majorities within the population trapped in poverty and excluded from formal social security systems. The African CHI movement was started out of a concern to either improve access to health care for a greater proportion of the population or to ensure a stable source of income for health-care provision or both. The first initiatives were developed under the direction of expatriate development aid workers who were most familiar with the history and operation of Europe's SHI systems. A well-known example is the provider-driven Bwamanda district hospital scheme in the Democratic Republic of Congo that commenced in 1986 with Belgian support. Also in 1986, the first community-based schemes emerged with the inauguration of the Mutuelle Pharmaceutique de Tounouma in Burkina Faso. Over time, different models and blends developed, first in West and Central Africa, followed later by East Africa.

Community Health Insurance in West Africa

From the early 1990s on, the West African CHI movement enjoyed increasing external support – often from organizations that had a strong attachment to the European SHI model. These organizations, such as the International Department of the Belgian Christian Mutualities, organized training sessions for scheme managers, designed technical manuals, and helped create and develop local support organizations. Gradually, governments and donors became interested in the potential of CHI to increase access to health care in adverse conditions. The movement gained strength and in 1998 several African countries, international partners, and local actors met in Abidjan to create the network La Concertation entre les acteurs du développement des mutuelles de santé en Afrique, currently known and referred to as La Concertation. This network supports and monitors the development of CHI schemes, mainly in francophone West Africa.

The rise in CHIs in this region has led to a sixfold overall increase in the number of schemes between 1997 and 2003, as documented by La Concertation in 2004. **Table 2** provides an overview count of the almost 600 CHI initiatives registered in 2003 in francophone

Table 2 Number of CHI schemes in francophone West Africa

	1997	2000	2003				
	Functional schemes	Functional schemes	Functional schemes	Starting up	In difficulty	All	Beneficiaries
Benin	11	23	42	11	0	53	41 428
Burkina Faso	6	26	35	50	4	89	14 873
Cameroon	18	20	22	14	2	38	15 947
Chad	3	4	7	0	0	7	1775
Guinea	6	27	55	44	10	109	84 820
Ivory Coast	0	29	36	1	3	40	527 670
Mali	7	22	51	16	4	71	469 815
Mauritania	0	0	3	4	0	7	13 055
Niger	6	12	9	3	1	13	49 868
Senegal	19	29	79	48	9	136	303 563
Togo	0	7	9	8	0	17	20 011
Total	76	199	348	199	33	580	1 547 825

Inventory by the *Concertation entre les acteurs du développement des mutuelles de santé en Afrique* (http://www.concertation.org), adapted from Ndiaye P, Soors W, and Criel B (2007) A view from beneath: Community health insurance in Africa. *Tropical Medicine and International Health* 12(2): 157–161.

West Africa. Forerunner Senegal ranks first in terms of number of schemes. A closer look at country level discloses not only different speeds of implementation, but also variations in the mode of implementation.

In Mali, the CHI movement benefited from the start of the Technical Union of Community Health Insurance Schemes, the Union Technique de la Mutualité Malienne (UTM). This federation offers urban communities a standard package (called *assurance maladie volontaire*) and rural communities a tailor-made CHI suited to local needs. The Union also acts as an interface between the movement and the government. Initially the UTM targeted organized formal urban workers, but now has extended its reach to include both the informal sector and the rural communities.

In Senegal, CHI schemes extended their remit in the opposite direction, expanding gradually from rural villages to urban and periurban settings and from the informal to the formal sector. New initiatives continue to emerge. Today formal workers are adopting the CHI concept as a welcome complement to bureaucratic social security arrangements with limited coverage. The Senegalese government supports the CHI concept and has provided a legal framework and a strategic plan for CHI development.

Guinea presents yet another particularity: A research project (the PRIMA project: Projet de Recherche sur le Partage du Risque Maladie) set out the stakes back in 1996. More recently the implementation of MURIGA (Mutuelles pour les Risques liés à la Grossesse et à l'Accouchement, i.e., CHI schemes for the management of pregnancy and birth-related risks, which differs from the classical CHI concept by focusing on a narrower target group), provides a possible entry point for yet additional risk sharing among populations.

Burkina Faso worked toward extending of CHI schemes through the medium of the health-care providers themselves, but today community-run CHI schemes are increasingly common. Approximately 40 CHI schemes, representing 20 000 beneficiaries, receive technical support and training from the Réseau d'appui aux mutuelles de santé. The Burkinian government endorses this third-party organization to enhance the negotiation capacity of the demand side, and eventually to contribute to a better-quality health-care supply.

Benin focused on the involvement of locally elected leaders. Cameroon, Niger, and Mauritania became involved only recently in CHI, but are fortunate in being able to rely on strong social and religious networks.

The bulk of West African CHI schemes have less than 1000 members within each scheme, in fact the majority of schemes only count a few hundred members. Moreover, most of them remain firmly linked to a single social setting, such as a village, a neighborhood, or a professional body. These features lead to high transaction costs and limited risk pooling with insufficient and unsustainable coverage of expensive risks, such as surgical interventions or prolonged medical treatment (HIV/AIDS being the most prominent example, but also hypertension, diabetes, etc.). Currently however, West African CHI managers show an increasing interest in creating unions, federations, and networks, in order to increase efficiency and common voice (Waelkens and Criel, 2007).

More than 60% of the West African CHI schemes handle activities in addition to health insurance, especially in Cameroon, Guinea, and Burkina Faso. The provision of microcredits (small loans for poor families) or health care is most likely to be associated with health insurance. This relation runs in both directions: 33% of microcredit schemes report health insurance as an associated activity.

In English-speaking West Africa, the case of Ghana is of particular interest. By 2002, 46 CHI schemes were active, but covered only a fraction of the population. In 2003, the government passed a Health Insurance Act, which significantly changed health financing across the entire country. The aim was to replace out-of-pocket payments (called cash and carry in Ghana) with health insurance, which would meet up to 20% of total health expenditure, while the remaining 80% would be underwritten by the government. This, it was intended, would facilitate less restrictive and more sustainable national health-care financing. In fact, the Health Insurance Act paved the way for scaling up CHI, as a basis for social health insurance in the long run. The act envisaged that every district would set up a district-based CHI scheme, the establishment of a National Health Insurance Council (NHIC, known as the Council) and the creation of a National Health Insurance Fund (NHIF, known as the Fund). The Council accredits and regulates both district-based and other CHI schemes, as well as commercial health insurance schemes. It also manages the Fund, whose main function is to subsidize district-based CHI schemes. The Fund is financed by a combination of earmarked levy proportional to income, a transfer from formal sector social security contributions, general taxation, and donations. By the end of 2005, 83 out of 138 districts boasted a CHI scheme. Most of these schemes provided coverage for between 20% and 40% of their target community. Enrollment at national level has reached 14.4% and is still rising. While implementation continues, some strengths and weaknesses can already be identified. Among the strengths, both cross-subsidies and tax allocations are seen as potentially effective innovations. Among the weaknesses, highly deficient health provision in deprived areas is recognized as an impediment to progress. In between, the combination of relatively low and differential individual contributions with a wide benefit package (first-line and referral care, but no antiretrovirals) is seen as attractive by some but as barely sustainable by others.

Community Health Insurance in East and Central Africa

In East Africa, CHI has recently been enjoying increased attention. In this part of Africa, both health-care providers and governments tend to play a prominent role in the launch and management of CHI schemes.

In Uganda for example, roughly a dozen CHI schemes are in existence. These were created in the late 1990s with the help of British bilateral aid. Nonprofit church-affiliated hospitals manage the majority of these schemes. Only recently, the community-based model – of the type that is common in West Africa – was introduced with support from the Centre International de Développement et de Recherche (CIDR), a French NGO with long-standing experience in West Africa. The importance of CHI is on the wane in Uganda, at least in the public sector where user fees were abolished in 2001. However, it is still a significant force in the private-nonprofit sector, which makes up half of all district hospitals in rural Uganda.

In Kenya, CHI was introduced in 1999–2000 as a result of the first Community Based Health Financing (CBHF) conference held in Uganda in 1998. These pioneering efforts were largely arranged by religious organizations. By 2005, Kenya boasted 32 schemes in various stages of development.

In Tanzania, user fees have progressively replaced financing from general taxation since 1993. As a result, a diversity of insurance configurations has emerged. The compulsory National Health Insurance Scheme (NHIS), which is restricted to civil servants and their families, covers only 3% of the population. A similarly compulsory National Social Security Fund (NSSF) was established for the remaining parts of the formal employment sector. Voluntary health insurance initiatives address the vast informal sector. Since 2002, these initiatives have received technical support from the Tanzania Network of Community Health Funds (TNCHF). There are approximately a dozen provider-driven CHI schemes, most of them based on church-related facilities, together with a few community-based schemes. Alongside these CHI schemes run district-based community health funds (CHF). While the 2001 CHF act made the creation of a community health fund obligatory for every district within a 2-year span, only 67 out of 129 districts had achieved a CHF by the end of 2005. Where a CHF scheme is in place, enrollment rises to approximately 10%. As in other CHI schemes, because of obvious problems in ability to pay, the poorest sectors of the community almost never join. In order to address this problem, the German Technical Cooperation is assisting in the development of a hybrid CHI and social assistance program. In this project, called CHFplus, district councils guarantee to meet the cost of insurance premiums for the very poor, following their identification by the local communities. This innovative concept could be of interest to policy makers and scheme organizers in Tanzania and elsewhere.

In Central Africa, the pioneering Bwamanda scheme in the Democratic Republic of Congo survived political instability, economic decline, and war. Subscription declined during wartime, but began to increase again beginning in 2003. Most impressively, the scheme reported a total of 114 465 members in 2004. A recent survey of 28 Congolese schemes highlighted evidence of a countrywide renewal in CHI activities since 2000, and to a great variety of CHI models (Atim and Criel, 2004).

In Rwanda, the government launched a health center-based CHI program in 1999 as part of the national reconstruction effort, following the 1994 genocide. With the assistance of USAID, 54 *Mutuelles* were implemented in three pilot districts, during 2000 and 2001. By 2005, 19 out of a total of 39 districts had a CHI scheme and a detailed legal framework was established. This determined state-driven approach yielded exceptional enrollment levels (up to 2.5 million people), but also contains inherent weaknesses: Cost-recovery rates are low, the benefit package at the referral level is limited, and peripheral management capacity and performance is frail. Moreover, the pushed-through CHI boom hardly takes account of preceding nongovernmental initiatives, such as prepayment arrangements organized by a number of nonprofit providers. Still, the current Rwandan approach includes promising novel features, such as the prepayment of premiums using microcredits at the community level.

Community Health Insurance in Asia

CHI in Asia began as part of a political process in the middle of the twentieth century. In China, the first medical cooperatives saw the light of day in a few communist-controlled rural areas as far back as the 1940s. This modest initiative eventually led to the nationwide implementation of the Rural Cooperative Medical System (RCMS) in the 1960s, which by the 1970s covered 90% of China's rural population. However, the RCMS collapsed following the market-oriented reforms of the early 1980s and by 2006 had not really recovered. In the Indian subcontinent, the Students Health Home was the first CHI scheme to be recorded, set up by the communist movement in West Bengal back in 1952. It was not until the late 1990s, however, that a crossover between the microfinance movement (which originated mainly as microcredit, but now encompasses a variety of products including microcredit, microsavings, and microinsurance) and CHI initiatives led to a spurt of CHI schemes in both

Bangladesh and India. Except for China and the Indian subcontinent, CHI in Asia – as in Africa – is a relatively recent introduction.

Community Health Insurance in China

The early Medical Cooperatives in the Shanxi, Gansu, and Ningxia provinces were established as a mechanism to help defray the cost of medical treatment and drugs. Initially set up as mutual prepayment funds, they subsisted on the peasants' voluntary contributions in the form of both cash and in-kind payments, as well as initial drug stocks provided by the ruling communist local governments. These initiatives proliferated and gained financial strength during the 1950s, when the communist state organized the agricultural workers into farmer cooperatives and consequently were able to introduce welfare funds at the community level. As an integral part of the collective system for agricultural production and social services, the Rural Cooperative Medical System became a nationwide structure of prepayment schemes for healthcare financing during the 1960s. Most villages funded their Cooperative Medical Scheme from three separate sources: Household health insurance premiums, the collective welfare fund, and state subsidies. Depending on the plan's benefit structure and the village's economic status, the household premium was usually fixed at between 0.5% and 2% of a peasant family's annual income. The welfare fund was a state-defined portion of the village's collective income from agricultural production. Subsidies from upper-level tiers of governments were typically earmarked to compensate health workers and purchase medical equipment. In 1965, the state explicitly encouraged the entire rural sector to adopt the Cooperative Medical Scheme as the mode of financing and organizing health-care services. The resulting community financing and organization model is believed by many to have contributed significantly to the achievements of the Chinese primary care of that era. Between 1949 and 1973, the infant mortality rate was reduced from about 200 per 1000 to 47 per 1000 live births and life expectancy increased from 35 to roughly 65 years. From the late 1960s until 1979, when the process of collectivization began to be reversed, the RCMS covered 90% of China's rural residents.

Due to market-oriented reforms, both the communal administrative structure that employed the health workers and the collective welfare funds (that once counted for 30–90% of the schemes' funding) disappeared. By 1984, population coverage had dropped to less than 5%. Between 1981 and 1993, the contribution made by the RCMS to national health expenditure fell from 20% to 2%. Despite several government-driven attempts to re-establish the RCMS in the second half of the 1990s, by the end of the century 90% of China's rural residents were uninsured (Carrin *et al.*, 1999). Still, the Rural Cooperative Medical System never disappeared entirely from the political agenda. In 2002, the Asian Development Bank made an appeal for its reinstatement, at least in central China's middle-income regions, a plea contingent on renewed and committed government support (Liu *et al.*, 2002). In 2003, China created a new RCMS, based on voluntary participation, co-funded by the local and central government, and managed on county level. Still expanding, the new RCMS covered 641 out of some 2000 counties by mid-2005 and is projected to cover the whole of rural China by 2008.

Community Health Insurance in the Indian Subcontinent

CHI in the Indian subcontinent emerged (though rarely as a stand-alone phenomenon) as an effort to improve access to health care and to protect households from catastrophic medical expenditure. Of the 49 Indian, Nepalese, and Bangladeshi health-related schemes listed in the International Labour Organization inventories (ILO 2003a, 2003b, 2005), all but three piggybacked onto existing organizations drawn from a spectrum that ranged from health-care providers to microfinance institutions, but consisted mainly of broad-spectrum development organizations. Typically, the resulting schemes took the form of NGOs and were able to build on a foundation of trust and financial capability. Most schemes are of relatively recent origin. Out of the 49 schemes mentioned, 30 were started after 1995 and so coincided with the shift of interest by the microfinance sector from microcredits to microinsurance.

The fact that most CHI schemes are NGO-owned still leaves room for organizational diversity. Where the NGO is also the health-care provider – as is more frequently the case in Nepal and Bangladesh than in India – the provider usually runs the scheme. Where the NGO has no health-care functions, it may act as an insurer for the community and purchase care from independent providers. In a third option, which became increasingly popular in India, the NGO purchases insurance – not care – from a formal insurance company. In this so-called partner-agent or linked model, augmented pooling can lead to wider risk sharing (Devadasan *et al.*, 2005). This gain may be overshadowed by several drawbacks: Where the premium and the benefit package is based on actuarial calculations, the premium may be prohibitive or the benefit package too limited. The resulting insurance product cannot be tailored to meet local conditions, while the patient still has to pay up front and reimbursement is often cumbersome. However, this model is still evolving: NGOs are improving their negotiating capacity and insurance companies are continuously adapting their products.

Across the whole Indian subcontinent, CHI focuses on the poorer sections of society: Small farmers, landless laborers, women's groups, self-employed vendors, in fact all communities within the informal sector. Enrollment ranges from a few thousand to several hundred thousand. Most of the Nepalese and Bangladeshi schemes focus on first-line health care, whereas in India the main benefit on offer is reimbursement of hospital costs. In all three countries – and particularly in Nepal and Bangladesh – there are considerable co-payments required. In most schemes, the providers operate either in the private not-for-profit or the private-for-profit sector, seldom in the public sector. Fee-for-service payment is ubiquitous and so is overprescribing. In this scenario, the need for provider regulation is obvious if cost escalation is to be kept under control. Though most of the operating NGOs lack technical expertise and a health-systems perspective, many of them have evolved mechanisms to manage risks (see **Table 3**). The lack of technical expertise led to the inception of microinsurance training centers in India – six by 2006 – encouraged by donors and the insurance industry.

Community Health Insurance in Indonesia, the Philippines, and Cambodia

CHI in Indonesia is mainly of historical interest. From the 1970s onward, the Indonesian government promoted the Dana Sehat (Health Fund) community schemes as an alternative form of health-care financing (Thabrany et al., 2003). The main motive for this top-down approach was to compensate on a nationwide scale for decreased access to care in low-income groups due to increased user fees. Despite renewed efforts to promote CHI, by 1998 only 1.9% of the Indonesian households were members of health funds. The lack of success associated with the Dana Sehat approach can be seen as a quintessential example of inappropriate scaling up, targeting, and implementation. Indeed, the concept was based on the embryonic experience of small NGO schemes during the late 1960s. The targeting of poor households in order to raise health-care finance proved misguided against a background where 80% of the household income is spent on food. Limited fund collection led to limited benefit packages, which in turn discouraged individuals from participation. Dropout rates from the first to the second year ranged from 60% to 90%. The Dana Sehat approach has now been almost completely replaced by a social assistance scheme (SSN), which enables the authenticated poor to access some basic and reproductive health services through a health benefits card.

CHI in the Philippines began life as an effort to improve access to health care among the poor. Many schemes are offshoots of community-based health programs initiated in the 1980s; most of them are cooperative-driven and are plagued by low enrollment (Yap, 2003). In addition, several local government-prompted schemes were set up in the 1990s. At the same time, CHI schemes (alongside health maintenance organizations) were activated by NGOs with external assistance. The Social Health Insurance Networking and Empowerment project (SHINE) anticipated an ongoing attempt to link and to frame these disparate efforts within the central Philippine health insurance corporation (PhilHealth), installed by law in 1995 and whose mission is to ensure universal coverage by 2010.

In contrast, CHI in Cambodia is still at the embryonic stage: The SKY scheme (Khmer acronym for health for our families) was only started in 1998. SKY was introduced by the French NGO GRET (Groupe de Recherche et d'Échanges Technologiques), based on an impact study among clients of a large microfinance program run by the same organization since 1991 (McCord, 2001). Initially offering only a limited-benefit package, the scheme had to overcome high dropout rates and was redesigned several times. In its current form, it offers both insurance for first-line care and hospital care after referral, and uses a vast array of risk-management strategies (see **Table 4**).

Membership has increased significantly since 2004, approaching 8% of its target population. Being the sole example within Cambodia and with still modest coverage, SKY is widely considered by CHI planners to be a case of special interest. Indeed, the scheme exhibits some features that, nowadays, are viewed as promising options in the field of CHI: It has achieved external financing for its administrative costs and has begun to link its activities with existing targeted social assistance programs

Table 3 Risk management in Indian CHI schemes

Risk	Methods used to mitigate risk	Methods not used to mitigate risk
Adverse selection	Definite collection period Definite waiting period Exclusion of pre-existing diseases	Household as enrolment unit Mandatory nature
Patient-induced moral hazard[a]	Co-payments Upper limits	Referral system
Provider-induced moral hazard	Fixed salary for providers	Case-based instead of fee-for-service billing
Fraud	Community checks ID cards for the insured	

[a]Moral hazard refers to a phenomenon according to which insured persons take undue advantage of the health services covered by the scheme because they know they are insured against the cost of such services (patient moral hazard). Moral hazard however also includes prescription abuse by health care providers, or the risk of over-prescription (provider moral hazard).

Table 4 Risk management in the Cambodian SKY scheme

Risk	Methods used to mitigate risk	Methods not used to mitigate risk
Adverse selection	Definite collection period	Mandatory nature
	Definite waiting period	
	Exclusion of membership outside definite groups	
	Exclusion of preexisting diseases	
Patient-induced moral hazard	Co-payments	
	Upper limits	
	Referral system	
Provider-induced moral hazard	Preselection of first-line providers	
	External assessment of first-line providers	
	Capitation payment for hospital care	
	Internal assessment of hospital care	
Fraud	ID passbooks, including the insured's medical history	

(the so-called health equity funds). While administrative cost subsidies are believed to deserve the consideration of international policy makers, it is the latter linkage of health care and social assistance programs that ensures that care reaches those too poor to insure and to that the efficiency of the targeted funds is increased.

Community Health Insurance in Latin America

CHI in Latin America is a marginal phenomenon, especially when compared to the venerable record of social health insurance and the recent expansion of commercial health insurance on the continent, despite the presence of mutual aid societies, which have existed since the nineteenth century. In the context of a highly inegalitarian society, segmented social protection systems and elitist private premiums, exclusion is common practice, also in health. It is the preoccupation with the excluded that gave rise to new CHI initiatives, without, however, really taking off.

Within a small number of case studies analyzed by the International Labour Organization, all such initiatives led to improved access to health care among their target populations, but only a minority were judged to be financially sustainable in the absence of external funding. Even so, most still exist and new schemes are being established. In the light of a growing regional commitment to universal social protection (ECLAC, 2006), it is pertinent to question if and how the scattered Latin American CHI efforts can contribute to this broader development goal.

Roundup of Current and Future Challenges

The growing interest in CHI should not divert the attention from the shortcomings and obstacles that have been reported by many observers. These include a lack of trust among potential members, limited operational capacity – certainly when managed on a voluntary basis – and the weak purchasing power of most schemes (Carrin et al., 2005). Above all, the perceived poor quality of the health care on offer deters people from investing scarce household resources in health insurance (Waelkens and Criel, 2004). Paradoxically, this key obstacle to enrollment is precisely one of the providers' deficiencies that CHI could in some degree counteract.

The advantages and disadvantages of CHI have been the subject of comments by observers representing a range of perspectives: The possible contributions of CHI to equitable health-care access, to health sector financing, to provider responsiveness, and to quality of care. Additionally, CHI can be regarded as a conduit for other developmental objectives aside from health. The increased social control and transparency observed in the presence of a well-implemented CHI scheme may boost sustainable development and democratization at community level. Eventually, CHI may contribute to poverty reduction (Waelkens et al., 2005). These are challenging issues indeed; the bottom line, however, is that our current knowledge remains insufficient to draw definite conclusions. While there is little doubt by now that a CHI scheme can improve access to health care for its members, the evidence on the broader impact of CHI in developing countries is still scanty. For the time being, research into CHI tends to concentrate on the technical and managerial aspects. A more comprehensive evaluation of CHI schemes spanning the full breadth of their sociopolitical, cultural, and economical contexts is needed to assess the performance and potential of CHI.

Equally, guidelines for the implementation of CHI focus on the technical and managerial aspects are needed. Yet, introducing CHI generates complex dynamics: It changes the relationship between patients and healthcare providers, influences the roles of the actors within the health system and the interactions between them, and may introduce new actors hitherto excluded from the decision-making process. Clearly, CHI staff need more than just technical and managerial training and support.

The time has come for research on CHI and implementation of CHI schemes to go hand in hand. Performance of CHI can only benefit from better information, which, in turn, will only be generated by action-oriented research taking into account the broader picture. Essential investigation into the contextual factors that determine the successful development of CHI still has its place. Beyond this, a series of questions remains unanswered:

- How can a better-organized demand side, in effect an insurance scheme, contribute to better quality of care?
- Which mix of interventions, on both the demand and supply sides of the health-care equation, can bring about improvements to the quality of health services?
- What are the broader social and political consequences of CHI?
- How can CHI be scaled up and integrated in a nationwide social protection system for health?
- How can CHI be linked to social assistance for the very poor?
- How can subsidies – whatever their source, be they domestically or externally funded – enhance the development and performance of CHI without damaging the internal dynamics?

CHI is too complex a subject for cavalier treatment. Hence the need to approach the issue from a medium-term perspective, resisting the temptation for quick gains. At best, CHI is one step on the road to sustainable universal coverage, and this needs time to develop properly.

See also: Comparative Health Systems; Health Inequalities; Resource Allocation: International Perspectives on Resource Allocation; Universal Coverage in Developing Countries, Transition to.

Citations

Atim C and Criel B (2004) Faisabilité de la mise en œuvre de mutuelles de santé en République Démocratique du Congo. *Mission report.* Kinshasa Democratic Republic of the Congo: Ministry of Public Health/Belgian Technical Cooperation; Antwerp, Belgium: Institute of Tropical Medicine.

Bennet S, Creese A, and Monasch R (1998) *WHO/ARA/CC/98.1 ARA Paper Number 15: Health Insurance Schemes for People Outside Formal Sector Employment.* Geneva, Switzerland: World Health Organization Division of Analysis Research and Assessment.

Carrin G, Ron A, Hui Y, et al. (1999) The reform of the rural cooperative medical system in the People's Republic of China: Interim experience in 14 pilot counties. *Social Science and Medicine* 48(7): 961–972.

Carrin G, Waelkens M-P, and Criel B (2005) Community-based health insurance in developing countries: A study of its contribution to the performance of health financing systems. *Tropical Medicine and International Health* 10(8): 799–811.

Criel B (1998) *Studies in Health Services Organisation and Policy, 9: District-Based Health Insurance in Sub-Saharan Africa; Part 1: From Theory to Practice.* Antwerp, Belgium: ITG Press.

Criel B and Van Dormael M (1999) Mutual health organizations in Africa and social health insurance systems: Will European history repeat itself? *Tropical Medicine and International Health* 4(3): 155–159.

Devadasan N, Ranson K, Van Damme W, Acharya A, and Criel B (2005) The landscape of community health insurance in India: An overview based on 10 case studies. *Health Policy* 78: 224–234.

Economic Commission for Latin America and the Caribbean (2006) Shaping the future of social protection: Access, financing and solidarity. *Proceedings of the 31st session of ECLAC, March 20–24, 2006,* Montevideo, Uruguay: ECLAC.

International Labour Organization (2003a) *An Inventory of Micro-insurance Schemes in Nepal.* Kathmandu, Nepal: International Labour Office in Nepal.

International Labour Organization (2003b) *Micro-Insurers: Inventory of Micro-insurance Schemes in Bangladesh.* Geneva, Switzerland: International Labour Office Strategies and Tools Against Social Exclusion and Poverty Programme (STEP).

International Labour Organization (2005) *India: An Inventory of Micro-insurance Schemes.* Geneva, Switzerland: International Labour Office Strategies and Tools against social Exclusion and Poverty Programme (STEP).

Kutzin J (1998) Enhancing the insurance function of health systems: A proposed conceptual framework. In: Nitayarumphong S and Mills A (eds.) *Achieving Universal Coverage of Health Care*, pp. 27–101. Nontaburi, Thailand: Ministry of Public Health Office of Health Care Reform.

Liu Y, Rao K, and Hu S (2002) *People's Republic of China: Toward Establishing a Rural Health Protection System.* Manila, Philippines: Asian Development Bank.

McCord MJ (2001) *Microinsurance: A Case Study of an Example of the Provider Model of Microinsurance Provision / GRET Cambodia.* Nairobi, Kenya: MicroSave-Africa.

Ndiaye P, Soors W, and Criel B (2007) A view from beneath: Community health insurance in Africa. *Tropical Medicine and International Health* 12(2): 157–161.

Segall M, Tipping G, Lucas H, et al. (2000) *IDS Research Report 43: Health Care Seeking by the Poor in Transitional Economies: The Case of Vietnam.* Sussex, UK: Institute of Development Studies.

Thabrany H, Gani A, Pujianto Mayanda L, Mahlil, and Budi BS (2003) *Social Health Insurance in Indonesia: Current Status and the Plan for National Health Insurance.* Presented at the Regional Expert Group Meeting on Social Health Insurance WHO/SEARO, New Delhi India March 13–15, 2003. New Delhi, India: WHO/SEARO.

Waelkens M-P and Criel B (2004) *Health Nutrition and Population (HNP) Discussion Paper: Les mutuelles de santé en Afrique sub-Saharienne: état des lieux et réflexions sur un agenda de recherché.* Washington DC: The World Bank.

Waelkens M-P and Criel B (eds.) (2007) *La mise en réseau de mutuelles de santé en Afrique de l'Ouest. L'union fait-elle la force? Enseignements d'un colloque international organisé à Nouakchott Mauritanie, 19 et 20 décembre 2004.* Antwerp, Belgium: ITG Press.

Waelkens M-P, Soors W, and Criel B (2005) *Extension of Social Security (ESS) Paper n°22: The Role of Social Health Protection in Reducing Poverty: The Case of Africa.* Geneva, Switzerland: International Labour Office Strategies and Tools against social Exclusion and Poverty (STEP).

Yap MEC (2003) *An Overview of Community Health Insurance Initiatives in the Philippines.* Presented at the Third Health Sector Development Technical Advisory Group Meeting WHO/WPRO, Manila, the Philippines February 17–19, 2003. Manila, the Philippines: WHO/WPRO.

Further Reading

Carrin G (2003) *Department Health System Financing Expenditure and Resource Allocation (FER), Cluster Evidence and Information for Policy (EIP), Discussion Paper n°1: Community-Based*

Health Insurance Schemes in Developing Countries: Facts, Problems and Perspectives. Geneva, Switzerland: World Health Organization.

Dror DM and Preker AS (2002) *Social Reinsurance: A New Approach to Sustainable Community Health Financing*. Geneva, Switzerland: International Labour Office.

International Labour Organization, Pan American Health Organization (1999) Synthesis of case studies of micro-insurance and other forms of extending social protection in health in Latin America and the Caribbean. *Regional Tripartite Meeting with the Collaboration of PAHO on the Extension of Social Protection in Health to Excluded Groups in Latin America and the Caribbean Mexico DF, Mexico November 29 – December 1, 1999, working document n°5*. Geneva, Switzerland: International Labour Office.

Moens F (1990) Design, implementations, and evaluation of a community financing scheme for hospital care in developing countries: A pre-paid health plan in the Bwamanda health zone, Zaire. *Social Science and Medicine* 30(12): 1319–1327.

Relevant Websites

http://www.ilo.org/public/english/protection/socsec/step/ – International Labour Organization, Strategies and Tools Against Social Exclusion and Poverty (STEP) Programme.

http://www.concertation.org/ – La concertation entre les acteurs du développement des mutuelles de santé en Afrique.

http://www.microinsurancecenter.org/ – microinsurance Center, independent institution promoting the partner-agent model.

http://www.phrplus.org/ – Partners for Health Reform plus, US Agency for International Development's project for health policy and systems strengthening and its successor http://www.healthsystems2020.org/.

http://www.masmut.be/masmut/website/ – Plateforme belge Micro Assurance Santé / Mutuelles de Santé (Belgian platform Community Health Insurance / Mutual Health Organisations).

http://www.who.int/health_financing/en/ – World Health Organization, Health financing policy.

The Demand for Health Care

G Mwabu, University of Nairobi, Nairobi, Kenya

© 2008 Elsevier Inc. All rights reserved.

Introduction

The information generated from health-care demand analysis has a number of potential applications. It can be used to improve access to health services because it shows the factors that affect health service utilization such as household income, distance to health facilities, service availability, health insurance, and prices of the services offered. Moreover, demand analysis can help identify factors that affect patients' perceptions of the quality of medical care, enabling policy makers to implement interventions to change patterns of health service usage in socially desired ways. These issues are important because health care helps the population only when it is used to maintain and promote health or to cure or prevent illnesses. Information on demand patterns could further be used to improve equity in health outcomes because it reveals social groups that are excluded from basic health care due to poverty or other factors. Such health care can then be delivered to vulnerable groups through targeted interventions. Thus, evidence on demand patterns provides policy makers with the information they need to address efficiency and equity issues in health care. Broadly conceived, health-care demand analysis includes investigations into behaviors and practices that improve health.

The article first reviews a unified model of health-care demand that links health service utilization to health production. The analytical and policy strengths of this model lie in the breadth of the issues it is capable of analyzing. It covers demand for marketable commodities, e.g., immunizations and medical treatments, and for non-tradeable inputs into health, such as behavioral changes that promote health. Next, related models of health-care demand are reviewed, emphasizing their policy value and estimation methods. The final section of the article provides perspectives on future research in the modeling of health-care demand.

The Unified Model of Health-Care Demand

Consumer Preferences, Budget Constraints, and Health-Care Use

The economic approach to the analysis of health-care utilization is based on three ideas. The first idea is that people know what they can do to maintain health and prevent or cure illnesses, and they are capable of ranking the actions that can be taken. In other words, people are endowed with the abilities or preferences for ranking health services. The second idea is that the material means that people possess, such as income and assets, limit the type and intensity of the actions they can take to maintain or promote health. This limitation arises from the fact that health services, like other goods, have prices that consumers must pay directly or indirectly given limited incomes or assets. The third idea is that, faced with this limitation, people try to do the best for themselves. Expressed strongly, the idea says that people make choices and behave in ways that enable them to maximize the benefits from health-care consumption given their income or wealth. This maximization hypothesis is the cornerstone of much economic analysis, including demand analysis. Not surprisingly, the hypothesis is the subject of intense debate in the health-care demand literature. Since individuals and households possess limited information about health care, the assumption that this care is optimally used to confront illnesses is too strong. For example, the assumption is contradicted by consumption behaviors that harm health, such as smoking, drug abuse, and unhealthy eating habits. Economists have to date not been able to respond convincingly to the persistent criticism that people do not possess the ability and the information required to engage in optimizing behavior. However, in order to derive the strong prediction of demand theory, that people respond to price incentives, a view on optimization assumption is required. Economists generally assume that people behave as if their purpose in life is to do the best for themselves using their scarce resources. This assumption permits a straightforward derivation of policy relevant prediction of demand models that is generally in agreement with everyday experience. For example, the models predict that people will reduce consumption of health-care services if health-care prices are increased, provided that other factors such as income and the disease environment remain the same. Policy makers can use estimation results from these models to set appropriate prices for health-care services. Indeed, information on demand parameters is essential for evidence-based financing of health services.

The Unified Model

The unified model of health-care demand was developed by Grossman (1972) and Rosenzweig and Schultz (1982). An important property of the model is that the production of health is embedded in the utility maximizing behavior of a household member. The household member is assumed to have preferences over health-neutral goods, health-related goods, and over the health status. To simplify the analysis, it is usually assumed that the household members share the same preferences about health care and other commodities. Under this assumption, all household members act as one unit when demanding health-care services so that the utility function of any member can be expressed as:

$$U = U(X, Y, H) \qquad [1]$$

where,

- X = a vector of health-neutral goods, i.e., commodities or services that yield utility, U, to an individual but have no direct effect on health status of the person demanding the goods, for example, bus transport or consumption of electricity;
- Y = a vector of health-related goods that impact on the utility of an individual and also affect his or her health status, e.g., quantity of smoking and alcohol consumption or sports activities;
- H = health status of an individual.

The health production technology of the individual is given by:

$$H = F(Y, Z, \mu) \qquad [2]$$

where,

- Z = a vector of health services or health investment goods, such as medical care and immunizations that affect health status directly;
- μ = a random component of health due either to genetic or environmental conditions.

The goods represented by vectors Y and Z in eqns [1] and [2] may also be viewed as health inputs into the production of health.

An individual acts as if his or her purpose is to maximize eqn [1] given eqn [2] subject to a linear budget constraint of the form:

$$I = XP_x + YP_y + ZP_z \qquad [3]$$

where,

- I is exogenous income;
- P_x, P_y, and P_z are, respectively, the vectors of prices of the health-neutral goods, X, health-related consumer goods, Y, and health investment goods, Z.

Notice from eqns [1] and [2] that the vector of health investment goods, Z, enters an individual's utility function only through H.

Equation [2] describes health production at the individual level. As noted previously, the health production function is imbedded in the utility function. Expressions [1]–[3] can be manipulated to yield the demand functions of the following general form

$$X = D_x(P_x, P_y, P_z, I, \mu) \qquad [4.1]$$

$$Y = D_y(P_x, P_y, P_z, I, \mu) \qquad [4.2]$$

$$Z = D_z(P_x, P_y, P_z, I, \mu) \qquad [4.3]$$

In the ensuing discussion, reference is made mainly to eqn [4.3] above, as it is the only direct demand function for health services in the equation system [4.1–4.3]. Equation [4.3] states that the empirical health service demand, i.e., the observed health service utilization pattern, is a function of exogenous prices, P, exogenous income, I, and μ. The term exogenous in this context means that over the relevant period, the household is powerless to change the key factors that determine health-care demand, namely, the commodity prices, income, and unobserved parameter μ. This demand function is to be understood as a quantity–price relationship. That is, the function depicts how the utilization of a particular health service is affected by its own prices holding other factors constant. Other relevant factors that can easily be incorporated in the equation include the time prices of using the health service in question and education, age, gender, and location of patients or their households.

Equation [4.3] can be used to estimate the effect of the price of a health service on the demand for that service; this is called the own-price effect. It can also be used to estimate the impact of the price of other goods on the demand for the health service, called the cross-price effect. An interesting cross-effect that can be estimated is the impact of the price of a health-neutral good on health-care demand. This cross-price effect, like all price effects, manifests itself through the budget constraint. It is possible to demonstrate through further manipulation of eqn [4.3] that efficacy of medical care is a key parameter in demand predictions (see Rosenzweig and Schultz, 1983). That is, in order to accurately predict the demand for health services, information is needed both on the effectiveness of medical treatments and on the estimated impacts of prices and incomes.

The estimates of the parameters of the unified model can reveal through eqn [2], the direct effects of medical care services (Z) on health, thus helping both policy makers and households to prioritize medical care expenditures. The estimates could further be used to assess the impacts of a whole range of behaviors (Y) on health. The unified demand model has been used to investigate determinants of birth weight in both developed and developing countries. For example, in the United States, Rosenzweig and Schultz (1982), showed that smoking during pregnancy and delay in using prenatal care reduce birth weight. African evidence generated using the model shows that tetanus immunization during pregnancy is associated with improvements in birth weight (Dow *et al.*, 1999).

Refinements and Extensions

In the framework presented in eqns [1]–[4], health-care demands and behaviors are inputs into the production of health. Thus, the amount of health produced and the quantities of the inputs used to produce it are determined by households in consultation with health-care providers.

As previously noted, the motivation for the unified model is to answer the policy question: How does utilization of health-care services affect health? In order to answer this question well, eqn [2] must be estimated using a special econometric technique known as the two-stage least squares (TSLS) method (Wooldridge, 2002). In the first stage of the technique, health-care demand equations are estimated using exogenous prices and incomes as explanatory variables. In the second stage, demands predicted from those first-stage equations are used to estimate the health production function (Wooldridge, 2002). This procedure permits a statistically correct identification and measurement of the effect of health-care services on health. Despite the attractiveness of the unified model, the data required for its estimation may not exist. Moreover, by making some reasonable assumptions about the correlation between health-care utilization and health status, much simpler demand models can be specified and estimated.

Reduced-Form Demand Models

Under the assumption that health-care consumption improves health, there is no need to estimate equation [2]. In that case, only the demand for health care, such as equation [4.3] needs to be estimated. The estimation can properly be accomplished using a simpler method such as the ordinary least squares (OLS). The demand specifications of this kind are known as reduced-forms because the underlying causal processes are not analyzed.

There are many situations where reduced-form demand functions for health care are appropriate to estimate. If it is known, for instance, that treatment for a particular disease such as tuberculosis is effective in curing the disease, the policy interest there is to identify the factors influencing the demand for TB treatment, rather than an assessment of its efficacy. Similarly, if the effectiveness of a particular vaccine is already established, the issue of policy interest is the estimation of demand for the vaccine, not whether the vaccine works. In reduced-form demand specifications where health status is included in the utility function, the health status can also depend on household characteristics such as education and gender. These characteristics are easy to incorporate in a reduced-form health-care demand, such as eqn [4.3].

Demand quantities based on the utility function of the form shown in eqn [1] usually reflect continuous health-care choices of households. That is, the households are assumed to continue to consume the same type of health care but in different quantities when its determinants such as prices and incomes change. However, in many situations, households shift completely from one form of health care to another when demand determinants change. These discrete changes in health-care demands are analyzed using probability models of choice.

Discrete Choice Health-Care Demands

A large literature exists on discrete choice health-care models (see Culyer and Newhouse, 2000; Sahn et al., 2003). The models have been used extensively to study health service utilization in developed and developing countries. Results from these studies show that changes in relative prices shift households from one health-care sector to another. In particular, an increase in user fees at government health facilities in developing countries has been shown to shift patients from these clinics to traditional and informal medications of low quality. The results suggest that health-care financing methods can have major effects on population health and should be designed with care. Information on health-care-seeking behavior obtained using discrete choice models of health-care demand can help in designing appropriate health-care financing policies. A related and consistent finding from the discrete choice demand literature is that the poor and the vulnerable groups are very sensitive to price changes. Thus, in the event of an increase in the cost of drugs or consultation, for example, health-care utilization by the poor is reduced proportionately more than that of the non-poor. This finding can be used to target public subsidies within the health sector in ways that improve equity in health service utilization. The literature further shows that service quality is a key determinant of patients' choice of medical facilities and of the intensity at which the facilities are used. Information on determinants of the quality of care can be used to increase health-care utilization by the population without changing the existing service costs. For example, the information can be used to encourage mothers to deliver at the health facilities rather than at home. Despite these advantages of discrete choice models, their estimation can be very demanding in data and skill requirements (see Culyer and Newhouse, 2000).

Information Imperfections and the Demand for Health Care

In the unified demand model and its variants, households are assumed to possess perfect information about all aspects of medical care, such as the prices being charged at different health facilities, and the quality or efficacy of the services offered. In a setting in which households are imperfectly informed about medical care, quality is an overriding determinant of demand. Health care is sought because it increases the probability of maintaining good health or of being cured or the probability of preventing an illness (see Leonard, 2003).

If households have little or no information about the benefits of health services, they might not use them even when provided free of charge. Thus, institutions that help households to learn about health-care quality can have an important impact on demand. The agency relationship that universally exists between the patient and a health-care provider is the prime example of an institution that ideally solves the information problem just noted. That is, since a health-care provider is trained in diagnosis and treatment of illness, she is knowledgeable enough to decide the type and quantity of care for the patient upon being consulted. However, even in a situation where the provider has full information about disease diagnosis and treatment, she cannot accurately predict the effect of treatment prescribed, because the patient might not comply with that treatment. As regards the patient, he too cannot tell whether the provider is using her medical expertise to the fullest extent possible or in his best interest. Thus, in practice, the standard agency relationship presented in the literature does little to assure either the provider or the patient as to the quality of care being provided. The reason is that health-care quality, i.e., the probability of prescribed treatment maintaining health or curing a disease, also depends on unobservable efforts of both the caregiver and the patient. Leonard (2003) has shown that an implicit contract between the caregiver and the patient that allows the cost of treatment to be paid after its effect on illness has been observed improves the standard agency relationship, thereby increasing the demand for health care. The outcome-contingent payment mechanism increases demand, both because it reduces the patient's risk of receiving ineffective treatment and because it provides an incentive for the caregiver to provide quality treatment so that she can be paid.

The market for health-care services offered by traditional healers, particularly in Africa, offers an excellent opportunity to study the effect of outcome-contingent payment mechanisms on health-care demand. The healers are able to enforce the implicit contract surrounding the outcome-contingent payment method because of the powers that social belief systems in some societies ascribe to them. For example, in many rural communities in Africa, healers are believed to have the power to harm patients who refuse to pay agreed fees after successful treatment. Because of their fear of this power, patients pay treatment fees voluntarily after being cured.

Leonard (2003) shows that poor households in rural Cameroon rely importantly on traditional healers for medical treatments. Patients from poor households preferred traditional healers partly because of the outcome-contingent contracts that offered them a form of credit, and partly due to the quality of the healers' services, as measured by the unobservable effort they devoted to treating long-lasting illnesses. As producers of health, patients and households work better with healers than with modern health caregivers to treat chronic illnesses.

One may doubt whether outcome-contingent payment systems are applicable in other settings. However, there is evidence that equivalent payment systems can be designed. For example, the Grameen bank model of credit extension to poor people, especially women, without them offering any collateral, which originally started in Bangladesh (Yunus, 2006), has some parallels with the outcome-contingent payment for traditional medicine in Africa. In a Grameen bank context, the peer pressure to honor a loan agreement and the social networks through which the borrower is monitored guarantee repayment, whereas in the traditional medicine context, credit repayment is ensured by the collective belief that the healer has the power to harm defaulters. In both cases, institutions play a role in repayment. In the African context, the debtor is anonymous, but the sharing of the common belief as to the powers of the healers leads to repayment. In the context of a *grameen* (i.e., village) bank, the debtor is known to peers and to other village members, and this puts pressure on the debtor not to defray the loan to avoid punishment such as ostracism from a group. The great lesson from the Grameen model of credit extension for health-care financing is that there are substitutes to collaterals in the credit market. Because nonpayment of credit by a group member can reduce creditworthiness of the whole group, the group has an incentive to devise mechanisms to help a lender recover a loan. Thus, group reputation, which is valued in the marketplace, serves as a collateral for credit. Yunus (2006) has strongly argued that institutions might exist or could be created that can allow extension of credit to beggars with a small risk of default.

The performance-based payment contracts in modern health-care financing systems in industrialized countries are not too different from the outcome-contingent contracts in agrarian, traditional settings because they rely on verification of the quantity and quality of health care provided and on application of commonly agreed rules for reimbursement, backed by an enforceable legislation. Under this system, the patient or his representative knows he would be legally compelled to pay if he defaults, so he pays. Similarly, the caregiver knows he would not be paid if his performance is found to be inadequate; so he tries to put forth a sufficient amount of unobservable effort. This situation is quite similar to the case of traditional medicine in Africa where outcome-based contracts are prevalent.

Time, Self-Control, and Behavioral Change

As noted previously, it is fairly straightforward to introduce the time cost in the unified demand model outlined in the section titled 'The unified model of health-care demand.' Patients often incur substantial opportunity costs in terms of the time they spend to travel to sources of treatment and to wait for treatment there. Thus, time costs affect health-care demand. However, in the models discussed so far, the effect of time on the health-care making process itself, is rarely analyzed. Instead, what is analyzed is the effect of the time cost on the outcome of that decision process. For example, if the outcome of the decision process is to seek health care outside the home, the time cost will determine the facility chosen, other things constant. Typically, empirical demand analysis of this kind (Sahn *et al.*, 2003) is conducted over short durations in a life cycle, such as 2 weeks or 1–3 months, i.e., the durations over which health service utilization data are available.

However, if health-care decisions are examined from the perspective of the life cycle of an individual, the length of time involved could alter both the benefits expected from health care and the ability to implement health-care decisions made in the previous period. For example, a smoker might decide to quit smoking today, but fail to implement this decision in subsequent periods, a behavior that is inconsistent with his rational decision-making processes at different points in time. People who display this type of behavior are, for obvious reasons, said to have time-inconsistent preferences. The reasons for this behavior might include the nature of time discount rates and attitudes toward risk. Since persons with time-inconsistent preferences lack self-control, with regard to consumption that is harmful to health, a study designed to generate information to help them change behavior should not focus on their demand for addictive substances, but on things that strengthen their decisions against addiction. In the case of smoking, such a study could investigate the effects of smoking bans on smokers' intentions to quit smoking. Persons who want to quit smoking but cannot do so for lack of self-control, would support bans on cigarettes or increases in cigarette prices (Kan, 2007), because such policies help them achieve their intentions. This is an example of how demand analysis can be used to uncover and implement policies that induce health-improving behaviors. A similar analysis can be extended to socially undesirable lifestyles, such as relationships involving multiple sexual partners that need to be understood when designing policies to control HIV/AIDS (Over *et al.*, 2006).

Conclusion and Perspectives on Future Research

This study has demonstrated how health-care demand can be linked to health production so that demand information can be used to design and implement strategies for improving health. Since the resources available to finance health-care consumption are scarce, it is important to assess effects of such consumption on health. Linking health-care demand estimates to health production facilitates such an assessment. The article has further shown how information asymmetries and risks in health care can be incorporated in the standard models of demand to improve their predictive powers and policy relevance. Future research on health-care demand should focus on these newer modeling efforts, using data from both household surveys and field experiments to test the hypotheses generated by the models.

Although the focus of the chapter has been on microeconomic aspects of health-care demand, macroeconomic models of health care would generate valuable information for formulating national-level policies to improve health. At the international level, research on demand for global public health goods, e.g., the protection against current pandemics such as HIV/AIDS and related diseases such as tuberculosis and cancer, as well the emerging contagious infections such as avian flu and severe acute respiratory syndrome is needed in view of a rapidly globalizing world.

See also: Demand and Supply of Human Resources for Health.

Citations

Culyer AJ and Newhouse JP (eds.) (2000) *Handbook of Health Economics*. Amsterdam, The Netherlands: the North-Holland.

Dow WH, Philipson TJ, and Sala-i-Martin X (1999) Longevity complementaries under competing risks. *American Economic Review* 89(5): 1358–1371.

Grossman M (1972) On the concept of health capital and the demand for health. *Journal of Political Economy* 80(2): 223–255.

Kan K (2007) Cigarette smoking and self-control. *Journal of Health Economics* 26: 61–81.

Leonard KL (2003) African traditional healers and outcome-contingent contracts in health care. *Journal of Development Economics* 71(1): 1–22.

Over M, Marseille E, Sudhakar K, et al. (2006) Antiretroviral therapy and HIV prevention in India: Modeling costs and consequences of policy options. *Sexually Transmitted Diseases* 33(10): S145–S152.

Rosenzweig MR and Schultz T (1982) The behavior of mothers as inputs to child health: The determinants of birth weight, gestation, and the rate of fetal growth. In: Fuchs V (ed.) *Economic Aspects of Health*, pp. 53–92. Chicago, IL: The University of Chicago Press.

Sahn DE, Younger SD, and Genicot G (2003) The demand for health care services in rural Tanzania. *Oxford Bulletin of Economics and Statistics* 65(2): 241–259.

Wooldridge JM (2002) *Econometric Analysis of Cross-Section and Panel Data*. Cambridge, MA: MIT Press.

Yunus M (2006) Nobel lecture. The Official Web Site of the Nobel Foundation, http://nobelprize.org/nobel_prizes/peace/laureates/2006/yunus-lecture-en.html.

Further Reading

Becker GS (1981) *A Treatise on the Family*. Cambridge, MA: Harvard University Press.

Deaton A (1997) *The Analysis of Household Surveys: A Microeconometric Approach to Development Policy*. Baltimore, MD: Johns Hopkins University Press.

Friedman M (1953) *Essays in Positive Economics*. Chicago, IL: University of Chicago Press.

Rosenzweig MR and Schultz TP (1983) Estimating a household production function: Heterogeneity, the demand for health inputs, and their effects on birth weight. *Journal of Political Economy* 91(5): 723–746.

Zweifel P and Breyer F (1997) *Health Economics*. New York: Oxford University Press.

Long Term Care, Organization and Financing

M Knapp and A Somani, London School of Economics and Political Science, London, UK

© 2008 Elsevier Inc. All rights reserved.

Introduction

Long-term care comprises a set of nonmedical as well as medical services delivered to individuals who have lost some capacity for self-care because of chronic illness or disability. It differs from other types of health care in that its primary goal is not to cure ill health but to allow individuals to achieve and maintain optimal levels of personal functioning. Promotion of quality of life is a core aim. Long-term care can therefore include provision of medical care, but tends to be more closely associated with an array of social, personal, and supportive services that provide help with domestic tasks (such as shopping, cleaning, preparing meals), personal care tasks (dressing, bathing), and personal concerns (safety). Specialized housing might be provided.

Most of the long-term care received by people who live at home is provided by family members or other informal (unpaid) carers. But, as we shall describe later, in most high-income countries, there has been a gradual shifting of the balance of care – away from the family and toward formal care services delivered by paid staff employed by health-care agencies, municipalities, voluntary (nonprofit, nongovernmental) organizations or private sector bodies.

Other key parameters of a long-term care system vary quite noticeably from country to country, again as we discuss later. The mechanisms used to finance long-term care can include collectively organized risk-pooling arrangements such as social insurance or tax-based funding, but across much of the world there is still heavy reliance on privately financed care, whether through out-of-pocket payments (user charges) or voluntary insurance policies. Another variable is the locus of care, with countries choosing to rely to differing degrees on residential forms of provision such as nursing homes, staffed care facilities and long-stay hospital wards. It is generally held to be preferable to provide long-term care in ordinary community settings, such as an individual's own home, although this is not always easy to achieve. Another relevant parameter is the balance between provider sectors, with some long-term care systems heavily reliant on public services and others dominated by services delivered by private and voluntary sector bodies.

Long-term care services are used by people with chronic health and related conditions. Older people are particularly heavy users of such services, and this pattern will undoubtedly persist given the aging of the world's population. We focus primarily on this age group.

Demographic Change

Population aging is a worldwide phenomenon. The challenge that this generates can be illustrated for some European countries (**Table 1**). Countries such as Germany and Italy, for example, are expected to see decreases in total population between 2004 and 2050, whereas the Irish population is expected to grow by more than a third, and the population of Sweden by 13%. Generally, high-income countries will see decreases in the population aged 15–64, conventionally the most productive ages in terms of contributions to national economies. Projected changes in the older population (age 65 and above) will be pronounced. For example, in the UK there were 9.5 million older people in 2004, projected to almost double to 17 million by 2050. Of more interest for long-term care systems is the expected growth in the old old age group. For example, again looking at the UK, there is a projected increase of 150% in the number of people aged 80 or above, but this pales by comparison to Ireland, Spain, the Netherlands, and Germany.

Central to many concerns about future long-term care arrangements is the demographic balance between dependent older people and the labor force. The ratio of the population aged 65 or older to those aged 15–64 is already quite high in Italy, Germany, France, and Spain, and by 2020 will be much higher (**Table 2**).

Why are these demographic patterns important? Use of long-term care and medical services is high among older people, and an aging population will inevitably put growing pressure on care services. This can be illustrated by projections of needs and expenditure for England using the Personal Social Services Research Unit (PSSRU) model (Wittenberg et al., 2006). The model has projected that the number of occupied residential places (in residential care homes, nursing homes, hospitals) would need to expand by 115% between 2002 and 2041 just to keep pace with demographic change, while care support for older people in their own homes would need to increase by 103%. But these needs could be much higher if the proportion of older people who are dependent increases (perhaps because people with high care needs survive into old age as a result of improvements in medical technology), or if quality of care improvements are demanded by future cohorts of service users, or family members are less able or willing to provide unpaid care for dependent older relatives (perhaps because of changing labor force participation patterns and geographical mobility).

The PSSRU model estimates that long-term care expenditure would need to increase by 325% in real

Table 1 Overview of the projected changes in the size and age structure of some European populations, in millions

	Population (total)			Older population (ages 65+)			Very old population (ages 80+)		
	2004	2050	% Change	2004	2050	% Change	2004	2050	% Change
Denmark	5.4	5.5	2	0.8	1.4	7	0.2	0.5	140
France	59.9	65.1	9	9.8	17.4	94	2.6	6.9	163
Germany	82.5	77.7	−6	14.9	23.3	105	3.4	9.9	187
Ireland	4.0	5.5	36	0.4	1.4	12	0.1	0.4	313
Italy	57.9	53.8	−7	11.1	18.2	89	2.8	7.2	158
Netherlands	16.3	17.6	8	2.3	4.3	26	0.6	1.6	191
Spain	42.3	43.0	1	7.1	15.0	99	1.8	5.3	199
Sweden	9.0	10.2	13	1.5	2.5	12	0.5	0.9	95
UK	59.7	64.2	8	9.5	17.0	93	2.6	6.5	150

From ECFIN (2006) The impact of ageing on public expenditure: Projections for the EU25 Member States on pensions, health care, long-term care, education and unemployment transfers (2004–2050). European Economy Special Report. http://ec.europa.eu/economy_finance/publications/european_economy/2006/eespecialreport0106_en.htm

Table 2 Ratio of the population aged 65 and older to population aged 15–64

	2005	2010	2015	2020
Australia	24.1	26.2	30.5	35.3
Canada	22.6	24.7	29.0	33.8
Denmark	28.6	31.6	36.5	40.9
France	37.0	38.9	45.5	51.4
Germany	37.5	41.2	42.2	45.2
Ireland	21.2	21.6	23.7	26.1
Italy	44.3	46.7	50.7	54.5
Japan	32.0	37.8	45.3	50.5
Netherlands	25.3	27.6	32.1	35.3
New Zealand	21.3	23.0	27.0	31.3
Norway	26.6	27.5	30.6	33.8
Spain	36.1	37.4	39.7	42.3
Sweden	33.5	36.7	41.6	45.5
US	20.9	22.2	25.1	29.1
UK	29.5	31.2	35.5	38.8

From OECD (2006) *OECD Factbook 2006: Economic Environmental and Social Statistics*. Paris: Organisation for Economic Co-operation and Development.

terms between 2002 and 2041 to meet demographic pressures and allow for expected real rises in unit costs. Projections of this kind are subject to uncertainty, of course, but they vividly illustrate why there is so much discussion of population aging and its implications.

Mixed Economy of Care

One of the complications in planning long-term care is that many older people have multiple needs. If a care system is well developed and adequately resourced it is likely that these needs will be identified, assessed, and addressed by a variety of agencies. Thus, for example, there might be roles for health services, social care, housing providers, social security agencies, and others in supporting older people. The financing arrangements could be very different between these agencies, with implications for who pays for what, and there could be the substantial challenge of coordinating care across organizational boundaries.

An added issue is that the care needed by older people and their families could be delivered by government (public sector), private (for-profit) or voluntary (nonprofit, charitable) organizations. Of course, most support and care is not provided through structured organizations at all, but by unpaid relatives and other individuals providing informal care. Most countries have a thriving mixed economy of provision – a mix of services delivered by a mix of agencies and individuals, each with potentially different motivations and funding bases. In understanding how long-term care systems operate, we therefore need to pay attention to the roles played by families, the types of formal service provided, and the ways that those services are financed. The next three sections address these topics in turn. We then consider a relatively new development in some long-term care systems – self-directed services.

Informal Care

Reliance on Unpaid Caregivers

Changing demographic patterns, family composition, labor force participation and geographical mobility are reducing the (potential) pool of family caregivers for older people. The substantial inputs of unpaid family caregivers (in terms of practical help, companionship, assistance in getting out, and general supervision) often go unrecognized. Yet without them either the state or civil society (voluntary/charitable) bodies would have to step in to provide formal care support, or older people or their families would have to purchase care themselves. The alternative would be poor and deteriorating quality of life for older people and others with long-term care needs.

The effects on caregivers can be considerable. On the positive side, most caregivers gain great satisfaction from their contribution to maintaining and improving the quality of life of the person they support, often a loved relative. However, more attention focuses on the negative aspects, and particularly the effects on health, stress, employment, and income. Caregiver health problems are particularly associated with supporting older people with high-level needs (Moise et al., 2004). One of the most tangible effects of caring is reduced opportunity to work and reduced income: Evandrou (1995) found that men and women who provide 20 or more hours per week of informal care have earnings from employment that are 25% lower than the earnings of employed noncaregivers.

Family caregivers, and particularly women, are absolutely the mainstay of all long-term care systems. Not surprisingly, most governments have therefore introduced a range of measures that seek to encourage families to continue to provide care for dependent relatives. Adequate and appropriate health and social services provided to older people, both in institutions and at home, are known to be a major factor in supporting the inputs of family carers and reducing the burden of care on their shoulders. Respite care is central to most countries' support programmes for caregivers: It offers families a break from their caring responsibilities, and could be offered in the home, or in a care facility (during the day or overnight for a few days). Financial support is available in some countries, through tax credits (as in Canada, Spain, the US), pension credits (as in Canada, Germany, the UK), or social care budgets (as in Australia, France, Sweden) or through self-directed payments (see the section titled 'Financing' below). Initiatives have also been taken to provide families with better general information, advocacy, education, and training about needs, how to meet them, and the availability of local support. Employment-friendly policies are also being introduced in some countries to help people combine a career with caring responsibilities.

Experience in Canada illustrates many of the practical and policy issues in relation to informal care. Unpaid caregivers provide more than 80% of the support needed by people with long-term conditions in Canada (Statistics Canada, 2002). Although men are providing more care than in the past, women still constitute the majority of caregivers. Data from Statistics Canada's 2002 General Social Survey reveal that 59% of people providing care to an older person in the preceding 12 months were women. According to Smale and Dupuis (2002), 92% of caregivers of older people in Canada are family members, 53% spouses, and 38% adult children of the person being supported. One in 25 caregivers said they had become economically inactive because of their caring responsibilities.

A mix of programs and policies is in place at federal, provincial, and territorial levels to support caregivers. One of the main ways of providing support is through provision of home care services, whether direct to care receivers or specifically to meet the needs of caregivers through, for example, respite services. These programs are largely the responsibility of provincial departments of health or social services, with the exception of veterans and members of First Nations, who fall under federal jurisdiction. While there have been calls for the development of a universal home care program, current federal health policy does not provide standards or guidelines for the development or delivery of home care services. As a result, home care programs vary widely across the country and meet the needs of caregivers with varying degrees of success.

One emphasis in Canada has been to use the tax system to provide financial support to those providing care to disabled or elderly relatives. There are a number of tax relief measures that can be claimed at the federal level, although a criticism that has been made is that these measures are least useful to those who most need them: Although women constitute the majority of caregivers, data from the 2000 tax year indicate that only 39% of Caregiver Credit claimants were women, which may be partly because many women caregivers do not have sufficient income to benefit from a nonrefundable credit (Shillington, 2004). While many caregivers meet some of the eligibility criteria for most tax deductions and credits, they rarely meet all, and so do not benefit from financial compensation policies. The complexity is also said to put off some potential beneficiaries.

The other national program offering financial compensation to caregivers is the Compassionate Care Benefit, an element of the Employment Insurance program. It came into effect in 2004 and provides temporary income support for eligible workers who need to take leave from work to provide care to a family member who is likely to die within the next 6 months. There are many significant restrictions on eligibility for receipt of this benefit: It is available, for example, only to close relatives who are eligible for employment insurance (so that, for example, self-employed persons are ineligible).

The provinces and territories have also used the tax system to provide financial assistance to caregivers. But tax credits available at this level, where they exist, largely parallel those found at the federal level, although amounts and eligibility criteria vary. There are also some sales tax exemptions for respite care.

Provision

Many of the needs of older people stem from deterioration in their health and are most usually appropriately met by health-care services. Other needs are more appropriately met by social care providers. But the boundaries between these sets of needs are hard to draw, and different patterns of service provision have grown up in different countries, influenced by national culture, financing arrangements, availability of skilled professionals and the caprices of day-to-day decision making. The distinction between health and social care has potentially important implications both for the level of cost (for example, needs may be excessively medicalized or specialist treatment underprovided) and for the balance of funding (if different eligibility criteria influence threshold levels of dependence, for instance). In turn, these could create (perverse) incentives: Cost-shifting is a problem in some countries, as is the risk of people falling between two separate care systems. Sweden is one country that appears to have solved long-standing problems such as hospital bed blocking and nursing home funding responsibilities, but new boundary issues have arisen there, concerning rehabilitation, home nursing, assistive technology and so on.

Although there are many differences between countries, there is a common core of (non-family) services that can be said to comprise long-term care, including needs assessment, counselling and advice, self-help support groups, respite care, crisis management, support centers, day programs, support for people in their own homes (so-called home care, including home help, meals, and community nursing), residential and nursing home provision, and – increasingly – a range of housing-with-support services (such as sheltered housing, extra-care housing and some retirement communities).

Institutional Care

The long-stay hospital ward for older people is gradually being phased out in many Western countries, although it remains an unwelcome feature of care systems in parts of

Eastern Europe. More policy attention in Western countries has therefore turned to the balance between institutional care (which now usually means residential and nursing home care) and home care.

An OECD (1996) study found suggestions of some convergence around a level of roughly 5% of older people supported in institutional settings, ranging from below 1% in Greece and Turkey (in the early 1990s or late 1980s) to above 6.5% in Canada, Finland, Luxembourg, the Netherlands, New Zealand, and Norway. Countries with an above-average level of bed provision were generally trying to reduce it and those below the average were generally trying to expand provision. Discussions on the appropriate balance of care have included arguments about relative effectiveness (for whom is residential/nursing home care more effective – in terms of promoting quality of life and other outcomes – and when?), relative cost (both in total and to various agencies, especially health and social care), and user and family preferences (themselves influenced by factors such as perceptions of quality, availability of informal care, the broader family-centered culture in certain societies, and personal cost).

One consequence of this shifting balance between institutional and other forms of care is that older people tend to get admitted to care homes when already quite dependent, for example at later stages of dementia. This can leave families carrying a heavy burden, and caregiver-related factors are common reasons for admission. Another consequence is that a high proportion of residents in care homes and other highly staffed congregate care settings today have dementia. Decisions on what is an appropriate balance of provision need to be thought through. For example, the availability of places in care homes has significant impacts on rates of delayed discharge from hospital in England (Fernández and Forder, 2007).

Home Care

The OECD (1996) found a great deal of intercountry variation in the provision of home care. For example, no more than 5% of all older people in Austria, Germany, Ireland, Italy, Portugal, and Spain were receiving home care at the time of the study, compared to more than 10% in Denmark, Finland, Norway, and Sweden. There was no evidence of movement toward a similar proportion. However, comparisons of home-based care are difficult to make across countries: "How much of this [observed] variation is due to differences in definitions of home care or other methodological issues, rather than due to the actual use of such services, is not clear" (Gibson *et al.*, 2003: 3).

Notwithstanding this difficulty, the extent and nature of development of what are sometimes called intermediate care arrangements (housing with various levels of care support) also vary considerably. A common phenomenon has been the transformation of most home care services from the traditional home help, focused on household chores, to services that concentrate on personal care. This transformation has often gone hand in hand with the development of intensively supported home care, often costing as much as a place in a care home. It is becoming increasingly common to find long-term care systems targeting available resources on people with the greatest needs (hence the development of intensive home care, for example), at the expense of low-level care for people with fewer needs. Indeed, collectively financed low-level support has virtually disappeared in some countries (such as England).

Provider Pluralism

Provider pluralism is another pervasive and increasingly visible feature of many long-term care systems. The public sector has often been the largest provider of formal services, but not-for-profit (voluntary) and for-profit (private) organizations have also been high-volume and/or high-profile contributors in the mixed economy of care (Kendall *et al.*, 2006). Responsibility for strategically coordinating or commissioning care still rests predominantly with public sector bodies, but increasingly it is nonpublic bodies that actually deliver services in the field.

Policy debates in some countries have kept services and financing distinct when discussing the future of long-term care (such as in the UK), although the two are obviously closely connected in practice. The sectoral balance of provision affects the balance of funding responsibilities: For example, charitable donations can be used to subsidize state or individual funding of services. The sectoral balance of provision may also affect the overall cost of care if one sector is demonstrably and consistently less expensive and/or more cost-effective than another.

Coordination

Good interagency coordination of long-term care is imperative if individual and family needs are to be met, which requires collaborative approaches to financing. Without effective coordination, yawning gaps could open up in the spectrum of support: Even in well-resourced care systems there are large numbers of people whose long-term care needs go unrecognized or unmet. Wasteful duplication of effort is another possibility. Countries, states, and municipalities differ in their service and agency definitions, responsibilities, and arrangements, and therefore in their interagency boundaries and the kinds of connected action that spans them. One of the major organizational resource challenges, therefore, is to coordinate service funding in ways that are effective, cost-effective, and fair. Cost shifting and problem dumping between agencies will not help individuals or families, but recognition of economic symbiosis could help decision makers fashion improved responses to needs through pooled budgets, jointly commissioned programs and other whole-system initiatives.

In some countries, such as the Netherlands and Scandinavia, there have been efforts to integrate housing and health/social care to improve service coordination and promote independence and self-care.

Quality of Care

Concern has been widely expressed about quality of care, how to improve it and how to assure it through appropriate regulatory mechanisms. There are inherent difficulties in measuring some aspects of quality, and service users with a moderate or high degree of cognitive impairment, for example, are unlikely to be able to participate as informed consumers using their voice to bring about change.

One factor working against quality improvements is the low status and high rate of turnover of staff. A number of countries are experiencing shortages of qualified or skilled staff for long-term care services, and particularly to work in services for people with dementia. One of the reasons is undoubtedly that rates of pay seem to be universally low, hindering recruitment and fostering turnover.

Financing

The main approaches to funding long-term care are out-of-pocket payments; voluntary insurance (sometimes called private insurance); tax-based support from general tax revenue; and social insurance. The last of these includes social health insurance but could be broader to include social care. All but the first are prepayment arrangements. They differ one from another in the personal–collective funding balance, extent of risk pooling, and nature of government intervention. Policy instruments applied to potentially any of these funding approaches include providing information and advice, regulation, subsidies, tax raising, transfer payments, and direct provision of services. All financing arrangements involve some redistribution over the life cycle, whether explicitly through contributions to long-term care or other insurance policies during the working years, or through tax or social insurance contributions (linked closely to employment) or through investment in housing equity.

Almost all high-income countries rely heavily on prepayment systems of revenue collection, widely held to be preferable to out-of-pocket payments when an individual's risk of needing long-term care is very uncertain, and, when the need arises, if the attendant costs (of care) and/or losses (of earnings) could be catastrophic. Prepayment contributions pool risks, and therefore redistribute benefits toward people with greater needs. They also have the potential to redistribute in favor of poorer individuals, either because need is inversely correlated with income, or purposively by making arrangements progressive so that poorer individuals pay proportionately less than wealthier individuals for equivalent care. Out-of-pocket-payment systems (from private savings, equity release and so on) generally do not have these same advantages.

Out-of-Pocket Payments

Although prepayment systems dominate, in many countries there are out-of-pocket charges for some services, whether as co-payments (a specific amount is paid for a service), co-insurance (an agreed percentage of cost is charged) or deductibles (an agreed amount is paid before insurance kicks in). There are various rationales for introducing out-of-pocket payments, including to raise revenue (if wealthier individuals can afford to pay, why not charge them?), to discourage unnecessary service use (moral hazard), and to create price sensitivity that might help direct service users to more cost-effective and appropriate treatments. But out-of-pocket payment mechanisms usually have undesirable impacts on access and equity, discouraging the use of essential as well as nonessential services, and delaying demand and utilization that might later mean substantially increased costs.

Voluntary Insurance

Voluntary insurance is taken up and paid for at the discretion of individuals (hence the label voluntary) or perhaps by employers on behalf of individuals. Insurance policies might be offered by public, quasi-public, for-profit or nonprofit organizations. Generally speaking, voluntary insurance is less important in European health-care systems than in the U.S., where it accounts for half of health-care expenditure (Center for Disease Control and Prevention, 2003). However, long-term care insurance has failed to establish itself even in the U.S., and has certainly not proved popular in countries where tax-based or social insurance arrangements are in place (Johnson and Uccello, 2005).

People individually purchasing insurance have lower bargaining power than when insurance arrangements are made by employers or the state, which in turn could affect the benefits covered. Inherent in voluntary prepayment systems are disadvantages such as adverse selection and cream skimming, where higher risk groups (such as those with chronic conditions) may find insurance unaffordable and lower risk groups may feel that their own premiums are too high. Insurance plans may also exempt existing conditions from the benefit packages, which could be a difficulty for long-term care. If there is no charge at the point at which a service is used there may be excessive utilization, the so-called moral hazard problem that might be addressed by introducing co-payments at point of use.

Tax-Based Financing

Many health and social care systems are funded from national, regional, or local taxes. If the tax that generates the revenue is progressive (as with income tax) and eligibility for benefits is not income-related, then long-term care financing will also be progressive. But long-term care financing could be regressive if financed from indirect taxes (such as sales or value-added tax), because poorer individuals often contribute larger proportions of their incomes. Generally, however, at least in discussions of health-care financing in high-income countries, tax-based systems are seen as the most progressive and equitable of all arrangements (Mossialos *et al.*, 2002), and the same would apply to long-term care.

Payments are mandatory, and scale economies can be achieved in administration, risk management, and purchasing power. Services (or cash payments in some countries – see the section on self-directed services below) are provided on the basis of need, and there is obviously also the potential to allocate or distribute services (or their cash equivalents under self-directed care arrangements) on the basis of income or assets. For those who advocate health or long-term care as a right, tax-based systems fit the bill, while those with conservative leanings might view such arrangements as erosions of personal responsibilities and freedom.

Tax-based systems have limitations. Funding levels may fluctuate with the state of the national economy: When an economy is not doing well, there is a tendency to cut back on publicly funded programs. Competing political and economic objectives make a tax-based system less transparent, and bureaucracy can add to inefficiency, perhaps reflected in long waiting lists (although there is also symptomatic underfunding). Service users may view tax-based systems as offering them limited choice, but uninsured individuals in an alternative financing system might argue that they face no choice whatsoever.

Social Insurance

Care systems based on social insurance generate their revenues from salary-based contributions administered and managed by quasi-public bodies. Employers also make contributions, and transfers are usually made from general taxation to sickness funds to provide cover for unemployed, retired, and other disadvantaged or vulnerable people. One of the most interesting financing arrangements is the system introduced in Japan in 2000, which have attracted worldwide attention. Mandatory long-term care social insurance was introduced in 2000, operated by the more than 3000 municipalities under central government legislation. (The decision was made to go with a social insurance rather than tax-based model on a number of grounds; see Ikegami, 2004.) The insurance is financed 50% from taxes (half from national taxes, a quarter each from local and regional taxes) and 50% from insurance premiums paid by people aged 40 and above. For people in employment, the premium is equivalent to 0.6% of income up to a ceiling, with employers and employees sharing this cost. For older people, premiums are deducted from pensions and are also income-related (Campbell and Ikegami, 2003). Co-payments amounting to 10% of care costs are paid.

Eligibility is based solely on need for everyone aged 65 and over and those aged 40–64 with aging-related disabilities. Insured people in need of care are assessed on application and classified into one of six care levels according to need. A fee schedule is set nationally according to the level of need. The role of a care manager was newly created with the introduction of the insurance system to draw up care plans reflecting individual needs. The scheme covers residential and home care services. Cash benefits are not paid – unlike in Germany, for example – partly to move care away from the traditional heavy reliance on female carers (particularly in a context of a declining ability and willingness of families to provide support; Ikegami, 2004), partly to help long-term care provision to expand (Campbell and Ikegami, 2003).

Tax revenues may also be called upon to cover deficits in social insurance funds, especially if the working population is too small to generate sufficient revenue to cover the population eligible to receive benefits. Enrollment is usually mandatory, and although premiums are not risk-adjusted, they tend to be linked to income so that pooling allows for redistribution according to both need and income. A disadvantage is that the link between financing and employment may constrain job mobility and hence economic competitiveness (at the national level).

Both tax-based and social insurance-dominated systems take account of ability to pay and cover vulnerable and low-income groups.

Comparing the Options

A number of criteria have been alluded to in describing the relative advantages of the different financing methods. Efficiency is obviously central – ensuring that the highest volume or best quality of care is achieved from a given funding base. Financing arrangements are obviously not desirable if they do not allow full assessment of individual needs, or embody inappropriate incentives to use residential care (or not to use it enough), or shift costs between agencies so that support arrangements are poorly coordinated or have heavy management or transaction costs.

Equity is also especially relevant as a criterion, looking at both the services and benefits received as well as funding contributions, and has been widely discussed in connection with long-term care financing options. Other criteria discussed include affordability, sustainability, independence, self-respect, dignity, choice, and social solidarity.

Governments of different political hues will give different emphasis to these and other criteria. What is common across many countries today is exploration of financing options that shift some of the burden away from the state, whether in tax-financed systems or because of the need to subsidize or underpin other financing arrangements.

Health and Long-Term Care Differences

Different financing arrangements can be employed for health and long-term care systems, or indeed for different services within these systems. In particular, there can be different regimes for charging users. In England, there is currently considerable tension between health care (which is free at the point of use) and social care (which is means-tested). People with dementia or other long-term conditions moving from a hospital ward to a nursing home might suddenly find themselves liable to pay (often substantial) charges for their care, even though their primary need is generated by a health problem.

Expenditure Levels

The OECD (2005) estimated public and private expenditure on long-term care as a percentage of GDP in 2000 (**Table 3**). (Public expenditure in this table is equivalent to general government expenditure as the term is used in national health accounting.) Total expenditure ranged from lows of 0.6% of GDP in Italy and Spain to greater than 2% in Scandinavian countries. The average of 14 countries covered by this OECD report was 1.25%. Generally, public sector spending on long-term care dominated private expenditure, except in Spain. However, these OECD data only include expenditure related to medical services and so underestimate total long-term care spending.

Self-Directed Services

A noticeable trend across some countries is the development of self-directed (or consumer-directed) services (Ungerson and Yeandle, 2007). The primary aim is to give more independence and choice to older people and thereby give them greater control over their lives. An increasingly common way to do so is to hand funding over to individuals to purchase their own care support. Voucher-like arrangements are also being used. The German long-term care financing system offers the devolved funds option, while in England there are opportunities for people assessed as eligible for state-supported long-term care to receive funding through direct payments or individual budgets (Knapp, 2007).

There are a number of reasons for these initiatives. Social work theory – which certainly exerts influence over long-term care systems in some countries – has long emphasized independence and empowerment, which gives normative professional credibility to devolved

Table 3 Public and private expenditure on long-term care as a percentage of GDP, 2000

	Total expenditure			Public expenditure[a]			Private expenditure		
	Home care	Institutions	Total	Home care	Institutions	Total	Home care	Institutions	Total
Australia	0.38	0.81	1.19	0.3	0.56	0.86	0.08	0.25	0.33
Canada	0.17	1.06	1.23	0.17	0.82	0.99	NA	0.24	0.24
Denmark	NA	NA	2.60	NA	NA	–	NA	NA	NA
France	NA	NA	1.10	NA	NA	NA	NA	NA	NA
Germany	0.47	0.88	1.35	0.43	0.52	0.95	0.04	0.36	0.4
Ireland	0.19	0.43	0.62	0.19	0.33	0.52	NA	0.1	0.1
Italy	NA	NA	0.60	NA	NA	NA	NA	NA	NA
Japan	0.25	0.58	0.83	0.25	0.51	0.76	0.00	0.07	0.07
Netherlands	0.60	0.83	1.44	0.56	0.75	1.31	0.05	0.08	0.13
New Zealand	0.12	0.56	0.68	0.11	0.34	0.45	0.01	0.22	0.23
Norway	0.69	1.45	2.15	0.66	1.19	1.85	0.03	0.26	0.29
Spain	0.23	0.37	0.61	0.05	0.11	0.16	0.18	0.26	0.44
Sweden	0.82	2.07	2.89	0.78	1.96	2.74	0.04	0.10	0.14
USA	0.33	0.96	1.29	0.17	0.58	0.74	0.16	0.39	0.54
UK	0.41	0.96	1.37	0.32	0.58	0.89	0.09	0.38	0.48
OECD average[b]	0.38	0.88	1.25	0.35	0.64	0.99	0.06	0.19	0.24

NA, not available.
From OECD (2005) *The OECD Health Project: Long-term Care for Older People*. Paris: Organisation for Economic Co-operation and Development.
[a]General government expenditure as the term is used in national health accounting.
[b]Average of: Australia, Canada, Germany, Ireland, Japan, Netherlands, New Zealand, Norway, Poland, Spain, Sweden, Switzerland, UK, and US.

purchasing or commissioning powers. There is also a belief that such arrangements can improve quality of care while being cost-effective. The approach appeals both to the political right because of its links to market mechanisms, and also to the center left because of its connections with choice and accountability in public services. From the user perspective, self-directed services can be attractive because of the empowerment offered and are clearly supportive of rights-based agenda. They might also help to break down barriers between sectors and budgets, because the funding can be used within the gray areas between health, social care, housing and so on.

However, there are potential drawbacks. Self-directed arrangements place considerable responsibility for finding, monitoring, and purchasing services on the shoulders of long-term care users, many of whom could be frail or cognitively impaired. Family carers might not be available to help. The funding transferred to individuals might be too little to allow them to access services they want or feel they need. Individual purchasers will have little bargaining power relative to service providers (compared to, say, large purchasers such as a municipality or social insurance fund), and there is the risk of exploitation by providers or financial advisers. Although brokerage (advisory, support) services are usually established in self-directed care systems, coverage or quality might not be adequate.

Conclusions

Across the world, populations are aging, and increasingly governments are worrying about the future affordability of long-term care, given the close correlation between age and the need for support in self-care and personal tasks. One area of concern is the availability of unpaid support by families and others, which remains the most common source of long-term care. The future supply of informal care is likely to be considerably lower than at present because of changing demography, growing labor force participation by women, and changing societal expectations. There is also growing recognition of the high psychological and opportunity costs of being a caregiver, and governments are gradually introducing information and advice, financial support, respite care, and employment-friendly policies.

Particular attention is also being paid to the organization of formal services provided by municipalities, voluntary organizations (civil society), and for-profit private companies. Historically there was quite heavy reliance in some countries on long-stay hospital services, nursing homes, and residential care facilities, but a common policy emphasis today is to try to substitute community-based services, on the grounds of quality of life, cost, and the personal preferences of older people. Home care services are themselves often being transformed from traditional home help models to personal care, and in some countries are being targeted on people with the greatest needs in efforts to avoid or delay admission into institutional facilities. There is also an observable tendency across a number of countries to develop long-term care arrangements that blur the boundaries between institutional and community-based provision, and between health and social care, while also developing specialist resources for conditions such as dementia.

As countries increase the resources devoted to long-term care, they wrestle with the challenge of how to finance services over the coming decades. One consequence has been to try to shift more of the funding balance away from collective responsibility and toward individual service users and their families. Nevertheless, there remains heavy reliance on prepayment financing arrangements (through taxation or insurance) that generally redistribute in favor of people with greater needs and lower incomes. While many governments are exploring ways to reduce their own financial responsibilities, at the same time there is growing government activity in regulating long-term care systems, providing safety net support, seeking to monitor care markets, and improving quality assurance mechanisms. Self-directed systems are being introduced in some countries, giving control over the selection and purchasing of services to the people who actually have long-term care needs, and this kind of arrangement seems likely to grow considerably in the future.

See also: Long Term Care for Aging Populations; Long Term Care in Health Services.

Citations

Campbell JC and Ikegami N (2003) Japan's radical reform of long-term care. *Social Policy and Administration* 37: 21–34.

Centers for Disease Control and Prevention (2003) *Health insurance coverage – National Center for Health Statistics.* http://www.cdc.gov/nchs/fastats/hinsure.htm (accessed September 2007).

ECFIN (2006) The impact of ageing on public expenditure: Projections for the EU25 Member States on pensions, health care, long-term care, education and unemployment transfers (2004–2050). European Economy Special Report. http://ec.europa.eu/economy_finance/publications/european_economy/2006/eespecialreport0106_en.htm (accessed September 2007).

Evandrou M (1995) Employment and care, paid and unpaid work: The socioeconomic position of informal carers in Britain. In: Phillips J (ed.) *Working Carers.* Aldershot, UK: Avebury.

Fernández J-L and Forder J (2007) Consequences of local variations in social care on the performance of the acute health care sector. *Applied Economics.* In press.

Gibson MJ, Gregory SR, and Pandya SM (2003) *Long-Term Care in Developed Nations: A Brief Overview.* Washington DC: AARP.

Ikegami N (2004) Opening Pandora's box: Making long-term care an entitlement in Japan. In: Knapp M, Fernández J-L, Netten A, and Challis D (eds.) *Long-Term Care: Matching Resources and Needs.* Aldershot, UK: Ashgate.

Johnson RW and Uccello CE (2005) Is Private Long-term Care Insurance the Answer? Issue in Brief No. 29. Chestnut Hill, MA: Center for Retirement Research at Boston College.
Kendall J, Knapp M, and Forder (2006) Social care and the nonprofit sector in the western developed world. In: Powell WW and Steinberg R (eds.) *The Nonprofit Sector: A Research Handbook*, Second edition, pp. 415–431. New Haven, CT: Yale University Press.
Knapp M (2007) Social care: choice, money, control. In: Hills J, Le Grand J, and Piachaud D (eds.) *Making Social Policy Work: Essays in Honour of Howard Glennerster*. Policy Press.
Mossialos E, Dixon A, Figueras J, and Kutzin J (eds.) (2002) *Funding Health Care: Options for Europe*. Buckingham, UK: Open University Press.
Moise P, Schwarzinger M, and Um MY (2004) Dementia care in 9 OECD countries: A comparative analysis. OECD Health Working Papers No. 13, OECD, Paris, France.
OECD (1996) *Caring for Frail Elderly People: Policies in Evolution*. Paris, France: Organisation for Economic Co-operation and Development.
OECD (2005) *The OECD Health Project: Long-term Care for Older People*. Paris, France: Organisation for Economic Co-operation and Development.
OECD (2006) *OECD Factbook 2006: Economic Environmental and Social Statistics*. Paris, France: Organisation for Economic Co-operation and Development.
Shillington R (2004) *Policy Options to Support Dependent Care: The Tax/Transfer System*. Prepared for Healthy Balance.
Smale B and Dupuis S (2002) Highlights report: preliminary results from the study on needs of caregivers of persons with Alzheimer Disease or a related dementia and community support services in Ontario. *Murray Alzheimer Research and Education Program*. Ontario, Canada: University of Waterloo. http://marep.waterloo.ca/projects.html.
Statistics Canada (2002) *General Social Survey (GSS)*. Ottawa, Canada: Statistics Canada.
Ungerson C and Yeandle S (eds.) (2007) *Cash for Care in Developed Welfare States*. Cambridge: Palgrave Macmillan.
Wittenberg R, Comas-Herrera A, King D, Malley J, Pickard L, and Darton R (2006) Future demand for long-term care, 2002 to 2041: Projections of demand for long-term care for older people in England. PSSRU Discussion Paper 2330. London: London School of Economics. http://www.pssru.ac.uk/pdf/dp2330.pdf.

Further Reading

Comas-Herrera A, Wittenberg R, Pickard L, Knapp M, and MRC-CFAS (2007) Cognitive impairment in older people: Its implications for future demand for services and costs. *International Journal of Geriatric Psychiatry*. Jul 2 [E-pub ahead of print].
Karlsson M (2002) Comparative analysis of long-term care systems in four countries, interim report. International Institute for Applied Systems Analysis: Laxenburg, Austria.
Merlis M (2000) Caring for the frail elderly: An international review. *Health Affairs* 19: 141–149.
Pickard L, Wittenberg R, Comas-Herrera A, Davies B, and Darton R (2000) Relying on informal care in the new century? Informal care for elderly people in England to 2031. *Ageing and Society* 20: 745–772.
Pickard L (2004) *Caring for Older People and Employment*. London: Audit Commission.
Wanless D, Forder J, and Fernández J-L (2006) *Securing Good Care for Older People: Taking a Long-Term View*. London: King's Fund.
Wiener J (2004) Home and community-based services in the United States. In: Knapp M, Fernández J-L, Netten A, and Challis D (eds.) *Long-Term Care: Matching Resources and Needs*. Aldershot, UK: Ashgate.
Wittenberg R, Sandhu B, and Knapp M (2002) Funding long-term care: The private and public options. In: Mossialos E, Dixon A, Figueras J, and Kutzin J (eds.) *Funding Health Care: Options for Europe*. Buckingham, UK: Open University Press.

Innovative Financing of Health Promotion

V Tangcharoensathien, P Prakongsai, and W Patcharanarumol, International Health Policy Program, Thailand
S Limwattananon, Khon Kaen University, Thailand
S Buasai, Thai Health Promotion Foundation, Thailand

© 2008 Elsevier Inc. All rights reserved.

Introduction

Health Promotion (HP) is one of the cornerstones for health development of the people (World Health Organization, 2006a). It represents a comprehensive social and political process of enabling people to increase control over and to improve their health (World Health Organization, 1986). Health promotion not only embraces actions directed at strengthening the skills and capabilities of individuals, but also action directed toward changing social, environmental, and economic conditions so as to alleviate their impact on public and individual health. With this comprehensive definition, the 1986 Ottawa Charter for Health Promotion called for countries and international organizations to reorient health services, fundamental conditions for example peace, shelter, education, food, income, social justice, equity, and their resources toward the promotion of health (World Health Organization, 1986). The 1997 Jakarta Declaration on Health Promotion reiterated the importance of mobilizing resources for health promotion (World Health Organization, 1997). The 2005 Bangkok Charter urged countries to make promotion of health a core responsibility of the governments, by giving priority to investments in health, within and outside the health sector, and to provide sustainable financing for health promotion (World Health Organization, 2005a). Despite the pivotal role of financing HP as highlighted by these charters, little is known on how much was spent on health promotion.

Much has been advocated on the role of HP and multisectoral community interventions in controlling chronic illnesses.

The following example highlights the success of the Finnish multiple approaches of HP in containing cardiovascular diseases (Vartiainen et al., 2000). In the 1970s, Finland had the world's highest death rate from cardiovascular disease, largely caused by widespread and heavy tobacco use, a high-fat diet, and low vegetable intake. In response to local concerns, a large-scale community-based intervention was organized, involving consumers, schools, and social and health services. It included legislation banning tobacco advertising, introducing low-fat dairy and vegetable oil products, changes in farmers' payment scheme, and incentives for communities achieving the greatest cholesterol reduction.

Death rates from heart disease in men have been reduced by at least 65% and lung cancer death rates in men have also fallen. Greatly reduced cardiovascular and cancer mortality has led to greater life expectancy, approximately 7 years for men and 6 years for women.

The effectiveness of these interventions was proven by scientific communities and synthesized by a WHO report (World Health Organization, 2005b). This report also set a global goal, by 2015, for all countries to reduce the death rates from all chronic diseases by 2% per year over and above existing trends during the next 10 years. This would result in the prevention of 36 million chronic disease deaths by 2015, most of which would occur in low- and middle-income countries (**Figure 1**). Achieving the global goal would also result in appreciable economic dividends such as economic gains from reducing mortality, and the reduction in countries' health expenditure. Although this goal is ambitious and adventurous, it is neither extravagant nor unrealistic, based on evidence and best practice of health promotion activities from countries that have implemented them.

To achieve this global goal, governments need to ensure the provision of adequate resources and show leadership to address the chronic disease problems in their countries. A series of low-cost, high-impact actions can be implemented in a stepwise manner even in a resource-poor setting. However, financial resources remain one of the major challenges. In developing countries, HP is generally funded by the government budget through conventional clinical prevention and health promotion services, very often on a hospital or clinic basis. For example, prenatal care, childhood immunization, and screening of blood cholesterol which the poor and the needy may not be able to access. Nevertheless, there is a need to explore alternative sources for financing HP and search for effective approaches to prioritize and implement the HP policy in developing countries across the world.

This paper synthesizes financing health care in general and HP in particular and reviews experiences of innovative financing of HP in selected countries that have a specific dedicated tax for HP. Finally, the paper draws on lessons from an in-depth case study in Thailand, a lower-middle-income country, of the Thai Health Promotion Foundation, which has been established since 2001, focusing on innovative financing and a multisectoral and multidisciplinary approach to HP.

Financing Health Care: A Global Review

The 2006 World Health Report (World Health Organization, 2006b) provides the level and profile of health expenditure among 192 member states in 2003. Total health expenditure (THE) was on average 6.2% of GDP (range from 4.6% in Southeast Asia to 7.5% in Europe),

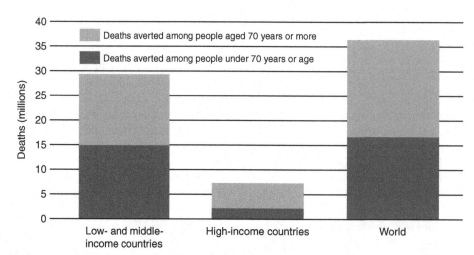

Figure 1 Estimated global deaths averted if the global goals are reached. From World Health Organization (2005b) *Preventing Chronic Diseases: A Vital Investment*. Geneva, Switzerland: World Health Organization.

and US $581.3 per capita (ranging from US $55.40 in Africa to US $1407.70 in Europe) (see **Table 1**). Poorer countries spent less on health; for example 31 out of 192 WHO member states spent less than US $20 per capita, more than two-thirds of which were members of the African Region.

An analysis of public and private financing sources of THE among different WHO regions in 2003 reveals a common trend of health-care finance between rich and poor territories. In **Table 2**, countries in poor regions, namely Africa and Southeast Asia, relied more on household out-of-pocket payment and external resources, compared to richer regions. Health receives a smaller share of government expenditure, and social security as well as prepaid health insurance are not well established and also have a smaller share. For example, total health spending for social security among countries in African and Southeast Asia regions in 2003 was 4.5% and 7.1% of general government health expenditure, whereas external resources were 15.6% and 10.6% of THE, respectively. In contrast, out-of-pocket spending accounted for a major share of private health expenditure in all regions. These findings support previous analyses of global health expenditure among 191 countries studied by the WHO (Musgrove et al., 2002; Poullier et al., 2002).

Financing Health Promotion

Based on information about National Health Accounts (NHA) available to the WHO, during the 5-year period from 1999 to 2003, there were a total of 120 data sets having complete information from which we can estimate expenditure on prevention and public health services. In this paper, expenditure on disease prevention and public health services is assumed as spending on HP activities.

Expenditure on prevention and public health services is classified as health-care function six (HC6, which includes the following details: HC.6.1, maternal and child health, family planning and counseling; HC.6.2, school health services; HC.6.3, prevention of communicable diseases; HC.6.4, prevention of noncommunicable diseases; HC.6.5, occupational health care; and HC.6.9 all other miscellaneous public health services) according to the International Classification of Healthcare Function by OECD Systems of Health Accounts (OECD, 2002). The analysis indicates that HC6, an average of the percentages computed for the 120 data sets, accounts for 2.94% of THE (range, 0.02–8.24%).

We assume that spending on HP is 2.94% of THE for those countries where information on HP is absent, in order to estimate expenditure on HP per capita. Results

Table 1 Total health expenditure as % of GDP and US$ per capita in 2003 by WHO regions

WHO region	Countries	THE (% GDP)	THE per capita (US$)	THE per capita <US $20 (countries)
African	46	5.0	55.4	23
American	35	6.8	469.3	0
Eastern Mediterranean	21	5.0	241.2	2
European	52	7.5	1407.7	1
Southeast Asia	11	4.6	69.9	4
Western Pacific	27	6.7	470.0	1
All	192	6.2	581.3	31

From World Health Organization (2006b) World Health Report 2006: Working Together for Health. Geneva: World Health Organization.

Table 2 Share of total health expenditure by sources and WHO regions, 2003

WHO region	GGHE, % THE	PvtHE, % THE	GGHE, % GGE	External resources, % THE	SocSec HE, % GGHE	Out-of-pocket spending, % PvtHE	Prepaid plans, % PvtHE
African	50.6	49.4	9.1	15.6	4.5	79.7	8.1
American	55.3	44.8	12.7	2.8	24.7	77.1	22.1
Eastern Mediterranean	53.9	46.1	7.4	5.1	14.1	83.1	13.6
European	66.2	33.9	12.7	1.7	48.3	84.6	11.0
Southeast Asia	53.2	46.8	7.4	10.6	7.1	85.3	2.2
Western Pacific	69.8	30.3	10.8	15.4	12.4	80.2	4.4
All	58.9	41.1	10.7	8.0	23.4	81.3	10.8

GGHE, general government health expenditure; PvtHE, private health expenditure; SocSecHE, Social Security health expenditure; THE, total health expenditure.
From World Health Organization (2006b) World Health Report 2006: Working Together for Health. Geneva: World Health Organization.

indicate a wide variation in HC6 spending across regions, from US $1.6 per capita in the African region, to US $36.9 in the European region (see **Table 3**).

This result, 2.94% of THE spent on HP, is slightly lower than 3.8% of THE (1.4–8.4%) among 13 high-income countries that are members of the Organization for Economic Cooperation and Development (OECD), as estimated by Tangcharoensathien et al. (2005), and much lower than 7.5% of THE (range, 3–12%) analyzed by Berman et al., for eight countries in Latin America (Berman et al., 1999).

Figure 2 illustrates expenditure on HP as percent of THE among the 120 data sets. Expenditure on HP has been more or less stable at 3% of THE over the 5-year period from 1999 to 2003, with no significant change.

Although the data from 120 data sets do not provide information on sources of finance for HP, a recent study in 14 OECD countries revealed that approximately 73.5% of expenditure on HP was financed by general government revenue (GGR), 12% by social health insurance (SHI), and 12.1% by donor resources (Tangcharoensathien et al., 2005). Out-of-pocket spending and private health insurance had a minor share of 2.3% and 0.1%, respectively. The above proportion of HP financed by GGR and SHI is simply applied to the estimated figure of US $16.7 per capita spending on HP, giving US $12.2 financed by GGR and US $2.0 by SHI.

After a comprehensive review of financing health care and HP, the following summary remarks can be made.

1. Globally, information on the level and sources of spending on HP is scarce, despite advocacy for more financial resources going to HP by several charters on health promotion.
2. Assessment of financing health care indicates that poor countries in Africa and Southeast Asia, facing resource

Table 3 Financing of prevention and public health services

		Available data set 1999–2003			2003	
WHO region	Members	Data sets	% Data set	HC6, average % of THE	THE of all members, per cap US$	Average HC6 of all members[a], Per cap US$
African	46	3	1%	2.2%	55.3	1.6
American	35	23	13%	4.5%	469.2	18.8
Eastern Mediterranean	21	0	0%	NA	241.1	7.1
European	52	79	30%	2.4%	1407.8	36.9
Southeast Asia	11	3	5%	8.1%	70.0	2.1
Western Pacific	27	12	9%	2.6%	470.4	13.4
All	192	120	13%	2.94%	578.4	16.7

NA, not available.
From World Health Organization (2006b) World Health Report 2006: Working Together for Health. Geneva: World Health Organization and details from NHA focal point in WHO Headquarters.
[a]Average spending on HP at 2.94% of THE was applied to data for those WHO members where information on HP was absent, especially for all WHO members in the Eastern Mediterranean region.

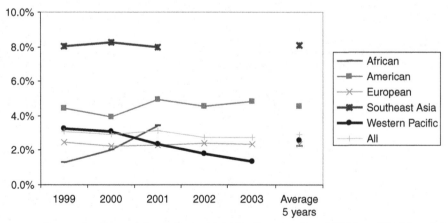

Figure 2 Average expenditure on health promotion as percent total health expenditure (THE) from 120 data sets in 1999–2003 according to WHO regions.

restrictions, spent merely US $55.4 and US $69.9 per capita, respectively, on the health of their population in 2003.
3. Spending on HP was much lower, given that only 2.9% of THE was used for HP; spending on HP was a mere US $1.6 and US $2.1 per capita, respectively, in countries in Africa and Southeast Asia.
4. This limited level of spending on health and very little on HP cannot meet the challenges of the current burden from preventable communicable and noncommunicable chronic diseases. This warrants further investigation into innovative financing of HP.

Review of Innovative Financing of Health Promotion

Many countries have had innovative health promotion strategies that conformed to WHO directions during the last two decades (World Health Organization, 1986, 1997). To fully implement the initiatives, governments in some countries have, through legislation, introduced the HP financing mechanism by means of dedicated portions of their revenues. Instead of transferring to the general revenue of the government, some portions, for example a tobacco excise tax, are earmarked for the HP Fund. As a result, financing of HP is ring-fenced and does not compete either within the health sector priority or between other social sectors in the general budgetary process, usually on an annual basis.

An earmark of so-called sin taxes from tobacco or alcohol has been commonly applied to fund the HP activities in many countries, such as the Health Promotion Foundations in Australia (since 1987), the Republic of Korea (since 1995), and Thailand (since 2001).

Some countries have also introduced additional levies on health insurance premiums to support HP activities such as the case in Switzerland (Health Promotion Switzerland, 2005). In Austria, the health promotion foundation is funded by an appropriation from treasury budgets (Fonds Gesundes Österreich, 2005). Several funds are administered and disbursed by the nongovernmental entities, especially in the form of health promotion foundations (Australia), though in some countries they are managed or governed by governmental agencies (Korea, the United States).

Historical development and characteristics of the innovative financing mechanism for HP are summarized country by country in chronological order of their fund establishment in these countries.

Australia

The Victorian Health Promotion Foundation (VicHealth) was the world's first health promotion foundation set up by using an additional levy on tobacco, which was directly earmarked to VicHealth in order to support activities in health promotion. VicHealth was established by the Victorian Parliament as part of the Tobacco Act in 1987, with funding from state government-collected cigarette tax. The governing board of VicHealth comprises parliamentary representatives from three major political parties and 11 ministerial appointments. This is a crucial strategy to ensure support from all political parties and ensure future sustainability of VicHealth under different ruling parties.

Logically, the VicHealth fund is generated from earmarked tax levied from tobacco products, while VicHealth's mandate is to promote health of the people, and support antismoking campaigns and tobacco control programs in the State of Victoria.

Since 1988, VicHealth has been used to buy out tobacco company's sponsorship of sports and art events. The Tobacco Act has banned billboards (since 1989), print media (since 1990), and point-of-sale advertising of tobacco (since 2000). All these proven effective actions against tobacco were the result of the VicHealth movement.

An impact of VicHealth on tobacco control is evident by a decline in the smoking rate of Victorian adults from 1986 to 2004 (31.5% in 1986 to 25.6% in 1991 and below 17% in 2005) (WHO Regional Office for the Western Pacific, 2004). VicHealth then moved to other major public health problems and active HP activities, for example, it funds breast cancer and cervical cancer screening campaigns, nutrition programs, health promotion in workplaces, and research in Alzheimer's disease and mental health. Each year VicHealth funds over 400 health promotion projects to hundreds of both large and small nongovernment and community-based organizations (VicHealth, 2005).

The South Australian government and the Australian Capital Territory (Healthpact) established health promotion funds in 1988 and 1989, respectively. Initially, funds were generated by tobacco licensing fees. The funds supported HP campaigns, in order to replace tobacco sponsorship of sports, arts, and racing events.

In Western Australia, the US $1.2 million tobacco tax increase in 1983 was allocated to a one-off Tobacco Tax Trust Fund. The Western Australian Health Promotion Foundation (Healthway) was formally established under the 1990 Tobacco Control Act in February 1991 (Healthway, 2004). Healthway avoids political interference by excluding members of state parliament from being associated with any payments made by the Foundation. It is governed by board members representing sports, arts, health, youth, and country interests.

In 1991, when Healthway was set up, the 15% increase in tobacco tax resulted in a 10% additional fund allocated to health promotion activities. Of the revenue of AU $17 million a year generated from tobacco tax, Healthway grants approximately one-third to health promotion projects and research, 30% to sports organizations, and 15% to arts organizations (Healthway, 2004).

In August 1997, the Australian High Court ruled that it was unconstitutional to earmark the state-based tobacco tax. Very unfortunately, this court decision ended the earmarked tobacco tax financing for health promotion foundations throughout Australia. As a result, Australian health promotion activities are at the present funded by a direct allocation from consolidated state government revenue (VicHealth, 2006).

After the High Court ruling, VicHealth managed to secure an increasing fund from the state government revenue, indicating high political support for HP. Health Promotion grants increased from AU $25.4 million in 2000–01 to AU $28.4 million in 2004–05 (VicHealth, 2005). A large portion of the Fund (84–87%) was grants provided to different agencies to move for HP; the operating expenditure was minimum (13–15%) (see **Table 4**).

Having reviewed the Australian cases, historically, they reveal a strong political intention by the State Parliament to provide an earmarked tobacco tax to fund HP activities and having their own governing structure for decision making. In response and accountable to the tobacco funding source, most activities primarily focused on anti-tobacco campaigns and then moved to other priority health problems. Working with several partners and using a variety of instruments including legislation, law enforcement, and public awareness campaigns led to many impressive results. This initiative brought down the prevalence of regular smokers in several states of Australia.

Estonia

In 1993, health promotion activities were formally launched in Estonia. The Ministry of Social Affairs decided to create a system for financing national and community-based health promotion projects. The funding was obtained from an earmarked share of the Estonian Health Insurance Fund (EHIF) and managed by a committee of experts making decisions on the funding as well as coordinating evaluation.

Since 1995, the EHIF has invested annually 0.3–1% of its budget for health promotion. In absolute terms, this amounted to €615 400 (€0.43 per capita) in 1995 and €865 400 (€0.62 per capita) in 2002 (The Estonian Health Insurance Fund, 2005).

In the Estonian case, financing HP was ring-fenced through an earmarked funding from the Health Insurance Fund. Though small in monetary terms, it has had an increasing trend in terms of the per capita HP budget. However, there is a need to investigate the nature of expenditure by the Estonia HP Fund.

The Republic of Korea

In 2001, health risk in the population of the Republic of Korea was high, for example the prevalence of smoking, heavy drinking, and obesity was 62%, 35%, and 32.6%, respectively, among Korean men. During the same period, lack of physical activity was also a serious health risk problem; 81.6% among women and 77.8% among men (Jung et al., 2005).

In response to these health risks, the National Health Promotion Fund (NHPF) was established under the National Health Promotion Act 1995. The Ministry of Health and Welfare was mandated to collect 150 Won (approximately US $0.15) for every pack of 20 cigarettes in 2000 (Jung et al., 2005). The earmarked tobacco tax increased to 354 Won in 2004, and around 500 Won at the end of 2004. The Fund plans to achieve 15 billion Won (approximately US $12 million) annually. A campaign against tobacco is one of the most active programs of health promotion in the Republic of Korea.

The Fund was administered by the Korea Institute for Health and Social Affairs (KIHASA; affiliated with the

Table 4 Financial statement of VicHealth 2000–2005

Income	2004–05	2003–04	2002–03	2001–02	2000–01
Health promotion grant	96%	95%	95%	95%	95%
Investment income	1%	2%	1%	1%	2%
Other	3%	4%	4%	4%	3%
Total income, %	100%	100%	100%	100%	100%
Total income, AU $1000	29 674	29 310	28 606	27 571	26 600
Expenditure					
Grants and associated expenses	84%	85%	86%	86%	87%
Business projects expenses	1%	2%	1%	0%	0%
Operating	15%	14%	13%	14%	13%
Total expenditure, %	100%	100%	100%	100%	100%
Total expenditure, AU $1000	28 804	30 672	29 116	26 808	27 277
Net result	870	–1362	–510	763	–677

From VicHealth (2005) Annual Report 2004–2005. Melbourne, The Victorian Health Promotion Foundation.

Ministry of Health and Welfare). Following a successful fund raised from the tobacco tax in 2002, approximately 3% of the fund (US $17 million) was allocated to HP activities, 14% for disease prevention and the majority, 65% was used for health insurance purposes (Korea Institute for Health and Social Affairs, 2006).

The Korea Institute for Health and Social Affairs, a governmental agency, is responsible for operating and making use of the fund and therefore it is likely that a decision on the use of the Fund is subject to political influence, for example the largest allocation for health insurance purposes is mostly for curative services.

Switzerland

Health Promotion Switzerland was established under Article 19 of the 1996 Sickness Insurance Act. Since 1998, activities of the Foundation have been financed in accordance with the Federal Health Insurance Act by annual contributions from all persons living in Switzerland. The Fund intends to stimulate, coordinate, and evaluate measures for health promotion and disease prevention. It has a governing Board, with 17 members, elected by the Swiss Federal Department of Home Affairs, and also federal and local government representatives. The Board has the support of an advisory committee of nine members, selected on the basis of personal capacity.

Since 1998, the activities of the Foundation have been financed in accordance with Article 20 of the Federal Sickness Insurance Act by annual contributions from all citizens in Switzerland. The contribution is currently SwF 2.40 per insured person per year (approximately US $1.80), which yields a total budget of around SwF 17 million per year (Health Promotion Switzerland, 2005). Contributions are collected by the sickness insurance provider via sickness insurance premiums. The annual amount of the contribution per person is set by the Federal Department of the Interior on request of the Foundation. The total SwF 11.8 million was invested in the 69 new HP projects contracted in 2004.

Switzerland was the second country, following Estonia, to earmark social health insurance contributions to a HP Fund, and the Fund is managed by a nongovernmental agency. A multisectoral approach was adopted by the Fund.

Austria

The Austrian Health Promotion Foundation was established by the 1998 Health Promotion Act. The Foundation receives grants-in-aid for each calendar year from the federal government's consolidated revenue from value-added tax. The Foundation operates on an annual budget of €7.25 million, serving as granting agency to promote and support projects and programs related to HP. The Foundation is governed by a 13-member board, and about half are government appointees. The remainder are candidates proposed by associations of local government officers, health professionals, and other interest groups. The Foundation supports activities to raise public awareness in health promotion and to create healthy living conditions and lifestyles, by funding over 500 projects (Fonds Gesundes Österreich, 2005).

United States

Similar to Australia, the U.S. demonstrated a strong relationship between an increase in tobacco tax and a major reduction in the prevalence of smoker and other tobacco-related chronic diseases. In Arizona, the smoking rate among the adult population dropped from 23.1% in 1996 to 18.3% in 1999, whereas the smoking rate among 18- to 24-year-olds decreased by 24% over the same period (American Lung Association, 2003). The incidence of lung cancer in California declined approximately 14% from 1988 to 1997. In Massachusetts, where in 2002 the cigarette excise tax rate was the highest in the US (US $1.51 per pack of 20 cigarettes), and had the highest increase (US $0.75 in the 2002 tax rate adjustment), the smoking rates in high and middle school children dropped by as much as 29.7% and 13% during the period of 1999–2002.

Facing budget constraints, legislatures in several states of the U.S. successfully raised significant amounts of state revenues by passing tobacco tax increase laws. However, spending on HP in some other states, especially on tobacco control, is still below the minimum amounts required by the US CDC's best practices. Maine, Delaware, Colorado, Hawaii, and Wyoming were the top five performers in tobacco control expenditure in 2006 (American Lung Association, 2006) (**Table 5**).

In 2006, there were 32 states (61%) in the US spending less than half of the benchmark on tobacco control, six states (12%) spent from 50% to 74%, and 11 states (21%) spent 75% to 100% of the benchmark (see **Table 6**). Interestingly, there were three states that spent over 100% of the benchmark on tobacco control.

In 1988, the primary source of financing tobacco control in California originated from the Proposition 99, which aimed to increase the state's tobacco tax by US $0.25 per pack. A 20% portion of the total revenue was further allocated to tobacco control and antismoking education, as well as research in tobacco-related diseases (5%). Spending on tobacco control efforts has been between US $85 and US $115 million, which falls short of the CDC minimum recommended amount.

In 2002, there was a push from a nongovernmental organization coalition to the Californian State Legislature to increase the US $0.87 current tax rate so as to earmark

Table 5 Top five highest and least states spending on tobacco prevention and control, against best practices recommended by CDC in 2006

US states	Total expenditure 2006, US$	CDC benchmark, US$	Ratio expenditure to benchmark
Five best performers			
1. Maine	15 785 699	11 190 000	141.1%
2. Delaware	10 851 501	8 630 000	125.7%
3. Colorado	26 404 214	24 550 000	107.6%
4. Hawaii	10 420 026	10 780 000	96.7%
5. Wyoming	7 043 151	7 380 000	95.4%
Five least performers			
1. Georgia	2 694 027	42 590 000	6.3%
2. Puerto Rico	1 083 264	25 197 000	4.3%
3. Tennessee	1 144 430	32 230 000	3.6%
4. Mississippi	611 761	18 790 000	3.3%
5. Missouri	857 000	32 770 000	2.6%

From American Lung Association (2006) *State of Tobacco Control 2006*. http://lungaction.org/reports/tobaccoprevention206.html (accessed September 2007).

Table 6 Percent distribution of US states actual spending on tobacco control against benchmark provided by American Lung Association, 2006

Percent actual spending to benchmark	Number of states	Percentage
0–24	19	36%
25–49	13	25%
50–74	6	12%
75–100	11	21%
100	3	6%
Total	52	100%

From American Lung Association (2006) *State of Tobacco Control 2006*. http://lungaction.org/reports/tobaccoprevention206.html (accessed September 2007).

for smoking cessation and tobacco-related research, heart disease prevention and cancer research, and health care for the uninsured.

Having learned from the precedent of earmarked tobacco tax set by California, in 1994 Arizona introduced a US $0.40 per pack increase in the cigarette excise tax, 23% of which was earmarked to tobacco control programs. The fund raised by tobacco tax has been managed by the state Department of Health Services since 1996, and has been used for programs such as antismoking campaigns among the youth, smoking cessation and counseling, and training and education. However, state legislature tried to cut the spending for health promotion activities to help balance the budget due to the loss of revenue dedicated to tobacco control.

In November 2002, the latest proposition pushed by NGO activists had successfully increased the Arizona State tobacco tax by US $0.60 (to a total of US $1.18 per pack) and reauthorized the 1994 tax for health promotion financing. In 2003, Arizona spent a total of US $18.5 million for tobacco control, which was still below the CDC recommendation.

In July 2002, the Massachusetts State Legislature increased the cigarette tax to the highest level in the U.S., namely U.S. $1.51 per pack, generating a state revenue of U.S. $222 million. At the same time, the legislature and governor reduced the spending on tobacco control from U.S. $48 million to U.S. $6 million, which is approximately one-sixth of the CDC recommendation.

Having reviewed innovative financing of HP in these countries, the following summary remarks emerge.

1. HP Funds in Australia, the U.S., and the Republic of Korea were rooted from a situation of very high smoking prevalence with an increasing trend and the economic loss from tobacco-related illnesses, both in medical care costs and loss of lives. For example, 23% of high school students and 10% of middle school students in the U.S. currently smoke (American Lung Association, 2004). The CDC estimates that each pack of cigarettes sold in the United States costs the country U.S. $7.18 in medical care costs and lost productivity (American Lung Association, 2004). It should be noted that VicHealth was also established by the Victorian Parliament as part of the 1987 Tobacco Act.

2. Based on this evidence, offsetting up an HP Fund is much influenced by the ideology of earmarking tobacco tax for a specific purpose.

3. The increase in tobacco tax was founded on strong evidence that increasing cigarette prices reduces youth smoking (The World Bank, 2000). Studies estimate that a 10% increase in the price of cigarettes would reduce teenage smoking by 7% and adult consumption by 4% (American Lung Association, 2004). Also, a 10% increase on cigarette prices worldwide would reduce consumption by up to 5% in high-income and by 8% in low- and middle-income countries, and low- and middle-income countries are more responsive to price increases (Ranson *et al.*, 2002).

4. In achieving earmarked tax from tobacco, it requires a legislative procedure. This is possible through the active engagement of civil groups and NGOs in such a campaign.

Table 7 summarizes country experiences on legislative framework, detailed funding sources, annual revenue, and population covered by each Fund.

Having reviewed the experiences in these countries, a matrix emerges on funding sources, for example, dedicated tax, earmarked contributions by insurance fund, and consolidated government revenue, as well as the organization and management of the fund, for example through an independent statutory body (e.g., a foundation or nongovernmental body) or merely through government agencies. Table 8 summarizes the experiences of the countries reviewed that fall into each group of arrangements and funding sources.

This matrix is a very useful framework for in-depth assessment of the performance of such innovative financing mechanisms, for example, sustainability of funding among three major sources, performance of downstream implementation of funding, and support activities.

Case Study on Innovative Financing of Health Promotion in Thailand

Historical Background

In the mid 1980s, health policy in Thailand gave high priority to reducing tobacco consumption (Supawongse and Buasai, 1997; Chantornvong and McCargo, 2001). In 1987, a nationwide campaign called Running Against Tobacco jointly organized by the Anti-Smoking Campaign Project (which later became the Anti-Smoking Foundation) and the Rural Doctor Society (a professional organization for the rural district doctors) raised significant public awareness on the health impacts of tobacco (Supawongse et al., 1998). This was the prime mover of the campaign against tobacco in Thailand.

Several important public health measures were introduced in the late 1980s, for example, the 1988 Executive Decree banning advertising of tobacco products and the 1989 Cabinet Decree on labeling tobacco as harmful products. In addition, the establishment of two important government agencies, the National Tobacco Consumption Control Board in 1989 and the Office of Tobacco Consumption Control under the MOPH in 1990 was the landmark of HP history (Chantornvong and McCargo, 2001). The Board and the Office served as an institutional umbrella for a systematic movement toward HP using tobacco as an entry point. The Office received an annual budget from the MOPH.

A 1992 act gave birth to the Health Systems Research Institute (HSRI), an independent public granting agency for health systems research (Health Systems Research Institute, 2004). HSRI receives an annual budget from the government. One of the major contributions of research granted by HSRI was evidence on epidemiology and trends of tobacco consumption, cost of tobacco-related illnesses, and evidence on income and price elasticity based on Thai household surveys (Buasai, 1993; Health Systems Research Institute, 1994; Sarntisart, 1995; Tungthangthum, 1997). This evidence serves as a platform for effective HP strategies.

The Tobacco Offices and HSRI facilitated a forum for intensive exchanges of experience, lessons, and visits of Thai and VicHealth on tobacco control in 1994–95. In the first biennial HSRI conference in February 1995, the VicHealth Chief Executive Officer was invited to deliver the VicHealth experience in Bangkok (Siwaraksa, 2005). One of the notable outcomes of this informal Thai–Australian collaboration is the confidence among the Thai partners on the feasibility of a dedicated-tax-for-health movement. As a result of convictions and commitments by Thai tobacco champions, many stakeholders were involved in a series of consultations, aiming to achieve a dedicated tobacco tax for health promotion. Finally a policy recommendation was made to the Government in 1996 on the possibility of founding such a mechanism (Siwaraksa, 2005).

In 1997, a working group was established by the Ministry of Finance (MOF) to investigate models of such a mechanism. The working group's recommendation endorsed a tobacco tax-funded health promotion foundation, and an appropriate and cost-effective mechanism to improve the health of the population. At the same time, the Alcoholic Policy Committee also recommended the MOF to create a financial mechanism in securing funds to minimize the problems related to alcohol consumption.

It took 2 years for dialogue and negotiation among stakeholders. At the end, in 1999, the MOF combined the two proposals to establish a health promotion foundation funded by tobacco and alcohol dedicated taxes. The dedicated tax is a major shift from conventional central pooling of all sources of government revenue to the Treasury, and a legislative endorsement was required. It took another 2 years for the drafting of a bill to be considered by the House of Representatives and the Senate. Finally the Thai Health Promotion Foundation Act 2001 was promulgated, and the Thai Health Promotion Foundation (ThaiHealth) came into force in October 2001.

Success factors for the founding of ThaiHealth are the knowledge-based movements by civic groups and political support by the MOF. Lessons learned from VicHealth were valuable and provided a context for this movement in Thailand.

The Priority

The mission of the ThaiHealth is to empower civic society and promote the well-being of the citizens, by acting as a catalyst and to provide financial support for projects that change social values, lifestyles, and environment conducive to health. Its mission is based on a broad definition of health and the application of the Ottawa

Table 7 A summary on country's experiences in using innovative financing for health promotion

Country/state	Organization	Legal framework	Funding sources	Annual revenue (2003)	Population covered, million (2003)
Australia, Victoria	Victorian Health Promotion Foundation (VicHealth) www.vichealth.vic.gov.au	Tobacco Act 1987 (Section 16)	State budget, initially from tobacco tax	US $16.2 m	4.6
Australia, Southern Australia	Department of Human Services Office for Recreation, Sport and Arts www.dhs.sa.gov.au	Tobacco Products Regulation Act 1987	State budget, initially from tobacco tax	US $9 m	2
Australia, Capital Territory	Australian Capital Territory Health Promotion Foundation (Healthpact) www.health.act.gov.au	Health Promotion Act 1995	State budget, initially from tobacco tax	US $1.4 m	0.3
Australia, Western Australia	Western Australian Health Promotion Foundation (Healthway) www.healthway.wa.gov.au	Tobacco Control Act 1990 (Section 15)	State budget, initially from tobacco tax	AU$17 m	1.9
Austria	Austrian Health Promotion Foundation (Fund for a Healthy Austria) www.fgoe.org	Health Promotion Act 1998	Federal consolidated revenue from value-added tax	€7.25 m	8
Estonia	Health Promotion Commission www.haigekassa.ee	Tobacco Excise Duty Act 1994 (Article 3); Alcohol, Tobacco, and Fuel Excise Duty Act 2000; Health Insurance Fund 2002	3.5% of tobacco tax, 3.5% of alcohol tax; 0.3–1% of health insurance fund	€0.8 m	1.4
Republic of Korea	Korea Institute for Health and Social Affairs under Ministry of Health and Welfare www.kihasa.re.kr	National Health Promotion Act 1995 (Chapter 3)	Tobacco tax (tax rate Korean Won 150 per pack) (3% allocated to health promotion and the rest to health insurance fund)	US $17 m	48
Switzerland	Health Promotion Switzerland www.gesundheitsfoerderung.ch	Sickness Insurance Act 1996 (Article 19)	Insurance premium and local government tax	SwF 17 m	7
Thailand	Thai Health Promotion Foundation (ThaiHealth) www.thaihealth.or.th	Health Promotion Foundation Act 2001	2% of tobacco and alcohol taxes	US $50 m	64
USA, Arizona	State Department of Health Services	Tobacco Tax and Health Care Act Arizona Revised Statutes, 1994	Tobacco tax (tax rate US $1.18 per pack) (23% of tobacco tax earmarked to health education)	US $18.5 m allocated to tobacco control	5.6
USA, California	State Treasury	California Revenue and Taxation Code, 1998	Tobacco tax (tax rate US $0.87 per pack) (in 1988, 20% earmarked to tobacco control)	US $108.1 m allocated to tobacco control	35.5
USA, Massachusetts		Massachusetts General Laws	Tobacco tax (tax rate US $1.51 per pack)	US $7.4 m allocated to tobacco control	6.4

Table 8 Matrix of funding sources and organization structure of the fund

Fund administrator and governing organizational structure	Funding sources		
	Dedicated tax from tobacco	Earmarked insurance contribution	Consolidated government revenue
Independent statutory body (Foundation, NGO)	VicHealth, Healthpact, Healthway (before 1997); ThaiHealth[a]	Switzerland, Estonia	VicHealth, Healthpact, Healthway (since 1997); Austria
Government organizations and agencies	Southern Australia (before 1997), Republic of Korea, Arizona, California		Southern Australia (since 1997); Massachusetts

[a]ThaiHealth includes earmarked tax from both tobacco and alcohol, as it moves beyond tobacco to the alcohol arena.

Charter. It plays in addition to the current players in HP, which invites collaboration and avoids resistance. ThaiHealth weaves different partners into networks who work closely together en route to national well-being.

Priorities include, for example, the introduction of health promotion, creating awareness of unhealthy behavior, supporting campaigns against tobacco and alcohol, and supporting research in HP (Thai Health Promotion Foundation, 2006). To achieve these goals, it employs four synergistic strategies; social mobilization, system development, healthy community development, and strengthening social capital.

The Governance

By law, ThaiHealth has two boards, the Governing Board and the Evaluation Board, appointed by the Cabinet. The Governing board has eleven members from the public sector (the Prime Minister is the chair, and ten other *ex officio*), and eight members from nongovernmental sectors selected on their personal capacities. ThaiHealth reports to the Cabinet and House of Representatives annually on achievement and performance.

ThaiHealth has eight clusters responsible for granting proposals and projects requested by partner agencies. Each cluster has an expert steering committee providing guidance, overseeing proposals and project implementation. According to the country's context, ThaiHealth usually has a common issue, which cuts across relevant clusters, for example, the Youth and Health issue in 2006.

Financial Profile

The total revenue of ThaiHealth in fiscal year 2005 was 2.32 billion Baht (approximately U.S. $57.9 million), with a 10% annual growth in nominal terms (Thai Health Promotion Foundation, 2005a). This is equivalent to U.S. $1 per capita, compared to an average U.S. $6.4 per capita (spent on conventional HP activities, mostly clinical preventive and promotion services) in 2000–02 (Tangcharoensathien *et al.*, 2005). Though per capita expenditure by ThaiHealth is small, it serves a catalytic function, engaging civil society and massive social mobilization.

The share of revenue from alcohol tax is nearly double that from tobacco. From the historical trend and current tax rate, ThaiHealth revenue is expected to increase from U.S. $57.9 million in 2005 to U.S. $116 million by 2020.

In 2005, ThaiHealth spent 2.52 billion Baht, slightly more than the current revenue; the deficit was absorbed by reserves. Of the total 2005 expenditure, 96% was grants to HP projects. ThaiHealth is a lean organization where operating and staffing expenditure were 2.5% and 1% of total expenditure, respectively.

Performance

We applied three dimensions of performance assessment of the health promotion foundation (WHO Regional Office for Western Pacific, 2004).

Relationship with partners

ThaiHealth was assessed by an external independent committee. Assessment indicated that it gathered the fragmented social capital and like-minded people across the country and interlaced them into a health promotion network, both area- and issue-based. For example, the Stop Drink Network, consisting of 144 partner organizations nationwide, worked jointly to reduce alcohol-related problems. Networking is a key success of the No Alcohol Campaign (Stopdrink Network, n.d.).

Project funding

In 2005, ThaiHealth supported over 700 projects. More than one-third of funded projects were on tobacco, alcohol, and prevention of road traffic injuries (34%), HP among specific populations (17%), and community capacity strengthening (16%) (see **Figure 3**).

The funding profiles conformed to the national priority and strategic plan. The Evaluation Board, however, identified some inconsistency of project plans and targets such as projects for community capacity strengthening and knowledge management in health promotion, particularly among these projects in the same geographical area (Thai Health Promotion Foundation, 2005b).

Impact on the population

National representative household surveys conducted regularly by the National Statistical Office include household consumption of tobacco. **Figure 4** illustrates the 1976–2003 prevalence trend of regular smokers among the population over 11 years old. Men had much higher rates than women. A decreasing trend was observed well before the existence of ThaiHealth in 2001, as a result of the tobacco campaign in the late 1980s. A stagnation of progress was observed in the early 2000s. Despite the strong enforcement of two tobacco laws – the 1992 Tobacco Product Control Act and the 1992 Non-Smoker Health Protection Act – much remains to be done to bring down smoking prevalence, especially among young adolescents.

ThaiHealth has demonstrated success in policy advocacy, public awareness, and national health promotion capacity building. Tobacco and alcohol supply control, regulation of alcohol advertisements, and road safety campaigns are examples of initial achievements (Thai Health Promotion Foundation, 2004). The 1.2 million

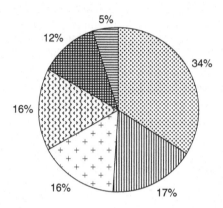

Figure 3 The distribution of HP programs funded by ThaiHealth in 2005. From Thai Health Promotion Foundation (2005a) *Annual Report 2005 Thaihealth.* Bangkok: Thai Health Promotion Foundation.

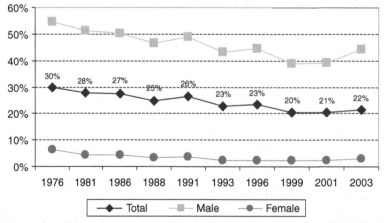

Figure 4 Trend of prevalence of regular smokers among population more than 11 years old, 1976–2003. From National Statistical Office, *National Health and Welfare Surveys in 1976–2003*. Bangkok, Thailand: Office of Prime Minister.

alcohol drinkers' intention to abstain from alcohol during the 3-month Buddhist Lent period in 2005 was evidence of a broad-based societal impact of ThaiHealth (Stopdrink Network, n.d.).

Lessons on success factors

Based on in-depth interviews of key stakeholders involved in the initiation and implementation of VicHealth, we identified three enabling factors: (1) organizational resilience to rapidly changing contexts and problems, (2) financial security, and (3) effective strategies.

ThaiHealth, a quasi-public agency, enjoys an autonomous status. It has corporate status and the legal capacity to sign contracts and fund projects, in a very flexible manner, while its social accountability is well in place, through the functions of the Evaluation Board, External Auditor, External Program Evaluators, and annual reporting mechanism to the Cabinet and the House of Representatives.

It allows full flexibility in coordinating multiple stakeholders, civil society, community-based organizations, individuals and partners in public and private sectors without rigid bureaucratic rules and regulations. A new set of skills is needed to manage ThaiHealth, especially setting strategic and program direction, engaging partners and networking, campaign skills and massive social mobilization, proposal reviews, and granting and implementation monitoring.

Dedicated tax from tobacco and alcohol ensures security and sustainability of the Fund. ThaiHealth receives transfer of tax on a daily basis from the Excise Department. Use of the Fund is approved by the Steering Committee and is free from political influence.

Finally, ThaiHealth plays a catalytic and complementary role to the existing health promotion players. The MOPH health promotion activities, mostly clinical preventive services, are delivered by health-care institutions and have little to do with other social determinants on health. ThaiHealth fills in the gaps and limitations faced by these partners.

Summary and Recommendation

Table 9 summarizes the differences in two models of financing HP, which are conventional and innovative financing mechanisms.

Although a majority of the burden of diseases can be mitigated by low-cost but effective health promotion interventions and consistent calls for increasing investment in health promotion by several charters, little is known on the actual level of financing health promotion.

Estimated spending on HP was low. If an estimated average 2.9% of total health expenditure was allocated for health promotion, the per capita expenditure on health promotion in 2003 was extremely low, U.S. $1.6 and U.S. $2.1 in countries in Africa and Southeast Asia, respectively. This is because expenditure on health was already low, and the proportion to health promotion was also low in low- and middle-income countries. This level of spending on HP cannot meet the challenges of current disease burden.

This article has investigated innovative financing models for HP, and lessons from high-income countries, except Thailand, a lower middle-income group. There is no such model for low-income countries. The historical evolution of innovative financing for health promotion reveals a close link with existing strong tobacco control measures, especially price increases and dedicated taxes for health promotion, as in Australia, the U.S., and Thailand. Another financing source is earmarking from social insurance premiums in countries that have achieved universal coverage, where social health insurance has been widely implemented. The limited role of social health

Table 9 Comparison of two models: conventional and innovative financing HP

	Conventional financing	*Innovative financing*
Source of finance	Government budget through annual budget cycle	Earmarked sin tax, social insurance contributions
Organization and management	Government agencies (federal and local)	Autonomous public agencies, corporate status and legal entity for grant signing
Governance and accountability	Mostly dominated by public agencies, bureaucratic inertia, conservative approaches	Multiple partners involved, civil society involved
Financial sustainability	Subject to political manipulation, priority, and decisions	Opportunity to increase tax for alcohol and tobacco, generate more revenue for the government and the fund, and halt consumption especially in the young adolescents
Deliverables	Conventional HP services, mostly clinical preventive services	Community-based, school-based, factory-based, social mobilization, campaign nature, through networking with partners and stakeholders
Organization and management	Less flexible, difficult to contract community-based organization, nongovernmental agencies	Exercise a full flexibility in management, campaign, contract and engage broad-base partners

insurance in low-income countries hampers their capacity to finance health promotion.

In all cases, achieving success in effective financing of HP requires legislation to endorse a fund and often an independent agency with greater flexibility in the organization and management of funding health promotion projects. These are concluded as indispensible characteristics of a successful health promotion fund.

Acknowledgments

We acknowledge institutional grants from Thailand Research Fund (TRF) and the Health Systems Research Institute (HSRI) to IHPP, which are mandated to strengthen the capacity in health systems and policy research in Thailand. Also, we are very grateful to the Ministry of Public Health for their support and collaboration. Contributions of partners in health promotion, tobacco and alcohol campaign in the movement of ThaiHealth are highly appreciated.

Citations

American Lung Association (2003) *State of Tobacco Control 2002: The Second Annual Report.* New York: The American Lung Association.
American Lung Association (2004) *State of Tobacco Control 2003 Fact Sheet.* http://www.lungusa.org/site/apps/nl/content3.asp?c=dvLUK9O0E&b=40408&content_id=%7B6D1769C3-A7E0-4AB6-ADBE-DA2BEB9BC90A%7D (accessed September 2007).
American Lung Association (2006) *State of Tobacco Control 2006.* http://lungaction.org/reports/tobaccoprevention206.html (accessed September 2007).
Berman P, Arellanes L, Henderson P, et al. (1999) *Health Care Financing in Eight Latin American and Caribbean Nations: The First Regional National Health Accounts Network.* Washington, DC: Partnerships for Health Reform.
Chantornvong S and McCargo D (2001) Political economy of tobacco control in Thailand. *Tobacco Control* 10: 48–54.
The Estonian Health Insurance Fund Estonian Health Insurance Fund. http://www.haigekassa.ee/eng/, from http://www.haigekassa.ee/eng/ehif.
Fonds Gesundes Österreich (2005) *Annual Report 2004.* Vienna, Austria: Fund for a Healthy Austria.
Health Promotion Switzerland (2005) *Annual Report 2004 – Executive Summary.* Bern, Switzerland: Health Promotion Switzerland.
Health Systems Research Institute (2004) *Annual Report 2004.* Nonthaburi, Thailand: Health System Research Institute.
Healthway (2004) Core Business of Healthway. http://www.healthway.wa.gov.au.
Jha P and Chaloupka FJ (eds.) *Tobacco Control in Developing Countries.* Oxford, UK: Oxford University Press.
Korea Institute for Health Social Affairs (2006) About KIHASA. http://www.kihasa.re.kr/html/english/sub02_01.jsp.
Musgrove P, Zeramdini R, and Carrin G (2002) Basic patterns in national health expenditure. *Bulletin of the World Health Organization* 80(2): 134–146.
National Statistical Office (several years) *National Health and Welfare Surveys.* Bangkok, Thailand: Office of Prime Minister.
Nutbeam D (1998) *Health Promotion Glossary.* Geneva, Switzerland: World Health Organization.
OECD (2002) A System of Health Accounts: Implementation. http://www.oecd.org/document/49/0,2340,en_2649_34631_32411121_1_1_1_1,00.html (accessed September 2007).
Poullier J, Hernandez P, Kawabata K, et al. (2002) Patterns of Global Health Expenditure: Results for 191 countries. Discussion Paper No. 51. Geneva, Switzerland: World Health Organization.
Ranson MK, Jha P, Chaloupka FJ, et al. (2002) The effectiveness and cost-effectiveness of price increases and other tobacco-control policies. http://www.worldbank.org/tobacco/tcdc/42T0448.pdf (accessed January 15, 2008).
Sarntisart I (1995) *The Impact of a Change in the Cigarette Excise Tax.* Nonthaburi, Thailand: Health Systems Research Institute.
Siwaraksa P (2005) *The Birth of The ThaiHealth Fund.* Bangkok, Thailand: Thai Health Promotion Foundation (ThaiHealth).
Stopdrink Network (n.d.) Over million decide to stop drinking [in Thai]. http://www.stopdrink.com/?content=ViewNews&id=132&type=5 (accessed September 2007).
Stopdrink Network (n.d.) Stopdrink Network partnership. www.stopdrink.com (accessed September 2007).
Supawongse C and Buasai S (1997) The evolution of tobacco consumption control in Thailand. *Health Systems Research Journal* 5(3): 25–26.
Tangcharoensathien V, Somaini B, Moodie R, et al. (2005) Sustainable financing for health promotion: Issues and challenges. Paper presented at the 6th Global Conference on Health Promotion, Bangkok, Thailand, August 2005.
Thai Health Promotion Foundation (2005a) *Annual Report 2005 Thaihealth.* Bangkok, Thailand: Thai Health Promotion Foundation.
Thai Health Promotion Foundation (Thai Health) (2006) *Vision and mission of Thai Health Promotion Foundation.* http://www.thaihealth.or.th/info/summaryreport/2549.pdf.
Tungthangthum S (1997) The political economy concerning cigarettes. *Health Systems Research Journal* 5(3): 190–203.
Vartiainen E, Jousilahti P, Jousilahti P, et al. (2000) Cardiovascular risk factor changes in Finland, 1972–1997. *International Journal of Epidemiology* 29: 49–56.
VicHealth (2005) Annual Report 2004–2005. Melbourne, Australia: The Victorian Health Promotion Foundation.
VicHealth (2006) Fact Sheet 1, VicHealth Funding Model. http://www.vichealth.vic.gov.au/assets/contentFiles/Fact%20Sheet_VicHealth%20Funding%20Model.pdf (accessed September 2007).
The World Bank (2000) Tobacco Facts 1: Price and Other Measures to Reduce Demand is Key to Tobacco Control. New York: The World Bank.
WHO Regional Office for the Western Pacific (2004) *The Establishment and Use of Dedicated Taxes for Health.* Manila, Philippines: World Health Organization.
World Health Organization (2005c) World Health Report 2005: Make Every Mother and Child Count. Geneva, Switzerland: World Health Organization.
World Health Organization World (2006b) Health Report 2006: Working Together for Health. Geneva, Switzerland: World Health Organization.

Further Reading

Jamison TD, Breman GJ, Measham RA, et al. (2006) *Disease Control Priorities in Developing Countries,* 2nd edn. Washington, DC: World Bank.
Siwaraksa P (2005) *The Birth of The ThaiHealth Fund.* Bangkok, Thailand: Thai Health Promotion Foundation (ThaiHealth).
Supawongse C and Buasai S (1997) The evolution of Tobacco Consumption Control in Thailand. *Health Systems Research Journal* 5(3): 25–26.
Tangcharoensathien V, Somaini B, Moodie R, et al. (2005) Sustainable financing for health promotion: issues and challenges. Paper presented at the 6th Global Conference on Health Promotion, Bangkok, Thailand, August 2005.
VicHealth (2005) The Story of VicHealth: A World first in Health Promotion. http://www.vichealth.vic.gov.au/assets/contentFiles/History_Book_Full_Version.pdf (accessed September 2007).
World Health Organization (2005a) *The Bangkok Charter for Health Promotion in a Globalized World.* http://www.who.int/healthpromotion/conferences/6gchp/hpr_050829_%20BCHP.pdf (accessed September 2007).
World Health Organization (2005b) Preventing Chronic Diseases: A Vital Investment. Geneva, Switzerland: World Health Organization.

ORGANIZATION OF HEALTH SERVICES

Health System Organization Models (Including Targets and Goals for Health Systems)

F C J Stevens, University of Maastricht, Maastricht, The Netherlands
J van der Zee, NIVEL, Netherlands Institute for Health Services Research, Utrecht, The Netherlands

© 2008 Elsevier Inc. All rights reserved.

Introduction

A health-care delivery system is the organized response of a society to the health problems of its inhabitants (Van der Zee et al., 2004). Societies differ significantly in the way they organize their response, and because of this they can be very well subjected to comparative analysis and research. This article describes health-care systems from a comparative perspective. It aims to answer the following three questions:

- What do we consider a health-care system?
- Why do health-care systems differ and how can we fruitfully group them?
- What health-care systems innovations can we expect in the future?

What Is a Health-Care System?

Usually, health care is rather loosely referred to as a system, without paying much attention to the term itself. Terms like sector and system are often used as synonyms, while the phrase 'health system' is habitually little more than shorthand for health-care (delivery) system. Philipsen (1995), in studying the neighboring but very contrasting health-care systems of Belgium and the Netherlands, noted that the term system should not be applied too loosely. Instead, for comparison reasons, he suggested using the term system as an essential analytic tool. Referring to the writings on systems of Parsons (1951) and Habermas (1981) he indicates that systems have four typical characteristics:

1. Functional specificity – systems have shared operational goals;
2. Structural differentiation – systems have a distinct division of labor between elements (persons, organizations);
3. Coherence among the composing elements – systems are subjected to coordination, planning, and organization;
4. Autonomy – systems are self-regulating to a certain degree, notwithstanding open borders to other systems (e.g., education, welfare, industry, legal system) and to the general environment.

These four systems characteristics are not just present or absent but vary in degree. Applied to health care, Philipsen suggests that one health-care system can be far more 'systematic' than another. In his two-countries comparison, he illustrates that according to the four characteristics, the Dutch health-care system was more 'systematic' than the Belgian one (Philipsen, 1985).

Such observations will be very familiar to students involved in comparative health (care) systems research. Countries vary considerably in the degree of central coordination of their health-care system, especially regarding the weaker or stronger role of the state (e.g., compare the UK and United States regarding coordination, planning, and organization). Also, the fuzzy boundaries between health care and social services make up, in degree of autonomy, a distinctive system characteristic. The boundaries between health and welfare are a notorious impediment for comparative analysis, specifically when studying health care for the elderly. So indeed, the 'system' concept and its features are a useful analytical tool for understanding international differences.

Why Do Health-Care Systems Differ?

As noted, health-care systems are societies' organized response to their health problems. So logically, when health problems vary between populations, it is likely that also their health-care systems vary. This is very obvious when contrasting health problems of countries at different levels of income (low-income, lower-middle-income, upper-middle-income, and high-income economies) (World Bank, 2007). Low-income countries are faced with many problems that impede health directly or indirectly. These include childhood diseases, negative maternal conditions, HIV/AIDS, malaria, and tuberculosis. Infectious diseases are the major cause of premature deaths and reduced life expectancy. In developed countries chronic diseases form the major causes of death. Consequently, the health-care systems in these two groups of countries are fundamentally different and thus pursue different approaches to health care: in developing countries the focus is mostly on hygiene and preventive care, whereas in the developed world the emphasis is on extensive curative care.

Besides observing such crude but evident health-related systems differences one also can, at least among high-income countries, differentiate between types of health-care systems that are *not* grounded in essential health problem differences. These systems differences have more or less grown historically. The essential difference between groups of health-care systems in high-income countries is grounded on their way of funding and the degree of governmental (state) influence on health-care delivery. Two typical groups are often dubbed after their founding fathers: Bismarck (Germany) on the one hand and Beveridge (UK) on the other. Bismarck, the first chancellor of united Germany 'invented' social security at the end of the nineteenth century and helped to create and foster mutual funds (sick funds) to protect the fund members against loss of income due to illness and disability. The social security system is mainly funded by earmarked, wage-dependent premiums. Beveridge, the founder of the British National Health Service (NHS) in 1948, created a state-dominated, tax-funded health services system for all British citizens that soon served as an example for many countries all over the world. Beside these two major types, two others should be mentioned. One is the market-based American health-care system, with limited government influence and funding. The other is the full-blown opposite of this, the health-care system in the former Soviet Union and its satellite countries (the Shemasko model, named after its founder) with strong governmental influence and extensive funding (Marrée and Groenewegen, 1997).

In the following sections of this article we first go deeper into the impact of societal transitions and the impact on differences between low-income countries and (lower and upper) middle-income countries on the one hand, and high-income countries and their health-care systems on the other (i.e., health care in a transitional perspective). Then we further elaborate on the basic elements of the four types of health-care systems prominent in high-income countries.

Health Care in a Transitional Perspective

To understand current health-care delivery systems from a longitudinal perspective three types of transition are significant: (1) the socioeconomic growth of a society, (2) its demographic expansion, and (3) its epidemiological development (**Figure 1**). Modern societies developed over the ages from agricultural economies through industrialization to service economies (Van der Zee *et al.*, 2004). They initially focused on survival and self-sustenance of the smallholder and his extended family, but later on developed into economies creating surpluses (wealth) and added value to products that could be traded. Commonly, the surpluses of these trades were used to institute new roles and occupations, which were not necessarily productive. Typical examples are priests, soldiers, tax collectors, and different kinds of healers. In this societal transition the surpluses were accumulated over long periods, in which stages of prosperity alternated with periods of hardship, due to war, food crises, and pandemics. As societies further developed and modernized, more structures and institutions came into existence that reduced the health and social risks of daily life. The widespread, kinship-based arrangements to cope with these risks were

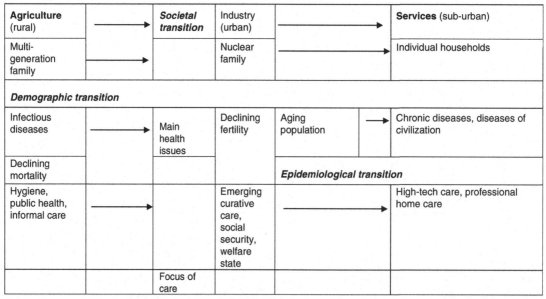

Figure 1 Health care and the societal, demographic, and epidemiological transitions. Adapted from Van der Zee J, Boerma WGW, and Kroneman MW (2004) Health care systems: Understanding the stages of development. In: Jones R, Britten N, Culpepper L, Gass DA, Grol R, Mant D, and Silagy C (eds.) *Oxford Textbook of Primary Medical Care*, vol. 1: pp. 51–55. Oxford: Oxford University Press.

gradually supplemented and replaced by collective arrangements (De Swaan, 1988).

In the wake of this societal transition a demographic transition took place, as it proved no longer essential to have many children as a provision against the risks of becoming dependent on kin when growing old or living in poverty. One of the later consequences was that fertility dropped.

In Europe, by the end of the nineteenth century, social security systems against loss of income due to accidents and disabilities came into existence, first in Germany, then later in other countries, including public pension schemes several decades later. In addition to these collective arrangements, financial surpluses were the foundations for economic growth and the expansion of educational and health-care facilities, which also generated more services and typical professions such as teachers, physicians, nurses, judges, lawyers, engineers, architects, and so on. In Europe, premium collection and taxes were the primary mechanisms and financial resources for these collective arrangements.

In the course of this modernization process the epidemiological transition took place, reflecting a gradual shift from the sheer necessity to overcome malnutrition and infectious diseases toward dealing with chronic diseases (primarily affecting the elderly). Today, health-care delivery systems in high-income societies are largely focusing on lifestyle diseases (obesity, diabetes mellitus), chronic diseases, and the subsequent changing needs and demands of an aging population. During the past century, in high-income countries, a dramatic shift in the cause of death has taken place, from infectious diseases and malnutrition to cardiovascular diseases and cancer. Chronic disease deaths now exceed mortality from infections and malnutrition.

In many high-income societies the societal, demographic, and epidemiological transitions took place during the course of many years. This went together with the coming into existence of more organized and institutionalized 'systems' of care, which replaced earlier fragmented services of competing health professionals and health institutions. In low- and middle-income countries we often see, in a shorter time frame, incomplete and more compressed transitions. This is manifested in less health-care systems coherence (i.e., coordination, planning, and organization). Organized health-care systems in lower-income countries – in particular on the African continent – were often copies of Western models and were habitually implemented and enforced as part of the colonization processes. In addition to this, many low-income countries inherited from colonial occupation health-care legislation that was not up-to-date. In the beginning, organized health care, with a strong emphasis on hospital care, was primarily oriented toward the military, civil servants, and settlers. It was only later that more community and primary health-care services came into existence for the local population. Today, health facilities are usually unequally distributed usually because of insufficient investments in human resources. Lower-income countries have three to four times less doctors and nurses than high-income countries per unit of the population, which is evidence that human resources is one of the most neglected components of health system development (Breier and Wildschut, 2006; Hongoro and McPake, 2004).

Access to clinical services is still primarily reserved for limited groups (armed forces, civil servants, and wealthy people). Health services are often organized through a set of vertical programs, addressing specific health problems. The advantage is that health-care delivery is assured; the disadvantage is that service provision is often fragmented and inefficient. Community health-care workers act as first-line contacts of the health system in these countries, where basic conditions for improving health often fail (e.g., poverty, protection of mother and child, birth intervals, education, basic maternity care, and immunization). Major health-care providers are the state and nongovernmental organizations.

In upper-middle-income economies, such as in South Africa, there is a high diversity of facilities with high-tech private hospitals for those who can afford it at one side of the continuum, and, for those who can't afford it, unqualified practitioners at the other, and everything else in between. Existing social insurance arrangements are mainly available and affordable for state employees (military, civil service). For example, South Africa has implemented mandatory insurance for civil servants, which can be seen as the kernel of a future social health insurance scheme. However, getting mandatory insurance for all formally employed, or setting up an affordable model for low-income beneficiaries, will take at least another decade, as there are many political and practical hurdles to tackle (McIntyre and Doherty, 2004). The ongoing debate includes what such health insurance plans should look like, for example, whether low-income countries should have a voluntary insurance plan, a private one, or a mix of both.

In low- and middle-income countries the bulk of health-care expenditure has to come from direct household (out-of-pocket) spending, taxation, and deficit spending. So what is often seen is a hodgepodge of facilities and means of health-care provision, formal, as well as informal, including a huge variety of traditional healers paid out-of-pocket or in kind.

The coming into existence of a modern health-care delivery system with a highly developed division of labor, a high degree of structural complexity, and means for coordination and planning requires extensive financial resources. Only affluent economies are able to put sufficient resources aside, and the extent to which these can be generated for health care signifies a nation's stage of economic development. Indeed, there is a strong association between health and wealth, not only at the level of the individual person, but on the macro level too. Put another way, the richer the country, the more health care is a 'system.'

As can be seen in **Figure 2**, the average life expectancy is plotted against per capita income in a large number of countries for the years 1900, 1930, 1960, and 1990, respectively (World Bank, 1993). From the early 1990s (see **Figure 2**), the highest health gain is found in the lowest income range, where societies move from 'poor' to 'less poor.' The initial increase in life expectancy is mainly due to reductions in infant mortality. But having reached a certain level of prosperity, life expectancy tends to stabilize. Evidently, in more affluent societies a point is reached beyond which substantial growth of life expectancy is unlikely to happen.

So, as **Figure 2** also demonstrates, the wealth of a nation has a major impact on health. At the beginning, when the wealth of a nation increases, its level of health improves, directly, by public health improvement, and indirectly by schooling and the increase of income level (in particular of mothers). Later, when economic wealth has further increased, lifestyle and chronic diseases tend to amplify. In affluent societies people are more likely to manifest unhealthy behavior and, as people grow older, the magnitude of chronic disease increases. Obviously, the overall impact of wealth on health is not linear. And because of this it is harder to improve on health in affluent societies than in poorer ones (provided, of course, resources for health care are sufficiently available and adequately distributed).

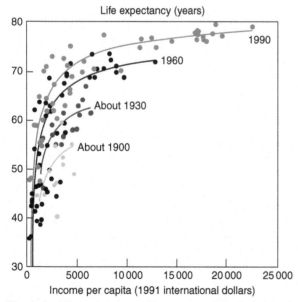

Figure 2 Life expectancy and income per capita for selected countries and periods. Reproduced from World Bank (1993) Investing in health, World development report 1993, p. 34. Oxford, UK: Oxford University Press.

The relationship between health and wealth is also reciprocal. Economic growth and wealth improve health, but good health stimulates economic growth as well. In mature economies a successful health-care sector encourages skilled employment, domestic production, building, and the consumption of service goods. Wealth also defines health-care targets. And again, the wealthier a nation, the more probable it is that it has a systematic health-care system.

Four Models of Health-Care Systems: Free Market, Social Insurance, NHS, and Socialist

Typically, high-income countries are characterized by public poverty and private wealth. There is an excess of energy consumption with environmental pollution as a resulting health threat. Pockets of relative poverty are manifested at the dark side of society's individualization, leading to problems of anomy, loneliness (in particular among the elderly), and suicide. Combating lifestyle-related illnesses, cost containment, unequal health-care access, preventing unnecessary or overtreatment, rationalizing pharmaceuticals and providing a dedicated mix of health and social services to the elderly are considered major health-care policy issues in all high-income societies. In time there has been a gradual extension of curative services from the wealthy to the population as a whole, with emphasis on specialist/hospital care and primary care as a counterbalance. Also, the focus has shifted from preventive to curative services, and later on again to preventive services (preventing lifestyle diseases).

Because of these similar health-care problems in high-income countries their health-care systems look more or less alike. They can be typified as mixed private–public systems, however, their origins differ. Based on their funding and degree of state intervention four models of health-care systems can be distinguished. These four models vary on a continuum between health care seen as a *commodity* to be bought on the free market on the one hand, and health care as a *public good* or *right*, independent of a person's income, on the other.

Free Market Model

The free market model applies when the state conducts a policy of noninterventionism and restricts its interference in health-care matters to the bare essentials, leaving the rest to private funding and corporate provision (e.g., health maintenance organizations, or HMOs). This is the typical situation in the United States, except for Medicaid (which is for the indigent) and Medicare (for the elderly) state interventions. Private insurance fills the gap to some degree, however, a large proportion of the U.S. population is still uninsured against health-care costs or loss of income due to illness and disability. The basic (original) model of the United States health-care system is a voluntary reimbursement model, with four actors playing a key role (Hurst, 1992). First-level (general practitioners, or GPs) and second-level providers (hospitals) deliver services to patients who will be reimbursed for their medical bill, in part or in whole. Patients pay a voluntary risk-related premium to voluntary insurers, who reimburse them for medical expenses. Typically, there is no, or minimal, interaction between insurer and provider. Only the patient interacts with both parties. The private reimbursement model has two major drawbacks (Hurst, 1992). One is that it does not have built-in incentives to restrict demand and supply. Therefore, it is often accompanied by cost sharing. Another drawback is that it does not have built-in mechanisms to prevent inequities. For reasons of profit maximization, private insurers have an incentive to select against poor risks. Moreover, access to voluntary insurance is only open to those who are willing or can afford to pay. This has enormous consequences for health-care insurance coverage in the United States. Whereas the vast majority of the Organisation for Economic Co-operation and Development (OECD) countries have achieved universal health-care coverage, the United States has the largest percentage of citizens without government-assured health insurance. The most recent figures show that, in 2005, 15% of the population (nearly 45 million people) were without health insurance. This varies between 8% for the population of Minnesota, and 24% in Texas (U.S. Census Bureau, 2007). This problem has been put on the political agenda again and again, but still has not seen any substantial improvements.

A second shortcoming is high spending. In 2004 U.S. health-care spending as a percentage of GDP was 13.3%, compared to 9.2% for neighboring Canada, and 8.1% for the average industrialized (OECD) country (OECD, 2006). United States per capita health spending continues to exceed per capita health spending in the other OECD countries, by huge margins. In the period between 1991 and 2001, the U.S. average annual growth in health spending was 3.1, compared to 2.1 in Canada and 3.0 for the OECD median. Despite managed care initiatives and government attempts at regulation, costs keep increasing in the United States (Anderson, 1997). Lack of (hospital) budget control, fragmented and complex payment systems that weaken the demand side and excessive administrative overhead may account for the high health-care spending (Reinhardt et al., 2004).

Social Insurance Model

The second health systems model is the social insurance system, founded in Germany just over a hundred years ago. Patients typically pay an insurance premium to the sick fund, which has a contract with first-line (GP) and second-line (hospital) providers. The role of the state is restricted to setting umbrella terms for contracts between patients, providers, and insurers. The social insurance system is funded by premiums paid and controlled by employers and labor unions. These, however, have little inference with the provision of services, which is left to the professions, specifically to the medical profession and to professionalized care organizations (e.g., home nursing, home help). Basically, continental European health-care systems originate from the German social health insurance model, founded at the end of the nineteenth century by the German Chancellor Wilhelm Bismarck. Earmarked premiums were paid to a sick fund, which was jointly controlled by employers and employees (labor unions). From this sick fund health-care provision from hospitals and from individual practitioners was paid.

For people with lower- and middle-class salaried incomes collective and enforced arrangements are available (sick funds). Founded in Germany, the social security model was quickly adopted by Czechoslovakia, and during the Austrian-Hungarian rule, by Austria, Hungary, and Poland. During the Second World War it was forced on the Netherlands (1941), and later on it was adopted by Belgium and France. The social insurance system survived two world wars and national socialism, and, in essence, still exists, although in a modified fashion, in Germany, the Netherlands, Belgium, France, Austria, Switzerland, Luxembourg, and Japan. Formerly it existed in other countries as well: Greece until 1982, Italy until 1977, Portugal until 1978, and in Spain until 1985 (Saltman and Figueras, 1997).

National Health Services (NHS) Model

The third model, typically found in the UK and Commonwealth nations, is the taxed-based National Health Services (NHS) model. First introduced in 1948, it is centralized and funded by means of taxation, while the state is responsible for the provision of institution-based care (hospitals). The medical profession has a rather independent position. Self-employed GPs are the gatekeepers in primary health care. Before visiting a hospital or a medical specialist one needs a referral from a GP. The NHS model leaves some room for private medicine. Until 1995 state hospitals and individual GPs were paid from this NHS taxation.

Through processes of diffusion and adaptation, the NHS model was first adopted in Sweden, and then by the other Scandinavian countries: Denmark, Norway, and Finland. At present, the NHS model applies to the United Kingdom, Ireland, Denmark, Norway, Sweden, Finland, Iceland, and outside Europe by Australia and New Zealand. Four Southern European countries adopted the tax-based model more recently: Italy, in 1978; Portugal, 1979; Greece, 1983; and Spain, 1986 (Saltman and Figueras, 1997).

Socialist Model

The fourth, most centralized systems model, the Soviet socialist model, was invented by Shemasko, a Minister of Health, and dates from 1920. It is characterized by a strong position of the state, guaranteeing full and free access to health care for everyone. This is realized by state ownership of health-care facilities, by funding from the state budget (taxes), and by geographical distribution and provision of services throughout the country. Health services are fully hierarchically organized. They are provided by state employees, planned by hierarchical provision, and organized as a hierarchy of hospitals, with outpatient clinics (polyclinics) as lowest levels of entrance. Among the nations that, until recently, had a health-care system based on the Soviet model were Russia, Belarus, the Central-Asian republics of the former USSR, and some countries in Central and Eastern Europe. Many former Soviet Republics, however, are in a process of transition toward a social insurance-based system.

The Cuban health-care system also underwent shortages following the collapse of the Soviet Union. But while Cuban secondary and tertiary care suffered from the crisis, the well-functioning universal and equitable health-care system from before the crisis remained largely intact, due to the government's support and grassroots organizations-based networks of solidarity (Nayeri and Lopez-Pardo, 2005). The Chinese health-care system, created in 1949, was also a typical example of now largely extinct twentieth-century communist societies. By the early 1980s the Chinese government virtually dismantled it (Blumenthal and Hsiao, 2005). Its way of financing was dramatically changed by reducing government's investments, the imposition of price regulation, and the decentralization and underfinancing of its public health system. China now has a private health-care system, with its typical failures: a large part of the population uncovered by health insurance (about 70%), unaffordable services for many, high national spending, overuse of (profitable) pharmaceuticals, and high-tech care (Blumenthal and Hsiao, 2005). Currently, the government is trying to repair the damage done, which ultimately may result in a mixed public–private system. Cuba and China prove, positive and negative, that government involvement in health care is essential to keep the health-care system intact, to protect patients, and to provide affordable access to services.

The four models make up a continuum in terms of their 'system' character, with state interventionism and centralized health care at one end, and noninterventionism at the other. Centralized systems provide the best mechanisms for cost control, while absence of state intervention appears less fruitful, as soaring costs in the United States make clearly evident. But the four health systems models are to be seen as pure types that can be found in many combinations and varieties. They further reflect stages and outcomes of a historical process, so that system models that came into existence in highly developed economies in the first half of the twentieth century can still provide useful options to choose from in developing countries or transitional economies, for example, in Eastern European societies.

Health-Care Delivery Systems Innovations

While the models presented reflect the major ones that can be found in high-income countries, none of them fully complies with only one of these. For example, in the 1960s and 1970s social insurance-based health-care delivery systems and the entrepreneurial system of the United States started to be faced with problems of rising costs. In the 1970s and 1980s the NHS delivery systems and Soviet-like delivery systems of Eastern Europe had problems of neglect, underfunding, and extensive bureaucracy, leading to private initiatives next to the NHS and to a flourishing black health-care market in Eastern and Central Europe. Since then, in particular in countries having social security-based health-care systems, this has led to more state regulation to curb the costs of health care. In other countries it resulted in the reversed situation of less state intervention, and in the introduction of different forms of managed competition (**Table 1**). For example, in Eastern Europe, after the fall of the Berlin Wall, there was a demise of state funding and state provision due to economic deficits. In the countries that have adopted the social insurance model there is more state regulation to introduce more planning and to curb the rising costs of health care. One of the consequences has been a more dominant position of hospitals in the delivery of health care. In the UK, however, there is a movement toward more decentralization, which was realized by a split between purchasers and providers, with GPs as the purchasers of hospital care (Saltman and Figueras, 1997).

Just like in other high-income societies, health-care reforms in the United States are essentially focusing on cost containment. Managed care initiatives, for example, HMOs, were developed to increase competition, to change methods of payment for medical services, and to curb the power of the medical profession. The fundamental model of the HMO is typified as a voluntary contract model (Hurst, 1992). It involves contractual relationships between insurers and independent providers, which give these providers an exclusive right to supply complete services, mainly free of charge. Patients pay a voluntary, risk-related premium to voluntary insurers who have contracts with providers. The difference with the

Table 1 Health systems models – their strengths, weaknesses, and innovations

Model	Definition of health care	Role of the state	Funding	Budget control	Strengths	Weaknesses	Major innovations
Socialist (Shemasko) (Communist countries; former Eastern Europe, Cuba)	Health care as state-provided public service	Very strong; owns facilities pays providers directly	Government funding	State/Party	Full and equal access, low costs, full coverage	Bureaucratism, rigidness, corruption	Total collapse (fall of Berlin Wall)
National Health Service (Beveridge) (UK, Australia, New Zealand, Canada, Nordic countries, Spain, Italy)	Health care as a guaranteed, state-supported consumer service	Strong; controls and finances facilities	Taxation	Ministry of Health	Equal access to comprehensive services, low costs	Bureaucracy, underfunding, rigidness	Referral market purchaser–provider split (GPs as hospital services purchasers)
Social Security (Bismarck) (Germany, Japan, Netherlands, France, Belgium)	Health care as a guaranteed, insured good	Intermediate; regulates the system	Earmarked premiums	Employers and employees	Client-friendly, professional autonomy, earmarked budgets	High costs difficult to control	Cost control by macro budgeting, introduction of market principles
Free Market (United States, South Africa, Switzerland)	Health care as a commodity	Weak (except for specific groups); providers are mainly private entrepreneurs	Private and state/federal government financing	For-profit insurers and government	Provider-friendly, professional autonomy, flexibility	Consumerism, high costs, fragmentation, unequal access and uninsured	HMO

Van der Zee J, Boerma WGW, and Kroneman MW (2004) Health care systems: Understanding the stages of development. In: Jones R, Britten N, Culpepper L, Gass DA, Grol R, Mant D, and Silagy C (eds.) *Oxford Textbook of Primary Medical Care* vol. 1. Oxford, UK: Oxford University Press.

voluntary reimbursement model is that insurers now have contractual relationships with providers. Managed care models are all aiming at controlling the costs of health care by monitoring the work of doctors and hospitals, and by limiting the use of second-level hospital care. In practice, this is often done by means of a 'case manager,' who, on behalf of the insurer, is authorized to decide whether the care to be rendered is effective and efficient. Another feature is that patients are only allowed to see a specialist after they have visited a general practitioner. This gatekeeper role of the primary care physician to the use of specialist care is similar to the role of GPs in European countries like Denmark, Norway, Italy, the Netherlands, Portugal, Spain, and the UK.

Health-Care Systems Environment: The Impact of Society

As noted in the introduction to this article, health-care systems have 'open' borders to their environment. So it goes without saying that health-care systems are impacted by the values and social structure of their societies (Helman, 1996). Based on history, traditions, belief systems, and so on, health-care systems reflect the way in which societies define and deal with health and illness. Health and health care are imbedded in value systems, which explains how in specific cultures health problems are dealt with. This may explain why, in some societies, health care is considered as a collective good for the benefit of all citizens, while in others, health care is considered more a 'commodity' – a calculable resource that can be bought or sold on a free market (Gallagher, 1988). The notion of health care as a commodity has not been rooted everywhere. Its most evident example can be found in the essentially market-oriented organization of the U.S. health-care system. But also in Europe it has become more widespread in political thinking, as a wide range of health-care reforms has shown (Saltman and Figueras, 1997). Regrettably, the cultural embedding of health care in societies is a well-acknowledged but rather underresearched topic (Saltman and Figueras, 1997; Stevens and Diederiks, 1995). There is surprisingly little empirical evidence grounding core values underlying health-care systems. But evidently, a society's emphasis on hospital care versus home care or care for the elderly, on individual responsibilities, or on the degree of solidarity between people reflect general value orientations that mirror societal priorities (Hofstede, 1991; Philipsen, 1980). As obvious differences in value orientations between North and South Europe, and between Europe and the United States show, it would be a useful endeavor for coming health services research to explain differences in health-care systems from a cultural perspective.

Conclusions: What Can We Expect in Future Developments?

As we showed in the previous sections, health-care systems in low- and middle-income countries differ considerably, as health problems do, from health-care systems in high-income countries. Future developments will differ accordingly.

Low- and Middle-Income Countries

One of the conclusions to be drawn from the famous World Bank graph (see **Figure 1**) about the relationship between 'health' (life expectancy at birth) and 'wealth' (average income per capita) in the period 1900–1990, is that 'we' all got substantially richer over those years. The corrected income figures for inflation and purchasing power quintupled between 1900 and 1990 (PPP, or purchasing power parities, is a technique to make financial data comparable over time and between countries by controlling for purchasing power differences). Many countries that were previously in the lowest income group can now be considered as middle-income countries. One of the health-care challenges in this economic stage is to introduce curative care for an ever-increasing number of citizens. As we pointed out, there are several ways to do so. One can introduce a (limited and partial) form of health services funded by taxes with a dominant role for the state in health-care funding and provision (the Beveridge model), stretching, as it were, available supply and resources as thinly as possible. Equity is the leading principle.

The other option is a pluralistic and gradual approach, where the state has the role of providing rules and laws regulating the system and leaves much to health-care insurers, providers, and consumers (the Bismarck or social security model). The latter model starts with some (economically) advanced groups in society (e.g., skilled workers) and with a limited benefit package. Later, in better economic circumstances, both the benefit package and the number of beneficiaries are extended until universal coverage (almost) will have been reached.

The current health-care systems in Europe are partially planned, such as the introduction of the NHS in the UK in 1948 and in Southern Europe at the end of the 1970s and beginning of the 1980s. But some were not planned: some developed incrementally by innovative adaptations while others were forced on a society (e.g., the German occupation spread Bismarckian principles in WWII).

Middle-Income Countries

Middle-income countries can consider the choice for a Bismarckian or Beveridgean as a serious and high-impact policy option instead of going into an incremental policy process and making a deliberate choice. A focus on equity and cost control and a positive attitude toward an active role of the state, makes a choice for Beveridge probable. Introducing earmarked health insurance premiums for a limited part of society (that is taxable anyway) creates more inequalities initially but might also stimulate economic growth, which, as we already stated, starts an upward cyclical process, gradually bringing the population as a whole under the social security-based health insurance coverage (De Swaan, 1988).

High-Income Countries

For high-income countries several processes take place simultaneously. First, internal changes occur in the Beveridgean and Bismarckian health-care systems such as splitting health-care purchasing and provision and creating an internal market in the British NHS, or increasing state influence in general in the Bismarckian health-care systems (Germany is a good example). Another example of several simultaneous processes is the introduction of managed care (HMOs) in the U.S. private insurance system. Last, there is the ultimate change to the system – the disappearance of it altogether – like the Soviet-based health-care systems in Eastern Europe. All these changes cause convergence, both in appearance and in performance (Van der Zee and Kroneman, 2007; on convergence, see also Stevens, 2001), especially in health outcomes of the systems.

Second, in spite of these long-term convergency trends Beveridgean health-care systems cost less than Bismarckian ones and better contain the costs (Saltman *et al.*, 2004; Van der Zee and Kroneman, 2007). But citizens tend to appreciate Bismarckian health-care systems more than Beveridgean ones. Kroneman and colleagues (2006) showed that the GP gatekeeping model may be responsible for these types of appreciation differences. Remarkably, health-care systems that have stronger system characteristics (e.g., more coordination, stricter labor differentiation) seem to have less popular support in general, with substantial exceptions.

Third, the European Union (EU) has its specific influences on the convergence of health-care systems. Case law produced by the European Court of Justice favored reimbursement of health-care cost due to purchasing health care in other EU-member states in spite of initial refusal by national health insurers or health-care authorities. The argument that such a liberal attitude (of the European Court of Justice) might hamper national health-care cost control, was countered by valuing the free movement of goods, services, and persons higher than national cost-control interests (under certain conditions). The case law started with the reimbursement of a set of spectacles, than went on by way of orthodontic services to specialized treatments; the end is certainly not yet there. New cases are in process.

Fourth and finally, voices get louder about the sustainability of both models (the NHS and the social security-based health-care system). Precisely due to the last decades' increases in wealth, some politicians are thinking aloud that the conditions under which governments created and extended welfare state arrangements (like universal health-care insurance and other social security elements) do differ substantially from current circumstances. Whether this will lead to shifting part of the responsibility to health-care consumers is not sure, however. The recent changes in the Dutch health insurance (with 62% publicly insured and 38% privately insured before 1 January 2006 and 100% publicly insured since) showed that an overwhelming majority (95%) of the formerly private patients, who had a wide variety of policy options, opted for a zero-deductible policy (De Jong and Groenewegen, 2007).

So what does all this mean for the future? First, we expect that for high-income countries (e.g., the members of OECD) NHS-type of health-care systems will have a tough future. These hierarchical, systematically organized systems – the most 'systematic' in Philipsen's (1985) terms that we discussed in the introduction – are superior in cost control, but they are not very popular. Social security-based health-care systems will fit better into the consumer-led, demand-led policy trend. But this will have a price tag, too; most probably at least a part of the cost burden will be shifted to individual households, as is already the case in the United States.

Second, we expect low- and middle-income countries to see a rift in the tendency to favor NHS-like solutions for their growing health-care systems, and we expect them to opt for some social security-based model. This happened in Eastern Europe, after the collapse of the Soviet system. Eastern Europe overwhelmingly returned to a Bismarck model (Marrée and Groenewegen, 1997). External factors, like EU case law, will stimulate further convergence of the European health-care systems.

For Europe, the challenge will be resisting the temptation to neglect the poorest groups in society; for the United States, the test will be to make the uninsured or partially insured join the health-care system. For the world, however, the effort will be to provide health-care services and health insurance for whole populations, including the very poor.

See also: Public/Private Mix in Health Systems.

Citations

Anderson GF (1997) In search of value: An international comparison of cost, access, and outcomes. *Health Affairs* 16(6): 163–171.
Blumenthal D and Hsiao W (2005) Privatization and its discontents—the evolving Chinese health care system. *New England Journal of Medicine* 353: 1165–1170.
De Jong J and Groenewegen PP (2007) *Percentage overstappers van zorgverzekeraar valt terug. Collectivisering zet door.* Utrecht,

The Netherlands: NIVEL, Netherlands Institute for Health Services Research.
De Swaan A (1988) *In Care of the State. Health Care, Education and Welfare in Europe and the USA in the Modern Era.* Cambridge, MA: Polity Press.
Gallagher EB (1988) Modernization and medical care. *Sociological Perspectives* 31: 59–87.
Habermas J (1981) *Theorie des Kommunikativen Handeln.* Frankfurt, Germany: Suhrkamp.
Helman CG (1996) *Culture, Health and Illness.* London: Wright.
Hofstede G (1991) *Cultures and Organizations. Software of the Mind.* London: McGraw-Hill.
Hongoro C and McPake B (2004) How to bridge the gap in human resources for health. *Lancet* 364: 1451–1456.
Hurst J (1992) *The Reform of Health Care. A Comparative Analysis of Seven OECD Countries.* Paris, France: Organisation for Economic Co-operation and Development.
Kroneman MW, Maarse H, and Van der Zee J (2006) Direct access in primary care and patient satisfaction: A European study. *Health Policy* 76: 72–79.
Marrée J and Groenewegen PP (1997) *Back to Bismarck: Eastern European Health Care Systems in Transition.* Aldershot, UK: Avebury.
McIntyre DE and Doherty JE (2004) Health care financing and expenditure—progress since 1994 and remaining challenges. In: Van Rensburg HCJ (ed.) *Health and Health Care in South Africa*, pp. 377–411. Pretoria, South Africa: Van Schaik.
Nayeri K and Lopez-Pardo CM (2005) Economic crisis and access to care: Cuba's health care system since the collapse of the Soviet Union. *International Journal of Health Services* 35: 797–816.
Organisation for Economic Co-operation and Development (OECD) (2006) *Health Data 2006: Statistics and Indicators for 30 Countries.* Paris, France: OECD.
Parsons T (1951) *The Social System.* New York: The Free Press.
Philipsen H (1985) Gezondheid en gezondheidszorg in België en Nederland (Health and health care in Belgium and the Netherlands). *Gezondheid en Samenleving* 5: 223–231.
Reinhardt UE, Hussey PS, and Anderson GF (2004) U.S. health care spending in an international context. *Health Affairs* 23: 10–25.
Saltman RB, Busse R, and Figueras J (eds.) (2004) *Social Health Insurance Systems in Europe.* Buckingham, UK: Open University Press.
Saltman RB and Figueras J (1997) European health care reform. *WHO Regional Publications, European Series.* Copenhagen, Denmark: World Health Organization, Regional Office for Europe.
Stevens FCJ (2001) The convergence and divergence of modern health care systems. In: Cockerham WC (ed.) *Blackwell Companion to Medical Sociology*, pp. 159–176. Oxford, UK: Blackwell Publishers.
Stevens FCJ and Diederiks JPM (1995) Health culture: An exploration of national and social differences in health-related values. In: Lüschen G, Cockerham W, and Van der Zee J (eds.) *Health Systems in the European Union. Diversity, Convergence, and Integration*, pp. 75–88. Munich, Germany: Oldenbourg.
US Census Bureau (2007) Statistical Abstract of the United States. Washington, DC; USA: http://www.census.gov/statab/www.
Van der Zee J, Boerma WGW, and Kroneman MW (2004) Health care systems: Understanding the stages of development. In: Jones R, Britten N, Culpepper L, et al. (eds.) *Oxford Textbook of Primary Medical Care* vol. 1, pp. 51–55. Oxford, UK: Oxford University Press.
Van der Zee J and Kroneman MP (2007) Bismarck versus Beveridge: A Beauty Contest between Dinosaurs. *BMC Health Services Research* 7:94.
World Bank (1993) *Investing in Health, World Development Report 1993.* Oxford, UK: Oxford University Press.

Primary Health Care

D Sanders, N Schaay, and S Mohamed, School of Public Health, University of the Western Cape, South Africa

© 2008 Elsevier Inc. All rights reserved.

Introduction

Building on the article by Bryant and Richmond which outlines the history of primary health care, this article aims to reflect on some of the successes and failures of its implementation over the past 30 years, and attempts a glimpse into the future in terms of some of the key challenges and opportunities.

The Alma Ata Declaration: Background, Focus, and Implications

The concept of primary health care (PHC) evolved during the 1970s, influenced by and influencing the basic needs approach to social development. Informed on the one hand by the disappointments experienced in implementing the basic health services approach, and on the other by the remarkable progress in improving health in China, as well as by the achievements of many small, mostly NGO-inspired, community-based health-care initiatives in developing countries (Newell, 1975), WHO and UNICEF elaborated the strategy of primary health care as the means to achieve *Health for All by the Year 2000*.

The concept of PHC had strong sociopolitical implications. It explicitly outlined a strategy that would respond more equitably, appropriately, and effectively to basic health-care needs and also address the underlying social, economic, and political causes of poor health. Certain principles were to underpin the PHC approach (PHCA), namely, universal accessibility and coverage on the basis of need; comprehensive care with the emphasis on disease prevention and health promotion; community and individual involvement and self-reliance; intersectoral action for health; and appropriate technology and cost-effectiveness in relation to the available resources.

The concept of social justice strongly informed the concept of PHC.

The implications of the PHCA were recognized, even at the time of the Alma Ata Declaration (WHO and UNICEF, 1978), to be far-reaching if the strategy were to be properly applied: the principles would have to be translated into changes not merely in the health sector but also in other social and economic sectors as well as in community structures and processes.

Some of the changes required would include the redistribution of existing resources (financial, material, and human) for health; a reorientation and a broadening of the skills of health personnel to enable them to respond to the challenges of implementing PHC and to work in teams as well as with other sector professionals and communities; and improved design, planning, and management of the health system to facilitate greater community involvement, intersectoral collaboration, and decentralization (adapted from Tarimo and Webster, 1994).

A Balance Sheet of PHC Implementation: Context and Progress

The Policy Context of PHC

In the 30 years since the Alma Ata Declaration there has been significant progress in global health with an overall increase in life expectancy. However, rapidly widening inequalities in health experience between and within countries – and even reversals in Africa and the former Soviet Bloc countries – give cause for concern.

These reversals are due to the emergence of new diseases, especially HIV/AIDS, and the resurgence of old ones such as TB, malaria, cholera, and dengue, as well as an alarming rise in the prevalence of noncommunicable diseases and violent trauma – especially among the poor in developing countries.

This disease pattern, and the widening inequalities in health experience, are a reflection of demographic changes together with rapidly widening disparities in socioeconomic status, structural unemployment, increasing pollution of the environment, social disruption, and its exploitation by the drug, alcohol, and tobacco trade (WHO, 1998b). Ultimately, this pattern is a reflection of growing inequalities in wealth between and within countries with the income gap between rich and poor being greater than ever before.

The situation outlined in the preceding paragraphs is a result of a complex history of uneven economic and social development extending over centuries, but progressing much more rapidly over the past 100 years or so, and more recently of what is termed *globalization*. The latter, ushered in by the debt crisis and structural adjustment programs of the 1970s and 1980s, has been underpinned by policies that have accelerated economic stratification and resulted in chronic underfunding of social services, including the public health infrastructure, especially in rural or peripheral areas.

The Declining Capacity of Health Systems

The decline in health expenditure since the mid-1980s, and the steady withdrawal by the state from provision of public health services, has resulted in diminished capacity of the health system to respond to the basic health needs of communities.

Technological innovation and globalization have greatly improved communications and information in all countries, and have thus created the potential for improved interventions in health care. However, the widening inequities between rich and poor and between industrialized and developing nations, coupled with the near-collapse of peripheral health services in many developing countries, has meant that such advances benefit only a minority.

Community-level care and programs have also suffered from a decline in support for community health worker schemes, occasioned by a complex of factors which have included observed limitations of such programs (Lehmann and Sanders, 2007), perceived threats by the medical establishment to their hegemony, and financial problems besetting developing country governments and communities.

With less and less money, ministries of health in developing countries have resorted to support from bilateral donors and global health partnerships (GHPs) and initiatives (GHIs), which now largely determine the main lines of action of health programs. This increased reliance on donor aid with its priorities is discussed later in this article.

Underfunded government services are, and are perceived to be, deteriorating in quality, with the result that communities are increasingly losing confidence in them and often turning to traditional and private practitioners. In many poor countries declining public sector wages have spawned corruption which has become institutionalized in many health facilities (Bassett et al., 1997).

Different Interpretations of PHC

A major fault line over the past period – and something which was in fact introduced in the Alma Ata document itself – has been the definition of PHC as both a 'level of care' and an 'approach.' These two different meanings have persisted and perpetuated divergent perceptions and approaches. Thus, in some industrialized countries and sectors PHC became synonymous with first-line, or primary, *medical care* provided by general doctors, with the result that PHC has been viewed by many as a cheap, low-technology option for poor people in developing countries (Tarimo and Webster, 1994).

Even in countries that embraced PHC as the key to *Health for All* (HFA), escalating foreign debt, global economic recession, and reductions in health and social sector spending in the 1980s bedeviled its implementation, leading to the following conclusion: "It was adopted several years too late for the political and social movements that could have provided support and served as a springboard for development".

As summarized above, global economic and social context and policies have been inimical to the implementation of an approach to PHC that emphasizes equity and participatory social development. Despite the above differences in interpretation of the concept of PHC and the changes in the economic and political climate there have been significant successes in implementing PHC. These have, however, been mainly in the development of peripheral health services, rather than in the facilitation of social development through the promotion of an intersectoral approach and community participation, which might lead to improvements in living environments and provision of job opportunities – a philosophy that was at the core of the Alma Ata Declaration.

In the following section we consider the progress that has been made in relation to implementing key aspects of PHC over the past 3 decades.

Progress in Implementing the Eight Program Elements of PHC

The Alma Ata Declaration suggested that primary health care, at the very least, should include a set of eight basic elements, namely: an adequate supply of safe water and basic sanitation; the promotion of food supply and proper nutrition; maternal and child health care, including family planning; immunization against the major infectious diseases; the prevention and control of locally endemic diseases and appropriate treatment of common diseases and injuries; health education; and the provision of essential drugs. Later, mental health was added as a ninth element of PHC.

Since the early 1980s there has been considerable progress in the coverage of populations with these essential elements of PHC, although the gap between availability in the industrialized and least developed countries is widening as is that between the rich and poor within countries.

In summary, there has been some progress in improving access to water supply and sanitation, although great differences continue to exist between and within countries and social groups. For example, in high-income areas in cities in Asia, Latin America, and sub-Saharan Africa, people have access to several hundred liters of water delivered to their homes, but slum dwellers and people in rural areas have access to less than 20 liters a day, and a little less than half the developing world's population (2.6 billion) is deprived of sanitation (UNDP, 2006). A welcome development over the past period, however, has been the shift in focus from water quality alone toward a more integrated approach to environmental improvement.

The nutrition situation in developing countries remains serious. According to data from the Food and Agriculture Organization, every day 799 million people in developing countries – about 14% of the world's population – go hungry (FAO, 2003). Clearly, progress in this area demands not only health sector interventions (e.g., treatment of infectious disease, supplementary feeding, nutrition education) but also effective intersectoral actions to improve living conditions and household food security (Mason *et al.*, 2006).

The most spectacular achievements have been in maternal and child health care and family planning, although maternal health has received far less attention than child health, with levels of maternal mortality and morbidity from largely preventable causes in developing (particularly the least developed) countries remaining unacceptably high. Maternal mortality is the highest in Africa where the lifetime risk of maternal death is 1 in 16 compared with 1 in 2800 in rich countries (WHO, 2005a).

Child health-care provision has increased greatly over the past 2 decades with the vigorous promotion of certain selected 'Child Survival' technologies: growth monitoring, oral rehydration therapy (ORT), breastfeeding, and immunization (GOBI). Of these, immunization has shown the most dramatic improvement, with global coverage of children under 1 year increasing from 20% (WHO, 1992, cited in Tarimo and Webster, 1994) in 1980 to 78% by 2005 (WHO, 2006). This impressive progress notwithstanding, there remain areas for concern. These include stagnation in immunization coverage since 1990, with the most difficult-to-reach population being the group experiencing a disproportionate burden of vaccine-preventable disease; the reappearance of diphtheria in the Newly Independent States as a result of vaccine shortage and poor program management; and only 57% coverage of pregnant women with tetanus toxoid vaccine being attained (WHO, 2006).

Acute respiratory infection (ARI) and diarrheal diseases are the two leading causes of death in children under 5 years of age globally. Since the early (in the case of diarrhea) and late 1980s (in the case of ARI) standardized case management guidelines have been developed with rewarding results: however, particularly in the case of diarrhea, the impact has been less than anticipated, due to interrupted and inaccessible supplies of oral rehydration solution, improper usage, and an unabated high incidence of diarrhea as a result of minimally improved environmental hygiene and persisting malnutrition (Werner and Sanders, 1997). Most deaths among under-fives are still attributable to just a handful of conditions and are avoidable through existing interventions, mostly pneumonia (19% of all deaths), diarrhea (18%), malaria (8%), measles (4%), HIV/AIDS (3%), and neonatal conditions, mainly preterm birth, birth asphyxia, and infections (37%) (WHO, 2005a).

Control of the three most common and serious communicable diseases, tuberculosis (TB), HIV/AIDS, and malaria, has proved elusive. TB exacts an annual toll of 8.8 million new cases and 1.6 million deaths worldwide (Maher et al., 2007); its prevalence has risen sharply over the past 2 decades as a result of HIV infection, deteriorating socioeconomic conditions, and poor-quality control programs, together with the emergence of multidrug-resistant organisms. Similarly, the HIV epidemic has spread rapidly to affect an estimated 40 million individuals (UNAIDS, 2006), most of whom live in developing countries. In countries hardest hit by HIV, for example, Botswana, Lesotho, South Africa, and Swaziland, there has been a dramatic impact on survival with over 10 years in life expectancy being lost over a short period of time. The malaria situation remains serious, particularly in sub-Saharan Africa where it imposes high mortality and morbidity levels and a major economic burden from lost productivity and escalating treatment costs as antimalarial drug resistance spreads. Every year, malaria causes approximately 1 million deaths (the majority of which are infants and children in Africa), and between 350 and 500 million people get sick with malaria (The Global Fund, 2006).

Current strategies for control of these diseases are multifaceted and remarkably similar. Given these synergies and the magnitude of the dual epidemics of HIV and TB, global partnerships like *The Global Fund to Fight AIDS, Tuberculosis and Malaria, The Stop TB Partnership,* and *Roll Back Malaria* were established.

Technologies employed in all three cases have evolved considerably in the past decade, for example, improved short-course anti-TB drug regimens, the syndromic management of sexually transmitted infections (STIs), increased access to antiretroviral therapy (ART), and geographic information systems to assist in targeting malaria vector control. However, sustained success in combating these diseases is unlikely without well-developed health systems, improved living and working environments secured through antipoverty measures and coordination with health-related economic and social sectors, and active participation by communities in such control campaigns. Indeed, a recent review has pointed out the lack of evidence for effectiveness of directly observed therapy – short course (DOTS) in the absence of a well-functioning health service and community engagement (Volmink and Garner, 1997).

The major noncommunicable diseases (NCDs) such as cardiovascular disease, cancers, diabetes, and mental illness, together with violence and injuries, contribute significantly to the burden of disease in developed and, increasingly, developing countries. The WHO estimates that currently 60% of all deaths are caused by NCDs. Reflecting increasing contamination of the food chain and the environment by chemical, hormonal, and radioactive pollution, most cancers are on the increase in both developed and developing countries, an exception being lung cancer, which is declining among men and the younger generations in developed countries as a result of reduced tobacco consumption; the reverse is generally true for women everywhere, as well as for developing countries where smoking is on the increase. Diabetes, too, has become much more common globally, reflecting inappropriate dietary patterns and exercise habits. Cardiovascular disease is now becoming more common in developing countries but has declined dramatically in most developed countries: here smoking reduction, particularly among men, has been a major factor.

The high prevalence of mental illness and the increasing incidence of violence and injury reflect marked changes in living and working environments which are characterized by rapid, squalid, and stressful urbanization, structural unemployment, and increasingly visible disparities within most societies. In recognition of the burden of mental disorders and their costs in human, social, and economic terms, the WHO developed a set of recommendations for action, many of which incorporated the principles of PHC (WHO, 2001).

The complex epidemiology of noncommunicable diseases reveals starkly the inadequacy of control measures based on a narrow medical-technical approach which in the past relied heavily on a combination of medical measures and individually directed health education. It is clear that a wide-ranging set of actions, involving a range of sectors and tied to more fundamental measures, is necessary for sustainable impact.

Thus it is that the understanding and application of health education, one of the elements of PHC, has evolved significantly from a preoccupation with individual behavior change toward a broader set of activities termed *health promotion*, whose scope has been elaborated at international conferences beginning with Ottawa (1986), and most recently in Bangkok (2005) and which incorporates individual as well as social action.

The final program element to consider is *essential drugs*. Since 1978, when the Action Program on Essential Drugs was established, great progress has been made. By 1990, 64 countries had installed operational essential drugs programs, 28 were developing such programs, and at least 68 had formulated national drug policies (Tarimo and Webster, 1994).

By 2002, at least 156 countries in total had adopted national essential drugs lists and over 100 countries had national policies in place or under development.

Despite this, however, approximately two billion people still do not have regular access to essential medicines (Quick *et al.*, 2002). At the same time the drugs bills for most countries and their health services remain massive, and wastage and irrational drug use in public and especially private sectors remain problems. Despite the introduction of an Essential Medicines List for Children, there is still a great need for comprehensive national policies and actions covering procurement and quality control, distribution, and rational prescribing and dispensing, as well as consumer education.

Progress in Health Systems Development

Support at the national level for the reorientation of existing facilities and personnel has been visible in many countries where large numbers of workshops on PHC have been organized for health workers, and organizational structures developed to facilitate PHC implementation. Logistic support for health services in terms of drugs, equipment, vehicles, and communications has frequently been inadequate, often determined by the overall level of development of the country, except where special (often donor-provided) resources have been allocated, as in the case of immunization and diarrheal-disease control programs (Tarimo and Webster, 1994).

In recognition of the fact that, almost a decade after Alma Ata, the activities of various programs and institutions largely continued to be piecemeal and poorly coordinated, and that health services often remained concentrated in particular areas, leaving large population groups with little or no access to health care, the concept of the district health system (DHS) was born. The DHS has been promoted as the unit within which the implementation of primary health care by the health and health-related sectors (public and private) and communities can be best organized and coordinated. District management structures were envisaged as a focus for decentralization of political power and resources, increased democracy, and equity.

Notwithstanding their potential as a mechanism for decentralized health systems management, Tarimo and Webster (1994) suggested that despite efforts over the previous 10 years or more, there were few countries where district health systems were functioning fully and effectively. In part this was seen as a result of many interventions being externally funded and based on 'blue print' models which did not create local ownership of the district system or a sense of commitment among those responsible for implementing the changes.

While the recognition at Alma Ata of the importance of health services research and operational studies has stimulated skills development, training materials production, and even health systems research studies, investment in and utilization of findings from these activities remain weak. Often this results from the lack of relevance of this research and/or the noninvolvement of decision-making cadres in its planning and conduct and the application of inappropriate methodologies.

Fiscal austerity, which has been a feature of the global economic crisis of the past 3 decades, demands greater value for money. Together with rising unemployment and changes in the labor market, changes in demographic and social trends, and rapid technological advances with major cost implications for health services, it has, over the past 2 decades, driven a process of health sector reform in industrialized and developing countries. The implications of this have been felt at the district level.

Although there is no consistently applied, universal health-care reform package, it essentially includes the following: the restructuring of national health agencies; better planning and more efficient implementation strategies and monitoring systems; the introduction of user fees for public health services; the establishment of health insurance schemes; introducing managed competition among service providers; and working with the private sector through contracting, regulating, and franchising different private providers (Cassels, 1995).

Whereas the above aims appear rational in their conception, the reform process has evolved at different rates and to different extents in different countries and it is difficult to generalize about the success of its implementation. It appears that in many, especially developing, countries the rhetoric of implementation often masks the truth that fundamental change has not occurred (Mills, 1998). Piecemeal approaches have sometimes aggravated inequities (as with user fees in several countries) (Kutzin, 1995), or have led to a deterioration of local health services as decentralization of responsibility has occurred, mostly without the accompanying decentralization of resources and enhancement of local capacity.

Furthermore, the focus on cost-effective and efficient 'delivery' of 'health-care packages' threatens to aggravate the neglect of the process of health development and reinforce the technicist emphasis seen with selective PHC.

The emergence in the 2000s of a plethora of GHPs or GHIs – such as the Global Alliance on Vaccines and Immunizations (GAVI), the Global Fund to Fight AIDS, TB and Malaria (GFATM), the World Bank Multicountry AIDS Program (MAP), and the U.S. President's Emergency Plan for AIDS Relief (PEPFAR) – have reinforced the selective approach to PHC: under pressure to show rapid results, they have developed country-wide, disease-specific funding mechanisms which are vertically implemented and managed. Although there is little evidence to date on the system-wide effects of the disease-specific GHIs, there is a concern that these target-driven, performance-based funding mechanisms may put pressure on countries to "pursue low-hanging fruit and focus on more easily reached target populations (Brugha *et al.*,

2005) and politically high-profile treatment campaigns, thereby exacerbating inequities and neglecting population-wide public health programs.

Although the rationale is compelling for decentralization of implementation and management of PHC to a self-contained geographic area, the DHS is potentially being misappropriated by those concerned with the technical aspects of management (e.g., information systems, management development) rather than with its role in developing comprehensive services within subdistricts (Tarimo and Webster, 1994). The DHS was, after all, conceived as a means to better organize and support integrated and comprehensive PHC.

In some contexts – particularly in hierarchical and nonegalitarian societies – there has been strong, and even violent, opposition to PHC efforts where they have been seen to be succeeding, and/or are perceived to be a subversive and even revolutionary social enterprise (Heggenhougen, 1984).

Progress with Human Resources for Primary Health Care

The successful functioning of health systems depends crucially on adequate numbers and competence of personnel who account, in most countries, for at least 70% of recurrent expenditure on health services. Consequently, not only does human resource development (HRD) assume a place of priority but is also a primary step in health systems development.

Since 1978 there has been a considerable expansion in health human resources, particularly at the 'auxiliary' or 'paramedical' level in developing countries and, especially in the immediate post Alma Ata period, in the community health worker cadre. Despite this, many poor countries, especially the least developed, have too few health workers to provide universal coverage, and in all countries there continues to be significant maldistribution of, and imbalances between, various types of health workers.

Teamwork to implement PHC is on the whole poorly developed and the motivation and competencies of health personnel require considerable strengthening, especially in the nonclinical domains. Also, greater involvement of traditional practitioners in the health system has been advocated in some countries: achievements in this regard have been limited, with the notable exceptions of China and India where progress largely antedated Alma Ata.

If education and training are to serve the development of comprehensive and integrated health systems, then the PHCA, with its clinical and public health components, needs to permeate much more strongly most health professional education. There is, however, in most tertiary health science educational programs an unfortunate separation between the clinical health care and public health components. The latter is often marginalized in the formal curriculum and, when present, is usually presented in an abstract and theoretical form. Indeed, the substantial failure of most tertiary education health science institutions to adapt their missions and activities to the challenge posed by HFA has probably been one of the most significant impediments to the successful implementation of PHC, and a major reason for the continued dominance of specialist and hospital-based health care in many countries.

There are also many aspects of the management of human resources which are critical to the functioning of the health system and to which insufficient attention has been given. These include satisfactory remuneration, positive work environments, and good supportive systems (Joint Learning Initiative, 2004) so as to specifically address the retention of skilled health workers in the context of their migration from low- to high-income countries, as well as the provision of ongoing support and supervision of health personnel. Neglect of these has contributed to demoralization and loss of personnel and inefficient and low-quality service provision in the public health sectors of many countries (Bassett *et al.*, 1997).

Summary

While progress in implementing the PHC strategy in developing countries has been greatest in respect to certain of its more medically related elements, the narrow and technicist focus characterizing what has been termed the *selective PHC approach* (Walsh and Warren, 1979) has at best delayed, and at worst undermined, the implementation of the comprehensive strategy codified at Alma Ata. The adoption in developing countries of certain selected interventions – such as ORT and GOBI – created the centerpiece of UNICEF's Child Survival Revolution, which, it was argued, would be the 'leading edge' of PHC ushering in a more comprehensive approach at a later stage. The relative neglect of the other PHC program elements and the shift of emphasis away from equitable social and economic development, intersectoral collaboration, and community participation, as well as the need to set up sustainable district-level structures, all suited the prevailing conservative winds of the 1980s (Rifkin and Walt, 1986). It gave donors and governments a way of avoiding the fuzzier and more radical challenges of tackling inequalities and the underlying causes of ill health.

A key thrust of later health sector reforms is the quest for technical efficiency. This aims to improve spending on health by proposing a 'package' of public health interventions and a 'package' of essential clinical services, the content of which is determined by what are regarded as cost-effective interventions. This approach is, in effect, a more elaborate version of the selective PHC approach, virtually neglecting intersectoral work and community involvement.

Proponents of the selective approach point to the impressive increases in immunization coverage, the declines in infant mortality in many countries, and the successful eradication of polio from the Americas. However, notwithstanding these successes, questions have been raised about the sustainability of mass immunization campaigns (Hall and Cutts, 1993), the effectiveness of health-facility-based growth monitoring (Chopra and Sanders, 1997), and the appropriateness of ORT when promoted as expensive and often inaccessible sachets or packets and without a corresponding emphasis on nutrition, water, and sanitation (Werner and Sanders, 1997). Evaluations at both national and provincial levels have found that it is only when core service activities (such as the child survival technologies, DOTS, and use of management guidelines for common diseases) are embedded in a more comprehensive approach (which includes strengthening health systems, engaging health-related sectors, and involving local communities) that real and sustainable improvements in the health status of populations are seen (Gutierrez et al., 1996).

The Revitalization of Primary Health Care

In advocating primary health care, the Alma Ata Declaration affirms that health is determined mainly by factors lying outside the medical or public health services. Countries that have achieved the greatest and most durable improvements in health are usually those with a commitment to equitable development that is broad-based and multisectoral. Good empirical evidence for this comes, for example, from a set of poor developing countries – the 'Good Health at Low Cost' examples of Sri Lanka, China, Costa Rica, and Kerala State in India. These countries demonstrated that investment in the social sectors, and particularly in women's education, health, and welfare, had a significant positive impact on the health and social indicators of the whole population (Halstead et al., 1985).

To realize the equity essential for a healthy society, evidence suggests that a strong, organized demand for government responsiveness and accountability to social needs is crucial. Tacit recognition of this important dynamic informed the Alma Ata call for strong community participation. To achieve and sustain the political will to meet all people's basic needs, and to regulate the activities of the private sector, a process that involves citizen participation is essential. In fact, analysts have noted that such political commitment was achieved in Costa Rica through a long history of egalitarian principles and democracy, in Kerala through agitation by disadvantaged political groups, and through social revolution in China (Halstead et al., 1985). Robust community involvement is important not only in securing greater government responsiveness to social needs but also in providing an active, conscious, and organized population so critical to the design, implementation, and sustainability of comprehensive health systems.

Given that the current global sociopolitical environment is markedly different from that of the late 1970s and is not generally supportive of a basic needs approach to social development, a number of strategies need to be employed – in different combinations depending on the particular situation – to revitalize PHC and drive forward the HFA initiative. Reflecting the dialectical relationship between strong, organized community demand and government responsiveness and accountability, these strategies are complementary and are 'bottom-up' (e.g., community-based program development) as well as 'top-down' (e.g., policy development and planning).

The PHC approach is based on the understanding that health improvement results from a reduction in both the effects of disease (morbidity and mortality) and its incidence, as well as from a general increase in social well-being. The effects of disease may be modified by successful treatment and rehabilitation and its incidence may be reduced by preventive measures. Well-being may be promoted by improved social environments created by the harnessing of popular and political will and effective intersectoral action.

Of particular relevance to the development of comprehensive health systems is the clause in the Alma Ata Declaration stating that PHC "addresses the main health problems in the community, providing promotive, preventive, therapeutic and rehabilitative services accordingly."

Comprehensive health systems include, therefore, both *therapeutic* and *rehabilitative* components to address the effects of health problems, a *preventive* component to address the immediate and underlying causative factors that operate at the level of the individual, and a *promotive* component which addresses the more basic causes which operate usually at the level of society.

For example, using the example of diarrhea in children, and starting with a disease focus, oral rehydration and nutritional support are required immediately, followed by a process of nutritional rehabilitation so as to restore the child to a state of well-being. However, these interventions need to be complemented with health education about the importance of hand washing, food hygiene, breastfeeding, and immunization. Coupled with such preventive measures ought to be broader, developmental interventions such as the promotion of improved child care, household food security, and access to water and sanitation so as to comprehensively address the root causes of diarrhea in children.

Strategies for comprehensively tackling such health problems can be grouped essentially under two, complementary headings: promoting healthy policies and plans, and developing comprehensive community-based programs. Success of these strategies depends on the creation of a facilitatory environment through such actions as advocacy, community mobilization, capacity-building, organizational change, financing, and legislation.

Developing and Promoting Healthy Policies and Plans

The choice between various policy options must be made on the basis of an ethical framework or a clear set of values and principles: these are essentially those enunciated in the Alma Ata Declaration with emphasis on *equity* in health and *participation* in decision making about matters that affect both individual and societal health.

Governments and international organizations have a responsibility to ensure the conditions and opportunities to enable present and future generations to exercise these rights. Public health problems, and therefore necessary responses, are becoming increasingly global. Consequently, the need for strong global leadership is crucial, along with a strong advocacy role. An agency, such as the WHO, should assume this responsibility: it should take the lead in analyzing and publicizing the negative impact globalization and neoliberal policies are having on vulnerable groups. It should spearhead moves to limit health hazards aggravated by globalization, including trade in dangerous substances such as tobacco, alcohol, and narcotics, and the arms trade. At the same time, WHO should demonstrate and promote the benefits of equitable development in the realization of HFA – which includes strong investment in the social sectors. It should vigorously promote health as a human right and give support to governments in building their capacities in policy, planning, and advocacy. At the time of writing this article, WHO is showing a renewed interest in PHC.

In a similar manner, governments should, in developing health policies and plans, give serious consideration to employing a process that engages as partners those sectors, agencies, and social groups critical to the achievement of better health. The first step is creating awareness of the need to make health objectives part of the broader process of socioeconomic development. Since 'health' and 'medicine' have become virtually synonymous in the popular consciousness, it is important to convey the understanding that ill health results from unhealthy living and working conditions, from the failure of society to equitably provide health-promoting conditions, and not merely from a biological organism. It then becomes obvious that health problems are the result of multisectoral failure and that their solution cannot lie in health care alone, but requires comprehensive and intersectoral actions. Such advocacy needs to be illustrated by a demonstration of health inequities and their social determinants, and needs to be directed in a user-friendly fashion at all prospective partners, especially underprivileged communities and their political representatives. The importance of addressing these factors and understanding the role of other sectors in health improvement has led to the appointment by WHO of a *Commission on Social Determinants of Health* in 2005. Here the media also have an important role to play.

The policy development process must be as transparent and inclusive as possible to secure broader understanding and greater ownership of the policies. Developing consensus by initiating a dialogue with the public and enlisting their support can contribute to the continuity and sustainability of policies for health. The setting of goals and indicators (for different levels) through a participatory process can be valuable in defining policy objectives more specifically, allowing progress to be monitored by partners and affected communities, and can assist in popularizing public health issues. Such processes can help focus partners on the scope and rationale for the policy, and on their roles in implementation, and become a rallying point around which civil society can mobilize and demand accountability.

Following a PHC approach, the formulation and implementation of health policies thus requires new alliances with different sectors, voluntary organizations, and public and private bodies. The health sector needs to take leadership in prioritizing health in other sectors: here the establishment of functional intersectoral structures is desirable.

The implementation of policies may require different actions at different levels. These include laws on financial and management instruments, and, importantly, on mechanisms to involve networks within civil society. Financing should be equity based to ensure that underprivileged groups are not excluded from health care for economic reasons. Resources should be allocated according to need rather than for services actually delivered. The monitoring and evaluation of progress in policy implementation ought to be done in such a way as to embrace a sense of accountability – with the progress toward goals being presented to elected bodies or displayed in the mass media.

The Development of Comprehensive, Community-based Programs

The implementation of PHC has too often focused on the (often facility-based) therapeutic and preventive components of comprehensive care, while the promotive aspect, which focuses on the broader social determinants of health, is often neglected. This gap urgently needs to be bridged, as they are clearly indivisible in the process of health development.

Much experience has been gained internationally in the development of comprehensive and integrated programs to combat undernutrition: these experiences can provide useful lessons for other programs (Mason et al., 2006).

The principles of comprehensive program development apply to all health problems, whether specific communicable (e.g, diarrhea) or noncommunicable diseases (e.g., ischemic heart disease) or health-related problems (e.g., gender-based violence).

Once the priority health problems in a district have been identified, the first step in program development is to conduct a situation analysis. This should identify the prevalence and distribution of the problem, its causes, and potential resources, including community capacities and strengths, which can be mobilized, and actions that can be undertaken to address the problem. The more effective programs have taken this approach, involving health workers, other sectors' workers, and the community in the three phases of program development, namely, assessment of the nature and extent of the problem, analysis of its multilevel causation, and action to address the linked causes.

Clearly, the specific combination of actions making up a comprehensive program will vary from situation to situation. However, there are certain principles that should inform program design, one of which is the deliberate linking of actions that address causative factors operating at different levels. So, for example, in a nutrition program any intervention around dietary inadequacy (immediate level of causation) should also address household food insecurity (underlying level of causation). Thus, the choice of food supplement should be based not only on its nutrient value but also on its availability, cost, and cultivability and/or purchasability. The careful choice of an appropriate food supplement should be reinforced as an educational action in order to positively influence food habits and feeding practices. Clearly this principle of linking therapeutic or rehabilitative (feeding), preventive (nutrition education), and promotive actions (improved household food security) could and should be applied to health programs other than nutrition.

In addition, a nutrition program will include a minimum of core health service activities (mostly facility based) including effective growth monitoring and promotion, the integrated management of childhood illness, the promotion of breastfeeding, the promotion of energy, and nutrient-dense weaning diets based on commonly available local foods.

Similar minimum or core service components can also be identified for other health programs, for example, activities in the Safe Motherhood Initiative, the integrated management of childhood illnesses (IMCI), DOTS, technical guidelines for the management of common noncommunicable diseases, and so forth. There is an advantage in standardizing and replicating these core activities in health facilities at different levels, thus reinforcing their practice throughout the health system.

The District Health System, Subdistricts, and Health Centers

As mentioned earlier, there are at a local level in most countries a number of health programs, often vertically organized and centrally administered, with specialized staff who perform only program-specific functions. The development of comprehensive programs that are integrated into a decentralized district service inevitably requires transformation of both management systems and health worker practice. Making the transition from a centralized bureaucratic system to a decentralized, client-oriented organizational culture calls for a significant investment in the reorientation and development of the existing management systems, structures, and capacity of health personnel. District-level staff must be trained in order to support decentralized development of comprehensive programs with clear roles, goals, and procedures.

To properly undertake the challenge of health development, health personnel need to be able to gather and use appropriate health information for planning programs as well as for monitoring and evaluating their implementation.

Interventions in this field are seen as a very cost-effective technical and financial investment (World Bank, 1993). However, there has not been adequate effort to develop, implement, and use locally relevant health and management information systems, and there is still transmission of raw data to the national level without informing district management. District-level staff therefore have to make major decisions based on estimates, and very often they lack the skills needed to do so. Even when routinely collected information is available and relevant, subdistrict and district managers often have difficulty in getting access to it because of resource constraints, unintelligibility of technical jargon, and general lack of empowerment. As a result, these personnel have only limited opportunity to learn from new ideas and from the data concerning their work.

There have been a number of attempts to set up appropriate information systems which have led to improvements in data collection, the improved relevance of information, and improved supervision. However, these have generally been small-scale projects which have not been replicated on a larger scale. There needs to be increased support for taking these small projects to scale and developing 'bottom-up' models of information systems that are relevant for the service provider, that support the management decisions of the district manager, and yet feed into the overall information needs of higher levels.

Where information for planning and program or system development or improvement is lacking, health systems research is an important tool to assist decision making (Tarimo and Webster, 1994). There is now significant experience in using the 'district problem-solving' approach, where health personnel identify priority health system problems and are guided in the development of research approaches to identify their causes and fashion appropriate solutions (Varkevisser *et al.*, 1991). Here there is an important opportunity for academic departments of public health to develop productive working relationships with the health sector and at the same time strengthen the relevance of their educational efforts.

Some district managers and district-level personnel will be based at the district center or hospital, but in most situations the majority will be located in health centers (HCs) or clinics in subdistricts. HCs are or should be the focal point within the DHS for comprehensive PHC: they should provide quality care as well as facilitate the promotion of the community's health. This implies that, apart from their clinical skills, the health center team should have the ability to identify and forge alliances with other health workers (e.g., general practitioners, traditional healers, community or village health workers), other sectors, and nongovernmental and community-based organizations and structures. For this, both subdistrict- and district-level staff need skills in advocacy, negotiation, and compromise (WHO, 1997a).

In the 1970s and 1980s an important role was given to community health workers (CHWs) in the implementation of PHC. Indeed, many of the 'model' PHC initiatives relied extensively on CHWs for their successful operation. One of the strongest features of CHWs is that they are not merely a technical means of extending basic health care to peripheral communities and households, but occupy an advocacy and social mobilization role, enrolling the conscious involvement of communities and other sectors in health development. As a result of a number of factors noted earlier, many of these programs have proved difficult to sustain, and CHW programs have disappeared from many countries or have been significantly weakened. In the recent past there has been renewed interest in CHWs and lay health workers, partly in response to the critical shortage of health-care personnel and partly as a result of the increasing health-care burden imposed by the HIV epidemic (Lehmann and Sanders, 2007).

Such HCs and clinics should, ideally, be managed locally by boards with a majority of local residents. This would allow them to identify, analyze, and take action in partnership with their communities on local public health issues. Such actions could include the formation of patients' groups on particular health issues (e.g., diabetes, hypertension), establishing health education groups, and working with other sectors such as housing, education, welfare, and transport to assess the potential for changing their operations so that they are more likely to promote health.

Monitoring Equity in Health and Health Care

Equity is core to the policy of *Health for All*. As noted earlier, reductions in public health and social services in many countries are one of the contributing factors leading to growing inequities in health. To more successfully advocate for equity in health and health care among international organizations, governments, donors, and professional organizations, ministries of health need to be able to demonstrate any social differentials in access to health resources or in health outcomes. Their capacity to routinely monitor equity in health and health care needs to be strengthened through the use of simple yet valid approaches, using where possible existing data sources from all relevant sectors (McCoy *et al.*, 2003).

Human Resource Development for Primary Health Care

Sufficient numbers and effective performance of health personnel in all phases of health systems development – policy development and advocacy, planning, implementation, management and evaluation – is fundamental to, almost a prerequisite for, the realization of HFA. In recent years there has been increased recognition of the importance of human resources for health (HRH), impelled primarily by Africa's health crisis and the inability of health systems to adequately respond. A large research and advocacy project, the Joint Learning Initiative (JLI), undertaken early in the decade, has resulted in greater attention to – and resources for – human resource development (Joint Learning Initiative, 2004).

In human resource planning, the dominant approach of employing 'norms' to calculate numbers of health personnel required needs to be supplanted by one that considers not only their numbers, but, more important, the competencies of personnel required to implement PHC (Green, 1992).

With regard to education and training of health personnel, the PHCA needs to inform both the curriculum content and the process and choice of venues of learning. There is accumulating evidence that problem-oriented and practice-based approaches result in more relevant learning, and in the acquisition of problem-solving skills, both necessary attributes for the successful development of systems based on the PHCA. If health workers are to contribute to a health system that enables people to assume more responsibility for their own health, then their training must expose them to the practice of comprehensive programming at the district level and to the social issues at the community level.

The above suggestions for education reform apply equally to all categories of health personnel, as well as to undergraduate and postgraduate training. It has long been acknowledged that nurses play a pivotal role in the

PHC team, and constitute the largest category of health personnel in most countries. Endorsement of such educational reforms and their fuller elaboration and promotion by countries' nursing leadership is critically important for progress toward HFA (WHO, 1997b).

In most countries, health science educational institutions have not resulted in curriculum reform along the lines described above. Although there are indications that some have embarked or will embark on such a course, there will probably still be a significant delay before sufficient 'new' graduates are available to work in and transform the health system. Clearly, if the implementation of comprehensive PHC is to be achieved during the next decades, the process of curriculum reform in the educational institutions needs to be accelerated and accompanied by a massive program of capacity development of personnel *already working* in the health system. In short, the current HFA imperative demands the rapid expansion of continuing education activities, whether through in-service learning programs conducted on site within a district, or through postgraduate training programs offered by academic institutions.

Any PHC-related training should also include personnel from other health-related sectors as well as community members: capacity development for these constituencies has generally been neglected and has weakened the growth of both community participation and intersectoral involvement in health development.

Human resource management problems referred to earlier cannot be solved within the health sector alone, but will require more fundamental interventions in the economy and in the public sector. However, some important intrasectoral measures should be promoted; these can be grouped broadly into incentives and regulations. Among the possible incentives are: continuing education, including the possibility of formal certification and qualification for promotion; additional pay and accelerated promotion as well as allowances for children's schooling for serving in remote and underserved areas; and honorary academic appointments carrying both financial and other privileges. Possible regulations include: limitations on the licensing of private medical facilities; control over public sector workers' involvement in private practice; and compulsory service in underserved areas for specified periods after graduation (Tarimo and Webster, 1994).

In implementing a PHC approach, health workers require a range of skills: they need to be able to work across disciplines and sectors, to be knowledgeable about both primary health care and public health, and to have a strong commitment to community participation. In addition, the day-to-day management of human resources – acknowledged to be critically important for the effective functioning of district health systems – is an area that also requires considerable investment and should be a priority training issue.

Conclusions

It is clear that progress toward Health for All has been uneven. Gains already achieved are under threat from a complex and accelerating process of globalization and neoliberal economic policies which are impacting negatively on the livelihoods and health of an increasing percentage of the world's population and the large majority in developing countries. Although the global PHC initiative has been successful in disseminating a number of effective technologies and programs that have reduced substantially the impact of certain (mostly infectious) diseases, its intersectoral focus and social mobilizing roles – which are the keys to its sustainability – have been neglected, not only in the discourse but also in implementation.

Government health ministries need to enthusiastically enter into partnerships with other sectors, agencies, and communities to develop intersectoral policies that address the determinants of inequities and ill health. The policy development process needs to be inclusive, dynamic, and transparent, and supported by legislation and financial commitments.

The time is long overdue for energetically translating policies into actions. The main actions should center around the development of well-managed and comprehensive programs involving the health sector, other sectors, and communities. The process needs to be structured into well-functioning district systems, which, in most countries, must be considerably strengthened, particularly at the household, community, and primary levels. Here comprehensive health centers and their personnel should be a focus of effort and investment and the reinstatement of community health worker schemes should be seriously considered.

The successful development of decentralized health systems will require targeted investment in infrastructure, personnel, and management and information systems. A key primary step is capacity development of district personnel through training and guided health systems research. Such human resource development must be practice-based and problem-oriented, and must draw on, and simultaneously reorient, educational institutions and professional bodies.

Clearly, the implementation and sustenance of comprehensive PHC requires inputs and skills that demand resources, expertise, and experience not sufficiently present in the health sector in many countries. Here partnerships with NGOs and expertise in various aspects of community development are crucial. The engagement of communities in health development needs to be pursued with much more commitment and focus. The identification of well-functioning organs of civil society, whether or not they are presently active in the health sector, should be urgently pursued.

In promoting the move from policy to action, the global health community needs to be much bolder in: advocating for equity and legislation to facilitate its achievement; pointing out the dangers to health of globalization and liberalization; and stressing the importance of partnerships between the health sector and other sectors to ensure that comprehensive PHC programs are developed. The WHO must assume greater responsibility for influencing other multilateral and bilateral agencies and donors, as well as NGOs and professional bodies, toward a common vision of PHC, and must argue for a major investment in health, especially in human resource development, without which HFA will remain a mere statement of intent.

See also: Alma Ata and Primary Health Care: An Evolving Story.

Citations

Bassett MT, Bijlmakers L, and Sanders D (1997) Professionalism, patient satisfaction and quality of health care: Experience during Zimbabwe's structural adjustment program. *Social Science Medicine* 45(12): 1845–1852.

Brugha R, et al. (2005) State of the art review. *Project Proposal: Experience of African Countries with Global Health Initiatives.* Submitted to European Commission – Brussels.

Cassels A (1995) Health sector reform: Key issues in less developed countries. *Journal of International Development* 7(3): 329–347.

Chopra M and Sanders D (1997) Is growth monitoring worthwhile in South Africa? *South African Medical Journal* 87: 875–878.

Food and Agriculture Organisation (FAO) (2003) *The State of Food Insecurity in the World 2003: Monitoring Progress Towards the World Food Summit and Millennium Development Goals.* Rome, Italy: Economic and Social Department, FAO.

Green A (1992) *An Introduction to Health Planning in Developing Countries.* Oxford, UK: Oxford University Press.

The Global Fund to Fight AIDS, Tuberculosis and Malaria (2006) *Malaria Information Sheet.* www.theglobalfund.org/en/files/malaria_information_sheet_en.pdf (accessed January 2008).

Gutierrez G, Tapia-Conyer H, Guiscafre H, Reyes H, Martinez H, and Kumate J (1996) Impact of oral rehydration and selected public health interventions on reduction of morality from childhood diarrhoeal diseases in Mexico. *WHO Bulletin OMS* 74(2): 189–197.

Hall AJ and Cutts FT (1993) Lessons from measles vaccination in developing countries. *British Medical Journal* 307: 1294–1295.

Halstead SB, Walsh JA, and Warren KS (eds.) (1985) *Good Health at Low Cost. Conference Report.* New York: Rockefeller Foundation.

Heggenhougen HK (1984) Will primary health care efforts be allowed to succeed? *Social Science and Medicine* 19(3): 217–244.

Joint Learning Initiative (2004) Global responsibilities. Chapter 4, *Human Resources for Health: Overcoming the Crisis.* Cambridge, MA: Harvard University Press.

Kutzin J (1995) *Experience with Organizational and Financing Reform of the Health Sector.* Geneva, Switzerland: Division of Strengthening Health Services, World Health Organization.

Lehmann U and Sanders D (2007) *Policy Brief: Evidence and Information for Policy, Department of Human Resources for Health,* pp. 1–6. Geneva, Switzerland: WHO.

Maher D, Dye C, Floyd K, et al. (2007) Planning to improve global health: The next decade of tuberculosis control. *Bulletin of the World Health Organisation* 85(5): 341–347.

Mason J, Sanders D, Musgrove P, Soekirman, and Galloway R (2006) Community Health and Nutrition Programs. In: *Disease Control Priorities in Developing Countries,* 2nd edn., Ch. 56. Washington, DC: World Bank Group.

McCoy D, Bambas L, Acurio D, et al. (2003) Global equity gauge alliance: Reflections on early experiences. *Journal of Health, Population and Nutrition* 21(3): 273–287.

Mills A (1998) *Reforming Health Sectors: Fashion, Passions and Common Sense.* Paper presented at Eighth Annual Public Health Forum, London, UK.

Newell KW (1975) *Health by the People.* Geneva, Switzerland: WHO.

Quick JD, Hogerzeil HV, Velasquez G, and Rago L (2002) Twenty-five years of essential medicines. *Bulletin of the World Health Organisation* 80(11): 913–914.

Rifkin SB and Walt G (1986) Why health improves: defining the issues concerning "comprehensive primary health care" and "selective primary health care". *Social Science Medicine* 23: 559–566.

UNAIDS (2006) *AIDS Epidemic Update.* www.unaids.org/pub/EpiReport/2006/2006_EpiUpdate_en.pdf (accessed 7 August 2007).

United Nations Development Program (UNDP) (2006) Beyond scarcity: Power, poverty and the global water crisis. *Human Development Report 2006.* New York: United Nations Development Program.

Varkevisser CM, Pathmanathan I, and Brownlee A (1991) *Proposal Development and Fieldwork: Designing and Conducting Health Systems Research Projects.* (Health Systems Research Training Series, vol. 2, PART 1), Geneva, Switzerland: WHO.

Volmink J and Garner P (1997) Systematic review of randomised controlled trials of strategies to promote adherence to tuberculosis treatment. *British Medical Journal* 315(7120): 1403–1406.

Walsh JA and Warren KS (1979) Selective primary health care: An interim strategy for disease control in developing countries. *New England Journal of Medicine* 301(18): 967–974.

Walt G (ed.) (1990) *Community Health Workers in National Programs: Just Another Pair of Hands?* Milton Keynes, UK: Open University Press.

World Bank (1993) *World Development Report: Investing in Health.* Oxford, UK: Oxford University Press.

World Health Organization (WHO) (1988) Learning together to work together for health. Report of a WHO Study Group on Multi-professional Education for Health Personnel: The Team Approach, (Technical Report Series, No. 769). Geneva, Switzerland: WHO.

World Health Organization (WHO) (1992) *EPI for the 1990s.* Unpublished document WHO/EPI/GEN/92.2). In: Tarimo E and Webster EG (1994) *Primary Health Care Concepts and Challenges in a Changing World: Alma-Ata revisited,* p. 7. Geneva Switzerland: World Health Organization.

World Health Organization (WHO) (1996) *Proceedings of the WHO Conference on European Health Care Reforms,* Ljubljana, Slovenia, June (Document EUR/ICP/CARE 01 02 01). Geneva, Switzerland: WHO Regional Office for Europe.

World Health Organization (WHO) (1997a) *Improving the Performance of Health Centres in District Health Systems,* (WHO Technical Report Series, No. 869). Geneva, Switzerland: WHO.

World Health Organization (WHO) (1997b) *Global Advisory Group on Nursing and Midwifery: Report of the Fifth Meeting,* Geneva, April 8–10 (WHO/HDP/NUR-MID/97.3). Geneva, Switzerland: WHO.

World Health Organization (WHO) (1998) *Health for All in the Twenty-first Century,* (Document A 51/5). Geneva, Switzerland: WHO.

World Health Organization (WHO) (2001) Mental health: New understanding, new hope. *World Health Report 2001.* Geneva, Switzerland: WHO.

World Health Organization (WHO) (2005) Make every mother and child count. *World Health Report 2005.* Geneva, Switzerland: WHO.

World Health Organization (WHO) (2006) *Progress Towards Global Immunization Goals – 2005. Summary Presentation of Key Indicators.* Geneva, Switzerland: WHO.

World Health Organization (WHO) UNICEF (1978) *Report of the International Conference on Primary Health Care Alma-Ata,* USSR, September 6–12. Geneva, Switzerland: WHO.

Demand and Supply of Human Resources for Health

G Dussault, New University of Lisbon, Lisbon, Portugal
M Vujicic, World Bank, Washington, DC, USA

© 2008 Elsevier Inc. All rights reserved.

Introduction

This article will show how economics can help understand the dynamics of the labor market in the health sector, and to respond, at least partially, to questions such as:

- Why are there important variations in the number and type of health workers, illustrated in **Table 1**, between countries with comparable epidemiological indicators, and, presumably, with comparable needs?
- Why are there also important variations within countries, with urban and richer areas, typically with healthier populations, having higher ratios? Dussault and Franceschini (2006) cite various examples: in Nicaragua, approximately 50% of the country's health personnel is found in the capital city, which comprises only 20% of the country's population. In Ghana, in 1997, 1087 of the 1247 (87.2%) general physicians worked in the urban regions, although 66% of the population lived in the rural areas. Richer countries, belonging to the Organization for Economic Cooperation and Development (OECD), report similar geographical variations.
- How many and what kind of health workers should a country have? Are there, or should there be, international norms to guide countries in responding to that question? When does a surplus or a shortage of health services providers exist? What determines the size and the composition of the health workforce in a given country? By health workforce we refer to all who deliver some health service. This includes qualified (doctors, nurses, dentists, pharmacists, technicians, etc.) as well as non-qualified (auxiliaries, community workers) personnel, formally recognized (through registration, certification, licensure, or some other mechanism) as well as nonrecognized providers (traditional healers, alternative practitioners, drug peddlers, etc.). What determines how the stock (the total number of individuals, active or not, in an occupational category) of workers changes over time?
- Why are some health workers unemployed in places where much unmet health needs exist? In Mexico, in 2000, it was estimated that 15% of all physicians are unemployed, underemployed, or inactive, and yet rural posts remain unfilled (World Health Organization, 2000). Kenya was reported to have 4000 unemployed nurses at the beginning of 2005 (Physicians for Human Rights, 2005). The observed unemployment does not mean that health needs in rural Mexico and Kenya have been met. It reflects the absence of willingness to work in remote and poor areas (Mexico) and restrictive policies of recruitment (Kenya).
- Why do rich and healthier countries import health workers from poor countries? Aiken et al. (2004) summarized the trends in migration of nurses from poor to rich countries and concluded that "predicted shortages and recruitment targets for nurses in developed countries threaten to deplete nurse supply and undermine global health initiatives in developing countries" (Aiken et al., 2004: 69). Why do some poor countries even encourage the export of their scarce human resources for health? Why do health workers want to migrate?

Available data suggest that health needs are not the only factor determining how many health workers will be available to the population of a country; then, which other factors are at play? Why do countries respond differently to similar health challenges? Answers to these questions are complex, because history, culture, politics, social structures, and the economy all play a role. These questions can be approached from various disciplinary angles. Sociologists, anthropologists, and historians will look at how culture shapes representations of health and disease and how to respond to health problems; they also try to understand how occupations and professions develop and interact and how they shape the division and the organization of labor in health. Public health specialists look at health needs, which they define as differences between the observed health status of a population, expressed in measurable terms (incidence, prevalence rates, standard mortality rates, etc.), and a health status targeted at a later time. From these, they derive service needs, which correspond to services needed to bridge the gap between the observed and the desired health status; from service needs human resources needs can be derived.

In an ideal world, needs-based planning of health services and of the health workforce would be desirable, but in real life, this is fraught with conceptual, methodological, and political difficulties. First, there is no univocal definition of what needs are and of how they should be

Table 1 Doctors and nurses/100 000 population ratios in selected countries, 2004 or latest available year

Country	Doctors/100 000 population	Nurses/100 000 population	Child mortality (2003)	GNI/capita (2004, $US)
High-income countries				
Belgium	418	1074	5	31 030
Canada	209	1009	6	28 390
Denmark	366	971	5	40 650
France	329	667	5	30 090
Ireland	237	1661	6	34 280
Italy	606	446	5	26 120
USA	548	772	8	41 400
Upper-middle-income countries				
Hungary	315	852	9	8270
Malaysia	70	135	7	4650
Mexico	171	221	28	6770
Poland	219	490	8	6090
Russian Federation	417	786	16	3410
Lower-middle-income countries				
Armenia	352	473	33	1120
Brazil	205	267	35	3090
Cuba	590	744	7	N/A
Philippines	116	442	36	1170
Thailand	30	161	26	2540
Low-income countries				
Bangladesh	23	12	69	440
Burkina Faso	3	26	207	360
Ghana	9	64	95	380
India	51	61	87	620
Nicaragua	164	107	38	790
Tajikistan	218	437	118	280
Vietnam	53	84	23	550

Sources: World Health Organization (2006) *World Health Report* 2006. Geneva, Switzerland: WHO (for workforce and mortality data) and The World Bank (2006) *World Development Report* 2006. Washington DC: The World Bank (for economic data).

measured. It is also difficult to say what the needs will be in 3, 5, 7 years, when the workers who start their training now will start providing services. Then, it is not always easy to say which services can better respond to health needs and which skills they require from health staff, nor how these skills are best acquired. Finally, the answers to these questions are not only technical: They are the object of negotiations between professional groups whose interests often diverge, as they occupy competing market niches.

This article proposes a review of the notions of demand and supply of health personnel, as they are defined by economists. It will look at their various dimensions and at the factors which influence them. It will remind policy makers that the health labor market has some particularities that are not found elsewhere and that these need to be taken into account by those seeking to influence it.

Demand, Need, and Supply of Health Workers

The observed differences in the availability of health workers, both within countries and between countries, can be explained by differences in the demand for and supply of health workers.

It is important to define the demand for health workers clearly, as this concept often carries very different meanings for different people and is a source of confusion in discussing shortages and surpluses of health workers in countries. The typical definition of demand that stems from the labor economics literature is the quantity of labor (or in the simplest sense the number of workers) employers are willing to hire at current levels of wages and other important variables such as worker productivity. This demand derives from the demand for health services expressed by individuals, organizations, or health planners and policy makers (Feldstein, 2004). There are many different types of employers in the health-care sector. The main ones include global level employers (e.g., multilateral organizations), a country's public sector (e.g., government-owned hospitals), a country's for-profit sector (e.g., for-profit clinics), the nonprofit sector (e.g., mission clinics), and individuals, e.g., sick people who seek care from health workers operating as self-employed entrepreneurs (Evans, 1984). A key result is that many factors other than the health-care needs of the population influence the demand for health workers (Vujicic and Zurn, 2006) (see **Table 2**).

Table 2 Factors influencing demand

Type of employer	Key factors influencing demand for health workers
Global public sector (WHO, World Bank, GFATM, GAVI)	Disease priorities, population health-care needs, donor aid levels, wages
Global for-profit sector	Profit expectations
Country public sector	Budget allocated to the health sector, budget allocated for salaries, population health-care needs, wages
Country for-profit sector	Profit expectations
Nonprofit NGOs (faith-based organizations)	Mission of NGO
Individuals	Household income levels, health status of individual, cost of using services

Demand differs from the concept of need for health workers, which can be defined as the number of health workers that are required in order to deliver some particular mix of health-care services to the population. The concept of need for health workers is normative – it is a judgment of what ought to be – and takes into consideration only the health-care needs of the population and no economic and financial factors that might constrain what is actually feasible. Financial, economic, and political factors can be thought of as driving a wedge between the demand for health workers and the need for health workers.

The important ingredient in defining the need for health workers is the method for determining what basket of health-care services ought to be provided to the population and by which types of health workers. This involves a great deal of priority setting on the part of policy makers to identify priority services (i.e., public health services versus tertiary care provision) as well as deciding on appropriate models of care and scopes of practice (i.e., should nurses be licensed to provide injections). For example, the Joint Learning Initiative (2004) has estimated that an extra 1 million health workers are needed globally based on a target health worker to population ratio. It is estimated that in Ethiopia 36% more physicians are required in order to expand ARV treatment to the government's target level (Kombe et al., 2005). To deliver an expanded essential health services package in Chad and Tanzania, it is estimated that an additional 400% and 200% of the current health workforce is needed, respectively. This estimate is based on a breakdown of the health-care services required and the labor requirements to deliver those services (Kurowski et al., 2003). How many health workers those countries will be prepared to employ, whether these are available or not, would represent the demand.

The supply of health workers can be defined as the number of health workers who want to work in the health sector given the current level of wages and other variables that affect labor participation decisions (e.g., working conditions). This is not necessarily the same as the number of people that have the necessary training to work in the health sector because some of these people will be retired or may not wish to be employed. It is also different from the number of full-time equivalent (FTE) workers that would correspond to the demand for health workers. This is because workers will not want to work the same number of hours or days for a variety of reasons. Other factors, such as the way work is organized (solo vs. team practice for example), individual skills, or personal preferences will also influence the calculation of FTEs.

With these concepts defined, it becomes clear that observed levels of health worker availability are not determined solely by the needs of the population but by the interactions of supply and demand.

Shortage, Surplus, Unmet Need, Overmet Need

The terms shortage and surplus of health workers are often used very loosely and can be a source of confusion. This is because the economic concept of shortages and surpluses differs from that used by policy makers. A shortage of health workers describes a situation where employers cannot hire as many health workers as they would like to hire and have the resources to hire. A surplus of health workers describes a situation where some health workers cannot find jobs, because employers have filled all of their vacancies and do not want to hire any more. The concepts of shortage and surplus, defined in this conventional economic way, simply describe the situation in the labor market for health workers.

The concepts of unmet or overmet needs, however, describe the extent to which the availability of health workers is sufficient to meet the needs of the population. This is often independent of the labor market situation, since factors beyond the needs of the population are important determinants of both demand and supply. Thus, it is quite possible (and often observed) that there is simultaneously a surplus of health workers (i.e., unemployment) and unmet needs. Indeed, many African countries have unemployed nurses and doctors, while having high mortality and morbidity rates that could be greatly reduced by making some basic interventions available. The distinction between shortages and unmet needs is important and has implications for policy makers, as will be illustrated in the section titled 'Policies to adjust demand and supply.'

Determinants of Demand and Supply

Demand and supply of health workers are not static. They vary over time, as a variety of factors influence the dynamics of the health labor market. The factors that determine the demand vary depending on where it originates. For the global public sector, levels of donor resources for specific health initiatives influence the demand for health workers to be used to address those priority diseases. For example, the large increases in external aid tied to HIV/AIDS has led to a sharp increase in demand for health workers who can provide HIV care. In the for-profit sector, the demand for health workers is driven principally by maximizing profit by delivering health-care services.

In the public sector, ministry of health hiring decisions are often influenced by political, economic, and social factors as much as by the health-care needs of the population, which are often only roughly estimated; these vary as the population grows older and as the epidemiological profile changes. The key economic factor is the budget allocated to the health sector and the proportion of it allocated to employment and the wages of health-care workers. The health sector competes with other sectors (e.g., education, defense) for government funding, as governments weigh – rationally or not – the benefits of increasing spending in the health sector against the benefits of spending in other sectors. For instance, in relation to the objectives of economic growth and poverty reduction, it is difficult to measure the marginal impacts of expenditure in the health sector (and within the health sector for human resources) respective to other sectors in the economy.

While recent studies have highlighted the positive impact on health outcomes of increased human resources for health capacity in settings where health workers are scarce (Anand and Barnighausen, 2004), the relative benefit of investing in human resources relative to other inputs (i.e., facilities, roads, clean water, and literacy) is not always apparent. Thus, policy makers must judge the extent to which additional resources for health ought to be devoted to human resources and this has an important impact on the demand for health workers.

The hiring decisions of governments – the main employers of both nurses and doctors in many countries – depend to a large extent on wages and the size of the hospital budget allocated to salaries. Empirically, governments tend to hire more personnel when budgets increase and are willing to lay off staff when budgets decrease. They also tend to respond to wage increases by reducing staff and by hiring more staff when wages decrease. Finally, the way the health-care delivery system is organized has an impact on demand. Alternative payment mechanisms, practice patterns, level of technology, and the type of health-care organizations available all affect the demand for health workers in a country.

The relevant decisions that are important in determining the supply of health-care professionals in a country are summarized in **Figure 1**. Several complex, often overlooked decisions affect the supply of health-care professionals: the purpose of **Figure 1** is to illustrate to policy makers the various policy options through which the supply of health-care professionals can be altered.

The decisions affecting the domestic supply of health-care professionals in a country can be divided into two groups: Education sector and employment sector decisions. Decision making in the education sector determines the number of health-care professionals graduating from various training programs each year as well as their education level. This sector is where human resources for health are produced. On the part of institutions, the main decision is how much capacity to provide for health-care training programs. On the part of individuals who are of school age, the main decision is whether to pursue an education in health or some other field such as teaching or engineering. Both of these decisions greatly influence graduation levels. To increase education output, there must be a sufficient number of individuals in the country who are interested in pursuing an education in the health-care field and are qualified to do so. Education capacity is affected by, for example, education spending by governments and training standards. The pool of candidates willing to pursue an education in health care is affected by, for example, population demographics and career opportunities in other sectors.

Within the health labor market, several decisions are critical. First, migration flows greatly affect the number of qualified health-care professionals within a country. Outflows of health-care professionals in developing poor countries – particularly in Africa – are perhaps the single biggest threat to the health-care system. Conversely, developed rich countries are increasingly relying on migrant health-care professionals to fill nursing and physician vacancies. The migration decision of health-care professionals depends on a complex set of push and pull factors, i.e., of factors in the country of origin that encourage people to leave, and factors in the destination country which attract potential migrants. Examples are poor/good working conditions, political stability/instability, poor/good conditions of security, etc. Migration flows and graduation levels jointly determine the number of individuals who are qualified to work as health-care professionals within a country. This pool

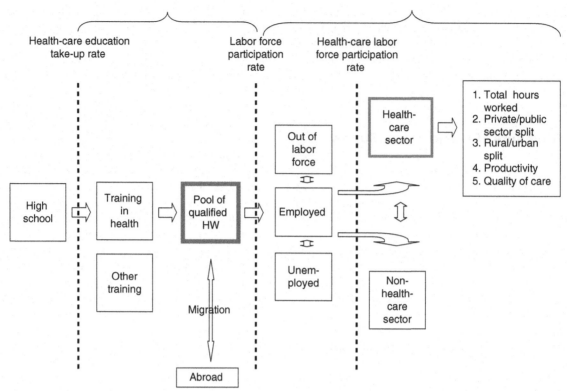

Figure 1 Determinants of the supply of health workers. Reproduced from Vujicic M and Zurn P (2006) The dynamics of the health labor market. *International Journal of Health Planning and Management* 21(2): 1–15. Copyright John Wiley & Sons Ltd. Reproduced with permission.

can be thought of as the potential supply of health-care professionals.

The labor force participation decision (whether an individual is willing to work) and the sectoral decision (whether an individual is willing to work in health care) jointly determine the number of qualified individuals willing to work in the health-care sector. Labor force participation depends on numerous factors such as age, gender, available wages, family situation, and the presence of another income-earner in the household. For those who have the necessary qualifications, the desire to work in the health sector depends on the attractiveness of working conditions and wages in the health-care sector relative to other employment opportunities.

Taken together, these decisions determine the number of individuals willing to work in the health-care sector – the supply of health-care professionals. Thus, altering the supply of health-care professionals in a country is not simply a matter of training more people in educational institutions. Certainly that has an impact, but several other factors are crucial as well. For a new worker to join the supply of health-care professionals, she has first to graduate, remain in the country, be willing to be employed, and, conditional on being employed, be willing to work in the health-care sector. Too often in the past, these labor market decisions have been ignored by policy makers.

Policies to Adjust Demand and Supply

The main message here is that it is not solely (or even principally) the health-care needs of the population that determine human resources for health outcomes in countries (i.e., employment level, skill mix, productivity). Rather, these outcomes are determined by the interaction of supply and demand in the labor market for health-care workers, and supply and demand are influenced by a wide variety of economic, social, and institutional factors. This characteristic of the health labor market has two important implications for policy makers. First, in order to adjust health workforce outcomes, such as employment levels, skill mix, geographic distribution, productivity, etc., policy makers need to design interventions that target either the supply of health-care workers or the demand for health-care workers, or both. Second, the particular menu of policy options will differ depending on the state of the labor market. When there are shortages, one set of options is appropriate, whereas when there are surpluses, a different set is likely to be more appropriate.

When there are surpluses – i.e. when there are few unfilled vacancies and employers are generally not interested in hiring more health workers – it is necessary to stimulate demand if one is aiming at increasing employment levels, for example to respond to unmet or neglected needs. Several policy options can be envisaged. In the government sector, lowering wages or increasing the resource envelope at the district and facility level is likely to stimulate demand for health workers. Negotiating lower wages is difficult as health care is highly unionized and has significant regulation and barriers to entry. It often involves highly publicized strikes and politically charged debate. However, wages can effectively be lowered by substituting lower paid health workers, either substituting cadres (e.g., shifting the skill mix away from physicians toward nurses) or contracting with private agencies where wages might be lower. In high-inflation settings, real wages can be lowered by negotiating fixed nominal wages that are not adjusted for inflation. From a purely economic point of view, all these measures may make sense, but they can be politically difficult to implement.

Increasing the level of resources in the form of higher budgets for salaries or increased block transfers to districts or facilities (depending on the financial set up in countries) can have a significant impact on the demand for health workers, which is very sensitive to changes in ministry of health, district, and facility budgets. These budgets often change as a result of factors unrelated to the health sector (e.g., wars, deficit reduction, shifts in political priorities, or donor resource flows), and managers adjust by increasing or reducing staffing levels. Recently, there has been debate on the degree to which governments in low-income countries can significantly increase salary spending in health in a fiscally sustainable way (Heller, 2005), or in the language of economists, whether they have the necessary fiscal space to do so. Another option is to shift resources from other sectors to health sector salaries, an exercise that is also politically perilous.

Reducing the cost of health-care services to households is also an effective way to stimulate demand for health care and, therefore, for health workers. Reducing or removing user fees or other financial barriers through national health insurance for example, has led to increased health service utilization in several settings.

When there are shortages of health-care workers – i.e., vacancies that are fully funded but cannot be filled – a different set of policy options is required in order to change employment levels. If the reason is that there are not enough workers available, it is necessary to stimulate supply. One option is to expand training capacity to increase the number of health workers, provided that graduates remain in the country; this means that increased production needs to be accompanied by retention measures. International migration flows have a tremendous impact on this type of policy. For example, Dovlo (2005) reports that in Ghana, between 1986 and 1995, 61% of doctors who qualified from one medical school left the country, and that in relatively wealthy Mauritius, the Ministry of Health estimated that 327 nurses (about 12.9% of the nurse workforce) migrated between 1998 and 2001. At the receiving end, rich countries have used in-migration as a method of filling vacancies. Middle-income countries, such as South Africa since 1996, and even poorer countries such as Ghana and Zimbabwe, more recently, have imported health personnel from Cuba, to compensate their own losses to other countries.

If the shortage is explained by the fact that workers are not willing to accept the terms of work, another set of policies is required. Higher wages, improved working conditions, better continuing education opportunities, improved management, and safer workplaces, make jobs more attractive to health-care workers. However, while wages tend to receive the most attention, the evidence has shown that improving other job characteristics is often a more cost-effective way to attract workers to vacant posts (Kingma, 2005). Since shortages occur in specific geographic areas and medical specialties (e.g., there are often shortages in rural areas but surpluses in urban areas), highly targeted interventions are often required. For example, most countries have some sort of incentive program to attract health-care workers to rural areas. These incentive programs often involve a financial bonus along with increased training opportunities that health workers in urban areas are not eligible for. In some cases, institutional factors might contribute to shortages, for example, when retirement age is at 60 or even 55 years of age. This can be addressed by policies that gradually extend minimal retirement age and facilitate the recruitment, on contract, of retirees who are still willing to work.

Finally, while the number, distribution, and skill mix of health-care workers are important outcomes for policy makers to target, it is equally important to monitor the efficiency and effectiveness of the workforce. The availability of services may be increased by enhancing workforce productivity. For example, in Tanzania staff productivity (defined as time spent on patient care, outreach activities, administrative tasks, in meetings, in training activities, on cleaning, preparatory and maintenance activities, and research) was 57%, on average, across all health workers. The potential productivity gain, defined here in terms of time devoted to health care-related activities, through improved staff management and optimized staffing levels was estimated to be between 26% and 37% (Kurowski et al., 2003). Other within-country and cross-country comparisons of aggregate workforce productivity indicators also show wide variation in service delivery per skilled health worker, indicating the scope for efficiency gains within the existing workforce (World Bank, 2005).

The advantage of this strategy is that it often requires far fewer resources than increasing the number of health workers. Under certain circumstances, improving data monitoring systems, enhancing workforce management practices, contracting health-care providers with some form of performance-based pay, can be effective in enhancing workforce performance, without increasing the number of workers employed, although the evidence is not conclusive (Liu and Mills, 2005).

Conclusion

In a perfect market, supply would equal demand and there would be no imbalances. A perfect market supposes that all actors are perfectly informed and that there are no obstacles to competition, conditions that are not met in health (Rice, 1998). For instance, it is difficult to define now what the health workforce needs will be in 5–10 years, which is the time required to train a physician. It is relatively easy to estimate how many will need to be replaced because of natural attrition (retirement, death), but, in times of high global mobility, it is more difficult to estimate losses to emigration. More difficult also, is to decide which skills will be needed, as needs tend to evolve rapidly. On the supply side, it is also difficult to say how many trainers, and with what skills, are needed. The rapid development of communication technologies challenges many of the assumptions on which demand for trainers was traditionally based.

Nor is competition between providers perfect, as access to the market is limited to providers with specific credentials. In a private market, there will be no or few incentives to produce certain services, such as health promotion and preventive services, nor is the assumption that educational institutions will spontaneously adjust to new needs likely to be confirmed. Issues such as gender equity are also unlikely to be addressed by the market. In an unregulated environment, the distribution of the workforce will tend to reflect the preferences of providers rather than those of consumers. This leads most health economists to conclude that some form of regulation is needed to ensure that the workforce will be adjusted to the needs of the population. In that perspective, a better understanding of the dynamics of demand and supply of health workers can be a powerful tool to help policy makers who are committed to improving access to good-quality health services to achieve their goals.

Citations

Aiken LH, Buchan J, Sochalski J, Nichols B, and Powell M (2004) Trends in international nurse migration. *Health Affairs* 23: 69–77.

Anand S and Barnighausen T (2004) Human resources and health outcomes: cross country econometric study. *The Lancet* 364: 1603–1609.

Dovlo D (2005) Wastage in the health workforce: Some perspectives from African countries. *Human Resources for Health* 3: 6.

Dussault G and Franceschini MC (2006) Not enough there, too many here: Understanding geographical imbalances in the distribution of the health workforce. *Human Resources for Health* 4: 12.

Evans RG (1984) *Strained Mercy*. Toronto, Canada: Butterworth.

Feldstein PJ (2004) *Health Care Economics*. 6th edn. Clifton Park, New York: Delmar Learning.

Heller P (2005) Back to basics: fiscal space what it is and how to get it. *Finance and Development* 42(2). http://www.imf.org/external/pubs/ft/fandd/2005/06/basics.htm.

Human Resources for Health and the Global HIV/AIDS Pandemic (2005) Testimony of Holly J. Burkhalter, Physicians for Human Rights, House International Relations Committee. April 13, 2005. Washington DC.

Joint Learning Initiative (2004) *Human Resources for Health: Overcoming the Crisis*. Cambridge, MA: Harvard University.

Kingma M (2005) *Nurses on the Move: Migration and the Global Health Care Economy*. Ithaca, NY: Cornell University Press.

Kombe G, Galaty D, Gadhia R, et al. (2005) *The Human and Financial Resource Requirements for Scaling Up HIV/AIDS Services in Ethiopia*. Bethesda, MD: Abt Associates.

Kurowski C, Wyss K, Abdulla S, et al. (2003) *Human Resources for Health: Requirements and Availability in the Context of Scaling up Priority Interventions in Low-Income Countries. Case Studies from Tanzania and Chad*. London: London School of Hygiene & Tropical Medicine.

Liu X and Mills A (2005) The effect of performance-related pay of hospital doctors on hospital behaviour: A case study from Shandong, China. *Human Resource for Health* 3(1): 11.

Rice T (1998) *The Economics of Health Reconsidered*. Chicago, IL: Health Administration Press.

Vujicic M and Zurn P (2006) The dynamics of the health labor market. *International Journal of Health Planning and Management* 21(2): 105–115.

World Bank (2005) *Global Monitoring Report 2005*. Washington, DC: The World Bank.

World Health Organization (2000) World Health Report 2000. Geneva, Switzerland: World Health Organization.

Further Reading

Chen L, Evans T, Anand S, et al. (2004) Human resources for health: overcoming the crisis. *The Lancet* 364: 1984–1990.

Figueras J, McKee M, Mossialos E and Saltman RB (eds.) (2006) *Human Resources for Health in Europe, World Health Organization on Behalf of the European Observatory on Health Systems and Policies*. Maidenhead, UK: Open Press University.

Joint Learning Initiative (2004) Human Resources for Health: *Overcoming the Crisis*. Cambridge, MA: Harvard University.

Martineau T and Martínez J (1999) Rethinking human resources: an agenda for the millennium. *Health Policy and Planning* 13(4): 345–358.

Vujicic M and Zurn P (2006) The dynamics of the health labor market. *International Journal of Health Planning and Management* 21(2): 105–115.

World Health Organization (2006) World Health Report 2006 (Working Together for Health). Geneva, Switzerland: World Health Organization.

Relevant Websites

http://www.africahrh.org.

http://www.capacityproject.org/index.php?option=COM-frontpage §itemid=1.

http://www.eldis.org/go/home&id=&type=Organisation – DFID, Health Systems Resource Guide.

http://www.human-resources-health.com – Human Resources for Health (online journal).

http://www.observatoriorh.org/eng/index.html – Pan American health Organization, Human Resources Observatories in Latin America and the Caribbean.

http://physiciansforhumanrights.org/ – Physicians for Human Rights.

http://www.who.int/hrh/en/ – World Health Organization, Department of Human Resources for Health.

The Private Sector in Health Care Provision, The Role of

A Harding, Center for Global Development, Washington, DC, USA
D Montagu, Institute for Global Health, University of California, San Francisco, CA, USA

© 2008 Elsevier Inc. All rights reserved.

Private clinics and hospitals and privately employed individuals provide a significant volume of health services in almost every country in the world. The extent of provision and the areas of involvement vary across countries; however, variations in the size of the private health sector cannot be systematically linked to the equity, quality, coverage, or other measures of health system performance, nor to the achievement of health policy goals. Despite this, private engagement in health provision remains a highly emotive topic. The reason for this derives in part from a widespread misunderstanding of private health-care delivery and the role it plays in health systems. This article will clarify the key definitions related to private service provision and summarize current knowledge on the role that the private sector plays in both high- and low-income countries. It will also present some of the most important issues that arise in discussions of private provision from public health and policy perspectives.

A source of confusion for students of public health is the often-complex overlap between financing and delivery of health services. The common perception is that public payment for health services necessarily implies public provision of health services. This is not the case, and misunderstanding of this basic point leads to highly erroneous conclusions about the health delivery systems of both low-income and high-income countries. This article focuses on private service delivery.

Private service providers are heterogeneous, encompassing world-class hospitals, unqualified drug sellers, and the whole range of providers in between. The role of the private sector varies by level of care, playing a limited role in in-patient care in most countries, and carrying more importance in the distribution and sale of pharmaceuticals, outpatient care, and informal care in low-income countries.

Background

Historically, health-care services were private in all countries until the rise of centralized governments in Europe and Asia in the eighteenth century. Governments' first interventions in health arose primarily to organize epidemic prevention and public health services, including mandatory hospitalization for tuberculosis, plague, leprosy, and other infectious diseases. With the rise of immunization options in the late nineteenth and early twentieth centuries, publicly supported health care expanded to prevention in many countries. Throughout this period, care and treatment of noninfectious diseases remained largely private, either for-profit or provided through religious charities. Government financing of care and treatment developed in parallel to the growth in government-supported education, and by the second half of the twentieth century, government-sponsored medical care had come to be seen as a central pillar of national social services.

Even where government financing of care is the strongest, in Western Europe and other high-income countries, service provision still often remains in the hands of private hospitals, clinics, and clinicians. Historical development and the institutional structure of the state appear more important in setting the public–private mix of care provision than national values. The social insurance systems of continental Europe, for example, based on the corporatist model of government, have established systems with extensive private provision, while ensuring equity of access through their funding arrangements (Saltman et al., 2004).

The Private Sector Today

It is necessary to look at three elements of service delivery to understand private provision of health-care services and how it is distinct from public provision: (1) the activity of providing services; (2) the facility in which provision takes place; and (3) the employment arrangements for individuals providing services.

Each of these may be private or public, and without distinguishing among them, it is difficult and sometimes meaningless to refer to service provision as public or private.

The organization of the activity or operation of providing health care can be public or private, with the distinction determined by the control of decisions about the activity, and control of funds generated by the activity. When clinics or hospitals are publicly owned, key managerial decisions (e.g., about hiring practices or services to be offered) are determined by government rules. Leftover funds generated by their operation belong to the treasury or public purse. When clinics or hospitals are privately owned, the organization itself determines the key decisions about its operation. The organization (or its owners) has a legal claim to leftover revenue. This makes the possession of the rights to leftover income and the responsibility for debts the clearest factors for determining to which category the organization belongs.

Much of primary health care, for example, is delivered by physicians who run their practice as a small business. They control the key decisions about how to run the practice. They are responsible for any debts, and are entitled to any profits.

The facility or premises within which services are being provided may be public or private. Public clinics are almost always located in publicly owned buildings. Private clinics and hospitals often do not own but rather rent their premises. Sometimes private clinics are located in publicly owned buildings. This does not make the business, or operation, any less 'private,' since they still decide how to run their practice, and leftover revenue remains with the organization or its owners.

The employment arrangements for health professionals can be either public or private. Most staff working within private health-care organizations are in private employment contracts. Most staff working in public facilities are on public employment contracts. These categories are not airtight, however. In a number of African countries, health ministries provide publicly employed health workers as a form of support to mission (nonprofit) hospitals. Public hospitals in high-income countries often have staff working under private employment contracts for the provision of specialized services. Hence, even once the public or private nature of a health-care organization has been determined, an examination of the employment arrangements within the organization may reveal a more complex picture. Public and private employment arrangements have different implications for incentives and hence the behavior of individuals working in health-care organizations.

Nonprofit Versus For-Profit

Another important distinction among private health-care activities is their organizational form, including their profit orientation. This distinction is important because it influences the behavior of the organizations and, in particular, may influence the degree to which behavior is likely to be more social versus opportunistic. There is also some evidence that they differ systematically with respect to efficiency and productivity, with for-profits exhibiting higher levels in some studies.

Many private health-care activities are organized as nonprofit entities. They can be distinguished from other service providers by the 'nondistribution constraint' – that is, even though they may generate a 'surplus' of revenue over expenditures, they cannot distribute this surplus to individuals in the form of profits. They can spend it in other ways, including higher wages or 'perks' to their employees and managers, training/education, research, community service, and subsidizing less profitable services. Nonprofit organizations are also distinct from for-profits in that they often pursue objectives other than the financial bottom line. It is important to keep in mind that only a small portion of nonprofit organizations are socially oriented. Many membership organizations (e.g., cooperatives of milk producers) or lobbying organizations (e.g., the National Rifle Association) are organized as nonprofits, but are pursuing the interests of their members and/or contributors rather than society at large.

For-profit organizations can be organized as either small businesses or investor-owned (Deber, 2002). The majority of private health-care providers are organized as small businesses (sometime referred to as 'proprietary'). Most private clinics and diagnostic labs, for example, are organized this way. While these organizations are run as a business, and the proprietor certainly takes home any profits generated, they do not have to generate a return on any investment by external shareholders. This difference is perceived to reduce the focus on the financial bottom line, allowing professional values and ethics to exert a greater influence. Hence, typically, policy makers are less concerned with quality skimping and patient 'cream-skimming' in the case of small health-care businesses.

Hospitals require very large amounts of capital investment, and therefore private hospitals are usually investor-owned. External investors are understood to prioritize return on investment – in either the form of distributed profits or appreciation of the value of the hospital. The focus on the hospital as a business often leads to concern by policy makers and regulators that profit maximization may reduce health-care quality or that unprofitable patients will be discouraged or turned away.

Private Health-Care Provision in High-Income Countries

In both high- and low-income countries, there is extensive private provision of health-care services. However, private providers play different roles and operate differently in the two groups of countries (Saltman et al., 2006). This section will characterize private provision in high-income countries. The next section will discuss low-income countries.

Primary health care is extensively delivered by physicians organized as small businesses in high-income countries, with the exception of Sweden, Norway, and Finland (see **Table 1**). In most of these countries, private providers play a coordinated role in the national health system, reflected in the public (or social) funding of the services. Funding is usually linked to the delivery of a specific package of services – both curative and preventive (e.g., immunizations, well-baby checkups). Hence, in the countries with predominantly private primary care systems, part of the package of core public health services is delivered by private providers. However, in a few cases, public funding is limited to public providers. As a result, patients who utilize private services must pay themselves (e.g., Spain, Portugal).

In high-income countries, a large portion of hospital service is provided by nonprofit organizations, many of which emerged from religious charities. Virtually the entire hospital sectors of Canada and the Netherlands are organized as a statutory class of nonprofit hospitals. The majority of hospitals in Belgium (99 of a total of 157) are nonprofit, as are 30% of hospitals in France. In Germany, 37% of hospital beds are nonprofit. The nonprofit hospital sector is important in Australia and the United States as well. For-profit (investor-owned) hospitals are less common, playing a substantial role in delivery in only Australia, the United States, Germany, and France.

This private provision takes place within a framework of extensive public or social funding, as well as extensive regulation and self-regulation, including accreditation (see **Table 2**). The result is that private provision is well-integrated into the system and performs relatively well in ensuring equitable access and reasonable levels of quality. This is not the case in low-income countries.

Private Health-care Provision in Low-Income Countries

Although there is broad agreement that the private sector plays an important role in the delivery of health services in low-income countries, there remains much debate on how to measure this role, and as a result, there is limited consolidated evidence. The role of private expenditure for health care changes relatively systematically, becoming less important as national income increases (Musgrove et al., 2002). The same cannot be concluded for private service provision, which appears to be unrelated to the level of private financing.

Low-income countries are characterized by ineffective regulation, small and often fragmented national service delivery programs, and the near total lack of public financing transfers to private for-profit providers. As a result, the role of private health providers varies greatly, reflecting a combination of historical and political priorities and the spontaneous demand of the population.

Consolidated information on providers is limited, and national data on private provision must be questioned, both because they do not include the informal or "less than fully qualified" providers (Berman, 1998) and because biases in reporting ignore the impact of dual employment, which can miss the private clinics of providers with concurrent public employment and also show providers as active in government facilities even if never present (Ensor and Witter, 2000; Hongoro and Kumaranayake, 2000).

As a result of the poor supply of data in low-income countries, utilization measures and payment data (from

Table 1 Countries with predominantly private provision of primary health care

Australia	Denmark	Netherlands
Austria	Estonia	New Zealand
Belgium	France	Norway[a]
Canada	Italy	Slovakia[b]
Czech Republic	Israel	United Kingdom

[a]Ovretveit J (2003) *The Changing Public-Private Mix in Nordic Healthcare – An Analysis*. Goteborg, Sweden: Nordic School of Public Health.
[b]Sedláková D, Hlavačka S, and Riesberg A (2003) Major reforms in Slovakia. *Euro Observer* 6(3).
Source: European Healthcare Observatory, *Health Care Systems in Transition* (most recent) country reports, except where noted.

Table 2 The five most important areas of interaction between government policy and private health service providers

1. Funding – Many governments use public funding of private providers to ensure access to services for the population. This may be implemented through set transfers or through a formal contract for services
2. Regulation – Certification standards, treatment requirements, and controls for medicines, procedures, and payment mechanisms all affect private provision
3. Training – National governments support private provision through medical education subsidies
4. Self-regulation oversight – Governments act to ensure minimum standards of quality in provision for professionals and facilities through oversight of self-regulation, usually performed by professional and provider associations
5. Accreditation – Review of an organization's compliance with established quality standards is undertaken by an external body

household surveys) are often used as a proxy. Demographic and health surveys provide an indication of the high importance of private providers as a source of health care across all income strata in low-income countries (Boone and Zhan, 2007), and national health accounts data offer some insight into the high importance of out-of-pocket expenditure for health care in the same countries. Neither data set alone is sufficient to describe the size, role, or distribution of private providers.

In an attempt to fill this void, Hanson and Berman (1998) measured clinic numbers and hospital beds in both public and private sectors across a number of countries. Using both published and unpublished surveys and government reports, we have recreated this assessment for 61 countries (see **Tables 3** and **4**). For countries with multiple data points, we examined changes over time. The trend differs by region, but in the rapidly growing economies of South and East Asia we note that for-profit providers and private hospitals are an increasingly important component of the health systems. This is supported by changes in health financing, illustrating that private out-of-pocket financing of health care in these same economies, notably China, India, Indonesia, Bangladesh, Vietnam, and the Philippines, is both large and increasing.

Tertiary Care

In sub-Saharan Africa, many national health programs were developed out of hospital and clinic networks created by European missionaries during the colonial period. As a result of this legacy, mission facilities are integrated into national health systems in a number of countries, receiving core funding from health ministry budgets as well as subsidized and free medicines, and incorporated into laboratory, referral, and vertical programs. In some South Asian countries, particularly Bangladesh, Cambodia, and Afghanistan, nongovernmental organizations (a special class of nonprofit organization, usually with a humanitarian or philanthropic focus) have taken on an important role with government support, extending the reach of national programs, again with core funding support through long-standing contracts.

More common are stand-alone for-profit hospitals, observed in almost all low-income countries and serving foreigners, wealthy nationals, and, increasingly, "medical

Table 3 Private sector importance in low- and middle-income countries

Country	Beds % private	Physicians % private	Hospitals % private
Albania			0%
Argentina	43%		
Armenia	9%		
Azerbaijan	0%		
Bangladesh	28%	50%	20%
Brazil	70%		68%
Burkina Faso		97%	
Cameroon		80%	
China	6%		2%
Costa Rica		24%	
Czech Republic	9%	74%	32%
Dominican Republic	38%		
Ecuador	23%		26%
Ethiopia		87%	
Honduras		62%	
Hungary	2%		
India	64%		93%
Indonesia	<50%		1%
Kazakhstan		2%	
Kenya			19%
Latvia	2%		7%
Lithuania	100%		
Malawi	0%	39%	0%
Mexico		48%	
Moldova			6%
Mozambique		14%	
Nigeria		21%	27%
Panama	14%		
Peru			49%
Poland	0%		9%
Rwanda	0%	77%	0%
St. Kitts/Nevis		20%	
St. Vincent/ Grenadines		22%	
Tanzania		7%	
Turkey	8%	14%	22%
Uganda		90%	
Venezuela			54%

Table 4 Private sector importance in high-income countries

Country	Beds % private	Physicians % private	Hospitals % private
Aruba	100%		
Australia	30%		
Austria	28%	51%	
Belgium	40%		63%
Bermuda	0%		
Cayman Islands	0%		
Cyprus	50%		
Denmark			0%
Finland	4%		41%
France	20%		38%
Germany	10%		
Greece	25%	18%	
Israel	50%		
Italy	22%		
Netherlands	100%		90%
New Zealand	48%	94%	81%
Norway	0%		
Portugal	23%		41%
Puerto Rico	56%	70%	
Spain	31%		
Sweden	19%		
Switzerland	20%	56%	
UK	5%		
US	95%		

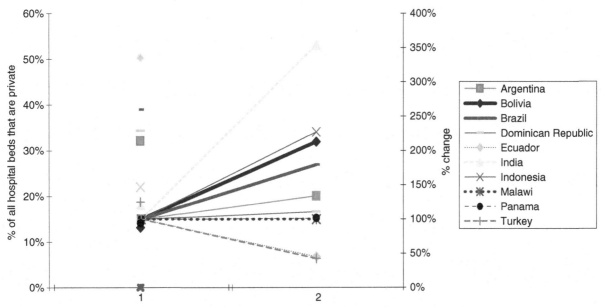

Figure 1 Baseline percent of all hospital beds that are private (late 1990s/early 2000) and percent change from baseline to second measurement (mid-2000s); all countries with two reported points in the past 15 years.

tourists" (Marcelo, 2003). Private hospital numbers are growing in many countries (**Figure 1**); in Indonesia, for example, they grew from 25% of all facilities in 1997 to more than half of all hospitals today (Thabrany, 2004). World Health Survey (WHS) data consistently shows evidence that in all low-income countries, the private sector is more important in outpatient than in-patient care (WHS, 2002).

Primary Care

Private clinics, pharmacies, consulting rooms, and home care make up the bulk of private practices in developing countries, and the majority of patient interactions with the private sector occur here (WHS, 2002). In China, for example, 70% of all ambulatory care clinics are private (Liu et al., 2006). There are conflicting arguments for when and why this is the case, but broad agreement that the reasons stem from a combination of accessibility, responsiveness, perceived quality, and opportunity cost (Castro-Leal et al., 2000).

Where data are available, they indicate that the private sector is often heavily involved in delivering priority preventative and curative treatments (e.g., public health priorities). In rich countries, this is by design and is linked to policies (e.g., payments, subsidies, regulations); in poor countries, it is often by default, based on demand and social concern, and sometimes is linked to nonprofit delivery. In most poor countries, immunizations are done by public providers, though some countries (e.g., India) give vaccines to private providers to promote coverage (Peters et al., 2002).

Nonprofits

In a number of African countries, religious missions formed the backbone of services during colonial times, and retain a significant role in current care provision. In these countries, mission facilities are *de facto* government providers, with regular subsidies for salaries and medicines, and full integration into the national reporting and referral systems. Aside from these special cases, however, nonprofits play a small role in overall health systems, for example, representing less than 2% of services in India and less than that in China.

Conclusions

The private sector plays a significant role in the delivery of health care in countries across all income levels (see (**Figure 2**). This role is higher for ambulatory care than for inpatient care, but beyond that, there are not clear patterns for variation in private sector size by national income, nor by national political leaning. There is some limited indication that the private sector is growing in importance in many places, and attention is increasingly, and appropriately, being paid to understanding how governments can work effectively with private individuals and institutions in order to promote public health goals.

In most instances, collaboration must be based upon an improved understanding of the private sector as a multifaceted grouping of actors, an acknowledgment of the

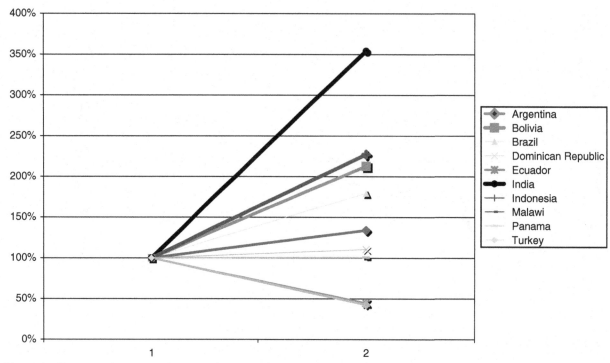

Figure 2 Change in percentage of all hospitals that are private: mid-1990s to mid-2000s.

motivation and capacity embodied by the sector, and the value of private care provision, as evidenced by health-seeking behavior of individuals from all wealth strata. Partnerships between private and public sectors have been developed in many countries, both rich and poor, to the benefit of both individual users and the public in general.

Contentious debates about private care provision take place relatively often in the context of development assistance for low-income countries, and to a lesser degree in discussions of health system changes in the United Kingdom and the United States. In most high-income countries, however, private versus public provision is not an explosive issue, both sectors having been incorporated into stable delivery systems with a range of national, insurance, and private financing sources. Where disputes over the role of the private sector develop, debate is often driven by larger political issues of system change (e.g., transition economies, health system decentralization) or reactions of local governments to escalating costs. The general lack of basic data on the efficiency, quality, and equity of private delivery arrangements limits the rigor of such debates, and hampers the development of appropriate policy and program planning. Further data collection and studies are needed to inform and support strategies that engage the private sector in the achievement of public health goals.

See also: Insurance Plans and Programs - An Overview.

Citations

Berman P (1998) Rethinking healthcare systems: Private healthcare provision in India. *World Development* 26(8): 1463–1479.

Boone P and Zhan Z (2006) *Lowering Child Mortality in Poor Countries: The Power of Knowledgeable Parents*. Center for Economic Performance Discussion Paper No. 751. London: London School of Economics and Political Science. http://cep.lse.ac.uk/pubs/download/dp0751.pdf (accessed October 2007).

Castro-Leal F, Dayton J, Emery L, and Mehra K (2000) Public spending on health care in Africa: Do the poor benefit? *Bulletin of the World Health Organization* 78(1): 66–74.

Deber RB (2002) *Delivering Healthcare Services: Public, Not-for-Profit or Private?* Discussion Paper No 17. n.p.: Commission on the Future of Healthcare in Canada. http://www.teamgrant.ca/M-THAC%20Greatest%20Hits/Bonus%20Tracks/Delivering%20Health%20Care%20Services.pdf (accessed October 2007).

Deber R, Topp A, and Zakas D (2004) *Private Delivery and Public Goals: Mechanisms for Ensuring that Hospitals Meet Public Objectives*. Background Paper. n.p.: World Bank.

Ensor T and Witter S (2000) Health economics in low income countries: adapting to the reality of the unofficial economy. *Health Policy* 57: 1–13.

Hanson K and Berman P (1998) Private health care provision in developing countries: A preliminary analysis of levels and composition. *Health Policy and Planning* 13(3): 195–211.

Hongoro C and Kumaranayake L (2000) Do they work? Regulating for-profit providers in Zimbabwe. *Health Policy and Planning* 15(4): 368–377.

Liu Y, Berman P, Yip W, et al. (2006) Health care in China: The role of non-government providers. *Health Policy* 77: 212–220.

Maarse H (2006) The privatization of health care in Europe: An eight-country analysis. *Journal of Health Politics, Policy, and Law* 31(5): 981–1014.

Marcelo R (2003) India fosters growing 'medical tourism' sector. *The Financial Times* July 2.

Musgrove P, Zeramdini R, and Carrin G (2002) Basic patterns in national health expenditure. *Bulletin of the World Health Organization* 80: 134–142.

Øvretveit J (2003) *The Changing Public-Private Mix in Nordic Healthcare – An Analysis*. Goteborg, Sweden: Nordic School of Public Health.
Peters DH, Yazbeck AS, Sharma R, Ramana GNV, Pritchett L, and Wagstaff A (2002) *Better Health Systems for India's Poor: Findings, Analysis, and Options*. Washington, DC: World Bank.
Saltman R, Busse R, and Figueras J (2004) *Social Health Insurance Systems in Western Europe*. Buckingham, UK: Open University Press.
Saltman R, Rico A, and Boerma W (2006) *Primary Care in the Driver's Seat*. Buckingham, UK: Open University Press.
Thabrany H (2004) Social health insurance in Indonesia: Current status and the plan for national health insurance. In: Sein T (ed.) *Regional Overview of Social Health Insurance in South-East Asia*, annex 3, pp. 101–162. New Delhi, India, Regional Office for South-East Asia, World Health Organization. http://www.searo.who.int/LinkFiles/Social_Health_Insurance_HSD-274.pdf (accessed October 2007).
World Health Survey (WHS) (2002) *World Health Survey, World Health Organization*. Geneva, Switzerland: WHS.

Relevant Websites

http://cep.lse.ac.uk/pubs/download/dp0751.pdf – Boone P and Zhan Z (2006) *Lowering Child Mortality in Poor Countries: The Power of Knowledgeable Parents*. Center for Economic Performance Discussion Paper No. 751. London: London School of Economics and Political Science (accessed October 2007).

http://www.teamgrant.ca/M-THAC%20Greatest%20Hits/Bonus%20Tracks/Delivering%20Health%20Care%20Services.pdf – Deber RB (2002) *Delivering Healthcare Services: Public, Not-for-Profit or Private?* Discussion Paper No. 17. n.p.: Commission on the Future of Healthcare in Canada (accessed October 2007).

http://www.gsdrc.org/go/topic-guides/service-delivery/non-state-provision – Governance and Social Development Resource Centre, Service Delivery. This site presents resources that consider how the use of private providers affects quality of and access by the poor to basic services. Also, there is discussion of the role of the state as regulator and the development of public-private partnerships in developing countries. Note that the website uses the term 'non-state' to refer to private provision.

http://www.south.du.ac.in/fms/idpad/index.html – IDPAP Project, Public-Private Partnership in the Provision of Health Care Services to the Poor. This site has an exhaustive literature review of published and unpublished materials on the role of the private health sector, with an emphasis on developing countries. It was assembled from 2003 to 2006.

http://www.psp.ki.se – Private Sector Programme in Health. The PSPH is a collaborative research program aimed at identifying policies and programs that will strengthen health systems' performance and their outcome in terms of improved health. The program explores the private health sector and how it can be involved in providing adequate health care to the population, particularly those in most need in low-income countries. The site provides access to useful material on the topic, including links to other websites.

http://www.searo.who.int/LinkFiles/Social_Health_Insurance_HSD-274.pdf – Thabrany H (2004) Social health insurance in Indonesia: Current status and the plan for national health insurance. In: Sein T (ed.) *Regional Overview of Social Health Insurance in South-East Asia*, annex 3, pp. 101–162. New Delhi: Regional Office for South-East Asia, World Health Organization (accessed October 2007).

http://www.psp-one.com/ – USAID, PSP-*One*. This is a project of the U.S. Agency for International Development (USAID), aimed at increasing the private sector's provision of high-quality reproductive health products and services in developing countries. This Resource Center is a clearinghouse for leading-edge knowledge, tools, and resources relevant to provision and use of quality private sector health products and services. It contains downloadable documents, links to resources and other websites, and citations of publications.

http://rru.worldbank.org/ – World Bank, Knowledge Services for Financial and Private Sector Development. This site offers best-practice public policy analytical materials and discussions for private sector–led growth and financial market development in developing countries. It provides links to expert analysis, powerful databases, quick solutions, and comprehensive 'how-to' guides. Site users will need to search for references to 'health' and 'healthcare'.

Competition in Health Care

P H Song, J D Barlow, E E Seiber, and A S McAlearney, The Ohio State University, Columbus, OH, USA

© 2008 Elsevier Inc. All rights reserved.

Economic competition describes market conditions based on the number of suppliers available to meet consumer demands and the ease of entry and exit of new firms into the market. In health care, competition exists among, within, and between providers, insurers, and pharmaceutical companies that provide health-care products and services to patients. It is a powerful force that continues to shape and impact health-care costs, quality, and access.

Principles of Competition

Market conditions including the number of sellers, type of product sold, barriers to entry, and consumer information determine the level of competition in a market. This level of competition can range from perfectly competitive to purely monopolistic. The highest degree of competition occurs in a perfectly competitive market. A perfectly competitive market assumes there are many individual suppliers of identical products, there are no barriers to entry or exit from the market and the availability of perfect information allows consumers to accurately determine which firm offers the best value.

Conversely, the least competitive market structure is a pure monopoly where there is one seller of a unique product in a market with high barriers to entry, allowing the firm to be a price-setter. A less extreme version of a pure monopoly is an oligopoly. An oligopoly is characterized by a few dominant firms in a market with substantial barriers to entry. The small number of firms causes the behavior of any one firm to significantly influence that of another. Collusive oligopolies are characterized by cooperation among the few firms in a market to inflate prices and maximize profits by acting together as a monopoly. In practice, firms are deterred from collusion due to anti-trust regulations. Monopolistic competition describes a market with many sellers selling a product that is differentiated across all firms. In this case, a firm with a highly differentiated product can gain significant pricing power in a particular market segment.

In health care, suppliers of goods and services include physicians, hospitals, pharmaceutical manufacturers, and private health insurance companies. Physicians offer treatment and diagnostic services to patients, while hospitals provide the use of their facilities and the resources consumed during the processes of treatment and diagnosis. Pharmaceutical manufacturers sell drugs used in treatment, and insurance companies sell various levels of insurance coverage to patients for the goods and services sold by physicians, hospitals, and pharmaceutical manufacturers. Purchasers of health-care goods and services include patients, employers who purchase health insurance on their employees' behalf, insurance companies, and the government.

Health care is a heterogeneous product by nature and it cannot typically be re-traded. No two physicians are exactly alike, and their services can only be purchased via direct interaction with the seller. Consumer preferences are also heterogeneous and this further differentiates the health services as a product, particularly in the physician services market. In addition, information in health care is highly asymmetric, with health-care providers acting as agents for patients. Finally, competition in health-care markets is marked by substantial barriers to entry created by government regulations, laws, licensure requirements, and capital investment costs. The U.S. health-care system is characterized by varying degrees of competition and is generally more competitive compared to the health-care systems of other advanced economies. The remaining sections explore the role of competition in the four major sectors of the health-care industry: physicians, hospitals, insurers, and pharmaceutical companies.

Physician Competition

In the United States, physician services were mostly unregulated until the formation of the American Medical Association (AMA) and the release of the Flexner Report in 1910. This report set strict standards for medical training in the United States, and states began to place greater scrutiny on the process of physician licensure. The early physician services market consisted of self-employed physicians who visited patients in their homes and owned solo practices that were paid by fee-for-service. Fee-for-service is a health-care reimbursement model under which a physician receives fees for each individual service provided, such as an office visit or a surgery. The introduction of many new and expensive technologies in the latter half of the twentieth century increased expenditures on physician services 50-fold (Raffel and Raffel, 1989) and generally increased the cost of providing medical care. Physicians today work in group practices to share costs, and only one-quarter of physicians operate their own individual practices. In addition, current physician reimbursement is no longer restricted to fee-for-service payment. Some physicians are employed by managed care organizations, which are health coverage plans that are responsible for both the financing and delivery of medical care. Physicians are also reimbursed on a number of different and often complex fee schedules. Fee schedules are lists of prenegotiated fees to be paid for specific services. Currently, the two primary buyers of physician services are the government and private insurers, which account for 83% of all expenditures on physician services. The major barrier to entry into the physician services market is medical licensure requirements. Licensure requirements vary by state but generally include a degree from an accredited medical school, internship or residency at an accredited institution, and the passing of a medical board exam. In addition, physicians' credentials are verified and reviewed before physicians are granted privileges to work at a particular hospital.

For purchasers of physician services, the presence of health insurance introduces moral hazard, which means that insured consumers bear only a small percentage of the actual cost of care, creating incentives for consumers to purchase unnecessary services. Thus competition for physician services is atypical compared to other markets because insured consumers are often less sensitive to the price of services. A lack of reliable information also makes consumers unaware of the quality of services; thus patients rely on their physicians to act as their agents in health-care purchasing decisions. While consumers may be able to assess their satisfaction with non-health-care products despite a lack of technical knowledge, such consumers may not be able to determine whether or not a bad medical outcome was due to substandard treatment (Newhouse, 2002), compounding the problem of quality assessment in health care.

With consumers often shielded from much of the cost of physician services and reliant on their physicians for purchasing advice, the presence of financial incentives for the physician to order inappropriate and unnecessary treatments has been studied at length. Supplier-induced demand is the hypothesis offered to explain this physician behavior (McGuire, 2000). Under this theory, consumers rely heavily on physicians to advise them on how frequently they should have office visits, medical tests, and appropriate treatments; thus physicians have the potential to control consumer demand and enhance these physicians' economic interests. The most compelling evidence of supplier-induced demand came from an early study that found that a 10% increase in surgeons per capita resulted in a corresponding 3% increase in surgeries per capita (Fuchs, 1978). However, more recent empirical studies have found much weaker support for supplier-induced demand (e.g., Escarce, 1992; Carlsen and Grytten, 1998).

As in the U.S. case, competition globally in physician services varies widely both across and within countries. For example, competition can vary by service environment, such as when hospital-based physicians earn a salary while their primary care counterparts operate in a competitive, fee-for-service environment. Alternatively, competition can vary by payer, with some physicians earning a salary working for the public sector while others are paid fee-for-service for patient visits at private clinics where patients pay entirely out of pocket. Combining these options, an individual physician may earn a salary in the public sector while moonlighting on a fee-for-service basis at a for-profit clinic. Most countries require licensing of physicians, but in many lower-income countries, informal or traditional providers compete with physicians who offer similar services. Quality varies widely among these informal providers, but this informal provider sector largely escapes regulation.

Hospital Competition

Until the development of the germ theory of disease, the introduction of new technologies in medical care, and the urbanization of America, hospitals were actually nonmedical institutions. Most medical care was performed outside hospitals, and hospitals were considered charitable institutions designed to improve the spirits of patients rather than impact their physical well-being. The years following 1880 saw hospitals grow from almshouses to technologically sophisticated centers for medical care innovation. Today, the hospital services industry is the largest of all medical care industries, and in 2003 it accounted for 36% of all U.S. health-care expenditures. The government sector accounted for the majority of hospital revenues in 2003, collectively purchasing 58% of all hospital services. This gives the government considerable influence concerning the allocation of resources in hospital services because of the significant market power they possess as the primary financer of hospital services through Medicare and Medicaid. Individual consumers, most of whom are shielded from the cost of services via insurance, account for only 3.2% of all hospital revenue and have relatively little direct impact on the market price for hospital care.

Certificate of need (CON) laws were historically considered a barrier to entry into the health-care market for hospitals as new or existing hospitals had to justify budgeting and expansion plans. While a large number of states have abolished or fundamentally revised their CON laws, building a new hospital today still requires substantial planning and capital investment resources, creating considerable barriers to hospital market entry.

One way in which hospitals have competed for market share has been through the acquisition of the latest technology and the construction of state-of-the-art facilities. This phenomenon has been called the medical arms race as hospitals race to acquire the latest and greatest technologies (Porter, 2006). The arms race was particularly intense under Medicare's cost-based reimbursement system, which reimbursed hospitals for a portion of their capital expenditures. Hospitals hoped to increase market share by offering access to the best possible equipment and facilities which attracted area physicians to direct their services to these hospitals. The building boom eventually created excess capacity, which led to the passage of Certificate of Need (CON) laws in many states to review the necessity of facility construction. In addition, the change in Medicare reimbursement from cost-plus to prospective payment that paid fixed fees for specific diagnosis-related groups meant that hospitals would no longer be reimbursed directly for the cost of building new facilities and acquiring new technologies. Many hospitals have since closed; as of 2003, 5800 of the 7000 hospitals that existed in 1980 were still in existence (Santerre and Neun, 2007).

Hospitals compete for market share by negotiating contracts with private insurance companies and managed care organizations. The effectiveness of each party in these negotiations is often determined by market penetration. As the presence of large managed care networks developed in the U.S. in the late 1980s, hospitals began to consolidate into large health systems to build bargaining power. Managed care organizations responded by doing the same, and the result was a boom in mergers and acquisitions. Two factors accelerated this trend toward mergers and acquisitions. One was the presence of Columbia/HCA, a for-profit hospital system known for the extraordinary number of acquisitions it made. Many hospitals feared that if they did not acquire hospitals in their area, Columbia/HCA would acquire them and threaten their market position. The second driving force was the perception that lone hospitals could no longer negotiate effectively with managed care organizations. As a result, many hospitals with strong market positions explored merger possibilities. In some cases, the government attempted to block hospital mergers, arguing that hospitals were exhibiting anticompetitive behavior. However, hospitals were successful in defending their mergers by contending that that consolidation would lead to lower costs through increased efficiency. Proponents of mergers between not-for-profit hospitals also argued that not-for-profits seek to maximize the welfare of their communities rather than to exercise market power, and that increased competition could adversely affect the amount of charity care provided by the hospitals to indigent patients (Gaynor and Vogt, 2000).

Accounting for the largest share of health expenditures, hospitals globally have experienced the greatest changes in their competitive environment. Early reforms focused on managerial decentralization, with policy makers frequently granting managerial autonomy to large hospitals with an expectation of increased efficiency. More recent reforms have sought to increase hospital competition through the creation of internal markets. These internal markets seek to separate payer from provider, even within the public sector. Rather than receive fixed budgets, public hospitals must compete to attract funding from public payers. Specific approaches vary across countries, with many reforms linking funding to the number of patients the hospital attracts. These volume-based contracts create incentives for hospitals to both improve quality and reform service mix to attract patients and funding. Some countries have extended contracting competition to primary care providers with physicians or groups of physicians competing to serve the primary care needs of a fixed population (Liu et al., 2007).

Competition Among Health Insurers

The growth of health insurance coverage is one of the most significant developments in the health-care field over the past decades. Private health insurance began to spread in the U.S. during the Great Depression as a number of hospitals began accepting premiums from local residents to cover any medical services provided. During this period, the American Hospital Association created Blue Cross insurance plans that allowed enrollees free choice among hospitals within a city. These insurance plans enjoyed a virtual monopoly position in the insurance market throughout the 1930s, but at that time premiums were very low. They grew more competitive following World War II when the federal government imposed wage and price controls. Unable to attract additional laborers with higher wages, employers offered benefits such as health insurance to circumvent the wage controls. The resulting boom in insurance coverage attracted commercial insurance companies to a market that had previously been dominated by the Blue Cross plans, thereby increasing competition. Today private health insurance is responsible for financing 36% of all health-care expenditures in the U.S. and provides coverage to 70% of the population (Santerre and Neun, 2007).

The U.S. market for private insurance is made up of many different health insurers that can specialize in group health insurance, individual insurance, or a combination of both. Group health insurance is purchased by employers on their employees' behalf, while individual insurance is purchased directly by a consumer. While the insurance market has many sellers, there is also high market concentration. It is estimated that out of 47 states and Washington D.C., the three largest health insurers accounted for more than 50% of enrollment in 43 states in 2003 (Robinson, 2004). Though the market for health insurance is relatively concentrated, many large employers choose to self-insure as an alternative to purchasing health insurance. This practice has grown because self-insured plans are exempt from paying premium taxes and from providing state-mandated benefits under the Employee Retirement Income Security Act of 1974 (ERISA). This can provide significant savings to firms that are large enough to have predictable medical expenses. Today most health insurance plans utilize provider networks to direct care and negotiate lower rates for services. The large expense of setting up these networks is seen as a barrier to entry for potential competition from new insurance companies.

Competition in the health insurance industry is much like an oligopoly with a large competitive fringe. A competitive fringe can be described as a large number of smaller firms with small market shares that compete with a few dominant firms. The smallest 50% of all group health insurers controlled 3% of the market in 2001. Since health insurers are purchasers of health services, the growing dominance of managed care and the increasing concentration of the insurance market have created concerns about monopsony power. Monopsony power exists when payers have enough buying power to drive price below a competitive level. Extreme monopsony would be one buyer and many sellers. Managed care firms with large market shares have substantially increased their bargaining power with hospitals and physicians. While a great deal of government attention has been paid to the anticompetitive implications of hospital mergers, regulators and courts have often regarded monopsony power as leading to reduced prices for consumers. Theoretically, the lower reimbursement tendered by a firm with monopsony power could force hospitals to reduce services to some unprofitable patients.

Private health insurance plans play substantially smaller roles outside of the United States. The U.S. system of voluntary, private health insurance is atypical among the higher-income, industrialized countries. Globally, competing, private insurers serve in a secondary role as supplements for government-sponsored social insurance programs or as insurers for affluent individuals in low-income countries.

Pharmaceutical Competition

The research-based pharmaceutical industry began during World War II when the U.S. military's demand for sulfa drugs and penicillin necessitated mass production of the items in lieu of handicraft methods. Chemical firms such as Merck were able to produce drugs in bulk form, and they were converted into dosage form by drug companies. This innovation increased potential profits and lured many new firms to the market after the war (Santerre and Neun, 2007). Today, there are over 700 pharmaceutical companies in the U.S.

The two main barriers to entry in the pharmaceutical industry are research and development costs and patents (Scherer, 2000). Because the introduction and approval of a new drug requires substantial investment in research and development, patents are awarded to protect the economic profits of the innovating firm over a period of time. Government patent protection grants the innovating firm the right to be the sole producer of a drug product for a legal maximum of 20 years. Without patent protection, drugs could be easily imitated and sold at a lower price by firms that have not invested resources in the research and development of the drug. The smaller profits that would be available in the absence of patents would reduce the financial incentive for firms to bear the cost and risk of undertaking potentially valuable research and development activities. When patents expire, innovating companies face competition from generic drug manufacturers. Generic drugs are products with the same active chemical ingredients as the original drugs that are sold with little or no advertising or promotion. However, when patents expire, brand loyalty can be a significant barrier to entry for a new firm. Generic drug producers are often able to offer sufficient discounts to gain market share because the FDA does not require them to carry out the extensive and costly tests required of innovating firms before a drug is approved. Instead, generic drug producers must demonstrate that their drugs have identical active ingredients and similar rates of absorption to the patent-protected drugs. These firms are also permitted to submit the required documentation to the FDA prior to the expiration of the patent so they can begin to sell the generic drug immediately after the patent expires. Generics tend to enter the market at 40–70% of the price of the original patented drug. As additional generic competitors enter the market, the price of the generic drug falls further while the original branded drug exhibits little price change.

Physician behavior is often presented as the explanation for the difference in price between brand-name and generic drugs. Pharmaceutical products can only be obtained legally with a physician's prescription, shifting the purchase decision from the consumer to the physician. Physicians are generally indifferent to the price of drugs and adhere to their prescribing preferences. The physician typically considers professional responsibilities and liability risk, but not necessarily cost when deciding about an appropriate pharmaceutical treatment. Further, consumers' purchases of prescription drugs, much like the purchase of other health services, are often reimbursed partially or wholly by insurance. With consumers partially or wholly insulated from the cost of prescribed medications and generally unable to assess the quality of the drugs they consume, the resultant demand for pharmaceutical products tends to be fairly unresponsive to price.

To combat these factors, many drug insurance plans use formularies, or lists of pharmaceutical products, that enumerate the medications physicians are allowed to prescribe under the individual insurance plan, thereby attempting to control the decisions of prescription-writing physicians and distributing pharmacists who also are advised to substitute generics for brand-name pharmaceuticals whenever possible. Government regulations have also attempted to encourage the use of generic medications in order to better contain drug costs.

Pharmaceutical markets are the most global dimension of health-care competition, with the sales of the top ten pharmaceutical companies approaching 50% of the world market (Busfield, 2003). Once in production, a patent-holding pharmaceutical firm faces low unit production costs for most compounds. These low marginal costs allow the drugs to be sold profitably at differing price levels in both wealthy and middle-income countries, assuming that drugs sold for lower prices in middle-income markets cannot be re-exported to higher-priced, wealthy markets. However, access concerns in the lowest-income countries led to the Doha Declaration on Trade-Related Property Rights and Public Health in 2001, stating that member countries of the World Trade Organization had the right to grant compulsory licenses during public health crises.

Conclusion

The objective of competition is to improve value for consumers as costs fall and quality improves. In the health-care industry, achieving improved value through competition has been complicated by imperfections in the health-care market such as incomplete information, highly differentiated products, government regulations, and lack of price transparency. Competition in health care has historically focused on the physician, hospital, or health plan level. Going forward, competition will likely also occur at the individual consumer level as patients are provided with more information about price and quality that may influence their health-care decisions. Consumer-driven health care, as it is currently described, relies on greater patient involvement and includes financial incentives for patients to select more efficient providers. Providers and health plans, in turn, will also be challenged to compete for patients based on both price and quality measures. However, the effectiveness of consumer-driven health care will rely largely on the adoption and use of information technology that facilitates the provision of accurate, timely, and useful information to patients about the price and quality of health-care services.

See also: Insurance Plans and Programs - An Overview; Provider Payment Methods and Incentives.

Citations

Busfield J (2003) Globalization and the pharmaceutical industry revisited. *International Journal of Health Services* 33: 581–605.
Carlsen F and Grytten J (1998) More physicians: Improved availability or induced demand? *Health Economics* 7: 495–508.
Escarce JJ (1992) Explaining the association between surgeon supply and utilization. *Inquiry* 29: 403–415.
Fuchs VR (1978) The supply of surgeons and the demand for operations. *The Journal of Human Resources Supplement: National Bureau of Economic Research Conference on the Economics of Physician and Patient Behavior* 13: 35–56.
Gaynor M and Vogt WB (2000) Antitrust and competition in health care markets. In: 1st edn. 1405–1487Culyer AJ and Newhouse JP (eds.) *Handbook of Health Economics* 1st edn Vol. 1, pp. 1405–1487. New York: Elsevier.
Liu X, Hotchkiss DR, and Bose S (2007) The effectiveness of contracting out primary health care services in developing countries: A review of the evidence. *Health Policy and Planning* 82: 200–211.
McGuire TG (2000) Physician agency. In: 1st edn. 461–536 Culyer AJ and Newhouse JP (eds.) *Handbook of Health Economics* 1st edn Vol. 1, pp. 461–536. New York: Elsevier.
Newhouse JP (2002) Why is there a quality chasm? *Health Affairs* 21: 13–25.
Porter M and Teisberg E (2006) *Redefining Healthcare: Creating Value-Based Competition on Results.* Boston, MA: Harvard Business School Press.
Raffel MW and Raffel NK (1989) *The US Health System: Origins and Functions,* 3rd edn. New York: Wiley.
Robinson JC (2004) Consolidation and the transformation of competition in health insurance. *Health Affairs* 23: 11–24.
Santerre RE and Neun SP (2007) *Health Economics: Theories Insights, and Industry Studies,* 4th edn. Mason, OH: Thompson Southwestern.
Scherer FM (2000) The pharmaceutical industry. In: 1st edn. 1297–1336Culyer AJ and Newhouse JP (eds.) *Handbook of Health Economics* 1st edn Vol. 1, pp. 1297–1336. New York: Elsevier.

Further Reading

Enthoven AC and Tollen LA (2005) Competition in health care: It takes systems to pursue quality and efficiency. *Health Affairs Web Exclusive W* 5: 420–433.
Gaynor M and Hass-Wilson D (1999) Change consolidation, and competition in health care markets. *The Journal of Economic Perspectives* 13: 141–164.
Ginsburg PG (2005) Competition in health care: Its evolution over the past decade. *Health Affairs* 24: 1512–1519.
Herzlinger RE and Parsa-Parsi R (2004) Consumer-driven health care: lessons from Switzerland. *Journal of the American Medical Association* 292: 1213–1220.
Porter ME and Teisberg EO (2004) Redefining competition in health care. *Harvard Business Review* 82: 64–76.

Public/Private Mix in Health Systems

C R Keane, University of Pittsburgh, Pittsburgh, PA, USA
M C Weerasinghe, University of Colombo, Colombo, Sri Lanka

© 2008 Elsevier Inc. All rights reserved.

General Considerations

The theme of public–private partnerships in public health and health-care systems has become remarkably prominent since the 1970s. More generally, the contrast between the role of public and private organizations in providing health services has become an extremely important part of discourse and debate internationally. Much of this discourse proceeds as if the distinction between public and private organizations, and their respective roles in health care, were clear and distinct. A broad definition of public organization is one with a mandate for delivering public goods. A narrower and more common definition of public requires that the organization be a governmental entity. Yet close inspection reveals a great diversity of definitions of public and private in health care and a great diversity of approaches to public and private partnership in public health. Moreover, the definitions of public and private are constantly evolving and, most interestingly, we see a constant hybridization of the public and private efforts in health care.

If the definitions of public and private in health care are so fluid, how and why is the literature on the ideal public–private mix so strident? The simplest explanation is that the terms public and private are always defined relative to each other, and that they refer to real opposing social movements in specific contexts. Those opposing movements are rooted in neoliberalism and its resistances, both of which have taken hold all over the world but always in a unique form, reflecting specific local political contexts (Leitner *et al.*, 2007). Therefore, one productive way to understand the meaning of public and private in health care and its underlying dynamics is to contextualize health care within various forms of the neoliberal agenda, which seeks to find market solutions to health-care problems, and the opposing movement of resistance, which seeks to preserve if not expand the public role in health care. While it is most common to advocate for public–private partnerships, some oppose this as a dilution of the unique public role in health. Still others enthusiastically promote privatization as a means of increasing efficiency and lowering cost of health services. The advocates of these opposing perspectives usually assume their audiences understand the meaning between public and private. In some cases, public is taken as synonymous with governmental, and private is reserved for nongovernmental. Others use private to denote for-profit organizations, with nongovernmental not-for-profits falling into a separate category, a third sector, that is not necessarily public or private. Reich (2002) notes that some international nongovernmental organizations, such as Médicins Sans Frontières and Helen Keller International belong to such a third sector, or civil society. These organizations are private in that they are not part of a governmental structure, but are public in the sense that their purpose is to promote the common good. He concludes that such nongovernmental organizations belong to civil society, a third sector (Reich, 2002: 3–4).

Reich's flexible approach to defining the public and private recognizes the inherently blurry boundaries between these categories and the pragmatic necessity of considering a third sector. Another example of a flexible and pragmatic approach to defining the public and private was taken in a conference on public–private partnerships for public health in Africa (Hursh-Cesar *et al.*, 1994). The conference concluded not only that a typology of the public and private in public health would necessarily vary from one country to the next, but also that the definitions could reflect the interests of those who have the power to define. Therefore, they believe it is important to ask "who would define the typology – the public sector or the private providers themselves? Would it clarify ownership and control of services?" (Hursh-Cesar *et al.*, 1994: 18–19).

Another approach to understanding public and private efforts in health care is to see these as outgrowths of basic human impulses for individual and collective well-being. Taking this general perspective, the private sector relies more on individual interests in preserving well-being and individual profiting from providing healing services to paying clients. The collective interest in preserving the health of a group is the basis for the development of public health services, meaning those that cannot be consumed individually but rather that benefit the public as a whole. The latter would include not only public goods such as clean water, clean environment, and safe collective food supplies, but also collective pooling of resources to ensure against the catastrophic loss associated with illness. Modeling private and public health in terms of individual and collective interests has the virtue of highlighting the conflicts between those interests. Classic examples of conflicts between individual and collective interests, also known as social dilemmas, include the likelihood that some individuals will free-ride on public generosity, taking advantage of collectively shared goods by not contributing or shirking one's responsibilities, for example not paying health premiums or taxes, or overutilizing services or a scarce public good such as clean water.

It is reasonable to assume that individual interest in well-being and individual strategies to preserve health probably existed well before our records of healing systems. Yet it is just as reasonable to assume that collective action for health also has a very long history, because the illness of any given individual has ramifications for every other member of the group, most obviously when disease is contagious. Yet different societies have different traditions for sharing public goods and, obviously, very different healing systems have evolved internationally. The modern health sector has roots in more ancient health and healing systems, which were themselves a mixture of both privately and publicly owned entities. Hence, the challenges of integrating the private and public sectors in health care is not a new phenomenon at all. Most contemporary healing systems include both private healers and at least some system for assuring collective health. Different societies have struck a different balance between private and public healing modalities, resulting in different types of complex health systems. Depending on the political ideology that has predominated, the health system developed in different ways in different nations. In certain countries, the state exercised their authority on the provision of health care to the people and developed a predominantly state-controlled service sector. In other countries, in contrast, the state has a minor involvement in managing health systems. In other societies, the political ideology affecting health care has changed, and the evolution of health systems has paralleled those broader ideological shifts.

Public health systems are not restricted to services provided by the governmental services or infrastructure, because private providers are inextricably part of public health systems. Private providers of many different types are in innumerable ways part of public health-care systems. In many countries at least, public health systems include dense networks of private and public providers of many different types that interact in complex ways on a daily basis. For example, when HIV-AIDS surfaced, public and private organizations often developed public–private partnerships to provide new services. HIV services, often carried out by private organizations, had to coordinate with HIV testing and reporting, the latter generally carried out by public providers and authorities.

No system is just an aggregate of the parts and, likewise, public health systems should not be seen as a list of services and functions. Public and private health providers interact in many ways. The great challenge is for the two sectors to find better ways to interact, to together become a viable system so that responses to public health crises, particularly sudden unanticipated ones, can be coordinated. One general model of understanding the ideal public–private mix, is the reinventing government approach popular in the United States, Britain, and several other nations. That model promotes many forms of promoting competition, including putting out competitive bids open to private and public providers, but also including many other ways of promoting competition. However, much of public health-care services may not benefit from such models, because public health involves provision of public goods that cannot be individually consumed, and also involves very high levels of professional expertise that does not thrive in competitive markets. Many public health and health-care organizations have actively been trying to get different stakeholders to share responsibility, not just turn it over to the private sector. The later concept is often referred to as a public–private partnership.

Public–Private Partnerships in Health Care

A public–private partnership (PPP) includes the following fundamental features:

- Includes at least two major partners, one representing a public entity established to deliver public goods and a second partner that is a nongovernmental organization, that intend to collaborate.
- The collaboration should lead to sharing of resources in improving the delivery of an intended public good.
- Both parties should be able to benefit by the collaboration while being accountable for the decisions made and outcomes achieved.

A simple partnership is often defined as the sharing of risks and rewards (included in items two and three above), while a public–private partnership (PPP) also needs to include explicit concern for meeting public needs and public accountability. It is important to note that some (e.g., Reich, 2002) define PPP as necessarily including a for-profit entity, while many others use a less restrictive definition that includes not-for-profits. Many parties in different capacities can be involved in the partnerships provided there is agreement on fundamental principles. Involvement of nongovernmental organizations (NGOs) between the partnerships of governments and private sector is commonly seen. NGOs can serve as facilitators of the partnership or as co-partners in pursuit of the objective of the partnership. The NGO may provide resources or expert guidance, as is the case of the World Health Organization. The best approach for public–private partnerships depends on factors such as:

- political ideology of the country or organization;
- organizational structure of the country or organization;
- primary focus (e.g., national, international);
- primary function – curative or preventive;
- modes of financing;
- possible private sector partners (e.g., are there sufficient private providers in the geographical area?);
- international agreements, e.g., GATS, TRIPS.

The political ideology of the government or the organization plays a major role in deciding the extent to which the private sector will be incorporated. Governments that insist on maintaining major responsibility for health may limit their partnerships to the outsourcing of nonclinical minor functions of the health services. A more liberal political setup would offer private sector to build joint ventures in hospital development and management.

The organizational structure of a country's public health system will spell out the possible mechanisms of integration of private stakeholders into the existing system for providing health services. For example, in a centrally controlled health system, partnerships need to be built at the center of decision-making if private stakeholders are to have a significant role in decision-making as well as in implementation.

Many consider certain international organizations such as the World Health Organization as more closely resembling public rather than private organizations. International organizations such as the WHO may negotiate partnerships with private partners with an international reach, as well as with private partners limited to one nation. The WHO has the competency and resources necessary to successfully undertake such large-scale partnerships. One of the best examples of the latter are the global partnerships developed with pharmaceutical companies producing vaccines against preventable infectious diseases. International organizations can partner with the pharmaceutical industry to purchase large quantities of vaccines, drugs, or other supplies. The purpose is to provide and distribute these products to underserved populations in less developed countries that cannot afford to buy them at the market prices. This guarantees a reliable market for the industry, through public provision of incentives for private research and development of drugs and vaccines. Such large-scale partnerships may reduce the cost of vaccines to populations in poor countries in a relatively short period of time. The international agency may withdraw its subsidy when the price of such drugs and vaccines has reached a level affordable by the recipient country.

Building public–private partnerships for preventing disease differs in many ways from more profit-oriented partnerships. For-profit private sector involvement in preventive efforts is generally low due to low financial incentive. However, the private sector involvement in preventive health efforts often has proven vital for long-term success. Elimination of vaccine-preventable illness in childhood in many countries was achieved with partnerships with private physicians. These private physicians collaborated with the public health authorities in reporting cases while the state provides free vaccines.

The mode of financing in public health is a key factor that determines the nature of many public–private partnerships. Funding to run public health systems could come from general national revenue, special taxes for developing the health sector, nominal user fees, social security systems, other health insurance systems, or foreign aid. Fiscal policies of the government or the organization will determine the extent of involvement of private investments and private sector participation in public enterprise. Policies for restricting private ownership in public facilities, public oversight of insurance systems, financial management in public health institutions, and payments for outsourcing of certain services in public facilities will all depend on the financing mechanisms.

Approaching the correct private partner is crucial for the success of any partnership. The private sector partner should be able to accommodate the common objective of improving the public good while attaining their own corporate objectives. For example, a private for-profit organization's incentives should not significantly differ from that of the public organization, or else the private entity may end up compromising the partnership. It is important not only to identify the explicit mission of both organizations, but also the implicit incentives. The private sector often expresses interest in certain subsectors that are more attractive to them financially, such as hospital services. However, it is often difficult to enroll partners for less attractive fields as preventive programs forcing the public sector to be more flexible on selection criteria. Private partners may believe they can turn a profit by restricting provision of needed services, especially if public monitoring is unfeasible or otherwise inadequate.

International trade agreements such as General Agreement of Trade in Services (GATS) currently influence public–private partnerships. State-operated services are not considered under the purview of the GATS agreement in that they provide noncompetitive and noncommercial services. The World Trade Organization may view some public–private partnerships as competitive and commercial depending on the nature of the arrangements under the partnership. Hence, the general rules of GATS, Most Favored Nation, National Treatment and Market Access, may apply to services provided by public–private partnerships in the health sector. These clauses are major concerns when deciding the nature of the partnerships in order to improve the health sector while safeguarding the national or organizational interest (**Table 1**).

Examples of Public–Private Mixes

The following are few examples of public–private mixes from both developed and less developed countries.

Public–Private Financing and Private Provision of Services in South Korea

South Korea employs public–private financing of primarily privately provided health care. Although publicly financed private provision is common in many other countries, the Korean case is a rather extreme example of private domination of provision. Over 90% of medical institutions are private, over 90% of total beds are private, and over 90% of specialist physicians are private. Moreover, the private provision is not strictly regulated and

Table 1 Examples of public–private partnerships at the national level hospital and preventive services

Hospital services
- Locating a private wing within a public hospital
- Private investment, constructing and leasing to operate a public hospital
- Private management of a public hospital
- Leasing a public hospital for private operation
- Outsourcing nonclinical services: Janitorial, catering, security, transport
- Outsourcing laboratory services
- Outsourcing clinical services that needs specialization and huge financial investments
- Leasing high-tech medical equipment and ambulance services

Preventive services
- Development and operation of health education projects by the private sector, funded by public sector
- Operation of screening programs by private sector, funded by public sector
- Involvement of private physicians and institutions in governmental programs: Childhood immunization, infectious disease reporting systems, other primary care services
- Health surveys, statistical analysis and clinical research conducted by private-sector experts under contract with government through research grants

patients have great freedom of choice (Jeong, 2005). The free-market approach there may be responsible for disparities between rural and urban regions in access. While 80% of the population lives in rural regions, 90% of the physicians and beds are in urban areas (Jeong, 2005: 135). Yet, on the demand side, the Korean government maintains a great deal of control over fee setting, while financing is funded through a mix of private and public sources (Jeong, 2005). The government public health system in South Korea has employed district health information systems since the early 1990s to help local authorities plan and manage comprehensive health-care services and to help the central government plan services nationally (Dongwoon and Heejin, 2003).

Tuberculosis Control in India

In India, the tuberculosis control program has used public–private partnerships to improve the accessibility and quality of services to the population in case reporting, screening, and providing treatment for diagnosed patients. As reported by Dewan and colleagues (2006), the partnership between the Indian government and private practitioners has increased the case notification rate.

Public–Private Mix in Canada

Private health care in Canada is essentially anything over and above what the public system will reimburse. What the public system will finance is regulated by the Canada Health Act. The Canada Health Act assures that all eligible people in the country have access to insured prepaid health services. This is essentially public health insurance. The Canada Health Act also assures that health-care coverage in the provinces is:

- Portable: Citizens that move from one province or territory to another do not lose coverage.
- Universal: All insured residents of a province or territory must be entitled to the insured health services provided by the provincial or territorial health-care insurance plan.
- Accessible: 'insured persons in a province or territory have reasonable access to insured hospital, medical and surgical-dental services on uniform terms and conditions.' (Overview of the Canada Health Act, Accessibility, Section 12: http://www.hc-sc.gc.ca/hcs-sss/medi-assur/cha-lcs/overview-apercu_e.html)

However, some provinces in Canada allow doctors to practice outside the public system, although many require that physicians charge the same or less than what the government would pay for the services under the publicly insured system. Many provinces are seeing an increase in health-care providers practicing outside the provincial system. For example, Quebec has seen significant growth in private, for-profit clinics. Some provinces, such as Ontario, have attempted to strengthen the public system.

Canada spent an estimated $142 billion on health care in 2005, according to Health Care in Canada 2006, a report released by the Canadian Institute for Health Information. Of that, just over $98.8 billion was spent by governments delivering public health care. Approximately $43.2 billion was spent on private health care. However, much of the health care is delivered by private providers while funded by the government. Many of Canada's privately run hospitals and clinics are funded through their provincial government. According to the former president of the Canadian Medical Association, 75% of health-care services are delivered privately, but funded publicly.

> Frontline practitioners, whether they're GPs or specialists by and large are not salaried. They're small hardware stores. Same thing with labs and radiology clinics ... The situation we are seeing now are more services around not being funded publicly but people having to pay for them, or their insurance companies. We have sort of a passive privatization.
> Dr. Albert Schumacher, 2006, CBC News Report

Several of the newer clinics now operate on a for-profit basis. Some have argued that a trend would damage the public health-care system. Yet in 2006, the Conservatives government proposed a mix of public and private health care, in which an expanded base of private providers would remain publicly funded and universally accessible. As a result, Canada has recently seen much debate about the pros and cons of shifting toward more private health care. Some argue that more private health would not threaten the public system, but rather will expand the health-care choices for those who can afford to pay for care over and above what is publicly financed. They argue the public system will be maintained and that more choice does not mean one system for the rich and one for those who cannot afford to pay extra.

Public and Private Health Insurance in the United States

The health care of most United States citizens is financed through a mix of public and private programs. The majority of citizens receive health-care benefits through private employers. Employment-based health-care coverage arose largely in the years after World War II, when many employers began to provide health-care benefits to workers in response to Federal Government wage controls.

Public funding for health care rose dramatically in 1965, when Congress established Medicare and Medicaid, through passage of the Social Security Act. The Medicare Program covered most persons aged 65 or older. The

Medicaid Program extended federally funded cash assistance programs for the indigent. Medicaid is funded jointly between the Federal and State governments. Each state administers somewhat unique Medicaid policies, although they are constrained by the general guidelines enforced by the Federal Government. Eligibility has expanded over the years (Rowland and Garfield, 2000). Congress established the State Children's Health Insurance Program (SCHIP) in 1997 to encourage States to extend Medicaid eligibility to a greater number of uninsured children (U.S. Department of Health and Human Services, 2001; Centers for Medicare & Medicaid Services, 2002).

Most of the recent proposed solutions to the problem of rising numbers of the uninsured have focused on making private insurance more affordable, rather than merely extending public coverage. Politicians and policy makers have recently proposed new mixes of public and private programs and policies, including tax credits for low-income uninsured and public funding for persons in very high-risk pools. These proposals generally modify or supplement, rather than replace, the existing private employment-based coverage. Payment for many types of health-care coverage by private employers has decreased. Employer-sponsored retiree coverage has decreased since the mid-1990s. The proportion of health-care costs paid for by private employers is likely to continue to decrease, and public coverage may not be able to cover the difference. As a result, the individual health-care consumer will share more of the burden in the form of increased co-payments and higher insurance premiums. That is, the proportion of private individual payments will increase as private employer-based payments decrease. Increases in premiums have led many individuals to drop health-care coverage entirely, contributing to increases in the numbers of uninsured.

Public policies emerge to fill in some of the gaps to private coverage, but then new private coverage policies emerge as potential solutions to the remaining gaps. For example, many significant gaps in Medicare coverage persist. One of the most important remaining gaps in Medicare is the lack of coverage for long-term care services. Thus most Medicare beneficiaries look to supplemental coverage from various public and private sources. Medicare covered 56% of personal health-care costs for its beneficiaries in 1997. Yet some personal health-care expenditures are for services not covered by Medicare such as long-term care and dental services. Even when services are paid for in part by the government, beneficiaries often must pay a portion of the costs. This co-payment requirement is also a substantial financial barrier to care for Medicare-covered services. For all these reasons, beneficiaries often are advised to seek out supplemental coverage. Beneficiaries with no supplemental coverage are much more likely to delay care due to cost compared with other beneficiaries (Shatto, 2001).

Changes in private and public health insurance, and changes in the relationship between them, are important for policy makers to understand.

Privatization of Public Health

Conventional wisdom has been that privatization is carried out when available financial resources are decreased. This rests on the assumption that decision makers believe private provision of services is cheaper if not more efficient, and that decision makers believe the cost or efficiency factor is more important than other considerations in deciding whether or not to privatize. Evaluation of the benefits and costs of public health service delivery, however, involves decisions that go far beyond short-term costs and benefits. Many public health services are oriented to prevention of disease or to preparedness for unexpected outbreaks. Such services cannot be evaluated simply in terms of simple measurements of health outcomes and costs. Moreover, although it is often touted as a way of avoiding governmental bureaucracy, the contracting out of public services often produces its own organizational complications (Sclar, 2000). Additional managerial time and resources in the form of paperwork, oversight capacity, and other transaction costs are associated with privatization (Keane *et al.*, 2001). This may explain why Rehfuss (1989) found that any costs savings due to privatization have generally been in single digit percentages. Thus there is preliminary evidence that public health privatization often does not have the conventionally expected effects on costs or efficiency. Nor is there good evidence that privatization is carried out as a response to declining resources. For example, a survey revealed that privatization of public health services in the Unites States resulted in increased time devoted to management and resulted in only modest costs savings, from the perspective of health department directors (Keane *et al.*, 2001).

Privatization of Public Health Department Services in the United States

Within the field of public health in the United States, there have been efforts to focus local health department (LHDs) on what has been considered the unique mission of public health, what the APHA in 1940 called 'desirable minimal functions' (Terris, 1949) and what since 1988 have been called core functions – assessment, assurance, and policy making – which have been further articulated into ten essential public health services. Since the 1970s, there has been an increasing emphasis in the managerial literature on the desirability of more tightly focusing organizations around their core mission. The core functions of public health represent an important managerial framework for defining the unique mission of governmental health departments (Koplin, 1990; Wall, 1998; Keane, 2005). Judging from references to the concept in publications as well as professional practice (Institute of Medicine, 1988; Baker et al., 1994), the core functions have become a central paradigm in the profession of public health. The concept of core functions directly bears on decisions to discontinue provision of services. Many believe that a critical issue confronting public health concerns the extent to which LHDs should withdraw from the direct provision of services, particularly for personal health care, in order to focus on the core functions (Wall, 1998).

Several decades ago, many LHDs in the United States began to increase their provision of personal health services, because they perceived that low-income populations did not have adequate access to such services from other providers (Wall, 1998). While some policy makers and public health officials believe that LHDs should focus exclusively on performance of core functions – assessment, assurance and policy making – and disengage from direct provision of personal health services, the vast majority of today's LHD directors use a more complex strategy in which they directly provide personal health services in when they believe the uninsured do not have adequate access to such services elsewhere.

Unfortunately, there are reasons to suspect that LHDs' capacity to provide personal health services has been eroding. Like many health-care providers, LHDs often have not received adequate funds to cover indigent care, despite increases in the numbers of uninsured. Many health-care providers, including LHDs, have become dependent on Medicaid revenues to enable them to provide care to the uninsured. Increases in Medicaid managed care, however, may have diverted Medicaid clients away from LHDs. Medicaid managed care is a privatization of the network formation aspects of Medicaid in that states contract with managed care organizations to provide care to a segment of the Medicaid population. Public health-care organizations such as LHDs are less likely to be included in managed care networks or designated as primary care providers. For these reasons, increases in Medicaid-managed care may have diverted Medicaid clients and revenues away from LHDs, a privatization of LHD Medicaid revenue. Thus, increased enrollment in Medicaid-managed care may be associated with a reduction of the ability of organizations, such as LHDs, to provide health-care services to the uninsured.

Two general types of privatization of health departments are occurring in the United States. One form of privatization occurs when a service once directly performed by an LHD is contracted out to a private provider. Another, less commonly recognized form of privatization occurs when an LHD becomes involved with a new service but contracts out (or otherwise delegates) the performance of the service from its inception.

By the end of the 1990s, more than one-half of health departments (57%) were delegating out the direct performance of at least one service that was formerly performed within the health department (Keane et al., 2001). About one-half (52%) had contracted out at least one public health service from the very inception of the service. Almost three-quarters (73%) of local health departments had privatized some public health service, whether a formerly in-house or not formerly in-house service. Indeed, most health departments have privatized more than one service, often a combination of services formerly performed in-house and services contracted out from their inception. LHDs that had privatized any given category of services were more likely to privatize services from the other service categories (Keane et al., 2001).

A total of 21% of all LHDs had discontinued provision of some personal health service. Discontinuation was defined as termination of all service provision by the LHD with no arrangement made for other providers to take over these services. Of all LHDs, 15% discontinued some HIV services, 5% discontinued some maternal and child health (MCH) services, and 5% discontinued other personal health services. Discontinuation of MCH services was significantly higher among LHDs that lost a large proportion of Medicaid clients to private providers (Keane et al., 2003).

A similar trend of privatization had occurred among public hospitals in the United States. Between 1985 and 1995, the total number of public hospitals declined by 14%. During those years, 165 public hospitals closed, and 293 public hospitals converted to private ownership, and 20 more public hospitals converted to private ownership but closed very soon afterward. This privatization of hospitals raises some of the same concerns associated with the privatization of public health departments. Even more so than health departments, public hospitals are often considered providers of last resort. For those who cannot receive health-care services elsewhere, public hospitals have served as a safety net, meaning that they generally serve the uninsured or underinsured without expectation of payment (Legnini et al., 1999). Therefore, closure and conversion of public hospitals may very well be associated with lower overall access for vulnerable populations, especially as the numbers of uninsured persons increase.

Problems and Difficulties Encountered in Mixing Private and Public

Public and private are historically viewed as two distinct domains despite numerous interconnections in operation. Thus, the main challenge is in getting these sectors together in defining a common agenda. This is particularly challenging given the fact that the basic objectives of each setup, the mandate they have, the organizational structure, the financing mechanisms, the management strategies, the nature of the employees, and the anticipation of outcomes by clients from the two sectors are different in many ways. Since harmonization of those different elements in the process of negotiation for a common agenda is needed in building a fruitful partnership; initial difficulties start from the stage of framing the policies of both sectors. Thus public–private partnerships require an attitude of transformation in policy making.

In framing the PPP, it is vital to define the ground rules of the partnership. Public–private partnership is not handing over the entire public responsibility to the private sector. It is rather a means of increasing the efficiency of the delivery of public goods and improving the sustainability of such services through a mutual arrangement of responsibilities to each party. Public and private sectors have their own strengths and weaknesses. Hence, the rationale is to utilize the optimal capabilities of each partner to produce a synergistic effect in achieving the objectives. Although privatization and public–private partnerships are two different entities, it is a prerequisite to define and frame the independent identities of the two sectors while explicitly presenting the extent of interaction of the sectors in achieving the common goal for the betterment of health of the people. Defining the responsibilities and stakes of both parties at the very beginning will help to minimize most of the problems relating to accountability, trust, and cooperation of public and other interested parties in the stage of actual operation.

In laying the policy framework and operational strategies for the partnership, the presence of a strong public sector is certainly an advantage. At the same time, the private partner needs to be involved in the decision-making process. Participatory decision making enables both parties to counterbalance each other's interests while harmonizing the power structure between the two. This provides shared responsibility for the decisions made and minimizes accountability issues in the long run. It is vital to assess the ability of the partners to sustain the commitment in the initial stages of negotiation. A regulatory process for public–private partnerships within the broader policies of the state with arbitration procedures needs to be in place. All actions in the partnership should ensure transparency and be accountable to the public. The private sector incentives and stakes in the partnership need to be explicit, as does the extent of control retained by the public sector. Legislative enactment of regulatory procedures and governance structure of the partnership will prevent any shift toward cessation of responsibilities of the public sector toward health. Such operational arrangements should alleviate most of the common problems encountered in public–private partnerships.

See also: Comparative Health Systems; Health System Organization Models (Including Targets and Goals for Health Systems).

Citations

Dewan PK, Lal SS, Lonnorth K, et al. (2006) Improving tuberculosis control through public-private collaboration in India: Literature review. *British Medical Journal* 332: 574–578.

Dongwoon H and Heejin L (2003) District health information systems in the public sector: Health centres in Korea. *Logistics Information Management* 16: 278–285.

Goody B, Mentnech R, and Riley G (2002) Changing nature of public and private health insurance. *Health Care Financing Review* 23(3): 1–7.

Hursh-Cesar G, Berman P, Hanson K, Rannan-Eliya R, and Rittmann J (1994) *Private and Nongovernment Providers: Partners for Public Health in Africa*. Conference Report, 1994, Nairobi, Kenya.

Institute of Medicine Committee for the Study for the Future of Public Health (1988) *The Future of Public Health*. Washington, DC: National Academy Press.

Jeong HS (2005) Health care reform and change in public private mix of financing: A Korean case. *Health Policy*. 74: 133–145.

Keane C (2005) The effects of managerial beliefs on service privatization and discontinuation in local health departments. *Health Care Management Review* 30(1): 52–61.

Keane C, Marx J, and Ricci E (2001) Perceived outcomes of privatization in local health departments. *Milbank Quarterly* 79(1): 115–137.

Keane C, Marx J, and Ricci E (2003) Local health departments' mission to the uninsured in the age of managed care: Results of a national survey. *Journal of Public Health Policy* 24(2): 130–149.

Legnini MW, Anthony SE, Wicks EK, Meyer JA, and Rybowski Stepnick LS (1999) *Privatization of Public Hospitals*. Washington, DC: Henry J Kaiser Family Foundation.

Rehfuss J (1989) *Contracting out in government: A guide to working with outside contractors to supply public services*. San Francisco, CA: Jossey-Bass Publishers.

Reich MR (2002) *Public-Private Partnerships for Public Health*. Cambridge, MA: Harvard University Press.

Rowland D and Garfield R (2000) Health-care for the poor: Medicaid at 35. *Health Care Financing Review* 22(1): 23–34.

Schumacher A (2006) *Health Care: Private Versus Public*. CBC News Report August 21, 2006. http://www.cbc.ca/news/background/healthcare/public_vs_private.html (accessed November 2007).

Sclar ED (2000) *You don't always get what you pay for. The economics of privatization*. Ithaca, NY: Cornell University Press.

Shatto A (2001) *The Characteristics and Perceptions of the Medicare Population. Data from the 1999 Medicare Current Benificiary Survey*. Baltimore, MD: Health Care Financing Administration.

Terris M and Kramer N (1949) Medical care activities of full-time health departments. *American Journal of Public Health* 39: 1125–1129.

U.S. Department of Health and Human Services (2001) *2001 HCFA Statistics* HCFA Pub. No. 0(3427).

Wall S (1998) Transformations in public health systems. *Health Affairs* 17: 65–89.

Relevant Websites

http://www.health-policy-systems.com/content/2/1/5 – Nishtar S, (2004) Public-private partnerships in health-a global call to action.

http://www.cbc.ca/news/background/healthcare/public_vs_private.html/ – Public vs. private health care in Canada-FAQs.

http://www.pitt.edu/~super1/lecture/lec16131/index.htm – Public-private partnerships in health: A Supercourse Lecture.

Provider Payment Methods and Incentives

R P Ellis and M M Miller, Boston University, Boston, MA, USA

© 2007 Elsevier Inc. All rights reserved.

Introduction

There are many ways that health-care providers can be paid. In India, government physicians are paid a salary and in Canada physicians are generally paid according to a government-regulated fee schedule. In the Netherlands, however, office-based physicians receive capitated payments for much of their revenue. Similar variations are seen in payments to hospitals, which may be paid using fixed budgets, detailed fee schedules, or episode-based systems. This article establishes a conceptual framework for thinking about methods of provider payment by focusing on payments to primary care doctors and to acute care hospitals. Both how payments are made and the market setting can affect the cost, quantity, and quality of care provided, so how payments affect incentives is also discussed. The section titled 'Performance-based payment systems' discusses recent payment systems that reward selected performance measures.

The focus of this article is on payments made to providers by social health insurance, private health insurance, other health plans, governments, and employers. These payments are not made by consumers, thus economists call them supply side payments. Demand side payments (often called cost sharing) are those made by consumers directly to providers. Cost sharing is discussed elsewhere in this encyclopedia. Clearly provider compensation and incentives are impacted by both supply and demand side payments, but this article focuses on supply side payments only.

There are four broad dimensions of provider payment. The first dimension is the type of information used to calculate payments. The second is the breadth of provider payment: Are doctors and hospitals paid narrowly for their own services, or are they paid broadly for bundles of related services, such as laboratory tests and other provider services? The third dimension of payment is the coarseness of the payment classification system used: Are there relatively few payment categories or are there many? The fourth dimension is the generosity of the payments: Are payments low or high? Each of these dimensions is discussed in the following sections, including how common payment systems use each element and the incentive properties of each method of payment.

Information Used for Provider Payment

Every provider payment system can be characterized by the information used to calculate provider payments. This information can be based on provider characteristics, patient characteristics, or the characteristics of the services provided. Each type of information can be conceptualized as forming a triangle, as displayed in **Figure 1**.

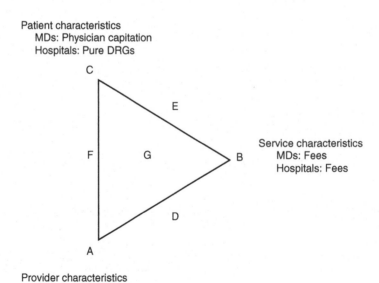

Figure 1 Three types of information available for provider payment.

Provider payments can either use information of one type as represented by the vertexes of the triangle, or payments can be based on hybrids of two or three types of information, as represented by the sides and interior of the triangle.

At one extreme, point A in **Figure 1**, payments only depend on the provider's own characteristics. For example, doctors can be paid a salary regardless of how many or which patients they see and regardless of what services they provide. These salaries may vary by provider characteristics, such as specialty, training, or experience. In many countries, including India and South Africa, public sector doctors are paid a salary. Even in the United States, doctors working for the federal Veterans' Administration and doctors in certain staff-model health maintenance organizations (HMOs) are paid a salary. Similarly, in many countries, hospitals receive 'block grants'; block grants are budgets based on hospital size or type without explicit regard to the number or type of patients seen or the services provided. Many public hospitals, including those in Spain and France, receive fixed annual budgets. Such hospital payment systems invariably adjust for variables such as the numbers of beds or population served, but these are still more correctly thought of as features of the provider and their market rather than patient or service characteristics. For a useful discussion of France's fixed budget system, see Sauvignet (2005).

Another payment system is represented by point B in **Figure 1**, in which payments are based solely on the health services provided. Fee-based and cost-based payment systems each pay providers according to the quantity of services given. Payments do not depend on who provides the services or who receives them. Under a fee system providers are paid for each service provided and hence are often called fee-for-service (FFS) payment. Fee payment systems can either allow the provider or the payer to set fee levels. Fee schedules set by the payer are the most common form of reimbursement for doctors; they are used in Canada, Germany, Norway, and the United States. Under a cost-based system, providers may be reimbursed at the end of the year for the cost of inputs (lab material, supplies, and staff salaries) regardless of how these inputs are used. In both cases, if providers use more resources to treat patients, revenues increase.

A third possibility (point C in **Figure 1**) is that provider payments are based exclusively on patient characteristics. A pure capitation system is a payment system based on patient characteristics. Under capitation, physicians receive a fixed amount of money for each patient they manage. Thus, a physician's gross income depends on the total number of people he or she cares for; the physician's income does not depend on the type of provider administering the service, the type of service being provided, or the quantity of services provided. Physician capitation payments were made during the 1990s to general practitioners in the United Kingdom and are used today in the Netherlands (Exter *et al.*, 2004). Similarly, hospitals can be paid according to a pure Diagnostic Related Grouping (DRG) payment system. Under a pure DRG payment system, a hospital receives a fixed amount determined solely by the patient's diagnostic group. Again, the hospital's revenue only depends on the patients' characteristics, not on the provider or service characteristics.

Payment systems are not limited to the three cases corresponding to points A, B, and C; providers can be compensated according to hybrids of different dimensions. Some systems are based on a hybrid of provider and service characteristics, corresponding to point D in **Figure 1**. The office physician payment system in Germany currently has features that make it appear this way. Although doctors receive FFS reimbursement, the total of all such payments is subject to a cap that varies by provider specialty. The payment caps work much like a salary, whereas the fee schedule is based on services actually provided (Busse and Riesberg, 2004). Alternatively, provider characteristics influence payments when fee schedules vary with the provider's training or specialty. For example, in the United States, a service provided by a doctor is often paid more highly than the same service provided by a nurse or other clinician. A different possibility arises when payment systems reflect not only what services are provided but also who receives them; this corresponds to point E in **Figure 1**, a payment hybrid of patient and service characteristics. For example, provider fees schedules may vary by insurance plan. In the United States, providers receive different compensation from patients with commercial insurance than from patients with Medicaid coverage. If the payment from commercial insurance exceeds the payment from Medicaid, and if a physician has enough business from commercially insured patients, then the physician has a reduced financial incentive to treat Medicaid patients. Similarly, in Germany, providers receive different compensation from patients in public versus private Sickness Funds. Finally, hybrids corresponding to point F in **Figure 1** are also possible, in which some compensation is based on both provider and patient characteristics.

Over the past two decades, payment mechanisms that combine provider, service, and patient characteristics have been developed. Payment systems combining all three of these dimensions are represented by point G in **Figure 1**. An example is the DRG payment system adopted in many countries, including the United States. In 1983, the U.S. Medicare program began using DRGs to standardize payments and help to control hospital costs. Although many adjustments were made, DRG payments are fixed prices per admission, with the payments reflecting patient characteristics (their diagnoses and age), health services provided (procedure codes), and provider characteristics (type of hospital). Australia, Germany, and several other countries have customized DRGs to their own needs.

Breadth of the Payment System

Separate from the issue of the information used to determine the payment system is the issue of how broadly or narrowly provider services are aggregated (**Figure 2**). Under a narrow system, doctors are paid explicitly for each procedure provided and separate payments are made for each laboratory test or procedure done by other providers. A broader payment system might bundle jointly performed procedures into one fee. A system might broaden even further to include associated fees for laboratory services. A still broader system might make payments to a doctor that include the cost of specialists, forcing the doctor to internalize the cost of all physician services.

Similar issues of the breadth of the provider payment system arise with hospital payment. Hospital DRG or per diem rates can narrowly cover only the room and board cost, or may include nursing services. Even more broadly, they may include hospital physician services. In the United States, certain DRG payments have even been broadened to include the cost of services provided after discharge. In some countries hospitals are even given responsibility for certain kinds of primary care services.

	Narrow ⟵		⟶ Broad
MDs:	Own time	Lab tests	Other specialists
Hospitals:	Room and board	MD inpatient services	Related outpatient services

Figure 2 Breadth of provider payment ('bundling').

This breadth of payments is often discussed in terms of 'bundling' of services. Recent trends in the United States have been toward increased bundling of payments. Similar innovations are being tried in many other countries.

Fineness of the Payment System

How many payment categories should be used? Should there be many gradations in payment (a 'fine' system), or is a simpler ('coarse') system appropriate (**Figure 3**)? In countries such as Taiwan and Korea, physician fee schedules are fairly coarse, with very few fee categories, while physician fee schedules in Australia and the United States are very fine, with many gradations in fee levels. In 2004, Germany reduced the fineness of its fee system.

Similar issues of coarseness and fineness arise with DRGs, capitation, and physician salaries. In the United States and many other countries, the DRG and capitation systems have become finer and finer, with increased distinctions made in payments. Coarse or fine gradations in payments are possible with each payment system.

The optimal fineness of the payment system reflects a trade-off between the potentially improved fairness and reduced selection incentives resulting from a fine system and the challenges of monitoring and administering a fine system. Coarser systems should in principle be easier to monitor. If the payer cannot easily distinguish what service was actually provided, or the patient characteristics are not readily observable, then it may not be worthwhile to make such distinctions for payment.

Generosity of Payments

Not only is the unit of payment important, but so is the overall generosity or level of payment. Empirical research

	Coarse ⟵	⟶ Fine
MDs:	Fixed fee per office visit	Fees vary by treatment intensity or duration
	Uniform salary per MD	Salaries adjusted by specialty or age
	Capitation using age/gender	Capitation using age, gender, diagnoses
Hospitals:	Simple per diem rate	Per diem varies by patient, department or service
	100 DRGs	800 DRGs

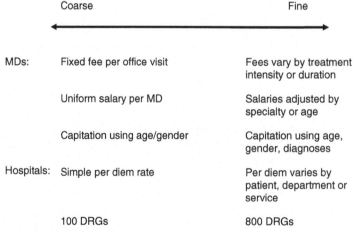

Figure 3 Fineness of provider payment (number of payment categories).

shows that relative prices as well as their levels matter. If payment levels to providers are set too low, this reduces the incentive for quality for almost any payment system. (This is discussed further in the section titled 'Incentives.')

Markets, Provider Competition, and the Delivery Structure

By defining what services, patients, and providers are eligible for payment, a provider payment system also inherently defines the degree of competitiveness in the market as well as the market boundaries. If the physician payments restrict which patients or services a doctor will be reimbursed for treating, this has important implications for incentives. Similarly, incentives are affected if some but not all hospitals receive DRG payments. A careful summary of all of the different ways of organizing health-care delivery markets lies well beyond the scope of this article; however, a brief discussion of delivery structure is important in determining incentives, costs, and outcomes.

Incentives

The previously discussed dimensions – the type of information used, the breadth, the fineness (or courseness), and the level of payments, as well as the market structure – all influence the incentives facing providers. Economists spend a great deal of time studying provider incentives because they generally believe the empirical evidence that providers respond to these incentives. This section describes the incentive effects of different payment systems commonly used around the world.

Incentives Created by Salaries and Fixed Budgets

Perhaps the easiest incentives to describe are those of salaried or fixed payment systems, where only provider information is used to calculate payments. Because revenues are fixed regardless of the volume of care rendered, physicians and hospitals have a financial incentive to inappropriately keep costs and costly effort at levels that are too low. Fixed revenues can also motivate physicians and hospitals to preferentially treat low-risk patients, to try to avoid high-cost patients, to make too many referrals, to minimize the number or intensity of services provided, and in general to underprovide quality. The one countervailing force is the possible threat to lose one's job, but countries that rely on salaried payments rarely fire salaried employees. Peer review and payer monitoring may also be effective at promoting quality. Payments based solely on provider characteristics do not tend to reward coordination of care across providers. Salaried or fixed hospital budget systems rely on provider altruism to ensure that appropriate and high-quality services are provided. However, if providers realize cost savings from preventive care, these payment systems may encourage providers to engage in preventive efforts.

Incentives Created by Fee-for-Service

The incentives of fee-based payments are very different from those of salaried or capitated payments. Newhouse (2002) carefully summarizes the conventional economists' and policymakers' views that FFS payment mechanisms create poor incentives for controlling cost or quantity. Fee-for-service rewards physicians with more revenue for rendering more services, whether these services improve the health or well-being of the patient. Under FFS reimbursement, services that have little or no value to the consumer may be provided merely because they increase provider net income. Overprovision is likely to be a problem if the fee for a particular service is more than the incremental cost of that service to the provider. Carrin and Hanvoravongchai (2003) mention several instances in which FFS payment systems caused the overprovision of services and thus caused a country's health-care costs to rise. For example, in 1987, when general practitioners in Copenhagen began to receive fees for some services, the provision of those services increased significantly. However, with fee-for-service, underprovision may occur if fees are too low relative to costs. For similar reasons, services not reimbursed through fees, such as preventative care counseling to the consumer (e.g., trying to change a patient's lifestyle or institute a smoking cessation program) receive little or no physician effort. Competition and consumer information also affect incentives of fee-based payments.

Incentives Created by Pure DRGs and Capitation

Under pure DRGs, hospitals have a financial incentive to discharge a patient early since they will not be reimbursed for the additional costs they incur on behalf of the patient. If payments are relatively generous, then hospitals may compete to attract more patients. However, hospitals may discourage patients with less generous payments. DRGs also create incentives to play the system for their own benefit; providers may 'upcode,' or classify patients into a higher DRG category, in order to receive a higher payment.

Capitation payments give physicians a fixed amount of money per patient, which creates a financial incentive to reduce costs per patient. Rather than necessarily managing care, capitation may instead result in providers competing to attract or select low-risk patients, using referrals, or providing preventative care. Here, how competition is regulated will clearly matter. Capitation creates an incentive to potentially use low-cost providers, increase outpatient services, reduce hospital admissions, and reduce days per admission. In addition, capitation creates incentives for the recipient of the capitated payment to increase the use of lower-cost alternative providers such as nurse practitioners and physician assistants, rather than physicians.

Incentives Created by Mixed Payment Systems

An alternative to pure DRGs and capitated payments is the mixed payment system originally developed in Ellis and McGuire (1986). Under Ellis and McGuire's payment system, hospital payments are based on both diagnoses and the level of services provided. The great attraction of a mixed payment system is that it can reward services somewhat, but not as excessively as a FFS payment. Partially using patient-based payments can reward providers for treating higher-risk patients and overcome provider incentives to select only the most profitable, easier-to-treat patients. The Netherlands has implemented a form of the Ellis and McGuire mixed payment system in that office-based doctors are paid partially on a fee basis and partially by capitation (Exter *et al.*, 2004).

Incentives and Fineness

The fineness of the payment system also affects provider incentives. A finer payment system tends to reduce cost variation within a payment category. This tends to create fewer incentives to select low-cost patients. However, with more classifications, there are greater monitoring problems and more incentives to play the system for their own benefit. Providers may upcode patients into a higher payment category to receive a larger compensation. In the literature, this is often referred to as 'DRG creep' when referring to hospitals and 'code inflation' when referring to procedure codes. Finer systems will tend to be more difficult to monitor since more patients will be near the margin in which upcoding can make a difference.

How coarseness/fineness and breadth/narrowness affect incentives is particularly apparent when payments go from physician fee schedules to DRG payments. This was illustrated in Korea when inpatient physicians switched from a relatively fine and narrow payment formula to a coarse and broad system. Until 1997, under the national health insurance program, a FFS payment system had been in place for approximately 20 years. The FFS payment system had led to a high volume of relatively low-intensity health care, characterized by frequent but short visits and hospital stays. Under the FFS system, inpatient physicians had financial incentives to choose treatments with greater profits, and hence extensively used medical supplies and pharmaceuticals and avoided hospitalizations. In 1997, in hopes of controlling quantity and selection, a DRG pilot program was introduced for voluntarily participating providers. By its third year, the pilot program covered nine disease categories with 25 DRG codes that depended on the severity of illness and age of the patient. The program began with disease groups that had low-expenditure variation, little disagreement among providers on treatment methods, low degree of uncertainty about treatment outcomes, high frequency of use, and lower possibility of DRG creep. Within each of these DRGs, patients were classified into three groups based on their length of stay: normal, outlier below a lower limit, and outlier above an upper limit. The pilot program succeeded in lowering expenditure on medical care, reducing length of stay, and reducing the use of antibiotics. Early evidence suggests that the program did not have a negative effect on the quality of care as measured by complications and reoperations (Kwon, 2003).

The effects of incentives were also demonstrated when the National Health Insurance was established in Taiwan in 1995. At this time, Taiwan switched from paying office-based doctors a salary to paying them according to a FFS schedule. Under FFS, a relatively coarse system of payment is used, based on a national fee schedule. The switch from salary to FFS was accompanied by an increase in the volume of services with shortened average visit length. According to one source, this led to misdiagnosis, improper treatment, and delays; the government responded by changing the fee structure so as to try to limit the number of patients each provider can treat during a given day (Cheng, 2003).

The U.S. Medicare system compensates providers according to a payment system that is finer (has more payment categories) than the systems in Korea and Taiwan. Under the U.S. Medicare system, hospitals receive a prospectively determined price depending on the patient's DRG. In 2006, the U.S. Medicare system had 559 DRGs. As mentioned above, providers have a financial incentive to select the most profitable patients within one DRG group. Even with numerous DRGs, Dranove (1987) discusses the large differences in costs that occur within one DRG in the U.S. Medicare system. In three Chicago-area hospitals Dranove (1987) finds that one-sixth of the DRGs have a standard deviation that exceeds the mean. Large differences in the cost of treating patients classified in one DRG encourage hospitals to prefer treating less costly patients within a DRG. Thus, Dranove concludes that a finer payment system is needed to avoid selection. One might worry that a finer U.S. Medicare system would create more incentives to upcode patients. The classic study of this phenomenon in the United States by Carter *et al.* (1990) found that upcoding or DRG creep accounted for less than one-third of the change in Medicare's Case Mix Index between 1986 and 1987.

Australia also uses a fine payment system to fund its public hospitals; the Australian National Diagnostic Related

Groups has 667 categories (Hilless and Healy, 2001). In January 2004, Germany implemented a fine DRG system to compensate hospitals. The German DRGs take the diagnosis, severity, patient's age, and the intervention performed into account. In 2005, there were 878 DRGs in Germany. Because the payment systems in Australia and Germany are relatively fine, on the one hand, there are fewer opportunities for providers to select low-cost patients. On the other, there are more opportunities for providers to upcode patients so as to increase payments.

Performance-Based Payment Systems

In recent years there has been a great deal of interest in payment systems that reward performance. For example, doctors may receive bonuses based on performance targets, such as high immunization rates, or low surgical complication rates. Other payment systems reward providers according to how well they perform relative to their peers on various cost or quality measures. In the United States, this has come to be called 'pay for performance,' often abbreviated P4P. P4P payment systems are commonly used by HMOs (Rosenthal et al., 2006). P4P systems calculate payments on patient characteristics, for broad sets of providers, using potentially fine (not coarse) distinctions among patient types.

There is mixed evidence on the impact of these performance-based payment systems. A recent study by Rosenthal et al. (2005) and a review by Dudley and Rosenthal (2006) provide up-to-date discussions of the challenges in the United States because of using P4P. Large demonstrations that are in progress in the United States and UK will also shed light on this new initiative.

There are many forms of P4P systems. Typically, primary care physicians are grouped into risk pools that share financial rewards and penalties; the size of the risk pool will influence a physician's responsiveness to incentives. Sometimes bonuses are shared among a large pool of physicians; in other cases, individual physicians are eligible for incentive payments. The size of the risk pool affects the intensity of incentives as well as the financial risk borne by providers.

Performance-based payment attempts to overcome the problem whereby doctors who provide inadequate care receive the same compensation as doctors who provide excellent care. Proponents of these systems argue that instead of paying doctors according to their characteristics, their patients' characteristics, or the type of service they provide, physicians should be paid according to their performance. Many believe that physicians will respond to performance incentives by providing higher-quality care.

For some medical conditions, such as diabetes and asthma, there are easily recognizable quality measures that gauge provider performance. For example, if bonuses are allocated to providers who track diabetics' blood sugar levels, then doctors will be more likely to have diabetic patients' blood sugar monitored. Similarly, asthmatic patients will receive high-quality treatment if physicians are given bonuses for prescribing the correct asthma medication. Performance-based payment can encourage providers to give high-quality care to patients with these two conditions.

However, there are challenges to performance-based payment systems. First, opponents argue that these programs increase selection. Because physician ratings are based on claims data, their ratings may not fully reflect a patient's risk factors. If so, bonuses create incentives for doctors to drop risky patients within a payment category. Many doctors oppose performance-based payment systems because their payments rely too heavily on their patients' risk factors as well as their patients' actions (e.g., whether their patients take their prescription or return for a follow-up appointment). Another concern is that only a relatively small number of performance measures are typically used. Incentives that do well on these measures may not carry over to other actions that are not measured or rewarded.

One widely cited study examined doctors who were offered bonuses if they complied with basic public health guidelines, including guidelines on preventative care. In 2003, California doctors were evaluated according to levels of breast cancer screening, cervical cancer screening, and hemoglobin testing. The top-rated doctors split a bonus pool of $3.4 million. Compared to doctors in Oregon and Washington who were not offered bonuses, California doctors offered more cervical cancer screening. Although the quality of care increased in all three areas, only for cervical cancer screening was the improvement greater in California than in Oregon and Washington; this may have been because the financial rewards to quality were too low or because substantial quality improvements take time. Physician groups whose performance was initially the lowest improved the most, whereas physician groups who had previously achieved the targeted level of performance improved the least (Rosenthal et al., 2005).

Bokhour et al. (2006) investigated the impact of P4P systems implemented in Massachusetts. This qualitative study interviewed 28 practice executives who noted that physicians viewed quality incentives as more aligned with their natural tendency to provide good quality of care. The study revealed that physicians appear to be motivated more by professional standards of quality than financial incentives.

P4P measures have also been introduced in other countries. Since 1990, general practitioners in the United Kingdom have commonly been paid according to targets. Initially, narrowly defined P4P target payments remunerated general practitioners if they delivered a minimum predetermined level of services or care. Kouides et al.

(1998) found that immunization rates rose 5.9% compared to a control group when PCPs received an additional 10% or 20% payment per shot for each immunization made over target rates. Ritchie *et al.* (1992) studied the effects of a lump sum payment received if a PCP immunized 70% of the eligible preschool population. However, according to their study, the target payment intervention did not have a significant impact on immunization rates. In 2004, the UK introduced a large P4P contract for family practitioners. This P4P payment system was much wider, with 146 quality indicators covering clinical care for 10 chronic diseases, organization of care, and patient experience. The National Health Service committed £1.8 billion ($3.2 billion) in additional funds for a three-year period; the program was intended to increase family practitioners' income by up to 25%. After the first year, the median reported achievement was 83.4% (Doran *et al.*, 2006).

In Haiti, nongovernment organizations (NGOs) provide basic health-care services including immunizations and prenatal care. Historically, these organizations were fully compensated for all their costs; therefore, they were not accountable for performance. In 1999, providers began operating under a performance-based payment system. Under this new system, a portion of each NGO's historical budget was withheld. Physicians could earn back the amount withheld plus a bonus if they met specific targets including a targeted 10% increase in child vaccinations. After the first year, the most striking result was the increase in immunization coverage in the NGO service areas. The doctors said that the shift in payment structure inspired them to question their model of service delivery; the possibility of earning bonuses sharpened their focus to achieving goals (Eichler *et al.*, 2001).

In 1998, the Cambodian government began an experiment that provided additional financial incentives for some health-care workers based on performance. Historically in Cambodia, government health-care providers received insufficient and irregular salaries, forcing them to seek alternative sources of income. Since this insufficient payment did not depend on performance, health facilities in Cambodia performed poorly. As detailed by Soeters and Griffiths (2003), after three years of implementation, when combined with monitoring, P4P improved use of health services and decreased total family health expenditure.

Similarly, a new output-based payment system was implemented in the Kabutare district of Rwanda in 2003. Before the introduction of the performance initiative, staff members received a fixed bonus in addition to their salaries. Under the new payment system, individuals kept their base salaries but an output-based remuneration replaced the fixed-bonus system. Meessen *et al.* (2007) found that productivity sharply increased between 2001 and 2003; average individual productivity increased by 53% under the new system.

There is evidence that performance payments need to be carefully designed and meaningful to have an impact. Hillman *et al.* (1998) could not reject that small financial bonuses did not affect compliance with cancer screening guidelines for a group of Medicaid physicians in Philadelphia. The authors attribute the insignificant result to the lack of awareness of the payments among physicians and to the difficulty of affecting treatment protocols when physicians have multiple payers.

At present the evidence is mixed on the effectiveness of P4P on quality and quantity of care. The theoretical and empirical research literature has not kept up with recent innovations, and many innovations are still being implemented that have not yet been validated or the incentives modeled. This remains an area promising possibly dramatic advances and worthy of significant new research.

Trends for the Future

This article shows that provider payment systems vary in a number of dimensions, all of which deserve consideration when considering reforms or study. Incentives created by provider payment vary according to each of these dimensions. Market characteristics, including provider competition, also influence incentives and outcomes in provider markets.

Other authors have noted recent trends in provider payment systems. Many countries have moved away from salary and fixed budget systems, which only reflect provider characteristics, and toward service- and patient-based payment systems. Because FFS payments may lead to the overprovision of services, sophisticated payers are using capitation or blends of different information so as to control costs.

Many countries are making their payment formulas finer, with more gradations of payment categories, and broader, with payments being made to few providers, who are in turn asked to manage or monitor other providers more carefully than an independent payer is able to. Trends toward P4P, with finely defined categories of information and broadly inclusive payments, reflect the latest movement toward patient-based payments. Whereas the evidence is mixed about whether P4P will ultimately be widely adopted, the desire to create incentives for cost-effective, high-quality accessible care suggests that elements of this approach will remain part of the provider payment strategy in the future.

Citations

Bokhour BG, Burgess JF, Jr., Hook JM, *et al.* (2006) Incentive implementation in physician practices: A qualitative study of practice executive perspectives on pay for performance. *Medical Care Research and Review* 63(supplement 1): 73S–95S.

Busse R and Riesberg A (2004) *Health Care Systems in Transition: Germany.* Copenhagen, Denmark: European Observatory of Health Care Systems.

Carrin G and Hanvoravongchai P (2003) Provider payments and patient charges as policy tools for cost containment: How successful are they in high-income countries? *Human Resources for Health* 1(6): 1–20.

Carter G, Newhouse J, and Relles D (1990) How much change in the case mix index is DRG creep? *Journal of Health Economics* 9: 411–428.

Cheng T (2003) Taiwan's new National Health Insurance program: Genesis and experience so far. *Health Affairs* 22: 61–76.

Doran T, Fullwood C, Gravelle H, et al. (2006) Pay-for-performance programs in family practices in the United Kingdom. *New England Journal of Medicine* 355: 375–384.

Dranove D (1987) Rate-setting by diagnosis related groups and hospital specialization. *RAND Journal of Economics* 18(3): 417–427.

Dudley RA and Rosenthal MB (2006) Pay for performance: A decision guide for purchasers. *Report Prepared for the Agency for Healthcare Research and Quality, U.S.Department of Health and Human Services* Contract No./Assignment No. 290-01 -0001/298 AHRQ. Publication No. 06-0047, April.

Eichler R, Auxila P, and Pollock J (2001) Promoting preventive health care: Paying for performance in Haiti. In: Brook PJ and Smith SM (eds.) *Contracting for Public Services: Output-Based Aid and Its Applications*, pp. 65–71. Amsterdam, the Netherlands: World Bank Publications.

Ellis RP and McGuire TG (1986) Provider behavior under prospective reimbursement: Cost sharing and supply. *Journal of Health Economics* 5: 129–152.

Exter A, Hermans H, Dosljak M, and Busse R (2004) *Health Care Systems in Transition: Netherlands.* Copenhagen, Denmark: WHO Regional Office for Europe on behalf of the European Observatory of Health Care Systems.

Hilless M and Healy J (2001) *Health Care Systems in Transition: Australia.* Copenhagen, Denmark: European Observatory of Health Care Systems.

Hillman AL, Ripley K, Goldfarb N, Nuamah I, Weiner J, and Lusk E (1998) Physician financial incentives and feedback: Failure to increase cancer screening in Medicaid managed care. *American Journal of Public Health* 88(11): 1699–1701.

Kouides RW, Bennett NM, Lewis B, et al. (1998) Performance-based physician reimbursement and influenza immunization rates in the elderly. *American Journal of Preventive Medicine* 14: 89–95.

Kwon S (2003) Payment system reform for health care providers in Korea. *Health Policy and Planning* 18(1): 84–92.

Meessen B, Kashala JPI, and Musango L (2007) Output-based payment to boost public health centers: Contracting in Kabutare district, Rwanda. *Bulletin of the World Health Organization* 85: 108–115.

Newhouse JP (2002) *Pricing the Priceless: A Health Care Conundrum.* Cambridge, MA: MIT Press.

Ritchie LD, Bisset AF, Russell D, Leslie V, and Thomson I (1992) Primary preschool immunization in Grampian: Progress and the 1990 contract. *British Medical Journal* 304(6830): 816–819.

Rosenthal MB, Frank RG, Li Z, and Epstein AM (2005) Early evidence with pay-for-performance: From concept to practice. *Journal of American Medical Association* 294: 1788–1793.

Rosenthal MB, Landon BE, Normand S-L T, Frank RG, and Epstein AM (2006) Pay for performance in commercial HMOs. *New England Journal of Medicine* 355: 1895–1902.

Sauvignet E (2005) *Le Financement du système de santé en France.* WHO/EIP/HSF Discussion Paper, No. 1, pp. 75–80.

Soeters R and Griffiths F (2003) Improving government health services through contract management: A case from Cambodia. *Health Policy and Planning* 18: 74–83.

Further Reading

Carrin G and Hanvoravongchai P (2003) Provider payments and patient charges as policy tools for cost containment: How successful are they in high-income countries? *Human Resources for Health* 1(6): 1–20.

Jegers M, Kesteloot K, De Graeve D, and Gilles W (2002) A typology for provider payment systems in health care. *Health Policy* 60: 255–273.

McGuire TG (2000) Physician agency. In: Culyer AJ and Newhouse JP (eds.) *Handbook of Health Economics*, pp. 461–536. North-Holland, the Netherlands: Elsevier.

Managed Care

S Glied and K Janus, Columbia University, New York, NY, USA

© 2008 Elsevier Inc. All rights reserved.

Introduction

Managed care has become an increasingly popular strategy for organizing the delivery of health-care services. Despite the regularity with which the term is used, there is no single accepted definition of managed care. Managed care may refer to a diverse array of arrangements, from those in which insurance and service delivery are fully integrated, such as staff and group model health maintenance organizations (HMOs); to those in which insured people are restricted to a defined set of providers, such as independent practice associations (IPAs); to arrangements in which the choice of providers is unrestricted but insurers provide incentives to use selected providers and monitor the care provided, such as preferred provider organizations (PPOs) that conduct utilization review (UR) of costly services. The term managed care is also used to describe management tools, such as utilization review or disease management, whether or not these tools are being used by managed care organizations.

Managed care is often thought of as a U.S. institution, operating in the private, voluntary insurance market and associated with the delivery of personal health-care services. Since the early 1990s, however, several countries, including Great Britain, the Netherlands, Germany, Israel, France, and several Latin American countries have formally incorporated elements of managed care into their health systems. Other countries are contemplating such changes.

Finally, managed care tools, although primarily associated with the delivery of personal health-care services, draw heavily on public health concepts. Managed care plans both finance care and attempt to manage the health (and expenditures) of their enrolled populations, unlike conventional insurers, which principally finance the care of individual patients. Managed care plans make use of epidemiology, prevention research, and cost-effectiveness analysis to achieve these population-oriented ends.

Elements of Managed Care

Managed care plans include a range of distinctive elements. Plans combine and modify these elements over time and across settings.

Provider Selection and Organization

Conventional insurers do not contract with specific health-care providers. Rather, they reimburse enrollees for care provided by any provider, often based on usual and customary payment rates. By contrast, most managed care plans do contract with a network of providers. Several of the earliest managed care plans were almost fully vertically integrated organizations, in which a limited number of hospitals and physicians were employees of organizations that took on insurance risk. These plans are often referred to as 'staff model' HMOs. Closely related to these plans are those (often referred to as 'group model' HMOs) in which a fixed group of physicians (and sometimes hospitals) contracts exclusively with an organization that takes on insurance risk. Most group and staff model HMOs are not-for-profit.

Several HMOs that use staff and group model approaches have recently been established in Switzerland. Germany and the region of Catalonia in Spain are experimenting with physician networks and integrated delivery approaches that follow this type of HMO model. Most U.S. plans today contract with independent providers, who may hold contracts with many managed care organizations and may also treat patients who hold conventional insurance. The most common form of this type of managed care is the PPO, in which plans negotiate discounted rates with a defined panel of providers and also permit members to seek care outside the network (though at higher coinsurance). Some European countries are considering the implementation of PPOs, but most plan to begin with the introduction of fully integrated delivery systems after experimenting with managed care tools in their traditional health-care systems.

Managed care plans have the opportunity to select the physicians, nonphysician providers, hospitals, and pharmaceuticals included in the plan. In principle, they make this selection by choosing the highest quality and lowest cost providers. There is only limited research examining the characteristics of providers who are selected into plans. In the United States, participating physicians are more likely to be board-certified than the national average; they may also have low-cost practice styles.

Paying Providers

Because managed care plans contract with providers, they can use a wider range of payment methods than can conventional plans. Plans may pay physician providers using salaries, fee-for-service, and capitation. They may pay hospitals using case rates, such as diagnosis-related groups, or *per diem* rates. Plans may also combine these mechanisms, as well as bonuses, including payment for performance, withholds for excessive service use, and other incentives, into tailored incentive schemes.

In fully vertically integrated plans, physicians are often paid using salaries. Many managed care plans pay physicians on a (discounted) fee-for-service basis. Denmark and the Netherlands use a mix of fee-for-service and capitation in their health-care systems.

Under capitation payment, providers receive a fixed periodic payment for each patient they enroll. They can earn more if they enroll more patients, as long as the capitation fee exceeds expected costs. If capitation payments are driven too low, physicians may refuse to enroll patients under capitated contracts, forcing a return to other payment forms.

Capitation arrangements vary according to the scope of services covered within the capitation contract. Under broad capitation arrangements, providers may also be financially responsible for the costs of services obtained through referral or hospitalization. If the scope of services is very narrow, providers paid a capitation fee have incentives to refer patients to other providers whose services fall outside the capitation fee. In consequence, capitation contracts with narrow service coverage often incorporate additional mechanisms to restrict referrals.

Plans can also combine these payment mechanisms. For example, plans may pay fee-for-service rates but withhold a portion of the payment if use exceeds a predetermined level. A recent trend in physician reimbursement is the use of pay-for-performance, which can be seen as a combination of a capitation base payment and fee-for-service payments tied to the achievement of agreed objectives. In these arrangements total reimbursement depends on the achievement of specific performance measures (clinical measures, patient satisfaction, and information technology implementation).

Pay for performance methods have garnered considerable interest outside the United States. Israel plans to make physicians accountable for quality of care and is contemplating putting physicians at financial risk for the health-care expenditures they generate. The UK introduced pay-for-performance for physicians in 2004. Family practitioners entered into contracts with the government that will provide additional payments for high-quality care.

Monitoring Service Utilization

Managed care plans may place limits on what providers can do. Through monitoring service use, plans can reduce the cost of care and may also improve (or reduce) the quality of care. The strategies used by plans may incorporate payment incentives, feedback mechanisms, and support services.

One way to monitor service utilization is through the use of 'gatekeeper' arrangements. Under these arrangements, enrollees can only use specialty services if they obtain a referral from a specified primary care physician or other designated referral source. Under gatekeeper arrangements, primary care doctors can be held responsible for the level of specialist use of their enrollees.

Gatekeeping has been applied in various countries (e.g., Germany and the Scandinavian countries); however, studies that evaluate its impact are rare and variable, particularly because of the heterogeneity of gatekeeping approaches. Some evidence suggests that health-care expenditures increased more slowly in countries with gatekeeping systems. In Switzerland studies have shown a decrease in costs by 7% to 20% as a result of gatekeeping.

Most managed care plans also monitor service utilization directly. Plans may refuse to pay for services unless authorization is obtained in advance. They may also monitor resources concurrent with use or retrospectively. Research suggests that UR may reduce hospital expenses by about 7% to 10% although the results are not unequivocal. Except as an element of gatekeeping, UR is not used widely outside the United States.

Many managed care plans use case management, especially for high-cost cases. Case management may involve using support services to ensure that medical care is delivered to patients in the least costly way. Case management may also use support services to improve the quality of care provided to patients. There is little evidence demonstrating the effectiveness of case management in reducing costs, although some evidence, including studies in both the United States and Europe, suggests that it may improve health-care quality in selected situations. A more recent innovation is disease management, in which the care of patients with a specific set of diseases is managed by a separate team. Disease management is an increasingly popular element of U.S. health insurance plans and has been introduced in Germany, the UK, and Switzerland. To date, there are few rigorous studies evaluating the effectiveness of disease management. Some evidence supports its role in the care of patients with type 2 diabetes.

Quality Monitoring

The emphasis in managed care plans on limiting unnecessary care through selective contracting, utilization management, and payment incentives, generated concerns that managed care undermined the quality of medical care. Plans, seeking to gain members, wanted to disprove this contention. At the same time, the ability of plans to measure outcomes within a defined population made it easier to assess the quality of care provided.

These developments generated a movement toward quality measurement. The U.S. National Committee for Quality Assurance (NCQA), a private not-for-profit organization, began accrediting managed care organizations in 1991. NCQA requires accredited plans to undergo rigorous evaluation and, beginning in 1992, to measure outcomes according to a standard based on the Health Plan Employer Data Information Set (HEDIS). The over 60 HEDIS measures include both clinical outcomes and patient satisfaction. NCQA and other organizations continue to refine quality measures, which are essential components in pay-for-performance initiatives.

Preventive Health-Care Benefits

Managed care plan contracts in the United States are more likely than other types of private insurance plans to cover preventive and maternity services. In all contexts, managed care plans tend to place a heavy emphasis on prevention. Managed care plans benefit from keeping their beneficiaries healthy as overall health-care costs to the plan may be reduced. Unfortunately, whereas many preventive health-care services are cost-effective, relatively few reduce medical care costs for the plan (at least in the short term). Moreover, plan members can, and often do, change plans well before the benefit of preventive interventions would be realized. Even if these benefits do not save money for managed care plans, offering generous preventive benefits may improve the health of their covered populations, helping them to attract additional members. Moreover, generous preventive care benefits may, themselves, be especially attractive to healthier than average populations.

Special Cases: Behavioral Managed Care and Pharmaceutical Benefits Management

Managed care principles have proven especially effective in the delivery of specific types of health care. For example, managed care arrangements have been used for the provision of disease-specific care and pharmaceutical benefits.

The most important of these 'carve-out' models of managed care is the managed behavioral health-care plan. Employers, governments, and some general managed care plans often contract with a separate behavioral health-care plan to provide management of behavioral health (mental health and substance abuse treatment) services to their enrolled populations. Behavioral health carve-out plans have several advantages over traditional indemnity insurers and general managed care plans. First, these plans contract with a specialized group of providers, who are generally quite distinct from general health providers. Specialized plans can develop expertise in the selection and monitoring of these providers. Second, this same specialized expertise makes behavioral health carve-out plans adept at monitoring mental health and substance abuse treatment. Indeed, utilization management has had its largest effects in this sector. Finally, contracting all behavioral health services to a single carve-out plan avoids problems of selection that often plague the delivery of mental health benefits in competitive insurance markets. Behavioral health conditions tend to be chronic and costly, leading to substantial self-selection into plans with generous benefits. In the absence of a specialized carve-out plan, general health insurers tend to avoid covering behavioral health services at all. The carve-out arrangement permits purchasers to maintain generous behavioral health benefits, while offering a choice of general health plans to the enrolled population.

Behavioral managed care has led to substantial reductions on spending for the combination of mental and general health care. In the absence of care management, most private insurers required much higher copayment rates and placed many more limitations on services for behavioral health than for general health care. Managed behavioral health plans have been able to constrain mental health spending while reducing copayment rates to parity with general health services.

The rise of behavioral managed care, however, also illustrates some of the problems that may occur in an environment where a plan is paid a fixed amount to care for an enrolled population. Capitated plans have an incentive to shift costs to other providers. In the case of behavioral managed care, plans are responsible for providing behavioral health services, but do not pay for any prescribed medications or for behavioral health-care services delivered through general health plans. This bifurcation of responsibility encourages behavioral health plans to promote the use of medication, rather than psychotherapeutic, management of behavioral health conditions. This cost-shift dampens (although it does not eliminate) the effect of managed behavioral health organizations on overall health-care spending. It also encourages general health plans to limit the provision of behavioral health services in general health care.

Pharmacy benefits management is a second common type of specialized managed care. General health plans and purchasers (including the U.S. Medicare program) contract with pharmacy benefits management firms to control the costs of prescription pharmaceuticals covered under insurance. Pharmacy benefits managers develop formulary lists, negotiate prices with drug companies, provide incentives to patients to choose less costly drugs (such as formularies with copayment rates that vary by drug cost category), monitor drug use directly, and work to educate physicians about the benefits of generic drug use ('counter-detailing'). Whereas pharmacy benefits management appears to lower the cost of drugs, some advocates have expressed concern that they limit access to necessary medications. Just recently, pharmaceutical benefit companies have expanded their scope of services to include disease management and other less drug-related and more health management–related services.

History of Managed Care

Managed care has a long history. The earliest mention of arrangements in which individuals (often employers) contracted with a number of physicians to provide services for a preset fee to a defined population dates back to 1849. The Kaiser Health plan, and other large prepaid group practices, emerged in the 1930s. For many years, the plans faced considerable opposition from organized medicine.

The United States

The federal government became interested in managed care in the late 1960s and, in 1973, the U.S. government passed the HMO Act, which provided incentives for HMO growth. Between 1970 and 1975, the number of HMOs increased from 37 to 183 and HMO membership doubled, though from a very low base.

In 1982, California relaxed laws that limited the ability of health plans to selectively contract with a subset of providers. This led to the emergence of PPOs and between 1981 and 1984, 15 other states passed laws encouraging the growth of PPOs. Almost immediately, growth in PPO plans escalated rapidly. By the late 1990s, about 85% of those receiving employment-based health insurance benefits were enrolled in managed care. Most were enrolled in PPOs and similar open-access plans, not in traditional HMOs with highly restrictive provider access. In 2005, a total of about 68 million Americans were enrolled in HMOs and 108 million were enrolled in PPO-type products.

Managed care has also grown in the U.S. public sector. Medicare permitted enrollment in HMOs from its inception, but plans had few incentives to participate. In 1983, only 1.5% of Medicare beneficiaries belonged to HMOs. From 1982 on, changes in Medicare legislation made managed care participation somewhat more attractive to Medicare beneficiaries, so that by 1990, 5.4% of Medicare beneficiaries belonged to HMOs. Further legislative action, and rising premiums for supplementary insurance, made managed care a more attractive option for Medicare beneficiaries during the 1990s. By 1996, one in eight Medicare beneficiaries belonged to a managed care plan. In 2005, 14% of Medicare enrollees belonged to HMOs.

Under Medicaid, a joint state-federal program, states have always been permitted to contract with managed care plans that could provide services to those who voluntarily enrolled. These voluntary plans attracted very few beneficiaries (only 1.3% of all beneficiaries in 1980) both because of difficulties in administering the plans and because Medicaid fee-for-service beneficiaries already received comprehensive services and had little cost sharing. Legislation in 1981 created the possibility of waivers for mandatory HMO enrollment. By 1991, nearly 10% of Medicaid beneficiaries were enrolled in managed care plans. Since then, states have been increasingly turning to managed care. By 1996, all states except Utah and Alaska used managed care as a component of their Medicaid programs, and nearly 40% of Medicaid beneficiaries were enrolled in managed care. The 1997 Balanced Budget Act eliminated the requirement that states seek a federal waiver to begin mandatory Medicaid managed care programs. While HMOs dominate the Medicaid managed care business, other forms of managed care are also in use. For example, California implemented a system of selective contracting for its Medicaid fee-for-service program in 1982.

The rapid growth of managed care, its effects on provider incomes and on the practice of medicine, and the restrictions placed on enrollees eventually generated a legal backlash against managed care. In 1995, 27 states required state-regulated insurers to permit 'any willing provider' to participate in a health plan, and some states require managed care plans to permit those holding coverage a free choice of provider or mandate that plans must offer a point-of-service option. Overall, by 1996, nearly one-third of the states had strong or medium-strong restrictions on the operations of state-regulated managed care plans. States are continuing to pass laws through the 2000s. Since 2000, legal restrictions on selective contracting, consumer interest in looser forms of care management, and legislation promoting the use of high-deductible plans as a response to rising health-care costs have all contributed to a flattening in the growth of managed care in the United States.

Changes in the market have also generated new organizational strategies for managed care plans. Today, vertically integrated plans are rare. Rather, under emerging models, health plans, medical groups, and hospital systems focus on those services they perform best while coordinating with other services primarily through contractual (rather than ownership) relationships. The consumer role has also changed, with a growing emphasis on consumer cost-sharing as a means of limiting the demand for services.

Europe

While managed care has a long history in the United States its implementation in other – mostly European – countries is rather recent. Initial European interest in managed care in the early 1990s focused on the introduction of managed care tools into frameworks of state-led medicine. Subsequent health-care reforms in the majority of European countries have paved the way for the development of new strategies and tools for managing health-care systems. Nonetheless, the formation of managed care organizations such as HMOs themselves is still in its infancy (except in Switzerland). In other countries, managed care organizations exist primarily as pilot projects.

In France, a health-care reform in 1996 introduced computerized medical records, practice guidelines, and incentives to encourage the use of primary care practitioners as gatekeepers. These developments enhanced managed care goals of price competition and selective contracting, but at the same time encountered the resistance of practicing physicians. To date, gatekeeping has not been used to constrain service use.

In Germany, health reforms that incorporate managed care elements date back to 1993, but only recently (2004) has legislation enabled organizations to form integrated delivery systems. Since 2000, physician networks, hospitals, and other licensed health-care providers have been formally permitted to cooperate to achieve 'integrated health-care delivery.' The legislation also permitted the introduction of a primary care physician gatekeeper system and the possibility that an integrated delivery system would take on budget responsibility.

Despite this enabling legislation, regulatory restrictions made it difficult to take any of the authorized steps. The 2004 Health Care Modernization Act has now removed these regulatory obstacles and has provided start-up funding for the development of managed care organizations. As of June 30, 2006, there were 2590 contracts in Germany for integrated health-care delivery approaches, covering 3.7 million insured persons. Most of these contracts, however, are quite narrow and cover only specific diseases, rather than taking on financial responsibility for care of a defined population.

The United Kingdom's National Health Service (NHS) has also incorporated several elements of managed care within its state-financed health-care system. The NHS has implemented incentives that make a substantial share of physician income dependent on performance.

Since 2003, integrated care approaches have been initiated in three regions (Torbay, Northumbria, and Eastern Birmingham).

Switzerland leads Europe in the development of managed care, subsequent to its 1996 health-care reform. Today, there are 19 HMOs (about 100 000 members) and several IPA-like physician networks (about 390 000 members) in existence. Similarly to the development in the United States, the emergence of managed care in Switzerland enhanced the demand for quality measurement and monitoring.

Latin America and the Developing World

Managed care and managed care tools have also made inroads in the health systems of middle-income and developing countries. In developing countries with an emerging middle class, managed care plans operating integrated delivery systems offer a private alternative to often limited government-funded health-care systems. Large employers may contract with these plans to provide employee benefits.

In Chile, Argentina, Brazil, and several other Latin American countries, managed care plans have been integrated more fully into the health system. Managed care plans may be offered by employers, selected by individuals, or may be an insurance option for beneficiaries of the national social security systems (usually limited to employed workers). Managed care is viewed as an attractive option by governments because it often brings an inflow of new investment funds to the health sector and allows the government to off-load the risk of health expenses to independent entities.

Effects of Managed Care

There has been a very substantial amount of research concerning the impact of managed care and of managed care tools. Despite this large volume of research, it is hard to come to definite conclusions about these effects. First, as discussed above, the term managed care incorporates many different combinations of mechanisms. Second, in most situations, managed care plans enroll different – often healthier – enrollees than do conventional plans. If managed care enrollees differ from enrollees of conventional insurance plans, differences in observed use at a point in time, growth in use over time, and outcomes may be a consequence of the underlying characteristics of the enrolled population, rather than anything the plans themselves do.

Third, managed care techniques control medical care costs, but, in many cases, they do so by adding administrative and managerial complexity, particularly in less integrated contexts. For example, implementing utilization review requires the insurer to hire skilled reviewers and forces physicians to communicate and often negotiate with these reviewers. These added administrative costs may reduce the overall social savings from the use of managed care tools.

Selection

Many studies in the United States have found differences in the characteristics of managed care and conventional insurance enrollees. On average, U.S. studies find that managed care plans in the private sector and in Medicare enroll beneficiaries who are 20% to 30% less costly than those who remain in conventional plans. In contrast, enrollees in German integrated delivery systems, which do not take financial responsibility for care but offer attractive care management programs for chronic populations, attract a population that is sicker than average.

Utilization

Many studies assess the effects of managed care on inpatient, outpatient, and total utilization. It is most valuable to study utilization across a broad range of services to address the possibility of cost shifting across services and from managed care entities to other providers. In early studies, managed care plans (generally staff and group model HMOs) reduced inpatient admission rates, had mixed effects on length of inpatient stays, and reduced total inpatient costs. The overall effect on inpatient days was a reduction of 5% to 25% for IPA plans and 35% for group and staff model plans. Similarly, analysis of integrated delivery models in the UK has found admission rates well below the national average.

The results of studies that compare PPOs with conventional plans are less clear. Some studies find that PPOs have lower costs, while others find that they have higher costs than competing arrangements.

By the late 1990s, even conventional fee-for-service plans adopted many aspects of managed care, including utilization review and price negotiation. In several studies conducted in the mid and late 1990s, there were no longer any differences between costs of inpatient (or outpatient) service use patterns in HMOs and traditional indemnity plans. Managed care plans, however, do tend to pay lower prices to providers than do conventional insurers.

Evaluations of physician networks in Switzerland that use the primary care physician as the gatekeeper also find that managed care models have lower costs than other plans. However, evidence varies as these networks are very heterogeneous (looser or closer networks with or without budget responsibility). Studies find risk-adjusted savings of 20% to 30% for HMOs and 7% to 20% for physician networks.

Quality

Most studies find few consistent differences between the quality of care provided in managed care plans and conventional insurance arrangements. To the extent that there is a pattern, managed care plans tend to perform better than conventional plans in the care of people with common chronic illnesses and worse in the care of those with serious, but less common, conditions. Subjective measures of quality, such as consumer satisfaction with care, tend to favor conventional insurance arrangements over managed care for most (but not all) populations.

Spillover Effects of Managed Care

Managed care may also have effects – positive or negative – on the delivery of care to those who are not managed care beneficiaries. If plans attract healthier than average populations, they may drive up costs for nonmanaged care plans. Conversely, if a lower-cost managed care practice style diffuses to nonmanaged care physicians, the effects of managed care may be compounded. Early studies of the effects of managed care on total costs were generally case studies, and most found no effect. More recent studies focus on the rate of cost growth in areas with high managed care penetration. Most, but not all, of the more recent studies find that increases in managed care penetration are associated with reductions in the rate of growth of total costs. Whereas these studies mainly support the hypothesis that managed care can reduce total costs, they do not yet conclude the issue.

Managed Care and Public Health

The managed care model alters the orientation of traditional health insurance plans in a direction that is more compatible with public health. Unlike traditional private health insurance plans, which paid bills for services organized and managed by individual physicians, managed care plans can be held responsible for defined populations of patients. Moreover, the growth of managed care has prompted a new emphasis on the measurement of population-level health outcomes for covered populations. To the extent that health promotion, disease management, and management of environmental risks help managed care plans to achieve measurable outcomes, they have an enhanced incentive to incorporate these activities among their functions.

Managed care plans can effectively work as adjuncts to the screening and data collection efforts of health departments, for example, by screening populations for lead and reporting abnormal levels. Plans have also been involved in the design and implementation of immunization and disease registries. Highly integrated plans have also been able to use their population level data to conduct important public health research.

Despite the potential for managed care to complement public health activities, the level of interaction between managed care organizations and public health departments in the United States has been limited. In a recent survey, only about one-half of U.S. local health departments had interacted with local managed care plans at all. Interactions between public health departments and managed care plans have been primarily around public sector (especially Medicaid) managed care plans. The providers in these plans are often traditional public health safety net providers.

Managed care plans cannot take over all public health functions. These plans are typically at risk for only a segment of a community, whereas public health has responsibility for the health of the community as a whole. Managed care plans have little, if any, incentive to invest in activities that benefit populations who are not enrolled in their plans, although a few are engaged in community-level public health activities.

Managed care also poses some dangers for health departments. Managed care plans face incentives to offload some of their costs onto public health departments and other public providers. This type of cost shifting, from a risk-bearing managed care plan to public entities, such as public health services, has been documented in the literature on managed behavioral health care. The growth of managed care – and the array of preventive activities that plans provide – may also reduce the funding base of traditional public health departments, making it more difficult for them to meet their community-level mandate.

Conclusion

Despite the recent backlash, managed care and managed care tools, are likely to remain an important part of the U.S. health-care system and a growing component of healthcare systems in other countries. Managed care could also contribute to the public health orientation of social health insurance systems. The tools of managed care, including the use of selective contracting and incentive payments, have applicability in both private and public health-care delivery. Just as managed care has built on public health approaches, public health may be able to adopt managed care strategies as it aims to provide more services with ever-tightening budgets.

See also: Competiton in Health Care; Insurance Plans and Programs - An Overview; Long Term Care, Organization and Financing; The Private Sector in Health Care Provision, The Role of; Provider Payment Methods and Incentives.

Further Reading

Draper DA, Hurley RE, Lesser CS, and Strunk BC (2002) The changing face of managed care. *Health Affairs* 21(1): 11–23.
Erdmann Y and Wilson R (2001) Managed care: A view from Europe. *Annual Review of Public Health* 22: 273–291.
Glied S (2000) Managed care. In: Culyer AJ and Newhouse JP (eds.) *Handbook of Health Economics*, pp. 707–753. Amsterdam, the Netherlands: North Holland Press.
Halverson PK, McLaughlin CP, and Kaluzny AD (1998) *Managed Care and Public Health*. Gaithersburg, MD: Aspen Publishers.
Janus K and Amelung VE (2005) Integrated health care delivery based on transaction cost economics – experiences from California and cross-national implications. In: Savage G, Chilingerian JA and Powell M (eds.) *Advances in Health Care Management Volume 5 – International Health Care Management*, pp. 121–160. Oxford, UK: Elsevier Publications.
Luft HS (1981) *Health Maintenance Organizations: Dimensions of Performance*. New York: Wiley.
Miller RH and Luft HS (1997) Does managed care lead to better or to worse quality of care? *Health Affairs* 16(5): 7–25.
Rodwin VG and Le Pen C (2004) Health care reform in France – the birth of state-led managed care. *New England Journal of Medicine* 351: 2259–2261.
Roland M (2004) Linking physicians' pay to the quality of care – a major experiment in the United Kingdom. *New England Journal of Medicine* 351(14): 1448–1454.
Stock AK, Redaelli M, and Lauterbach KW (2007) Disease management and health care reforms in Germany—does more competition lead to less solidarity? *Health Policy* 80(1): 86–96.
Sullivan K (2000) On the 'efficiency' of managed care plans. *Health Affairs* 19(4): 139–148.
Wickizer TM and Lessler DS (2002) Utilization management: Issues, effects and future prospects. *Annual Review of Public Health* 23: 233–254.

Relevant Websites

http://www.healthpolicymonitor.org – Health Policy Monitor, Bertelsmann Foundation (international information on managed care developments).
http://www.kff.org/insurance/ – Henry J. Kaiser Family Foundation (managed care enrollment statistics).

Economic Models of Hospital Behavior

X Liu, National Institutes of Health, Bethesda, MD, USA
A Mills, London School of Hygiene and Tropical Medicine, London, UK

Published by Elsevier Inc.

Glossary

Average variable cost The total variable cost divided by output. The average variable cost curve will generally be u-shaped because increasing returns in the short run initially reduce average variable costs.
Demand curve A graph that shows the amount of a good or service that consumers are willing and able to buy at various prices, holding other factors constant.
Endogenous variable A variable that is identified within the workings of the model. Also termed a dependent variable, an endogenous variable is in essence the 'output' of the model. It should be compared with an exogenous variable; this is the 'input' to the model.
Exogenous variable A variable that is identified outside the workings of the model. Also termed an independent variable, an exogenous variable is in essence the 'input' to the model. It should be compared with an endogenous variable; this is the 'output' of the model.
Fixed cost Production expenses that are independent of the level of output. Fixed costs could include buildings and equipment, loan repayments, and administration.
Indifference curve A curve that graphically depicts various combinations of goods that generate the same level of utility to a consumer. In other words, a consumer is 'indifferent' among any of the bundles because they all provide the same satisfaction.
Marginal cost The amount spent on producing one extra unit of product or service. The marginal cost is the increase in total cost when one more unit is produced.
Marginal revenue The income received from the production and sale of one extra unit of product or service.
Marginal utility The satisfaction gained from the consumption of one extra unit of a good or service.
Monopoly The situation in which one firm produces the entire output of a market.
Objective function This expresses what factors or variables are important for a utility maximizer.
Oligopolistic firms A situation in which a few producers dominate the market and their output accounts for a large proportion of the total market output.

Price elasticity of demand Measures the responsiveness of demand to a given change in price. It equals the percent change in demand divided by the percent change in price.
Price taker Firms whose output does not influence price. This is particularly apparent in perfectly competitive markets.
Utility The satisfaction of wants and needs obtained from consumption of goods and services.
Utility function This expresses utility as a function of the factors that determine the total utility.
Variable cost Production expenses that are dependent on the level of output. In other words, if output increases, then variable costs increase.

Introduction

Hospital behavior models can be used to explain a hospital's past behavior and provide experiences and lessons for policy making regarding hospital regulation and payment. They can also be used to predict future behavior under changing external factors, one of which is the transformation of the payment system. A good hospital payment system can be designed only if the change in hospital behavior as the payment system changes can be predicted with reasonable accuracy. This is one of the major reasons why so many attempts have been made to model hospital behavior over the past 30 years.

Modeling hospital behavior is complex, and no single model is likely to be able to explain hospital behavior. Hospital behavior is associated with hospital objectives, and the latter are related to hospital types. In other words, different types of hospital may have different goals and be financed differently, and their behaviors may also differ. The categorization of hospitals can provide the basis for considering the development and utilization of hospital behavior models. On several dimensions, hospitals can be divided by ownership, into private and public hospitals; financial objectives, into for-profit and nonprofit hospitals; educational responsibilities, into teaching and nonteaching hospitals; level of care, into primary, secondary, and tertiary hospitals; degree of service specification, into general and specialized hospitals; and employee status of their doctors, into staff model hospitals (in which doctors are the employees of the hospitals) and non-staff model hospitals (doctors are not employees, but practice medicine in the hospitals under contract).

Given the range of hospital types, the generalization of their objectives is difficult, a representative and typical hospital cannot be identified, and developing a single model for predicting hospital behavior is problematic (McGuire et al., 1988). An important first step to understanding the overall picture of hospital behavior is to identify the alternative objectives mentioned in the literature and relate them to the main hospital types. Ownership and financial objectives are commonly considered the most important influences on objectives.

The aims of this article are to review the available models of hospital behavior and discuss their potential uses in the development of hospital payment systems. Following this brief introduction, we review the major models of hospital behavior. In the third section, we provide perspectives for future research. A glossary is provided for those unfamiliar with economic language.

Economic Models of Hospital Behavior

Since there is no consensus on the objectives of hospitals, various models have been developed in association with particular hypothesized objectives that fit particular types of hospitals and special applications. This section reviews the major available models of hospital behavior.

Profit-Maximizing Model

Profit maximization is recognized as the single most important objective of for-profit hospitals (Davis, 1971; Feldstein, 1979). Indeed, many hospitals are built explicitly to earn a profit and would not otherwise enter the medical market. These hospitals include for-profit proprietary hospitals, private nursing home industries (such as those in the United States), joint venture hospitals, and joint-stock hospitals.

Feldstein (1979) and Jacobs (1991) developed similar models of hospital behavior, in which they assumed:

- the hospital's objective is to maximize profit;
- the hospital provides a single product or multiple products measured by a single output indicator;
- all the hospital's revenue comes from service charges;
- the hospital is a price taker rather than a price setter because the price is set by an independent administrative agency or because the hospital operates in a competitive situation in which the best price it can get for its product is the price prevailing in the market;
- to produce the product, the hospital incurs both fixed and variable costs, and the average variable cost is assumed to fall initially and subsequently rise as output increases.

With the preceding assumptions, the central questions become what quantity of output will be supplied, and how will this quantity vary when prices and costs vary?

The model predicts that a profit-maximizing hospital will produce services to the point where the marginal cost (MC) equals the marginal revenue (MR), in this case, the price of the hospital's output (P). As long as the marginal revenue (price) exceeds the marginal cost, the hospital as a profit maximizer will always try to expand output, because the additional revenue from the additional output exceeds the additional cost, and the hospital can earn more profit by expanding the output. As shown in **Figure 1**, at a MR or price at P0, P1, and P2, given the MC curve, the hospital will produce Q0, Q1, and Q2 amount of services. The hospital will not expand output to the point where the marginal cost exceeds the marginal revenue (e.g., at a price of P3, the hospital will not produce Q4 amount of services), because more output would mean less total profit.

A change in marginal cost will affect the quantity of supply. An increase in the marginal cost of a given amount of output will reduce the quantity of supply, at constant prices, and vice versa. The implication is that a profit-maximizing hospital will reduce its output to raise profits if input prices increase.

The model also predicts that a hospital will increase output if the price of output increases, and vice versa. The supply curve of the hospital will be the marginal cost curve. The quantity supplied will be where the price equals the marginal cost.

According to the model, if the output price is so low that the hospital would be better off producing nothing, the hospital will close. The criterion the hospital will use to decide whether to continue to produce is not whether it incurs a loss, but whether it can minimize its loss. It is assumed that if the hospital closes, it has to incur the loss of its total assets (equal to the total fixed cost). If the price is lower than the average total cost (ATC) but higher than the average variable cost (AVC), the hospital will incur a loss but will not close because the surplus over AVC makes a contribution to the fixed cost. If the price is lower than the AVC, continuing operations means incurring losses that exceed the fixed cost, and the hospital will close. Thus, the shut-down point is where the price equals the AVC, below which there will be no reason for a profit-maximizing hospital to continue operations.

Quantity-Maximizing Model

For most hospitals, profit making is not a stated goal, or at least earning profit is not their major objective. These hospitals include public hospitals and private nonprofit hospitals. For the nonprofit hospitals, many health economists support the hypothesis that quantity maximization is their major objective (Rice, 1966; Brown, 1970). Thus this model assumes that the hospital is an output maximizer (Rice, 1966; Jacobs, 1991), not a profit maximizer. This model is assumed to be appropriate for nonprofit hospitals, the predominant type in almost every nation. Other assumptions are the same as in Jacobs' profit-maximizing model, in particular, that the hospital is a price taker.

According to this model, total costs are directly related to output. The slope of the total cost curve increases as output expands, reflecting the effect of diminishing marginal productivity on marginal costs. The revenue curve is drawn with a slope that decreases as output increases. This reflects decreases in the marginal revenue associated with a declining price elasticity of demand, which occurs as the quantity produced and sold increases. As is shown in **Figure 2**, the total surplus (TS) or profit is equal to total revenue (TR) minus total cost (TC). The quantity-maximizing hospital will expand its output to the point at Q3, where the firm just breaks even, that is, where the total cost (TC) equals total revenue (TR), or the price (P) equals the average total cost (ATC) in **Figure 1**. The output of a nonprofit output-maximizing hospital will be higher than the output of a profit-maximizing hospital.

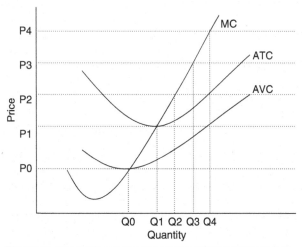

Figure 1 The profit-maximizing model: Relationship between prices and output.

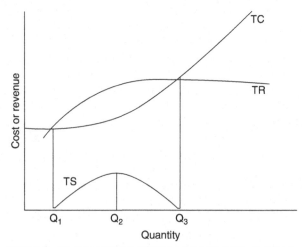

Figure 2 The quantity-maximizing model: Quantity of output supplied.

Revenue-Maximizing Model

The hospital as a sales- or revenue-maximizing entity was suggested by Steven Finkler (1983), based on the theory of sales maximization. According to this theory, a business always tries to increase the total number of sales (or total revenue) until the break-even point, while Finkler argues that hospitals will keep expanding their roster of services, even when losing money, and that if there is a break-even constraint, nonprofit hospitals will not offer products with insufficient demand even if they do not make a loss.

The revenue-maximization model (Finkler, 1983) assumes the following:

- Nonprofit hospitals pursue a policy of revenue maximization or sales maximization, because the hospital executives are rewarded on the basis of revenue rather than profits. Although sometimes it is said that managers are rewarded for the quality and quantity of hospital services, that is problematic because quality is difficult to define and measure, and quantity is also difficult to measure because of the multiproduct nature of hospitals.
- Hospitals are oligopolistic firms, faced by a downward-sloping demand curve. It is further assumed that demand for each hospital product is finite, even at a price of zero, because of patients' limited need and costs such as travel and time costs. Finkler argued that a hospital cannot maximize revenue simply by offering to mend an infinite number of broken legs.

Demand for or revenue from hospital services are functions of service price and the number of medical doctors affiliated with the hospital. The more doctors, the greater is the demand for that hospital. This is particularly true in the United States where the hospital's inpatients are referred by its affiliated doctors. In addition, the higher the price, the less is the demand for the hospital.

The model predicts that the hospital, as a revenue maximizer, will produce as many types of products and as much of each product as possible, as long as total revenue is maximized and the hospital can still break even, and that some products will be offered at a loss if their effect on demand for other products produces a profit greater than or equal to the loss. In particular, increasing demand is dependent on attracting more affiliated doctors, which requires offering a wide range of services. Although a new product may be offered at a loss, its introduction may increase the profitability of existing products through attracting more affiliated doctors and hence increasing demand and revenue.

Utility-Maximizing Model

Supporters of utility maximization argue that hospital behavior is guided by more than one or many factors of importance to the hospital (Newhouse, 1970; Lee, 1971; Hornbrook and Goldfarb, 1983). Some authors include only quantity and quality; others include many variables, such as profit, number of hospital admissions, emergency capacity, case mix, and quality of care, in what is called the hospital's objective function. Utility maximization seems to be the only objective that has the potential to cover comprehensively the objectives of all types of hospital. The utility-maximizing model includes several submodels, which are briefly described in the following sections.

Lee's model

Lee (1971) focused on hospital administrators, postulating that they attempt to maximize their own utility, which is a function of salary, prestige, security, power, and professional satisfaction. He further argues that the determinants of utility are directly related to the number and types of sophisticated inputs and services used by the hospital, which enhance the hospital administrators' income, security, and prestige. This model predicts that the pursuit of conspicuous production will result in unnecessary duplication of facilities and overhiring of staff.

Feldstein's model

Feldstein (1971) took a different approach, introducing, in his utility function, a trade-off between the quantity and quality of hospital services. This model is based on the simplified assumption that, given a fixed budget, hospital decision makers face a trade-off between quantity and quality of services. The model also assumes that the utility of the decision maker is a function of quality and quantity and that there are different combinations of quality and quantity with the same level of utility to the decision maker. The model implies that different hospitals will have different sets of indifference curves, reflecting differences in their valuation of the trade-off between quality and quantity. It predicts that hospitals will choose different production patterns in terms of the quality and quantity of services depending on their valuation of the trade-off between quality and quantity.

Cromwell's model

Cromwell (1976) extended Feldstein's model above by imposing a payment constraint, that is, prospective payment, based on inpatient days or per case. After the imposition of the prospective payment system, the hospital will be paid a reduced fixed amount per case or per inpatient day. The revenue ceiling imposed by the prospective payment does not allow the hospital to provide care that is more expensive than the value of the inputs needed to provide the initial amount of quality per unit of services. At the new equilibrium, the hospital will produce more units of service, but at a lower level of quality. This model predicts that the imposition of prospective payment will provide the hospital with an incentive to reduce service quality and increase service quantity, as defined by the payment system.

Goldfarb-Hornbrook-Rafferty's model

In contrast to earlier utility models, Goldfarb, Hornbrook, and Rafferty (1980) explicitly recognized the multiproduct and multigoal nature of the hospital. The model assumed that hospital decision makers attempt to maximize utility, which is a function of the number of admissions, case mix, quality, and profit, subject to the constraints of reimbursement policies, technology, patient availability, and general resources. It is also assumed that hospital decision makers face trade-offs between the components of the objective function, and that they equalize the marginal utility of each of the components of the objective function.

Rosko's model

Rosko (1982) extends Cromwell's model by considering marginal slack as a variable in the administrator's utility function. The model predicts that, as the slack increases, the quality and quantity of services would decrease and the cost per unit of service would increase. The model also predicts that the imposition of revenue constraints in the form of *per diem* prospective payments would reduce slack and thus improve internal efficiency.

Sloan-Steinwald's model

Similar to Goldfarb's model, this model, as developed by Sloan and Steinwald (1980), assumes that the hospital's utility is a function of a service composite, which incorporates both the quality and quantity dimensions of the output; amenities, including those provided to patients and physicians; and profit. It is argued that different types of hospital may place different weights on the objectives. For-profit hospitals may emphasize profit, while nonprofit hospitals may place more weight on service mix or amenities. It is noteworthy that both Sloan-Steinwald's and Goldfarb's models take profit as a variable for the nonprofit hospitals. Nonprofit hospitals do have an incentive to earn profits (Rosko and Broyles, 1988) because of changes in hospital payment systems and the trend toward hospital corporatization.

Executive-Benefit-Maximization Model

This model focuses on hospital executives, rather than physicians. Its assumptions are as follows (Jacobs, 1991):

- The executives or administrators of the hospital have considerable control over hospital behavior, and the behavior of the executive can be taken to represent the behavior of the hospital as a whole.
- The behavior of executives is driven mainly by pecuniary incentives in for-profit hospitals.

- Executives in nonprofit hospitals are paid a fixed salary, and hospital profit cannot be translated into executive pay. Their behavior in nonprofit hospitals is driven mainly by nonpecuniary incentives, such as good office furniture, a relaxed work atmosphere, and high status due to high quality of care.

In a for-profit hospital, greater profit can be expected from a smaller commitment of resources for a given amount of output. For a nonprofit hospital, there will be a trade-off between executives' nonpecuniary benefit and hospital profit. The nonpecuniary benefits of executives will increase costs for a given amount of hospital services, and reduce profit.

This model predicts that productivity and profitability would be lower in nonprofit hospitals than in for-profit hospitals. The former hospital type is expected to have higher service quality and a more complex case mix than the latter hospital type, which may want to minimize its costs by reducing quality and avoiding accepting more costly cases.

The Application of Hospital Behavior Models

A major objective in developing models of hospital behavior is to predict changes in hospital behavior that will occur with changes in exogenous factors. One of these factors is how and how much the hospital is reimbursed.

To be applicable to the design of hospital payment, a model must meet five prerequisites:

1. objective captivity: The model must be able to include all of the endogenous variables that are important to the hospital;
2. argument measurability: The variables included in the model should be operationally defined and measurable with reasonable validity;
3. trade-off testability: The trade-offs between variables must be identified and estimated;
4. utility estimatability: The relative importance of the variables must be quantifiable, namely, the marginal utility attached to each variable must be examined;
5. effect predictability: The effect of payment systems and other exogenous factors on the quantity of the variables and their utility contributions should be predictable.

If these five prerequisites can be met, hospital behavior will be predictable. Although the current hospital behavior models suffer numerous limitations and none of the models can meet all these requirements, these models have guided the prediction of hospital behavior and the estimation of the effect of hospital payment reforms.

Due to the complexity of hospitals, generalizing about the objective function of hospitals is difficult. Profit maximization models are said to fit best for-profit hospitals, but it is generally thought that other objectives are also important to hospitals. Although some of the modelers of nonprofit hospitals recognize that the hospital's major objective is to maximize the quantity of service provision subject to breaking even, others argue that more objectives should be included in the hospital's objective function. In addition, the current models suffer from measurement problems in terms of the valid measurement of variables that describe the hospital's objectives and the utility values of different variables in the objective function.

In general, therefore, empirical studies of hospital behavior are far from conclusive. Further efforts are needed to ensure models reflect real-world situations and to make them of practical use in predicting hospital behavior.

Perspectives for Future Research

Although limited in their applicability, the models reviewed above have provided sound foundations for future research, which should focus on four areas.

First, the identification of the hospital's objective function should be based on empirical investigations of different types of hospitals. All groups that influence hospital objectives (e.g., administrators, board of trustees, medical staff, the hospital owner) should be investigated in terms of what is important to each of them and how differences are reconciled.

Second, further efforts should be made to improve the measurement of the variables in hospital objective functions. If perfect measures are difficult or impossible to develop, they must be able at least to reflect the concepts with reasonable validity. In addition, efforts should be made to standardize measurement, at least at the national level. If one approach to measurement of a variable is not suitable for all hospitals, different approaches can be developed so that measures are appropriate for different types of hospitals.

Third, the relative utility contribution of each unit of an endogenous variable should be investigated. This information can be directly used to roughly predict hospital behavior. For instance, if there are three variables in the hospital objective function, A, B, and C, and the relative utility contribution of each unit of the three variables is 1, 2, and 3, if the change in an exogenous factor is predicted to reduce utility by 3 units, the hospital will be expected to produce 1 more unit of C or 1.5 additional units of B, or any combination of B and C to maintain the original level of utility. The related actions (behavior) of the hospital to realize this adjustment can be predicted.

Fourth, for the longer term, more sophisticated analysis should be conducted, involving the measurement of the marginal utility of each variable and exploration of the trade-offs between different variables. The best combination of different variables should maximize the total utility of the hospital. The solution of the best quantity combination of variables will involve complicated procedures of linear programming and the construction of simultaneous models.

Acknowledgments

This article is an adaptation of chapter 9 of the book *Public Ends, Private Means: Strategic Purchasing of Health Services*, edited by Alexander Preker, Xingzhu Liu, Edit Velenyi, and Enis Baris. The publication of this article does not mean NIH or FIC's endorsement or recommendations for the use of any products, services, materials, methodology, or policies stated therein. Conclusions and opinions are those of the individual authors only and do not reflect the policies or views of their affiliated institutions.

See also: Demand and Supply of Human Resources for Health; Insurance Plans and Programs - An Overview; The Demand for Health Care.

Citations

Brown M (1970) Economic analysis of hospital operation. *Hospital Administration* 15(60): 67–74.
Cromwell J (1976) Hospital productivity trends in short-term general nonteaching hospitals. *Inquiry* 11(2): 181–187.
Davis K (1971) *Economic Theories of Behavior in Nonprofit, Private Hospitals*. Washington, DC: Brookings Institute.
Feldstein M (1971) Hospital cost inflation: A study of nonprofit price dynamics. *American Economic Review* 61(5): 853–872.
Feldstein PJ (1979) *Health Care Economics*. New York: John Wiley and Sons.
Finkler SA (1983) The hospital as a sales-maximizing entity. *Health Service Research* 18(2): 117–133.
Goldfarb M, Hornbrook M, and Rafferty J (1980) Behavior of the multi-product firm: A model of the nonprofit hospital system. *Medical Care* 18(2): 185–201.
Hornbrook M and Goldfarb M (1983) A partial test of a hospital behavior model. *Social Science and Medicine* 17(10): 667–680.
Jacobs P (1991) *The Economics of Health and Medical Care*. Gaithersburg, MD: Aspen.
Lee ML (1971) A conspicuous production theory of hospital behavior. *Southern Economic Journal* 38(1): 48–58.
McGuire A, Henderson J, and Mooney G (1988) *The Economics of Health Care: An Introductory Text*, pp. 152–249. London: Routledge & Kegan Paul.
Newhouse J (1970) A model of physician pricing. *Southern Economic Journal* 37(2): 174–183.
Rice R (1966) Analysis of hospital as an economic organism. *Modern Hospital* 106(4): 88–91.
Rosko M and Broyles R (1988) *The Economics of Health Care: A Reference Handbook*. Westport, CT: Greenwood Press.
Rosko MD (1982) Hospital response to prospective rate setting. Doctoral Dissertation, Temple University.
Sloan A and Steinwald B (1980) *Insurance, Regulation, and Hospital Costs*. Lexington, MA: DC Health and Co.

Further Reading

Folland S (2006) *The Economics of Health and Health Care,* 5th edn. New York: Prentice Hall.

Frank S (2002) Not-for-profit ownership and hospital behavior. In: Culyer AJ and Newhouse JP (eds.) *Handbook of Health Economics,* pp. 1141–1174. Amsterdam, the Netherlands: Elsevier.

Harrison TD and Lybecker KM (2005) The effect of the nonprofit motive on hospital competitive behavior. *Contributions to Economic Analysis and Policy* 4(1): 1368–1368.

Preker A, Liu X, Velenyi E and Baris E (eds.) (2007) *Public Ends, Private Means: Strategic Purchasing of Health Services.* Washington, DC: World Bank.

Essential Drugs Policy

H Haak, Consultants for Health and Development, Leiden, The Netherlands

© 2008 Elsevier Inc. All rights reserved.

Introduction

Governments around the world have always been concerned with securing and sustaining access to medicines for their populations (the terms medicines, drugs, and pharmaceuticals, are used here interchangeably, although preference is now given to the term medicines, to avoid confusion with the term hypnotics). This concern has often posed a challenge because medicines often represent significant monetary value and because numerous stakeholders are involved in their procurement, management, prescription, and use. Views about medicines are often strong and sometimes polemic.

Even though pharmaceuticals play a key role in health care – and major resources are spent on them – according to the World Health Organization (WHO) (2000) they are often unavailable, unaffordable, unsafe, and/or improperly used. These problems are common around the world. Health systems are challenged by the rising costs of medicines, difficult choices regarding conventional and new therapies, and inequities in access (Govindaraj *et al.*, 2000). Pharmaceutical expenditures in developing countries represent between 20–50% of total health-care expenditures (WHO, 1998). This figure is much higher than the average spent in industrialized countries. Access to pharmaceutical products is strikingly imbalanced between rich and poor countries and also within countries.

The politics of pharmaceuticals are complex. Governments have many – sometimes contradictory – obligations to protect health, safeguard jobs, and ensure a strong economy (Almarsdottir and Traulsen, 2006). Balancing these different obligations requires skill and careful management of the political dimensions. Unfortunately, policy makers do not always seem to be aware of the distinct features of pharmaceuticals and pharmaceutical policies, which may explain the frequent failures in access to pharmaceuticals in countries around the world.

Pharmaceuticals Are Unique

An issue that often complicates discussions on pharmaceutical policy is the mistaken belief that pharmaceuticals are like any other commodity. One study by Smith (1983: 112) identified 27 "latent functions" of pharmaceuticals. These include symbolic and social functions in patient-doctor interactions as well as broad political functions (e.g., poor people claiming rights to health and pharmaceutical care) and economic functions (e.g., interests in strengthening pharmaceutical industries). The multifaceted nature of pharmaceuticals contributes to the complexity of pharmaceutical policy decision making. Assuming that pharmaceuticals can be viewed as any other commodity without considering their context may result in ineffective policy decisions. Discussions of pharmaceutical policy are often further complicated because it elicits debates about basic social values such as the roles of the market and the state, and the relative importance of efficiency and equity (Reich, 1995).

Pharmaceutical Policies Are an Integral Part of Health Policies

Pharmaceutical policies cannot be isolated from broader health policies and need to fit within the framework of health-care systems. Most governments would see the goals of national pharmaceutical policy as having to be consistent with broader health objectives (WHO, 2001). Despite this intertwined role, pharmaceutical policy is fundamentally different from health policy and its development requires a different set of tools and knowledge (Traulsen and Almarsdottir, 2005a). Differences include the actors involved, their interests, the different power relations between them, and the influence of specific configurations of international forces. These differences have an impact on all aspects of pharmaceutical policy development and implementation.

Pharmaceutical Policy Literature

Pharmaceutical policy means different things to different people (Traulsen and Almarsdottir, 2005a). Searching the literature on 'pharmaceutical policies' or 'drug policies' results in an avalanche of papers, as both phrases are added as keywords in almost any paper that refers to medicines.

As well, the pressure of increasing prices of medicines has resulted in a narrowing of the discussion of pharmaceutical policy to one of cost. Much of the current literature is about pharmaceutical budgets, pricing of individual medicines, and whether inclusion of individual medicines in reimbursement schemes can be justified.

The literature on the advantages and disadvantages of specific medicines in defined disease conditions is substantial. Much of this literature is considered relevant by the authors for 'pharmaceutical policy development' (i.e., policy content). As this literature generally does not discuss the pharmaceutical policy process, however, it will not be part of the analysis and conclusions of this article.

A number of pharmaceutical policy papers describe specific experiences of policy implementation and change in particular countries. These papers are extremely useful, but they do not always compare the experiences of pharmaceutical policy implementation in different contexts. The relevance of these papers is therefore limited to policy development in comparable systems.

Actors in Pharmaceutical Policy Development

In most settings, there are many actors involved in pharmaceutical sector regulation and policy making. These actors may include various ministries (health, finance, and industry), scientists, health professionals, nongovernmental organizations (NGOs), pharmacists, and consumers. In addition, activists, industry representatives, and drug wholesalers and retailers may claim a role in policy and regulation decisions. Some of these players are discussed here.

Governments and Their National Drug Regulatory Agencies

Governments are generally considered to hold the legal power to develop policies for production and delivery systems of pharmaceuticals. Most governments have also created national drug regulatory agencies, which ensure quality through national drug registration systems, and which – at least in theory – restrict the number of pharmaceuticals circulating within national borders. While not all countries have the capacity to actually enforce such registration schemes, registration status may nevertheless influence the procurement of medicines for public health-care systems. Stakeholders naturally lobby governments for pharmaceutical policies favorable to their interests.

Stringent Drug Regulatory Agencies

Some drug regulatory agencies have gained an important transnational drug regulatory role. When such agencies have international relevance it is because their decisions have assumed an impact beyond their respective, national stakeholders. The countries included in this category are the regulatory authority member countries of the Pharmaceutical Inspection Cooperation Scheme (PIC/S) and/or the International Conference on Harmonization of Technical Requirements for Registration of Pharmaceuticals for Human Use (ICH). The countries include all European Union member countries, the United States, Australia, Canada, Iceland, Japan, Liechtenstein, Malaysia, Norway, Singapore, and Switzerland. Although not a medicines registration agency, the European Medicines Agency (EMEA) has an increasingly important role in international pharmaceuticals registration decision making. The decisions of these 'stringent' drug regulatory agencies are important, as they have implications for the range of products that can be procured using the resources of some of the large international donors and financing mechanisms, include the Global Fund to Fight AIDS, TB, and Malaria (Global Fund), the President's Emergency Plan for AIDS Relief (PEPFAR), and the President's Malaria Initiative (PMI).

International Development Agencies

Intergovernmental organizations such as the WHO and the World Bank have traditionally aspired to play a key role in guiding pharmaceutical policy development. Their input is noticeable in several of the documents quoted here. The WHO's focus is on meeting the pharmaceutical needs of disadvantaged populations (WHO, 2004). The WHO's framework for national pharmaceutical policy development was essentially the only comprehensive framework for national pharmaceutical policies until the late 1990s and is outlined later (see the section 'The World Health Organization's perspectives on pharmaceutical policies').

The World Bank has recently assumed a more active role in pharmaceutical sector development in member countries (Govindaraj et al., 2000). Until the late 1990s, the agency's main focus in the sector was on ensuring adequate procurement practices and capable supplies systems. As Traulsen and Almarsdottir (2005b) stated, software components of pharmaceuticals supplies – such as pharmaceutical policy development and correct (i.e., rational) use of medicines – was often only an afterthought. The revision of the World Bank's strategies was stimulated by the continuing challenge of rising costs, new pharmaceutical therapies, and persistent inequities in access to pharmaceuticals (see the World Bank's conceptual thinking outlined in a later section, 'The World Bank's perspectives on pharmaceutical policies.')

International Pharmaceutical Industry

In 2006 the world pharmaceutical market was worth an estimated $608 000 million at ex-factory prices. The North American market (the United States and Canada) was the world's largest market with a 47.7% share, with Europe at 29.9%, and Japan at 9.3%. Shareholder value tends to be the decisive factor in its decisions at the corporate, national, or international levels, more than public health considerations about the populations served. The pharmaceutical industry has a strong interest in pharmaceutical policies that are favorable to increased sales of its products. The application of the principles underlying 'essential medicines' approaches (see the section 'The World Health Organization's perspectives on pharmaceutical policies') is generally not in the pharmaceutical industry's interest, and it has traditionally opposed policies restrictive to the introduction of the latest and more expensive pharmaceutical solutions. Its powerful lobby, especially in the United States, has often succeeded in influencing national- and international-level pharmaceutical policy decisions, while its considerable financial and legal power has often led to the defeat of its opponents. Its power is, however, by no means a guarantee for victory. In 1997, for example, 39 pharmaceutical companies unsuccessfully sued the South African government for perceived violation of international property rights. Support of the internationally operating AIDS advocacy movement and worldwide press coverage resulted in the industry's admission of defeat (*The Economist*, 2001).

International Nongovernmental Organizations and Activist Groups

International NGOs and activist groups have gained an increasingly strong role in influencing decision making on pharmaceutical regulations and policy. Groups in this category include organizations such as Health Action International, Social Audit, Healthy Skepticism, and others (see the section 'Relevant Websites'). Some special initiatives by international NGOs have also had important repercussions for national pharmaceutical regulations and policy frameworks. Such initiatives include the Médecins Sans Frontières Access Initiative, the Clinton Foundation HIV/AIDS Initiative, and the Consumer Project on Technology (see the section 'Relevant websites'). Assisted by rapid, Internet-based information sharing, these groups not only gained an increasingly authoritative voice in pharmaceutical policy debates, but also managed to have an impact on some national and international pharmaceutical policy discussions and thereby affected their content. AIDS activists pressured the World Trade Organization (WTO) to consider public health needs in the adoption of intellectual property rights and also successfully pressured the WHO to include patented AIDS medicines in its Model List of Essential Drugs – this was unheard of until that time. Activist pressure has led to remarkable battles in the pharmaceutical arena.

Patient Organizations

Patient organizations have traditionally tried to influence decisions on treatment policies, thereby also affecting pharmaceutical policy decisions. Until recently most patient organizations were independent, but more recently a new set of patient organizations has emerged with pharmaceutical industry funding. The independence of these industry-funded 'patient organizations' has been questioned, and some consider them to be marketing mechanisms in disguise (Herxheimer, 2003).

Health Insurance Industry

Health insurance companies are not expected to make national pharmaceutical policy, but their influence on policy making may be large, because of their reimbursement policies and the size of the populations they insure. Especially in countries in which the private sector has large responsibilities in health insurance, their influence may be significant.

Information Networks

A set of internet-based pharmaceutical policy discussion forums emerged with the growth of the Internet during the 1990s. The best known of these is the E-drug discussion forum (see the section 'Relevant Websites'). Established in 1994, E-drug membership now also includes staff from international agencies and the multinational pharmaceutical industry. It is not uncommon for highly controversial issues to be discussed in the E-drug forum. Novartis, for example, justified its decision to sue the Indian government in an open letter found at the website E-drug for what Novartis considered patent infringements of its profitable product Glivec (Novartis International, 2007). Similarly, an industry-sponsored effort led to a lengthy debate on whether expensive, patented antiretrovirals (ARVs) had an impact on access to these products in developing countries (Attaran, 2003). Information networks have clearly come to play a key role in rapidly circulating information to selected groups of opinion and decisions makers.

World Trade Organization

The WTO is not an actor in the pharmaceutical sector in the strict sense of the word. The WTO has, however, worked on strengthening patent protection of costly pharmaceutical products, so it has often been perceived as such. Patent issues have played a controversial role in securing access to and cost containment of modern pharmaceuticals in both developing and developed countries. The pharmaceutical industry has tried to defend its position that patents ultimately improve access of populations to high-quality pharmaceutical care, an argument that has been met with skepticism by many health-care professionals and activists. The WTO's meeting in Doha, Qatar, in 2001 reached agreement to allow developing countries to override certain patent laws and facilitate the use of less expensive generic drugs. In Article 31(f) of the Agreement on Trade-Related Aspects of Intellectual Property Rights (TRIPS), the WTO allowed countries to issue licenses to manufacturers other than the patent holder to produce patented medicine (so-called 'compulsory licensing'). The article also allowed the import of patented pharmaceuticals if they were less costly in another country ('parallel importing'). The key principle of the TRIPS agreement was that trade agreements should be interpreted and implemented to protect public health and promote access to medicines for all. The United States refused to support a more detailed plan saying that it failed to protect patents on drugs for noninfectious diseases and that it would undermine research and development (Laing, 2003).

Given the (research-based) pharmaceutical industry's strong influence on U.S. foreign policy, the United States has started to establish bilateral free trade agreements (FTAs) to enforce patent protection in individual countries after failing to work out the details of the TRIPS agreement. These FTAs are often dubbed 'TRIPS-Plus' agreements, as their patent protection arrangements go well beyond the original TRIPS agreement. Some countries (e.g., Australia) had to accept the decision to provide a seat to brand-name industry representatives in the medicine selection committee of its pharmaceutical benefit scheme (PBS) (Hughes, 2004). These players (and others) influence drug regulatory and policy decisions to varying degrees, and the dynamics are rarely static. The balance of power tends to shift continuously. In studying the literature it becomes clear that pharmaceutical policies can and should be different, and that a one-size-fits-all approach for all pharmaceutical policies, and in all countries and health systems, is not recommended.

Key Concepts in Pharmaceutical Policy Development

Since the mid-1970s, the WHO has urged countries to establish national pharmaceutical policies (WHO, 2001). Initially considered appropriate only for countries with limited health resources, more recently pharmaceutical policy development has been seen as relevant in industrialized nations as well. The increased cost of pharmaceuticals has played an important role in changing this perception.

The World Health Organization's Perspectives on Pharmaceutical Policies

The WHO, in its role as technical assistance agency to governments, considers a national pharmaceutical policy as presenting

> a commitment to a goal and a guide for action. It expresses and prioritizes the medium- to long-term goals set out by a government for the pharmaceutical sector, and identifies the main strategies for attaining them. It provides the framework within which the activities of the pharmaceutical sector can be coordinated. It covers both the public and the private sectors, and involves the main actors in the pharmaceutical field. It includes drug legislation and regulation, essential drugs selection, drug registration, pricing policy, and public sector procurement. (WHO, 2001: 7)

WHO literature (Quick *et al.*, 1997; WHO, 1998, 2000, 2001, 2004) prioritizes a number of problems that in its view determine poor access to medicines:

- *Unaffordable medicine prices*, especially for newer products, such as ARVs, artemisinin-based antimalarial medicines, and other recently launched products.
- *Irrational use of medicines*, for example, the WHO estimates half of all medicines are inappropriately prescribed, dispensed, or sold and that half of all patients fail to take their medicine properly.
- *Unfair health financing mechanisms*, leaving poor households to cover the cost of essential medicines they need, placing the heaviest burden on those least able to pay.
- *Persistence of unreliable medicine supply systems*, causing irregular and unsustainable supply of medicines. Inefficient procurement systems pay up to twice the global market price for pharmaceuticals and lead to waste of resources.
- *Greatly varying quality of medicines*, especially in low- and middle-income countries. Counterfeit and substandard medicines are circulating globally. An estimated 50–90% of samples of antimalarial medicines in WHO-member countries failed quality control tests and more than half of sampled ARVs did not meet international standards.
- *Lack of new medicines for diseases that typically affect the poor*, especially 'neglected' diseases. Most research and development of medicines is focused on medical conditions of the richest 20% of the global population.

Table 1 Key components of a national pharmaceutical policy

Legislative and regulatory framework	Financing strategies
• legislation and regulations	• roles of government
• drug registration and licensing	• medicines financing mechanisms (public financing, user charges, health insurance)
• pharmaceutical quality assurance	
• regulation of prescription and distribution	Rational use of medicines
• pharmaceutical promotional activities	• medicines information systems
Selection of medicines	• rational prescribing by health personnel
• principles of medicines selection	• rational use by consumers
• selection process, criteria, and levels of use	Human resources in pharmaceutical sector
• application of traditional medicines in allopathic health systems	• human resources development
Supply systems	• training strategies
• programming and budgeting needs	• motivation and continuing education
• procurement mechanisms	
• supply system strategies and alternatives	
• storage and distribution functions	

Reproduced from Quick *et al.* (1997) (eds.) *Managing Drug Supply*, 2nd edn. West Hartford, CT: Kumarian Press.

To achieve major improvements, the WHO notes that a pharmaceutical policy should be based on the essential medicines concept. This concept is believed to be the most cost-effective way of guaranteeing access to the majority of the global population (WHO, 2004). Key features of the essential medicines concept are:

- Selection of products as 'essential' based on national health priorities, and proven therapeutic effectiveness;
- Careful quantification of needs;
- Efficiency in procurement and supply mechanisms;
- Promotion of rational drug use.

Key components of a national pharmaceutical policy are summarized in **Table 1**.

The WHO's priority is to expand access to essential medicines, particularly for low-income and disadvantaged populations and for the priority diseases of HIV/AIDS, tuberculosis, and malaria. More recently, the WHO also started to place greater focus on financing, supply systems, and quality assurance. It is currently broadly agreed that the WHO's essential medicines concept is potentially applicable in any country, in public and private sectors, and in rural or urban settings. The large-scale application of essential medicines selection and the use of generic medicines by health maintenance organizations (HMOs) in the United States exemplify this.

The WHO claims that efforts of its own organization, countries, and other actors to update national pharmaceutical policies have increased access to essential medicines for people in countries from roughly US$2.1 billion in 1977 to an estimated US$3.8 billion in 1999 (WHO, 2000).

The World Bank's Perspectives on Pharmaceutical Policies

The World Bank's view on pharmaceutical policies is congruent with that of the WHO, but there are differences that have important implications for pharmaceutical policy making. A recent World Bank discussion paper presented the following reasons for the agency becoming more involved in pharmaceutical policy debates (Govindaraj *et al.*, 2000):

- *Significant public and private expenditures:* Pharmaceuticals represent a significant proportion of government and private, out-of-pocket expenditures in many developing countries. The policy implications of these large public and out-of-pocket expenditures are many.

- *Inadequate regulatory capacity:* Governments in developing countries often lack adequate institutional capacity to regulate pharmaceutical activities effectively and have difficulty in assuring the quality of pharmaceuticals in the public sector and on the private market.

- *Inadequate access to essential medicines:* Inefficient use of pharmaceutical resources in many developing countries has substantially reduced access to essential medicines and potential health benefits. A significant portion of pharmaceutical expenditures in developing countries is wasted due to inefficiencies associated with the procurement and management of supplies. Problems in some countries are compounded by widespread corruption in public sector procurement and distribution systems, including the health sector.

- *Limited access to new medicines:* There is limited funding for new pharmaceutical products in developing countries, resulting in limited access for groups who might benefit therapeutically. The limited access is compounded by the tendency of pharmaceutical companies to set prices close to those of industrialized countries.

- *Globalized product patents affecting developing countries' purchasing power:* Patent protection is believed to provide an impetus to research and development investments, but globalized patent protection may also reduce access if those products are marketed at high monopoly prices in developing countries.

- *Limited incentives for research and development of new medicines:* Developing countries represent a relatively small proportion of the global pharmaceutical market, providing limited market incentives for the development of new medicines specific to diseases of those countries (including many tropical diseases).

The World Bank believes that these pharmaceutical policy issues have created market failures and failures in good governance, resulting in poor access to pharmaceutical products and, consequently, in poorly functioning health systems. In line with this analysis, the World Bank proposed a number of directions for pharmaceuticals in its lending and advisory activities (Govindaraj et al., 2000). Of key importance is that the World Bank should become more involved in pharmaceutical policy dialogues with client governments on sustainable pharmaceutical reform. Such policy dialogues may target comprehensive national drug policy reform, or focus on specific subcomponents, such as drug financing, management of drug supplies, pharmaceutical pricing, or selection of drugs to be included in national essential drug lists and/or reimbursement packages. Moreover, pharmaceutical sector assessments should become an integral part of World Bank lending activities, especially when pharmaceutical procurement is involved, and outcomes help to determine the poverty focus as well as the institutional and political context of reforms. In addition, the following propositions were made:

- Restrict World Bank support for pharmaceutical procurement to projects that promote policy and systems development and target the poor: Drug procurement should only be financed in situations in which the lending is linked to institutional development, capacity building, and specific poverty alleviation initiatives. Sufficient attention should be paid to the careful selection of pharmaceuticals, appropriate delivery to and storage within the recipient health system, and stringent monitoring and assurance of quality through inspection and product testing, as well as to the cost-effective management of the purchasing of goods.
- Control corruption and increase transparency and accountability in all World Bank pharmaceutical lending activities: As pharmaceutical procurement and handling typically involve significant amounts of money, there is a high potential for corruption in the pharmaceutical management chain, from selection of drugs to be procured, to nontransparent contracts, or illegally selling publicly procured drugs. Corruption in the pharmaceutical sector not only means inefficiencies and waste in the health system, but may also result in health risks for the population.
- Create incentives for pharmaceutical research and development targeted at critical diseases of the poor: As the World Bank has financed initiatives such as the UNDP/World Bank/WHO Special Programme for Research and Training in Tropical Diseases (TDR), the Medicines for Malaria Venture (MMV), and the International AIDS Vaccine Initiative (IAVI), collaboration with the private sector is recommended, to stimulate the development of medicines for critical diseases of the poor.
- Expand access to drugs through public-private partnerships and encourage the use of the private sector as a technical resource: A number of public-private interactions aim at increasing access of populations to needed drugs, such as single-drug donation programs of the private sector, efforts to create incentives for the pharmaceutical industry to enter underserved markets (e.g., The GAVI Alliance), and strategies to implement tiered pricing for new drugs. These efforts are believed to offer opportunities to increase access of populations to drugs. In addition, it is believed that the private sector – both for-profit and nonprofit – may be used as a technical resource in defined areas.

Assessing Pharmaceutical Policy

Sound pharmaceutical policy development needs a solid understanding of the problems at hand. This requires evaluations of past policies in a given country context and careful studies of the impacts of possible future policy options. Policy analysis as a discipline is considered as a multidisciplinary social science – drawing particularly from the fields of political science, economics, and sociology (Buse et al., 2005). Research into pharmaceutical policy has similarities with general policy analysis and evaluation. The knowledge base for good pharmaceutical policy making needs to be broad with varied approaches (Almarsdottir and Traulsen, 2006).

Proper pharmaceutical policy making is guided by questions like, 'What works?,' 'What does not work?,' 'Why?' or 'Why not?,' and 'How does it work, and at what cost/benefit?' In particular, users' views on pharmaceutical policies should be studied. Answering these key questions requires using varied approaches ranging from highly quantitative and experimental methodologies to purely qualitative ones. International collaboration between policy makers and other stakeholders is of key importance in these efforts (Almarsdottir and Traulsen, 2006).

Nevertheless, the concept of systematically using evidence in health and pharmaceutical policy making and implementation is relatively new, and its value is not always appreciated. As Traulsen and Almarsdottir (2005a) pointed out:

> Although evidence-based decision making has become routine in medicine and is taking its place in insurance benefit design, there is no comparable trend toward evidence-based policy. Despite rigorous research, numerous health policy publications in the peer-reviewed literature, timely conferences, and methodological advances through professional societies, appeals to evidence as the basis for legislators' decisions are uncommon.

This important conclusion highlights the current challenges of using evidence in pharmaceutical policy making and implementation. Pharmaceutical policy evaluation and analysis is not necessarily difficult, but there are several potential problems (Almarsdottir and Traulsen, 2006):

- *Choosing inappropriate or poor assessment methodologies.* Inappropriate or poor methods and designs are often selected based on the experience of the researcher (or the lack thereof) rather than on the most appropriate for the study in question. Qualitative research often does not have a place in pharmaceutical policy research and evaluation.
- *Not being transparent about assessment designs.* Given the sensitive nature of pharmaceutical policy, full openness about methods is a precondition to using assessment results to develop new policies.
- *Using evaluation questions and policy options that are too narrow.* Pharmaceutical policy analysis and evaluation should be broad and include the full spectrum of options available for policy.
- *Using bias and self-censorship.* Bias and self-censorship may distort study outcomes and be caused by preconceived ideas or financial obligations with funders. Special care must be taken to avoid industrial or political bias.
- *Failing to estimate the effectiveness of pharmaceutical policy interventions* outside of clinical settings.
- *Not applying social science methods* in pharmaceutical policy development.

Although pharmaceutical policy research is slowly gaining ground, it continues to be one of the lower priorities in formulating and evaluating policy. More research data is needed on policy making and on how research data is used. Almarsdottir's and Traulsen's study (2006) joins other calls for putting a stronger focus on using research in analysis, as opposed to basing policies on opinion-based approaches.

Strategies to Develop and Change Pharmaceutical Policies

Pharmaceutical policy development may address the formulation of comprehensive national policies or be limited to specific subcomponents. According to Mossialos *et al.* (2004), common objectives of pharmaceutical policies have been to:

- Enhance quality of care;
- Improve access to pharmaceuticals;
- Improve efficiency in the sector;
- Define roles and responsibilities in the sector;
- Contain expenditures.

These objectives sometimes conflict and policy changes may be difficult to implement. The focus of policy change in developing countries has often been on improving access and quality of care. In industrialized countries the focus has frequently been on containing costs while maintaining access and quality. These different objectives make it difficult to compare policy change processes between developing and industrialized countries.

A recurrent theme of many pharmaceutical policy papers is that effective change strategies include carefully designed mixes of interventions by governments, health delivery systems, health training institutions, professional societies, pharmaceutical companies, and consumers. Such interventions include strengthening regulation, educating medical or pharmaceutical professionals or the general public, and economic interventions to make adequate practices also financially attractive. Available intervention theory appears to agree that multifaceted interventions (e.g., implementing changes in drug reimbursement schemes, accompanied by dissemination of well-tested manuals and broad information campaigns to the medical profession and the general public) are more likely to succeed than small-scale, narrowly focused actions (e.g., mailing printed educational materials only) (Govindaraj *et al.*, 2000; Quick *et al.*, 1997). Another common theme is that professional education is often expected to bring about substantial change. It is now generally recognized, however, that strategies relying heavily on training do not always result in major improvements (Quick *et al.*, 1997; Radyowijati and Haak, 2003).

Pharmaceutical policies are most successful when they include an implementation plan that involves all stakeholders, a human resource development plan, and a monitoring and evaluation plan. A pharmaceutical policy implementation plan will also need sufficient resources to achieve effective change.

Political Management of Change

Designing policies on the basis of careful study of current realities and examples of comparable systems is of major importance. Equally, if not more important, is careful management of the change process. Health and pharmaceutical policy development reform teams tend to focus on the technical rather than the political change process (Reich, 2003). Authoritative policy content–oriented literature is often believed to play a key role in generating changes in pharmaceutical policies. International agencies regularly publish technical literature that they expect governments and technical assistance agencies to consider in their policy development work. As Haak and Claeson argued (1996), however, providing scientific information to change policy may have limited impact. Pharmaceutical policy reforms are often contested because they may change the costs and benefits of different stakeholders, including domestic and international pharmaceutical producers, physician groups, and governments. Some of these stakeholders (e.g., the pharmaceutical industry) are relatively well organized, while others (e.g., patients) may be less able to use political influence. A few patient organizations are well organized and may be able to make their voices well heard in the policy process. The political change process may, in fact, be far more important than the power of individual players, and this process should, therefore, be handled skillfully.

A number of factors are important in the policy change process:

- Policy making is characterized by debate, disagreement, and conflict (Traulsen and Almarsdottir, 2005). Such disagreements should not be considered a complication but a natural occurrence that can, and should be, managed. Negotiation and interaction should take place among all key players in the pharmaceutical sector (Grund, 1996). Such negotiations may be complex and time-consuming.
- Shared values among various interest groups may be used to make policy development successful. The interests of a politically weak group (e.g., consumers) can often be protected if their goals coincide, at least partially, with those of more powerful interest groups (e.g., pharmacists).
- Winner-takes-all approaches should be resisted. The perspective of various interest groups (government, health-care system, providers, patients, public) should be incorporated in pharmaceutical policy making and create a situation in which no one party simply wins or loses.

Politics are bound to be played in all stages of the development policy cycle, including defining problems, defining solutions to be considered, shaping proposals for policy, policy adoption, and policy implementation. There are political limits to trying to implement radical changes in any policy (Reich, 1994), so it is important that these limitations are understood early. Evidence suggests that major policy reform in the health sector is feasible provided it is well defined and well timed. Evidence also suggests that political conditions for policy reform can be shaped by skilled leaders (Reich, 1995).

Explicit political strategies may be employed to enhance the political feasibility of reform (Reich, 2003). Strategies may include helping supporters, weakening arguments of opponents, increasing the commitment of allies or nonmobilized players, decreasing commitment of opponents, and changing the nature of the issue. Support from domestic and international interest groups can be solicited. It may be necessary to enter into bargains and negotiate trade-offs to obtain this support. The consequences of each trade-off in the formulation and implementation of pharmaceutical policies should be carefully considered. Many pharmaceutical policies are usually, not surprisingly, the result of long and painstaking negotiation processes in which several concessions are made by all parties.

Reich (1995) proposed to analyze relevant political conditions so as to shape political factors to achieve policy reform. A method known as political mapping was proposed to help policy makers manage the political dimensions of pharmaceutical policy reform and improve its political feasibility. Reich further argued that health sector reform is a profoundly political process so applied political analysis is required to determine feasibility and enhance the probability of success (1995). An important benefit of political analysis is that it acknowledges that politics are part of policy making, and that it cannot be ignored.

Good timing and careful political maneuvering may allow policy change to occur as was shown by the adoption of a major pharmaceutical policy overhaul in Bangladesh (Reich, 1994). On the other hand, poor timing and failing to take a gradual approach may create social turmoil. In Korea, for example, poor timing and swift radical change in prescribing and dispensing regulations resulted in social tensions (Kim et al., 2004).

Monitoring Pharmaceutical Policy Change

The impact of pharmaceutical policies must be monitored as they evolve. Progress toward achieving targets should be assessed in each policy area and strategies adjusted accordingly. Indicators for monitoring national pharmaceutical policies have been developed by the WHO (Brudon-Jakobowicz et al., 1999), although they may need to be adapted to match particular contexts. Monitoring needs to be carried out using both quantitative and qualitative research methodology. Obviously the actors responsible for policy implementation have a key role in monitoring progress, but independent oversight of the process cannot be left behind.

Policy Enforcement

Although less popular in pharmaceutical policy discussions, pharmaceutical regulation without active enforcement assures neither quality of health care nor of pharmaceutical products. Enforcement of regulations is a problem in many countries, in particular in low-income countries. Many problems in pharmaceutical sectors have their root in financial incentives in their manufacture, importation, supply, prescription, and sales. Sometimes these financial incentives become barriers to evidence-informed policy making, for example, generics of ARV drugs not being registered to protect the interests of the brand-name industry, or mono-component artemisinin medicines not being de-registered, despite the WHO advice to do so. In other cases, regulations are adopted, while enforcement is left behind (e.g., not monitoring the sales of banned pharmaceutical products in pharmacies). Voluntary guidelines and self-regulation, often selected as an acceptable compromise, are rarely effective on their own.

Conclusions

Pharmaceutical policy development is a challenge for governments and health-care systems. The issues are complex; there are many stakeholders with multiple social, economic, and political interests. Agencies, such as the WHO and the World Bank, have supported countries in the development of pharmaceutical policies, through provision of information and examples of 'best practices.' The expectation was that this would result in improved policy making. Evidence-based pharmaceutical policy making has not yet become sufficiently common, however, even though evidence-based decision making is common practice in many other fields of medicine.

The evidence suggests that to stand a chance of being effective, pharmaceutical policy approaches must be based on clear, verifiable data and tailored to individual environments. Carefully designed mixes of actions by several stakeholders are more likely to result in effective system changes than a narrow range of activities. A clear implementation plan and a budget are also key factors in successful pharmaceutical policy development.

Teams responsible for reforming health and pharmaceutical policy development tend to focus on the technical rather than on the political aspects of the change process. However, as politics play a role at all stages of the development and implementation of any policy, politics cannot be ignored. It is important to realize the necessity of managing, rather than ignoring, political factors. Negotiation and concession-making aimed at reaching agreements with all relevant stakeholders should be accepted as part of the whole developmental process.

Furthermore, effective implementation relies on the presence of sound frameworks for monitoring and enforcement. These are especially important in the implementation of any newly designed policy.

To summarize, pharmaceutical policy change is feasible. However, improved access to medicines and containment of their soaring costs – the goals of responsible pharmaceutical policy design – can only be achieved by applying the evidence-based, politically sensitive, new approaches described in this article. Without these, the impetus to improve pharmaceutical policy will remain mere words on paper.

See also: Agenda Setting in Public Health Policy.

Citations

Almarsdottir AB and Traulsen JM (2006) Studying and evaluating pharmaceutical policy – becoming a part of the policy and consultative process. *Pharmacy World and Science* 28: 6–12.

Attaran A (2003) Reply to Dr. Srinivas from Dr. Attaran (cont'd). http://www.essentialdrugs.org/edrug/archive/200304/msg00011.php (accessed November 2007).

Brudon-Jakobowicz P, Rainhorn JD, and Reich MR (1999) *Indicators for Monitoring National Drug Policies. A Practical Manual.* 2nd edn. Geneva, Switzerland: World Health Organization.

Buse K, Mays N, and Walt G (2005) *Making Health Policy.* Milton Keynes, UK: Open University Press.

European Federation of Pharmaceutical Industries and Associations. The Pharmaceutical Industry in Figures. Key Data – 2007 update. http://212.3.246.100/Objects/2/Files/infigures 2007.pdf.

Govindaraj R, Reich MR, and Cohen JC (2000) World Bank pharmaceuticals. Internal discussion paper (unpublished).

Grund J (1996) The societal value of pharmaceuticals: Balancing industrial and healthcare policy. *Pharmacoeconomics* 10: 14–22.

Haak H and Claeson ME (1996) Regulatory actions to enhance appropriate drug use: The case of antidiarrhoeal drugs. *Social Science and Medicine* 42: 1011–1019.

Herxheimer A (2003) Relationships between the pharmaceutical industry and patients' organisations. *British Medical Journal* 326: 1208–1210.

Hughes T (2004) Big Pharma vs. Australian Pharmaceutical Benefits Scheme. http://www.bmj.com/cgi/eletters/329/7475/1169#85148 (last accessed November 2007).

Kim HJ, Chung W, and Lee SG (2004) Lessons from Korea's pharmaceutical policy reform: the separation of medical institutions and pharmacies for outpatient care. *Health Policy* 68: 267–275.

Laing R (2003) Whose interests does the World Trade Organization serve? *The Lancet* 361(9365): 1297.

Mossialos E, Walley T, and Mrazek M (2004) Regulating pharmaceuticals in Europe: An overview. In: Mossialos E, Walley T and Mrazek M (eds.) *Regulating Pharmaceuticals in Europe: Striving for Efficiency, Equity and Quality.* Milton Keynes, UK: Open University Press.

Novartis International (2007) Perspectives from Novartis: An open letter. http://www.essentialdrugs.org/edrug/archive/200702/msg00008.php (accessed November 2007).

Quick JD, Rankin JR, Laing RO, O'Connor RW, Hogerzeil HV, Dukes MNG, and Garnett A (eds.) (1997) *Managing Drug Supply,* 2nd ed. West Hartford, CT: Kumarian Press.

Radyowijati A and Haak H (2003) Improving antibiotic use in low-income countries: An overview of evidence on determinants. *Social Science and Medicine* 57: 733–744.

Reich MR (1994) Bangladesh pharmaceutical policy and politics. *Health Policy and Planning* 9: 130–143.

Reich MR (1995) The politics of health sector reform in developing countries: three cases of pharmaceutical policy. *Health Policy* 32: 47–77.

Reich MR (2003) Introduction to political analysis. Flagship course on health sector reform and sustainable financing. USA: Boston13–31 January 2003.

Smith MC (1983) *Principles of Pharmaceutical Marketing.* Philadelphia, PA: Lea and Febiger.

The Economist (2001) Drug-induced dilemma. *The Economist* 19 April 2001 (available in Google).

Traulsen JM and Almarsdottir AB (2005a) The argument for pharmaceutical policy. *Pharmacy World and Science* 27: 7–12.

Traulsen JM and Almarsdottir AB (2005b) Pharmaceutical policy and the lay public. *Pharmacy World and Science* 27: 273–277.

WHO (1998) *Health Reform and Drug Financing: Selected Topics.* WHO/DAP/98.3 Geneva, Switzerland: World Health Organization.

WHO (2000) Medicines Strategy 2000–2003: *Framework for Action in Essential Drugs and Medicines Policy.* Geneva, Switzerland: World Health Organization.

WHO (2001) How to Develop and Implement a National Drug Policy. 2nd edition. Geneva, Switzerland: World Health Organization.

WHO (2004) *Medicines Strategy 2004–2007: Countries at the Core.* Geneva, Switzerland: World Health Organization.

Further Reading

Abraham J (1995) *Science, Politics and the Pharmaceutical Industry*. London: Routledge.
Avorn J (2005) *Powerful Medicines: The Benefits, Risks, and Costs of Prescription Drugs*. New York: Vintage Books.
Brody H (2007) *Hooked: Ethics, the Medical Profession and the Pharmaceutical Industry*. Lanham: Rowman and Littlefield.
Cohen JC, Schuklenk U, and Illingsworth P (2006) *The Power of Pills: Social, Ethical and Legal Issues in Drug Development, Marketing, and Pricing*. London: Pluto Press.
Davis P (ed.) (1996) *Contested Ground: Public Concern and Private Interest in the Regulation of Pharmaceuticals*. Oxford, UK: Oxford University Press.
Goozner M (2004) *The $800 Million Pill: The Truth Behind the Cost of New Drugs*. Berkley, CA: University of California Press.
Hansson O (1989) *Inside Ciba Geigy*. Penang: International Organization of Consumers Unions.
LeCarre J (2001) *The Constant Gardener*. London: Hodder and Stoughton.
Medawar C (1992) *Power and Dependence: Social Audit on the Safety of Medicines*. London: Social Audit.
Moynihan R and Cassels A (2005) *Selling Sickness*. Sydney, Australian: Allen and Unwin.
Permanand G (2006) *EU Pharmaceutical Regulation*. Manchester, UK: Manchester University Press.
Reynolds-Whyte S, van der Geest S, and Hardon AP (2002) *Social Lives of Medicines*. Cambridge, UK: Cambridge University Press.
Silverman M, Lydecker M, and Lee PR (1992) *Bad Medicine: The Prescription Drug Industry in the Third World*. Stanford, CA: Stanford University Press.

Relevant Websites

http://www.clintonfoundation.org – Clinton Foundation.
http://www.cptech.org – Consumer Project on Technology.
http://www.essentialdrugs.org – E-drug Discussion Forum.
http://www.efpia.org/Content/Default.asp – European Federation of Pharmaceutical Industries and Associations.
http://www.haiweb.org – Health Action International – Europe.
http://www.healthyskepticism.org – Healthy Skepticism – Countering Misleading Drug Promotion.
http://www.accessmed.msf.org – Médecins Sans Frontières – Campaign for Access to Essential Medicines.
http://www.socialaudit.org.uk – The Social Audit website.
http://www.worldbank.org – The World Bank.
http://www.who.int/medicines – World Health Organization – Medicines.
http://www.wto.org – The World Trade Organization (WTO).

Long Term Care in Health Services

J Brodsky, Myers-JDC-Brookdale Institute, Jerusalem, Israel
A M Clarfield, Ben-Gurion University, Beersheba, Israel

© 2008 Elsevier Inc. All rights reserved.

For the most part long-term care (LTC) has not been among the main concerns of health policy makers. Cost-containment issues, perhaps an excessive focus on specialized medical care, and the fact that families have always been and remain the major providers of LTC have contributed to a slow development of public long-term care services (WHO, 2000). However, demographic transitions are resulting in dramatic changes in health needs around the world. Care for the chronically ill and for those with disabilities and a steep rise in the numbers of elderly are a growing challenge in practically all societies.

Definition and the Target Population in Need of LTC

LTC includes activities undertaken for persons who are not fully capable of self-care on a long-term basis by informal caregivers (family and friends), formal caregivers, and volunteers.

The target population includes those who suffer from any kind of physical or mental disability requiring assistance with the activities of daily living.

LTC encompasses a broad array of services such as personal care and assistive devices that are designed to minimize, restore, or compensate for the loss of independent physical or mental functioning.

Disability also results in difficulties in accessing health care and in complying with health-care regimes, and it affects the ability of the individual to maintain a healthy lifestyle to prevent deterioration in functional status. Therefore, LTC includes efforts to ensure access to acute, chronic care and rehabilitation services and to prevent deterioration of the functional capacity of the disabled (such as, for example, preventing bedsores and preventing depression). The central role of the family in providing LTC requires significant efforts to inform and guide the families (WHO, 2002).

The Uniqueness of Long-Term Care

Whereas more traditional health care is concerned with cure and recovery, LTC attempts mainly to contribute to alleviating suffering, maintaining the best possible quality of life, reducing discomfort, improving the limitations caused by diseases and disability, and maintaining the best possible levels of functioning (Larizgoitia, 2003).

An additional significant difference between LTC and the acute sector is that the provision of LTC is heavily based on unspecialized, labor-intensive, and relatively unskilled providers. Professionals (physicians, nurses, social workers, and others) are involved to a degree that is significantly less than that in acute care. LTC allows lay volunteers, in particular the family, to take part in its implementation. Indeed, in most countries, care is still predominantly a family task – mainly performed by women. Despite the increasing role of the government, nongovernmental organizations (NGOs) and the private (for-profit) sectors in service provision, informal care has remained the dominant form of care (Wiener, 2003). However, the increasing proportion of women in the labor market and the declining ratio between those needing care and those who are potential caregivers are raising questions of whether informal care will maintain its predominant role.

Issues in the Organization and Provision of LTC Services

All developed countries have established LTC programs under the auspices of health and welfare services, and many developing countries are in the initial stages of some development. Programs usually include some combination of health, social, housing, transportation, and support services for people with physical, mental, or cognitive limitations. However, there is no single paradigm and there are a number of different approaches in the organization and provision of LTC. An understanding of the nature of the variance among countries is important to provide insight for development of care policies.

Countries differ in the way they have resolved basic design issues. Among the most central issues are the nature of entitlements, targeting and finance; service delivery strategies; and issues of integration between LTC and health and social services.

Nature of Entitlements, Targeting and Finance

Among the most significant key policy design issues are the principles of eligibility for publicly subsidized LTC services and the nature of entitlements. Underlying these issues are two fundamental decisions:

1. Who does a country decide to support – everyone or only the poor?
2.. Should access to services be based on an entitlement (insurance principle) or subject to budget constraints (tax-funded principle)?

Such questions also arise in the provision of acute care. What is unique, however, to LTC is the additional possibility that the family might at least in part meet these needs for many individuals. Thus, underlying this determination is society's view of the appropriate and expected roles of the people with disabilities and their families.

The choice among different options is often between selective (or means-tested) and universal approaches to service provision. Support for the poor is obviously based on a concern for their inability to purchase these services and can lead to an exclusive focus on this group. Even if such is one's primary goal, this can lead to a strategy that supports the nonpoor, if it is believed that including them in a more universal program is the best way to mobilize support for the poor and to avoid the problems associated with programs for the poor, such as low quality. Support for the broader population can have several rationales, including:

- The catastrophic potential nature of LTC costs when broad segments of the population may find it difficult to pay; when resources are depleted, they become a burden on public programs;
- Concern with the broader social costs of care provision and an interest in easing the burden on families (particularly women);
- Reducing utilization of more costly acute care (particularly hospitalization) services by substituting LTC and in part by medicalizing it.

A second key question is whether access to LTC services should be based on an entitlement or subject to budget constraints. An entitlement program means that, irrespective of available budgets, everyone who fulfills the eligibility criteria must be granted benefits.

Entitlement programs are generally financed through insurance-type prepayments, whereas nonentitlement programs are usually financed through general taxation. A prepayment is generally viewed as granting a right to a service.

It should be kept in mind that an entitlement approach can influence the targeting of services. With contributory entitlement, strict income testing is unlikely to be adopted so as to prevent exclusion from benefits for the many who contribute to financing the program. Nonentitlement programs, focused primarily on the poor, will usually have a relatively strict means test.

The decision to adopt an entitlement approach and a contributory finance system has implications for additional eligibility criteria. The nature of family availability and support will not typically be taken into account in an insurance framework.

A third implication is that under an entitlement system, benefit levels are set relatively lower because family support is not a criterion, and benefits will be provided to many who might already be receiving significant family support. Setting low benefit levels also reflects concern with cost control. In an entitlement system, cost is not easily predictable or defined because it is determined by the number of eligible applicants.

We can illustrate the variation in these fundamental design issues by using a couple of examples. On the one hand, in the UK, provision of LTC is normally income tested and provided on a budget-restricted basis. On the other hand, Scandinavian countries (e.g. Sweden) have a policy commitment to maintaining high levels of services to the entire population and not only for the poor, even though services are financed through general taxation. There are user charges related to income, but given the high level of pensions, this has not been a significant barrier for those who need LTC services. Most Canadian provinces are somewhere in between countries like the UK and the Scandinavian countries with respect to targeting the poor (UK Royal Commission on Long-Term Care, 1999).

The Medicaid program in the United States is an interesting example of a system that while focusing on the poor and financed by general tax revenues provides an entitlement subject to a strict means test.

In recent years, a number of countries have adopted a broader insurance-based approach and a full entitlement. This model includes Germany, Austria, Holland, Israel, and more recently Japan (Brodsky et al., 2000).

Service Delivery Strategies: Balancing Care in the Home, in the Community, and in Institutions

Another element of variation among countries is reflected in the actual package of services offered to people with disabilities. There is no universally agreed-upon package of LTC services. For one thing, countries are in different stages of economic development, and some can afford a more comprehensive package than others. In addition, countries have different sociodemographic and epidemiological patterns, cultures, and values, which can all play an important role in defining the needs and priorities. For example, in Sweden most families do not feel obligated to look after older parents, believing that this is just as much the role of government. In contrast, in Israel much more is expected of family members (and less by government).

One of the most important distinguishing dimensions among services is the location in which these services are to be provided, collectively referred to as a continuum of care: home-based, in ambulatory settings in the community, or in a LTC institutional setting.

Home-based programs
Such programs may include

- Home health services – include skilled medical/nursing care, health promotion, prevention of functional deterioration, training and education, facilitation of self-care, and palliative care;
- Personal care – care related with activities of daily living (ADL) (e.g., bathing, dressing, eating, and toileting);
- Homemaking – assistance with instrumental activities of daily living (IADL) (e.g., meal preparation, cleaning, and shopping);
- Assistive devices, physical adaptations of the home, and special technologies (alarm systems).

Ambulatory settings
Ambulatory settings in the community can provide a different package of services, which may be more health related or more social related. For example, some models of day-care provision focus on health-related services such as monitoring of health status and rehabilitation, whereas others focus on providing the disabled person opportunities for recreation and socialization.

Institutional services
This model includes a wide range of institutions which provide various levels of maintenance and personal or nursing care. There are LTC institutions aimed mainly at addressing housing needs and providing opportunities for recreation and socialization, whereas others (usually referred to as nursing homes or skilled nursing homes) address health-related needs. The first type serves the moderately disabled, whereas the second type the more severely disabled.

Assistive living, service-enriched housing, and sheltered housing
This model includes special housing units that offer independent living but also services and care to an extent, which, in some cases, comes close to a modern, noncustodial institution. These kinds of sheltered accommodations are now substituting the traditional residential homes, and to some extent also nursing homes.

Whereas almost all industrialized countries offer a broad package of services, the absolute level and the relative importance of the service mix vary. There is also noticeable convergence. In most industrialized countries, the share of the older population (over 65) in institutions varies between 5 and 7%. This percentage does not appear to have grown dramatically in recent years despite continued aging of older populations, and in some countries such as Canada and Holland, it has even declined.

Partly because of the rising cost of institutional care, a focus on community care has taken place in many industrialized countries. 'Aging in place' is perceived as preferred by the elderly and, in the majority of cases, as a less expensive alternative to institutional care. One of the hopes of those planning various LTC programs was that their broader availability would reduce costs by reducing acute care hospital utilization and the demand for long-term institutional care. In Japan and Canada, for example, there is an overuse of acute beds by those needing LTC. As a result, reforms have been introduced in Quebec. The Netherlands is one of the countries in which the level of institutional care has been particularly high. The Dutch government has actively implemented experimental programs aimed at reducing institutionalization.

Although the infrastructure of supportive services has grown, the expectation of diverting a significant number of disabled elderly people from nursing homes has been somewhat scaled down in many countries. The extent to which the various LTC programs have influenced patterns of referral to institutions has depended in part on the extent and type of community care available. When such services are limited, they are less likely to offer an alternative to institutionalization, particularly for the more severely disabled elderly.

More recently, some countries have highlighted the potential of health services such as post-acute care and rehabilitation in delaying or preventing long-term institutionalization. Over and above the availability of community services, other factors may affect an elderly client's ability to choose between community and institutional services, including the supply of beds and the level of copayments for institutional care. In Germany, for example, a copayment of 25% is levied on people entering LTC to keep such care from becoming financially preferable to home care. Japan has made similar efforts to damp down institutional demand.

There is a wide variation in the provision of home care. For example, home help (nursing and assistance in activities of daily living) has been estimated to be provided to between 5 and 17% of the population, depending on the country (OECD, 1999).

In some countries, greater individual flexibility in choice of care delivery has been considered, for example, the provision of cash benefits in addition to or instead of services in-kind. There are three basic forms of provision: services in kind (e.g., Israel); cash allowances without restrictions which enables a client to use the funds as he or she sees fit (e.g., Germany and Austria); and cash allowances with a restriction to purchase services (e.g., experimental programs in Holland and the United States).

Long-Term Care Assessment

Assessment in LTC serves multiple purposes: to determine eligibility for services, develop the most appropriate care plan according to clients' needs, monitor clients' status over time, and assess services' outcomes in relation to functional needs or maintaining maximum function and enhancing the quality of life of people with disabilities and of their families. At a health-service level, measures may be used to monitor quality of care, allocate resources based on case mix, and even to plan for the development of appropriate resources (Berg and Mor, 2001). The desired characteristics of an assessment instrument will vary relative to the objective of the assessment, but the same instruments can sometimes be used for multiple purposes. Comprehensive assessment should address different domains of impairment (e.g., cognitive status, strength, sensory and perceptual deficits), disability (e.g., measures of activities of daily living), and health-related quality of life (e.g., mental health and emotional well-being). For each domain, there is no single best measure. There is general agreement as to the types of domains and indicators that should be included in assessment for long-term care, although the relative weights to be placed on these various domains are more debatable.

There are numerous available assessment instruments that focus on particular aspects of LTC. **Table 1** gives selective examples of some of the most established instruments developed in the United States and Europe. Some of these instruments are quite culturally specific and would need to be adapted not only to other languages but also to other cultures and worldviews.

In the United States, Medicare and Medicaid authorities, along with the development of managed care, have given a tremendous push to research in this area (Shaughnessy *et al.*, 1994). One of the best-known LTC assessment tools is the Minimal Data Set (MDS). Its main aim is to provide a reliable, uniform, and universal set of data across settings and for different purposes, which are used to inform care planning to provide a basis for external quality surveys and internal continuous quality improvement and in the case mix adjusted reimbursement systems. Although MDS began in institutions in the United States, it has since been expanded for home care and other settings, and has been used in both English- and non-English-speaking countries.

Issues of Integration between LTC and Health and Social Services

A major concern involves the continuum of care between the acute and LTC systems, and between the health and social service systems. However, one of the major problems in many countries is fragmentation of such services (Clarfield *et al.*, 2001). The interest in integration arises out of a number of concerns for the quality and efficiency of care. These include the ability to provide for coordinated care packages, consider alternative services in the most optimal way, and ease the access to services by offering one easily identified source of provision. Nevertheless, it is by no means simple to provide integrated LTC because services are the responsibility of many jurisdictions, and the various components tend to work in parallel with separate funding streams and budgets.

Links between LTC and acute health systems can encourage continuity of care. These connections may

Table 1 Long-term care: Examples of assessment instruments

Assessment domain	Examples of indicators	Examples of standardized measures
Activities of daily living (ADL)	Ambulation; toileting; continence; personal hygiene; dressing; mobility; locomotion	Katz Index; Barthel Index; Functional Independence Measure (FIM); Mobility Assessment
Instrumental activities of daily living (IADL)	Meal preparation; housekeeping; shopping; laundry; management of oral medications; use of transportation; basic finances	PSG Scale
Health status	Skin condition; pain interfering with activity; nutritional status and significant weight loss; pressure ulcers; falls	Minimum Data Set (MDS); the Mini Nutritional Assessment (MNA)
Cognitive status	Cognitive functioning: memory; decision making; language; orientation	Mini-Mental State (MMSE); The CERAD Assessment Packet
Emotional/behavioral status (affect)	Anxiety level; level of social interaction; level of social participation; behavioral problems; depression	Geriatric Depression Scale (GDS); Neuropsychiatric Inventory (NPI); the CERAD Behavior Rating Scale for Dementia (BRSD)
General quality of life measures and measures of well-being	Multidimensional indicators including health, mental, emotional, social status	SF-36; General Health Questionnaire (GHQ); Philadelphia Geriatric Center Morale Scale (PGCMS)
Family/caregiver strain	Caregiver burden (physical, emotional, economic, social); effect of caregiving on the relationship between caregiver and care receiver; abuse	Burden Interview (BI); Caregiver Social Impact Scale; Caregiving Appraisal Scale (CAS); Cost of Care Index (CCI)

reduce acute hospital stays and create an incentive to provide adequate home health care and rehabilitation, especially if the health-care providers can enjoy the benefits of reduced institutional long-term care. At the same time, there are concerns about linking LTC with primary health care that generate interest in independent models of LTC. The impact of integration on incentives to provide adequate LTC are neither certain nor easily predictable. Within health systems, there is concern for a preference toward addressing acute care needs over those that are more chronic or function related. A related concern is for the overmedicalization of LTC services if provided in a medically oriented system and the consequences of higher costs as a result. In addition, in the United States, for example, the integration of acute and LTC has depended on integrating medical and social care funding streams. There is a belief that such integrated funding is the basis for program integration. However, although such linkage is necessary, it is insufficient. Successful integration requires a major reorganization of the programmatic infrastructure, which can then be reinforced with funding approaches (Kane, 2003).

In general, most developed countries have not fully integrated LTC within the acute system. Some countries have made an effort to partially integrate components of LTC (e.g., Germany), where it is administratively but not financially integrated. Other countries have implemented demonstration projects that fully integrate acute and LTC such as the PACE program in the United States and the SIPA program in Quebec (Béland et al., 2006).

The PACE – program for all-inclusive care of the elderly – was implemented experimentally in one neighborhood in San Francisco in the 1970s and has been expanded to some 36 locations throughout the United States. The model enables the resources for acute and long-term care to be pooled. Disabled elderly who join the program receive a variety of services under one roof. Those eligible for the program are disabled elderly who are eligible to enter long-term care facilities from Medicaid, but who remain in their homes. The program is funded on a capitation basis by Medicare and Medicaid.

SIPA – French acronym for system of integrated care for older persons – is an integrated system of social, medical, and short- and long-term hospital services offered in both the community and institutions to vulnerable elderly persons. It has been implemented in Canada. Its distinguishing features are community-based multidisciplinary teams with full clinical responsibility for delivering integrated care through the provision of community health and social services and the coordination of hospital and nursing home care; all within a publicly managed and funded system.

In the absence of integrated systems, many countries have been experimenting with various coordinating mechanisms such as care management.

Conclusions

Care for people with disabilities is a major challenge in industrialized as well as in developing countries. We have shown that although almost all industrialized countries offer a broad package of services, their level and mix vary among countries. In some areas there seems to be more convergence, whereas in others, policies have taken a different route and differ on principles of targeting, entitlement, and finance. There is much to be learned from the experience of industrialized countries in defining the range of options and in learning from some of the disadvantages and advantages of these systems. Unfortunately, the ability to learn from the experience is limited by the lack of adequate systems for monitoring outcomes and evaluating implementation, as well as in difficulty in 'comparing apples and oranges.' As LTC programs continue to develop, it is hoped that more attention will be given to systematic and comparative evaluations.

See also: Comparative Health Systems.

Citations

Béland F, Bergman H, Lebel L, *et al.* (2006) Integrated services for frail elders (SIPA): A trial of a model for Canada. *Canadian Journal of Aging* 25(1): 25–42.

Berg K and Mor V (2001) Long term care assessment. In: Maddox (ed.) *The Encyclopedia of Aging*, 3rd ed., pp. 631–633. New York: Springer.

Brodsky J, Habib J, and Mizrahi I (2000) *Long-Term Care Laws in Five Developed Countries*. Geneva. Switzerland: World Health Organization, WHO/NMH/CCL/00.2.

Clarfield AM, Bergman H, and Kane R (2001) Fragmentation of care for frail older people – an international problem. Experience from three countries: Israel, Canada and the United States. *Journal of the American Geriatric Association* 49(12): 1714–1721.

Cummings JL, Mega M, Gray K, Rosenberg-Thompson S, Carusi DA, and Gornbein PH (1994) The neuropsychiatric inventory: Comprehensive assessment of psychopathology in dementia. *Neurology* 44: 2308–2314.

Folstein MF, Folstein SE, and McHugh PR (1975) Mini mental state: A practical method for grading the conginitive state of patients for the clinician. *Journal of Psychiatric Research* 12: 189–198.

Golberg DP and Hillier VF (1989) A scaled version of the general health questionnaire. *Psychological Medicine* 9: 139–145.

Heyman A, Fillenbaum G, and Nash F (eds.) (1997) Consortium to Establish a Registry for Alzheimer's Disease: The CERAD experience. *Neurology* 49 (suppl 3, whole issue).

James LM, Mack J, Patterson M, and Tariot P (1999) Behavior rating scale for dementia: Development of test scales and presentation of data for 555 individuals with Alzheimer's disease. *Journal of Geriatric Psychiatry and Neurology* 12(4): 211–223.

Kane R (2003) The interface of LTC and other components of the health and social services systems in North America. In: Brodsky J, Habib J, and Hirschfeld M (eds.) *Key Policy Issues in Long-Term Care*, pp. 63–90. Geneva: World Health Organization.

Katz S, Ford AB, Moskowitz RW, Jackson BA, and Jaffe MW (1963) The Index of ADL: A standardized measure of biological psychosocial function. *Journal of the American Medical Association* 185: 914–919.

Keith RA, Granger CV, Hamilton BB, *et al.* (1987) The Functional Independence Measure (FIM): A new tool for rehabilitation. *Advances in Clinical Rehabilitation* 1: 6–18.

Kosberg JI and Cairl RE (1986) The cost of care index: A case management tool for screening informal care providers. *The Gerontologist* 26(3): 273–278.

Larizgoitia I (2003) Approaches to evaluating LTC systems. In: Brodsky J, Habib J, and Hirschfeld M (eds.) *Key Policy Issues in Long-term Care*, pp. 227–242. Geneva: World Health Organization, ISBN 92 4 156225 0.

Lawton MP (1975) The Philadelphia Geriatric Center Morale Scale: a revision. *Journal of Gerontology* 30(1): 85–89.

Lawton MP and Brody EM (1969) Assessment of older people: Self-maintaining and instrumental activities of daily living. *Gerontologist* 9: 179–186.

Lawton MP, Kleban MH, Moss M, *et al.* (1989) Measuring caregiving appraisal. *Journal of Gerontology* 44(3): 61–71.

Mahoney FJ and Barthel DW (1965) Functional evaluation: The Barthel Index. *Medical Journal of Rehabilitation* 14: 61–65.

Morris JN, Fries BE, Steel K, *et al.* (1997) Comprehensive clinical assessment in community setting: applicability of the MDS-HC. *Journal of the American Geriatric Society* 45(8): 1017–1024.

OECD (1999) *A Caring World*. Paris, France: Organization for Economic Cooperation and Development.

Poulschock SW and Deimling GT (1984) Families caring for elders in residence: Issues in the measurement of burden. *Journal of Gerontology* 39(2): 230–239.

Royal Commission on Long-Term Care (1999) *With Respect to Old Age: Long-term Care – rights and Responsibilities*. United Kingdom: The Stationery Office.

Shaughnessy PW, Crisler KS, Schlenker RE, *et al.* (1994) Measuring and assuring the quality of home health care. *Health Care Financing Review* 16(1): 35–67.

Sheikh JI and Yesavage JA (1986) Geriatric Depression Scale (GDS): *Recent Evidence and Development of a Shorter Version. Clinical gerontology: A Guide to Assessment and Intervention*, pp. 165–173. New York: The Haworth Press.

Tinetti ME (1986) Performance-oriented assessment of mobility problems in elderly patients. *Journal of the American Geriatric Society* 34(2): 119–126.

Vellas B, Guigoz Y, Garry PJ, *et al.* (1999) The Mini Nutritional Assessment (MNA) and its use in grading the nutritional state of elderly patients. *Nutrition* 15(2): 116–122.

Ware JE, Jr. and Sherbourne CD (1992) The MOS 36-Item Short-Form Health Survey (SF-36). *Medical Care* 30(6): 473–483.

WHO (2000) *WHO Study Group on Home-based Long Term Care*. Geneva, Switzerland: World Health Organization, Technical Report Series, No. 898.

WHO (2002) *Lessons for Long-term Care Policy*. Geneva, Switzerland: World Health Organization, WHO/NMH7CCL/02.1.

Wiener J (2003) The role of informal support in long-term care. In: Brodsky J, Habib J, and Hirschfeld M (eds.) *Key Policy Issues in Long-term Care*, pp. 3–24. Geneva, Switzerland: World Health Organization.

Zarit SH, Reever KE, and Bach-Peterson J (1980) Relatives of the elderly: Correlates of feelings of burden. *The Gerontologist* 20: 649–655.

Further Reading

Brodsky J, Habib J, and Hirschfeld M (eds.) (2003) *Long-Term Care in Developing Countries: Ten Case Studies*. Geneva, Switzerland: World Health Organization.

Brodsky J, Habib J, Hirschfeld M, and Siegel B (2002) Care of the frail elderly in developed and developing countries: The experience and the challenges. *Aging Clinical and Experimental Research* 14(4): 279–286.

Feldman PH and Kane RL (2003) Strengthening research to improve the practice and management of long-term care. *The Milbank Quarterly* 81(2): 179–220.

Jacobzone S (1999) *Ageing and Care for Frail Elderly Persons: An Overview of International Perspectives*. Paris: Organization for Economic Cooperation and Development (OECD), Labour Market and Social Policy– Occasional Papers, No. 38.

Ikegami N and Campbell JC (2002) Choices, policy logics and problems in the design of long-term care systems. *Social Policy and Administration* 36(7): 719–734.

Kane RA, Kane RL, and Ladd R (1998) *The Heart of Long-Term Care*. New York: Oxford University Press.

Kodner DL (2004) Following the logic of long term care: Toward an independent but integrated sector. *International Journal of Integrated Care* 4. http://www.ijic.org (accessed November 2007).

Morris JN, Fries BE, Steel K, et al. (1997) Comprehensive clinical assessment in community settings: applicability of the MDS-HC. *Journal of the American Geriatrics Society* 45(8): 1017–1024.

OECD (1996) *Caring for Frail Older People, Policies in Evolution*. Paris, France: Organization for Economic Cooperation and Development, Social Policies Studies No. 19.

Pacolet J, Bouten R, Lanoye H, and Vesieck K (1999) *Social Protection for Dependency in Old Age in the 15 EU Member States and Norway*. Luxemburg: Employment & Social Affairs ~ Social Security and Social Integration, European Commission, Office for Official Publications of the European Communities.

Stone R (2000) *Long-Term Care for the Elderly with Disabilities: Current Policy, Emerging Trends, and Implications for the Twenty-First Century*. New York: Milbank Memorial Fund.

Relevant Websites

http://www.cdc.gov/ – Centers for Disease Control and Prevention.
http://www.medicare.gov/ – Medicare, U.S. Department of Health and Human Services.
http://www.oecd.org/document/ – Organisation for Economic Co-operation and Development.http://www.archive.official-documents.co.uk/ – Official-Documents.co.uk.
http://www.nia.nih.gov/ – National Institute on Aging, U.S. National Institutes of Health.
http://www.who.int/topics/longterm_care/en/ – World Health Organization, health topics, long-term care.

Long Term Care for Aging Populations

E Stallard, Duke University, Durham, NC, USA

© 2008 Elsevier Inc. All rights reserved.

Long-term care (LTC) encompasses a wide range of health and social services including skilled and intermediate nursing care, assisted living, custodial or personal care, adult day care, respite care, home health care, and hospice care; LTC generally does not include care in short-stay hospitals (Actuarial Standards Board, 1999).

The primary use of LTC is among people with limitations in one or more activities of daily living (ADLs) or instrumental activities of daily living (IADLs), and people with cognitive impairment (CI), where the expected duration of the limitation or impairment is at least 3 months. Some people use LTC throughout their lives; more generally, the use of LTC increases exponentially with age, making it a significant health and financial risk for the elderly. Use of LTC is associated with developmental disabilities and mental illnesses, chronic diseases, injuries, disabling conditions, physiological frailty, and dementia. LTC use rates are high in the period preceding death. Recovery from conditions requiring LTC declines with age; higher recovery rates among the elderly occur at ages 65–74 and lower rates at ages 85+.

LTC financing varies substantially between and within countries, and according to the LTC user's income, assets, and social support networks. This article focuses on LTC in the United States.

LTC Surveys

The population using LTC can be defined narrowly based on ADL limitations and more broadly using IADL limitations and/or CI. Variations in operational implementations of each definition can yield vastly different estimates of the size of the population using LTC and its change over time. Wiener *et al.* (1990) reviewed the measurement of ADL status in 11 national surveys and found that the prevalence of ADL limitations among noninstitutionalized persons in the 1984 National Health Interview Survey Supplement on Aging (NHIS-SOA) was 62% of that in the 1987 National Medical Expenditure Survey (NMES) and 56% of that in the 1984 National Long-Term Care Survey (NLTCS).

Freedman *et al.* (2002) reviewed the quality and consistency of disability trends in seven national surveys and assigned the best ratings to the NLTCS and to a combination of the National Health Interview Survey (NHIS) and the National Nursing Home Survey (NNHS). The NLTCS used a nationally representative stratified list sample of elderly Medicare enrollees aged 65+ years; the NHIS used a complex area-probability sample of the civilian noninstitutionalized population, covering all ages; the NNHS used a stratified two-stage list sample of nursing homes, covering all ages. The combined NHIS-NNHS sample, in theory, overlaps and extends to all ages the elderly sample of the NLTCS.

Rogers and Komisar (2003) used the combined 2000 NHIS-NNHS to estimate that 9.5 million persons had ADL or IADL limitations, of whom 3.5 million were younger than age 65 and 6.0 million were aged 65+. Manton and Gu (2001) used the 1999 NLTCS to estimate that 7.0 million persons aged 65+ had ADL or IADL limitations. The 1.0 million person difference at age 65+ was the difference between the estimates of the size of the noninstitutionalized LTC population: 4.5 million in the NHIS versus 5.5 million in the NLTCS.

Kinosian (2006) performed detailed comparisons of ADL limitations in the NHIS and NLTCS and found that the 1999 NHIS estimate for noninstitutionalized persons was 72.4% of that in the 1999 NLTCS; in contrast, the 1999 NNHS estimate for institutionalized persons was 99.6% of that in the 1999 NLTCS. Blackwell and Tonthat (2003) reported estimates for noninstitutionalized persons in the 1999 NHIS that were 82.8% of the 1999 NLTCS estimates.

The above comparisons indicate that the estimates of the size of the population using LTC will depend on the source of the data used in making the estimates, even when using data that are judged to be of high quality and reliability. Time differences in the relative sizes of the NHIS and NLTCS estimates can produce trend differences in the rates of change of the sizes of the population using LTC.

NLTCS

The best source for details on the use of LTC in the US is the NLTCS. Its purpose was to measure LTC disability and the use of LTC services among the U.S. elderly aged 65+ at multiple points in time. It included six closely related surveys conducted in 1982, 1984, 1989, 1994, 1999, and 2004. LTC disability included ADL and IADL limitations, cognitive impairment (CI), and institutionalization. The six waves constituted a nationally representative longitudinal sample of 49 274 Medicare enrollees aged 65+. Beginning in 1984, each wave added a replenishment sample of approximately 5000 persons who had passed their 65th birthday since the closing date of the sample drawn for the prior wave. The replenishment sample ensured that each wave contained a representative cross-sectional sample of approximately 20 000 elderly Medicare enrollees. The response rates were generally 95% or higher, except for 2004, which dropped to 91%.

The NLTCS employed a two-stage sampling of Medicare enrollment files. The first stage consisted of a short screener interview to assess the inability of a community resident to perform nine ADLs and seven IADLs without help or to determine that the respondent was a resident of a nursing home or a similar LTC institution. Help meant assistance from another person or special equipment needed to perform the activity. The IADLs were recognized as being limited only when the inability to perform the activity was the result of a disability or health problem. A community resident screened in if the duration of the ADL and/or IADL limitation was expected to be at least 3 months. Institutionalized persons screened in without any additional conditions.

The second stage consisted of a detailed in-person assessment that was given to new and prior screened-in persons, institutionalized persons, and certain supplemental samples of persons who screened out at the first-stage assessment. The ADLs and IADLs were modified in the second stage to facilitate the detailed assessment of the nature of the limitations. One ADL was dropped and one was moved to the IADL list, where it was separated into two component activities. These changes yielded seven ADLs and nine IADLs.

The nine IADLs were light housework, laundry, meal preparation, grocery shopping, outside mobility, travel, managing money, taking medication, and making telephone calls. An IADL limitation was recognized only when caused by a disability or health problem. A tenth IADL, heavy housework, was also assessed but was not part of the screener criteria.

The seven ADLs were eating, inside mobility, transferring, dressing, bathing, toileting, and continence. The NLTCS questions allowed the ADL limitations to be classified according to the following hierarchy:

1. needs, but does not receive, help with ADL;
2. performs ADL with special equipment;
3. uses standby help with/without special equipment;
4. uses active help with/without special equipment;
5. unable to perform ADL.

Questions were also asked about the elapsed (but not expected) duration of the ADL limitations and the frequency of help. Beginning in 1994, questions were asked about whether the help actually received on specific ADLs was enough to meet the respondent's needs, and if not, the frequency at which such insufficiencies occurred.

Continence was included in the first-stage screener interview and as part of the toileting module in the second-stage detailed interview; however, it did not trigger the toileting ADL nor was it included as part of the standard set of six flap-item ADLs designed to identify disabled persons in the NLTCS.

The NLTCS did not screen for CI in the first-stage assessment. The second-stage detailed interviews employed the Short Portable Mental Status Questionnaire (SPMSQ; Pfeiffer, 1975) in 1982–1994 and 2004, and the Mini Mental State Exam (MMSE; Folstein et al., 1975) in 1999. In addition, CI can be inferred when a proxy interview was listed as resulting from senility or Alzheimer's disease.

Health Insurance Portability and Accountability Act

Clarification of the tax treatment of LTC expenses (including LTC insurance) was included in the Health Insurance Portability and Accountability Act of 1996 (HIPAA). HIPAA introduced rules under which LTC expenses could qualify as income-tax-deductible medical expenses. HIPAA required that a licensed health-care practitioner certify that the LTC care recipient is a chronically ill individual on account of one or more of three possible triggering criteria (Internal Revenue Service, 1977):

1. ADL Trigger: The individual is unable to perform without substantial assistance from another individual at least two out of six ADLs (bathing, dressing, toileting, transferring, continence, and eating) for at least 90 days due to a loss of functional capacity. Substantial assistance means hands-on or standby assistance. Hands-on assistance means the physical assistance of another person without which the individual would be unable to perform the ADL. Standby assistance means the presence of another person within arm's reach that is necessary to prevent injury to the individual while the individual is performing the ADL.
2. Cognitive Impairment (CI) Trigger: The individual requires substantial supervision to protect him or her from threats to health and safety due to severe cognitive impairment. Severe cognitive impairment means a loss or deterioration in intellectual capacity comparable to Alzheimer's disease or similar irreversible dementia with a measurable impact on memory, orientation, or reasoning. Substantial supervision means continual supervision (including cueing) that is necessary for the individual's health/safety.
3. Similar Level Trigger: The individual has a level of disability similar to that described in the ADL Trigger, as determined under regulations developed in consultation with the Department of Health and Human Services (DHHS). This trigger is currently inactive, but may at some future date be activated using, for example, some combination of ADLs and IADLs.

By 2002, 90% of all LTC insurance policies sold in the US complied with the HIPAA requirements for tax qualification (Coronel, 2004). These rules are the *de jure* criteria for classifying LTC expenses as medical expenses, making it reasonable to consider their use in public health and public policy research.

LTC Disability Estimates

Table 1 displays the population distribution of the HIPAA ADL and CI Triggers by ADL and IADL disability levels among the U.S. elderly in 1999, based on data from the 1999 NLTCS. The cumulative totals at the bottom of the table indicate that 4.75 million elderly met at least one of the two HIPAA triggering criteria: 2.96 million met the ADL Trigger, 3.44 million met the CI Trigger, and 1.65 million met both triggers.

The implementation of the HIPAA ADL Trigger in this article followed the standard NLTCS protocol in accepting as ADL-disabled all cases that met the personal assistance criterion for ADL limitations in the detailed questionnaire without further considering whether the expected disability duration would be at least 3 months. Expected 3-month duration was queried on the screener questionnaire, but only for newly screened-in cases; for previously screened-in cases, expected 3-month duration was queried, if at all, at the time they screened in.

Thus, the determination that the expected duration was at least 3 months was incomplete in the NLTCS detailed interview; some cases (e.g., institutionalized persons; the healthy subsamples) were automatically screened in or were otherwise designated for detailed interview without explicitly meeting the expected 3-month duration criterion (Wolf et al., 2005).

The standard NLTCS protocol may have a small bias when used to estimate HIPAA ADL prevalence rates. Among the reasons for this opinion are the following:

1. The HIPAA ADL prevalence rate based on two or more ADL impairments in the NLTCS detailed questionnaire would be approximately 15% lower if one eliminated all cases whose disability duration was less than 3 months (Stallard and Yee, 2000). Multiple decrement analysis of these same cases showed that the relative risks of ending the disability episode with institutionalization or death versus recovery or improvement were 1.3 at ages 68 and 70, 2.3 at age 75, 2.9 at age 80, 4.8 at age 85, and 6.3 or higher at ages 90 and over. With the highest absolute numbers of cases that met the two or more ADL impairment criteria occurring at age 81, these relative risks imply that roughly one-quarter of the 15% reduction in prevalence that would result from the elimination of cases with less than 3 months' duration of disability would be due to recovery or improvement. Hence, the bias induced by failing to screen for expected 3-month duration could be as large as 3.75%.
2. The 3-month minimum duration in the HIPAA ADL Trigger is neither a waiting period nor a qualification period; it is an expectation that may or may not be realized. HIPAA certifiers might assume that the age-specific average durations for two or more ADL disability episodes (in the range 36–26 months at ages 65–90) (Stallard and Yee, 2000) applied to each individual case, implying that the bias associated with the standard NLTCS protocol could be zero.
3. Alternatively, HIPAA certifiers might rely on model-based (or expert-opinion-based) estimates of the expected individual durations, in which case the bias would be non-zero only if the durations from initial disability to recovery/improvement were predictable and the model (or expert) yielded at least some predicted durations below 3 months; the bias would reach the upper limit of 3.75% only if the model reproduced the distribution of durations without error. Under these conditions, the bias associated with

the use of the standard NLTCS protocol is likely to be substantially less than the upper limit of 3.75%.

The estimates for the CI Trigger depend on the scoring range selected for the MMSE. An individual with an MMSE score in the range of 0–23 of a possible 30 points was classified as cognitively impaired in **Table 1**. An alternative classification would use the range 0–15. The upper bounds of 23 and 15 correspond to the midpoints of the ranges for mild (21–25) and moderate (11–20) dementia identified by Perneczky et al. (2006) using the Clinical Dementia Rating instrument. The impact of the alternative classification rule can be seen in **Table 2**.

The number of persons meeting only the CI Trigger declined from 1.79 million to 571 000. The total number meeting the CI Trigger declined from 3.44 million to 1.93 million. The number meeting the ADL Trigger was unchanged at 2.96 million. The number meeting at least one of the triggers declined from 4.75 million to 3.53 million.

Although the HIPAA CI Trigger uses the terms severe cognitive impairment with a measurable impact, HIPAA did not provide guidance as to the specific cut-points one should use for standard tests such as the MMSE. As a consequence, there may be substantial variation in estimates of the size of the LTC population when different tests of cognitive functioning or different cut-points on the same tests are employed. The remainder of this article employs the criteria in **Table 1**.

The cumulative totals at the right side of **Table 1** show the distribution of the 2.96 million persons who met the HIPAA ADL Trigger. Of these, 2.00 million had four or more ADL limitations and 830 000 had six ADL limitations; and, of these, 62% and 72%, respectively, were also cognitively impaired.

The number of persons with any ADL or IADL limitation, including limitations in inside mobility, was estimated as 6.79 million. The number of nondisabled persons meeting the CI Trigger was 564 000 (108 000 in **Table 2**). Since the NLTCS did not screen for CI, this may be an underestimate of the true number. Thus the total number with any CI, ADL, or IADL limitation was at least 7.35 million.

Table 1 Distribution of HIPAA triggers by ADL/IADL disability level, United States 1999, age 65 and above, in 000s

ADL/IADL disability level	HIPAA trigger				Total	Right cumulative total
	None	CI trigger only	ADL trigger only	ADL & CI trigger		
Nondisabled	27 861	564			28 426	35 211
IADL only or inside-mobility	2001	895			2897	6785
1 ADL	598	327			925	3888
2 ADLs			324	214	539	2963
3 ADLs			237	190	427	2425
4 ADLs			205	231	435	1998
5 ADLs			318	415	733	1563
6 ADLs			229	601	830	830
Total	30 461	1786	1313	1651	35 211	
Right cumulative total	35 211	4750	2963	1651		

CI trigger is defined as a score in the range 0–23 on the MMSE, senility, or Alzheimer's disease.
Source: Author's calculations based on the 1999 National Long-Term Care Survey.

Table 2 Distribution of modified HIPAA triggers by ADL/IADL disability level, United States 1999, age 65 and above, in 000s

ADL/IADL disability level	Modified HIPAA trigger				Total	Right cumulative total
	None	CI trigger only	ADL trigger only	ADL & CI trigger		
Nondisabled	28 317	108			28 426	35 211
IADL only or inside-mobility	2583	313			2897	6785
1 ADL	776	149			925	3888
2 ADLs			402	137	539	2963
3 ADLs			296	131	427	2425
4 ADLs			273	163	435	1998
5 ADLs			389	344	733	1563
6 ADLs			249	581	830	830
Total	31 677	571	1608	1355	35 211	
Right cumulative total	35 211	3534	2963	1355		

CI trigger is defined as a score in the range 0–15 on the MMSE, senility, or Alzheimer's disease.
Source: Author's calculations based on the 1999 National Long-Term Care Survey.

An area of potential discrepancy in estimating the LTC population involves differences between the list of ADLs in HIPAA and the list used in the NLTCS flap items, which forms the set traditionally used in published reports based on the NLTCS (Manton and Gu, 2001).

Five of the six HIPAA ADLs are the same as the traditional six flap-item ADLs in the NLTCS. HIPAA's ADLs include continence, but not inside mobility. The flap-item ADLs include inside mobility, but not continence. Because continence was measured in the NLTCS, the NLTCS can be used to generate estimates of the population meeting the HIPAA LTC criteria in addition to estimates of the population meeting the traditional NLTCS disability criteria. The former are shown in **Tables 1** and **2**; the latter are shown in **Table 3**.

The flap-item ADLs in the NLTCS are triggered by the use of special equipment in addition to the use of personal assistance. The largest difference occurs under the column heading None, where 1.14 million persons having two or more flap-item ADLs are classified as not disabled by the HIPAA LTC triggers. The total number of 7.08 million with any ADL or IADL limitations is only 4.3% higher than the corresponding number (6.79 million) in **Table 1**. The 4.61 million with two or more ADLs in **Table 3** is 56% larger than the corresponding number (2.96 million) in **Table 1**.

Table 4 provides a direct comparison between the two sets of classification rules. The 16 000 with one HIPAA ADL that were nondisabled on the traditional flap-item ADLs and IADLs were all due to incontinence.

Table 3 Distribution of HIPAA triggers by traditional NLTCS ADL/IADL disability level, United States 1999, age 65 and above, in 000s

NLTCS ADL/IADL disability level	HIPAA trigger				Total	Right cumulative total
	None	CI trigger Only	ADL trigger Only	ADL & CI trigger		
Nondisabled	27 600	530			28 131	35 211
IADL Only	714	382			1096	7080
1 ADL	1006	358	9	2	1375	5984
2 ADLs	564	294	54	90	1003	4609
3 ADLs	373	156	181	123	834	3606
4 ADLs	183	66	271	200	720	2773
5 ADLs	20		359	433	812	2053
6 ADLs	1		438	802	1241	1241
Total	30 461	1786	1313	1651	35 211	
Right cumulative total	35 211	4750	2963	1651		

CI trigger is defined as a score in the range 0–23 on the MMSE, senility, or Alzheimer's disease.
Source: Author's calculations based on the 1999 National Long-Term Care Survey.

Table 4 Distribution of HIPAA ADL/IADL disability level by traditional NLTCS ADL/IADL disability level, United States 1999, age 65 and above, in 000s

NLTCS ADL/IADL disability level	HIPAA ADL/IADL disability level								Total	Right cumulative total
	Nondisabled	IADL only or inside-mobility	1 ADL	2 ADLs	3 ADLs	4 ADLs	5 ADLs	6 ADLs		
Nondisabled	28 115		16						28 131	35 211
IADL only		1090	5						1096	7080
1 ADL	255	800	309	11					1375	5984
2 ADLs	49	565	244	130	14				1003	4609
3 ADLs	5	314	211	203	84	17			834	3606
4 ADLs	3	121	125	150	233	71	18		720	2773
5 ADLs		6	14	44	86	329	304	29	812	2053
6 ADLs			1		9	19	411	801	1241	1241
Total	28 426	2897	925	539	427	435	733	830	35 211	
Right cumulative total	35 211	6785	3888	2963	2425	1998	1563	830		

Source: Author's calculations based on the 1999 National Long-Term Care Survey.

LTC Demographics

Table 5 displays the distribution of the HIPAA LTC triggers by age and sex among the U.S. elderly population.

Among males, 434 000 met both the ADL and CI Triggers, with the largest number of those aged 75–84. Among females, 1.22 million met both the ADL and CI Triggers, with the largest number of those aged 85+. Among the 6.1% of males who met the ADL Trigger, 49% simultaneously met the CI Trigger; among the 10% of females who met the ADL Trigger, 59% simultaneously met the CI Trigger.

Certain patterns of change over age can be more readily assessed using the percentage distributions shown in **Table 6**. For example, the relative frequency of ADL Trigger cases meeting the CI Trigger increased with age for both sexes, but the increase was larger for females. Moreover, the percentage of females meeting any HIPAA trigger was larger at all ages for females and the relative excess increased with age from 8.1% at age 65–74 to 43% at age 85+. This latter increase was attributable to the absolute excess of 10.7% of females at age 85+ meeting both the ADL and CI Triggers.

Tables 7 and **8** stratify the population counts and percentage distributions in **Tables 5** and **6** by community residence versus residence in an LTC institution, where an LTC institution was a nursing facility or similar setting having a health professional (e.g., registered nurse, licensed practical nurse, licensed vocational nurse, psychiatrist, etc.) on duty for 24 h each day (including weekends).

The age–sex group with the largest number of institutional residents was females aged 85+ with 656 000 of the total 1.44 million. The next largest group was females aged 75–84, followed by males aged 75–84.

Among institutional residents, 92% met at least one HIPAA LTC trigger, the only notable discrepancy occurring among males aged 65–74, where 80% met at least one trigger. For females aged 65–74, the corresponding value was 89%. For both sexes, the value increased with age, reaching 97% for males aged 85+ and 93% for females aged 85+. These results indicate that the HIPAA LTC triggers were reasonably successful (i.e., their overall

Table 5 Distribution of HIPAA triggers by sex and age, United States 1999, age 65 and above, in 000s

Sex	Age	HIPAA trigger				Total	Right cumulative total
		None	CI trigger only	ADL trigger only	ADL & CI trigger		
Male	65–74	7700	206	140	101	8147	14 594
	75–84	4456	286	184	191	5117	6447
	85+	918	139	132	142	1331	1331
	Total	13 074	631	456	434	14 594	
Female	65–74	9342	248	221	120	9931	20 616
	75–84	6306	529	294	426	7556	10 685
	85+	1739	378	341	671	3129	3129
	Total	17 387	1156	857	1216	20 616	
Total		30 461	1786	1313	1651	35 211	
Right cumulative total		35 211	4750	2963	1651		

CI trigger is defined as a score in the range 0–23 on the MMSE, senility, or Alzheimer's disease.
Source: Author's calculations based on the 1999 National Long-Term Care Survey.

Table 6 Percent distribution of HIPAA triggers by sex and age, United States 1999, age 65 and above

Sex	Age	HIPAA trigger				Any trigger	Total (in 000s)
		None	CI trigger only	ADL trigger only	ADL & CI trigger		
Male	65–74	94.5	2.5	1.7	1.2	5.5	8147
	75–84	87.1	5.6	3.6	3.7	12.9	5117
	85+	69.0	10.4	9.9	10.7	31.0	1331
	Total	89.6	4.3	3.1	3.0	10.4	14 594
Female	65–74	94.1	2.5	2.2	1.2	5.9	9931
	75–84	83.5	7.0	3.9	5.6	16.5	7556
	85+	55.6	12.1	10.9	21.4	44.4	3129
	Total	84.3	5.6	4.2	5.9	15.7	20 616
Total		86.5	5.1	3.7	4.7	13.5	35 211
Right cumulative total		100.0	13.5	8.4	4.7		

CI trigger is defined as a score in the range 0–23 on the MMSE, senility, or Alzheimer's disease.
Source: Author's calculations based on the 1999 National Long-Term Care Survey.

Table 7 Distribution of HIPAA triggers by institutional status, sex, and age, United States 1999, age 65 and above, in 000s

Institutional status	Sex	Age	HIPAA trigger None	CI trigger only	ADL trigger only	ADL & CI trigger	Total	Right cumulative total
Community	Male	65–74	7687	200	128	71	8085	14 243
		75–84	4441	272	143	100	4956	6158
		85+	913	127	88	73	1201	1201
		Total	13 041	599	359	244	14 243	
	Female	65–74	9332	238	176	93	9839	19 532
		75–84	6280	514	210	217	7220	9693
		85+	1695	351	178	249	2473	2473
		Total	17 307	1103	563	559	19 532	
	Total		30 349	1701	922	803	33 775	
LTC institution	Male	65–74	13	6	12	31	61	351
		75–84	15	14	41	91	160	290
		85+	4	12	44	69	129	129
		Total	32	32	96	190	351	
	Female	65–74	10	10	46	27	93	1085
		75–84	26	16	84	209	336	992
		85+	43	27	164	421	656	656
		Total	80	53	294	658	1085	
	Total		112	85	390	848	1436	
Total			30 461	1786	1313	1651	35 211	
Right cumulative total			35 211	4750	2963	1651		

CI trigger is defined as a score in the range 0–23 on the MMSE, senility, or Alzheimer's disease.
Source: Author's calculations based on the 1999 National Long-Term Care Survey.

Table 8 Percent distribution of HIPAA triggers by institutional status, sex, and age, United States 1999, age 65 and above

Institutional status	Sex	Age	HIPAA trigger None	CI trigger only	ADL trigger only	ADL & CI trigger	Any trigger	Total (in 000s)
Community	Male	65–74	95.1	2.5	1.6	0.9	4.9	8085
		75–84	89.6	5.5	2.9	2.0	10.4	4956
		85+	76.0	10.6	7.3	6.1	24.0	1201
		Total	91.6	4.2	2.5	1.7	8.4	14 243
	Female	65–74	94.9	2.4	1.8	0.9	5.1	9839
		75–84	87.0	7.1	2.9	3.0	13.0	7220
		85+	68.6	14.2	7.2	10.1	31.4	2473
		Total	88.6	5.6	2.9	2.9	11.4	19 532
	Total		89.9	5.0	2.7	2.4	10.1	33 775
LTC institution	Male	65–74	20.5	10.1	19.0	50.3	79.5	61
		75–84	9.6	8.7	25.3	56.4	90.4	160
		85+	3.4	9.2	34.2	53.2	96.6	129
		Total	9.2	9.1	27.5	54.2	90.8	351
	Female	65–74	10.9	10.7	49.3	29.1	89.1	93
		75–84	7.9	4.7	25.1	62.3	92.1	336
		85+	6.6	4.2	25.0	64.2	93.4	656
		Total	7.4	4.9	27.1	60.6	92.6	1085
	Total		7.8	5.9	27.2	59.1	92.2	1436
Total			86.5	5.1	3.7	4.7	13.5	35 211
Right cumulative total			100.0	13.5	8.4	4.7		

CI trigger is defined as a score in the range 0–23 on the MMSE, senility, or Alzheimer's disease.
Source: Author's calculations based on the 1999 National Long-Term Care Survey.

sensitivity was 92%) in meeting their goal of identifying severely disabled elderly persons, assuming that residence in an LTC institution was a valid indicator of severe disability.

Meeting a HIPPA LTC trigger, however, does not necessarily imply institutional residency. **Table 9** displays the age, sex, and HIPAA LTC-Trigger-specific institutionalization rates for the data displayed in **Table 7**.

Among those meeting any HIPAA LTC trigger, 31% of females and 21% of males (28% combined) were institutionalized.

The institutionalization rates varied significantly depending on the specific triggers that were met. Among those meeting both the ADL and CI Triggers, 54% of females and 44% of males (51% combined) were institutionalized; among those meeting only the ADL Trigger, 34% of females and 21% of males (30% combined) were institutionalized; and among those meeting only the CI Trigger, 4.6% of females and 5.1% of males (4.8% combined) were institutionalized.

The overall institutionalization rates were 5.3% for females and 2.4% for males (4.1% combined); these rates increased significantly across the three age groups, from 0.8% to 9.7% for males and 0.9% to 21% for females. Within the HIPAA LTC triggered groups, the highest institutionalization rate (63%) was for females aged 85+ meeting both the ADL and CI Triggers; the next highest rate (49%) was for females aged 75–84 meeting the same triggers.

Table 10 stratifies the institutionalization rates in Table 9 by marital status. Among those meeting any HIPAA LTC trigger, 15% of married females and 12% of married males (13% combined) were institutionalized. For the same conditions, 35% of unmarried females and 34% of unmarried males (35% combined) were institutionalized. Among those meeting both the ADL and CI Triggers, 35% of married females and 26% of married males (30% combined) were institutionalized. For the

Table 9 Percent institutionalized by HIPAA triggers by sex and age, United States 1999, age 65 and above

Sex	Age	HIPAA trigger					Total
		None	CI trigger only	ADL trigger only	ADL & CI trigger	Any trigger	
Male	65–74	0.2	3.0	8.3	30.4	10.9	0.8
	75–84	0.3	4.9	22.0	47.4	21.9	3.1
	85+	0.5	8.5	33.5	48.5	30.3	9.7
	Total	0.2	5.1	21.2	43.8	21.0	2.4
Female	65–74	0.1	4.0	20.7	22.6	14.0	0.9
	75–84	0.4	3.0	28.7	49.1	24.7	4.4
	85+	2.5	7.2	48.0	62.8	44.1	21.0
	Total	0.5	4.6	34.3	54.1	31.1	5.3
Total		0.4	4.8	29.7	51.4	27.9	4.1

CI trigger is defined as a score in the range 0–23 on the MMSE, senility, or Alzheimer's disease.
Source: Author's calculations based on the 1999 National Long-Term Care Survey.

Table 10 Percent institutionalized by HIPAA triggers by marital status, sex, and age, United States 1999, age 65 and above

Married	Sex	Age	HIPAA trigger					Total
			None	CI trigger only	ADL trigger only	ADL & CI trigger	Any trigger	
Yes	Male	65–74	0.0	0.0	4.6	11.1	3.9	0.2
		75–84	0.0	2.6	13.3	32.6	14.4	1.7
		85+	0.2	1.6	30.7	24.3	19.9	5.7
		Total	0.0	1.6	13.6	25.9	12.3	1.1
	Female	65–74	0.0	4.8	6.5	19.4	8.4	0.4
		75–84	0.1	3.4	10.4	42.2	18.1	2.2
		85+	0.9	8.9	15.7	39.9	23.8	5.9
		Total	0.1	4.5	9.2	35.4	14.9	1.2
	Total		0.0	2.7	11.9	29.8	13.3	1.1
No	Male	65–74	0.8	6.9	40.4	47.7	23.8	2.9
		75–84	1.3	8.6	41.2	75.0	35.9	7.3
		85+	0.9	13.4	36.4	73.6	39.7	14.2
		Total	1.0	9.5	38.8	66.8	34.1	6.4
	Female	65–74	0.2	3.5	30.6	24.7	17.8	1.5
		75–84	0.6	2.9	38.0	51.0	26.8	5.5
		85+	2.7	7.1	50.0	63.9	45.1	22.6
		Total	0.7	4.6	42.5	57.1	34.8	7.9
	Total		0.8	5.7	41.8	58.6	34.7	7.5
Total			0.4	4.8	29.7	51.4	27.9	4.1

CI trigger is defined as a score in the range 0–23 on the MMSE, senility, or Alzheimer's disease.
Source: Author's calculations based on the 1999 National Long-Term Care Survey.

same conditions, 57% of unmarried females and 67% of unmarried males (59% combined) were institutionalized. The highest rates of institutionalization were among unmarried males aged 75–84 (75%) and 85+ (74%) meeting both the ADL and CI Triggers.

Home and Community-Based LTC

Table 11 displays the usage rates among community residents of personal assistance within the week prior to the NLTCS detailed interview, where the assistance stemmed from a disability or health problem and details of the nature and amount of the assistance were provided.

The personal assistance rates were very low for persons who met neither HIPAA LTC trigger: 3.8% of married persons and 6.5% of unmarried persons (4.9% combined) had such assistance; unmarried females had the highest rates of assistance (6.9%) and married males the lowest (2.8%).

The specificity of the HIPAA LTC triggers can be estimated as the percentage of persons among the estimated 29.88 million community residents meeting neither HIPAA LTC trigger who had no personal assistance due to a disability or health problem within the prior week, assuming that the lack of such assistance was a valid indicator of the absence of severe disability. The number of such persons was 28.85 million, implying a specificity of 97%.

In contrast, personal assistance rates were substantial for persons meeting any HIPAA LTC trigger: 72% of married persons and 69% of unmarried persons (70% combined) had such assistance; married females had the highest rates of assistance (72%) and unmarried males the lowest (68%).

The highest personal assistance rates were for persons meeting both the ADL and CI Triggers: 96% of married persons and 91% of unmarried persons (93% combined) had such assistance; married males had the highest rates of assistance (98%) and unmarried males the lowest (86%). The assistance rates for females meeting both the ADL and CI Triggers were the same (92%) for married and unmarried women.

The personal assistance rates were almost as high for persons meeting only the ADL Trigger: 92% of married persons and 93% of unmarried persons (92% combined) had such assistance; unmarried males had the highest rates of assistance (95%) and married females the lowest (91%).

The personal assistance rates were substantially lower for persons meeting only the CI Trigger: 42% of married persons and 50% of unmarried persons (47% combined) had such assistance; unmarried males had the highest rates of assistance (54%) and married males the lowest (41%). These declines suggest that the current implementation of the CI Trigger may overestimate the number of cases that meet the HIPAA certification requirements. However, because the modified CI Trigger used in Table 2 would only raise the marginal percentage in Table 11 from 47% to 55%, it follows that the use of

Table 11 Percent of community residents reporting personal assistance within the prior week due to a disability or health problem; by HIPAA triggers by marital status, sex, and age, United States 1999, age 65 and above

Married	Sex	Age	HIPAA trigger					Total
			None	CI trigger only	ADL trigger only	ADL & CI trigger	Any trigger	
Yes	Male	65–74	1.4	36.5	94.3	100.0	71.1	4.4
		75–84	4.3	45.5	91.2	99.0	71.3	10.9
		85+	9.6	37.1	85.9	94.8	71.6	24.3
		Total	2.8	41.1	91.7	98.0	71.3	7.9
	Female	65–74	3.8	38.1	84.3	81.9	64.1	6.3
		75–84	7.4	44.7	96.3	97.0	75.7	14.2
		85+	10.4	69.2	100.0	100.0	89.2	24.3
		Total	5.1	43.9	91.2	92.2	72.1	9.4
	Total		3.8	42.2	91.5	95.8	71.6	8.5
No	Male	65–74	1.7	48.2	100.0	91.1	61.9	6.1
		75–84	5.7	45.0	91.5	78.2	59.4	12.1
		85+	17.8	73.3	97.1	86.5	82.7	33.5
		Total	5.3	54.0	95.2	86.3	67.7	12.5
	Female	65–74	3.2	36.0	93.7	82.3	62.5	6.9
		75–84	7.0	44.4	92.0	89.7	63.1	15.2
		85+	17.6	59.3	92.1	95.9	78.3	37.8
		Total	6.9	48.6	92.4	92.0	69.4	16.1
	Total		6.5	49.8	92.9	91.3	69.1	15.3
Total			4.9	47.3	92.2	92.9	70.1	11.5

CI trigger is defined as a score in the range 0–23 on the MMSE, senility, or Alzheimer's disease.
Source: Author's calculations based on the 1999 National Long-Term Care Survey.

more stringent MMSE scoring criteria would not resolve the overestimation.

The relatively low frequency of personal assistance among those meeting only the basic or modified CI Triggers was attributable to subgroups of persons identified in **Tables 1** and **2** as CI Trigger Only who were free from IADL and ADL limitations and whose marginal rates of personal assistance were only 8.4% and 6.6%, respectively, for the two forms of the CI Triggers. Among married persons meeting these same criteria, the rates of personal assistance were similarly low at 6.3% and 6.6%, respectively. These calculations suggest that some forms of assistance provided to persons meeting only the CI Trigger may not be captured by the NLTCS survey instruments.

Eliminating the CI Trigger Only persons who were free from IADL and ADL limitations would raise the marginal percentages among those meeting only the basic or modified CI Triggers to 67% and 68%, respectively. The marginal percentages would increase further to 79% and 80%, respectively, if the IADL-only groups were eliminated (leaving a residual group with exactly 1 ADL limitation). These calculations indicate that ADL and IADL assistance provided to persons meeting only the CI Trigger is captured by the survey instruments.

Table 12 displays the percentages using paid personal assistance among community residents with any personal assistance within the week prior to the NLTCS detailed interview. The numerators of the percentages in **Table 11** were the denominators of the percentages in **Table 12**.

The use of paid personal assistance was substantial for persons who met neither HIPAA LTC trigger but who had personal assistance: 13% of married persons and 34% of unmarried persons (25% combined) had paid assistance; unmarried males had the highest rates of paid assistance (37%) and married males the lowest (11%). Of course, these percentages would be reduced substantially if one multiplied them by the corresponding values in **Table 11** to produce the marginal usage rate of paid personal assistance among all persons who met neither HIPAA LTC trigger.

The use of paid personal assistance was 8–10% higher, absolutely, for persons who met any HIPAA LTC trigger: 23% of married persons and 42% of unmarried persons (35% combined) had paid assistance; unmarried males had the highest rates of paid assistance (46%) and married males the lowest (21%).

The use of paid personal assistance was an additional 9–11% higher for persons who met both the ADL and CI Triggers: 34% of married persons and 51% of unmarried persons (45% combined) had paid assistance; unmarried females had the highest rates of paid assistance (52%) and married males the lowest (32%).

The use of paid personal assistance for persons who met only the ADL Trigger was similar to the use for those who met any HIPAA LTC trigger: 23% of married persons and 44% of unmarried persons (34% combined) had paid assistance; unmarried males had the highest rates of paid assistance (51%) and married males the lowest (20%).

Table 12 Percent of community residents reporting paid personal assistance among those with any personal assistance within the prior week due to a disability or health problem; by HIPAA triggers by marital status, sex, and age, United States 1999, age 65 and above

Married	Sex	Age	HIPAA trigger					Total
			None	CI trigger only	ADL trigger only	ADL & CI trigger	Any trigger	
Yes	Male	65–74	0.0	12.0	8.9	13.0	10.4	7.3
		75–84	5.1	9.3	28.3	40.7	26.5	18.9
		85+	47.6	11.7	31.1	32.2	28.0	33.9
		Total	10.9	10.5	20.1	31.6	21.2	17.9
	Female	65–74	9.3	9.0	38.4	20.0	26.8	16.7
		75–84	19.7	10.7	13.7	44.5	21.8	20.8
		85+	13.6	22.0	44.1	49.8	40.2	30.8
		Total	14.0	11.6	26.8	37.7	26.0	19.9
	Total		12.7	10.9	22.9	33.8	23.1	18.8
No	Male	65–74	9.5	48.9	21.9	41.9	43.4	34.3
		75–84	36.0	63.1	52.0	22.7	53.1	46.1
		85+	47.8	26.6	56.6	61.6	42.9	44.9
		Total	36.9	45.0	51.0	43.0	46.4	42.8
	Female	65–74	27.1	19.8	44.1	37.2	35.4	31.8
		75–84	40.2	28.4	48.7	47.6	39.8	40.0
		85+	29.9	32.2	37.9	57.9	43.7	39.4
		Total	33.7	29.1	42.9	52.0	41.0	38.4
	Total		34.3	32.8	44.4	50.9	42.0	39.2
Total			24.9	26.5	33.6	44.6	34.6	30.9

CI trigger is defined as a score in the range 0–23 on the MMSE, senility, or Alzheimer's disease.
Source: Author's calculations based on the 1999 National Long-Term Care Survey.

The use of paid personal assistance for persons who met only the CI Trigger was substantially lower than for persons who met the HIPAA ADL trigger, and was close to the use for persons who met neither HIPAA LTC trigger: 11% of married persons and 33% of unmarried persons (27% combined) had paid assistance; unmarried males had the highest rates of paid assistance (45%) and married males the lowest (11%).

Table 13 displays the average number of hours of help per week among community residents reporting personal assistance within the week prior to the NLTCS detailed interview. The numerators of the percentages in **Table 11** were the denominators of the averages in **Table 13**.

Hours of help were missing for about 8% of the respondents in the numerators of **Table 13**; these missing values were assumed to be equal to the cell-specific means for the nonmissing values. The weekly hours of help were substantial for persons who met neither HIPAA LTC trigger but who had personal assistance: Married persons had an average of 20 h and unmarried persons an average of 13 h (combined average was 15 h); married males had the highest average (25 h) and unmarried females the lowest (12 h). These averages would be reduced substantially if one multiplied them by the corresponding values in **Table 11** to produce the marginal hours of help among all persons who met neither HIPAA LTC trigger.

The weekly hours of help were substantially higher for persons who met any HIPAA LTC trigger: Married persons had an average of 49 h and unmarried persons an average of 46 h (combined average was 47 h); married males had the highest average (52 h) and unmarried males the lowest (44 h).

The weekly hours of help were highest for persons who met both the ADL and CI Triggers: Married persons had an average of 63 h and unmarried persons an average of 68 h (combined average was 66 h).

Among those meeting only the ADL Trigger, married and unmarried persons both had an average of 50 h. Among those meeting only the CI Trigger, married persons had an average of 25 h and unmarried persons an average of 16 h (combined average was 19 h).

Table 14 displays the average number of paid hours of help per week among community residents reporting paid personal assistance within the week prior to the NLTCS detailed interview. The numerators of the percentages in **Table 12** were the denominators of the averages in **Table 14**.

Hours of help were missing for about 4% of the respondents in the numerators of **Table 14**; these missing values were assumed to be equal to the cell-specific means for the nonmissing values.

The weekly hours of paid help were lowest for persons who met neither HIPAA LTC trigger but who had paid personal assistance: Married persons had an average of 8 h and unmarried persons an average of 10 h (combined average was 9 h); unmarried females had the highest average (10 h) and married females the lowest (8 h).

The weekly hours of paid help were substantially higher for persons who met any HIPAA LTC trigger: Married persons had an average of 19 h and unmarried persons an average of 38 h (combined average was 33 h);

Table 13 Average hours of help per week among community residents reporting personal assistance within the prior week due to a disability or health problem; by HIPAA triggers by marital status, sex, and age, United States 1999, age 65 and above

Married	Sex	Age	HIPAA trigger					Total
			None	CI trigger only	ADL trigger only	ADL & CI trigger	Any trigger	
Yes	Male	65–74	23.8	23.7	61.9	51.8	53.6	43.7
		75–84	23.9	26.4	55.4	72.8	53.1	42.9
		85+	28.0	44.9	53.0	42.8	47.2	40.8
		Total	24.7	28.4	56.9	60.4	52.0	42.7
	Female	65–74	14.5	33.4	41.7	50.6	42.9	28.3
		75–84	14.6	14.4	40.9	78.8	46.3	31.5
		85+	28.2	20.2	47.6	58.0	44.7	38.3
		Total	15.8	20.0	41.9	67.3	45.1	31.2
	Total		19.8	25.4	50.1	63.1	49.1	37.3
No	Male	65–74	6.2	11.6	19.8	105.4	41.0	27.6
		75–84	16.6	18.3	69.8	44.6	46.3	32.5
		85+	13.6	20.6	57.0	56.4	44.3	30.9
		Total	13.7	17.6	58.1	68.2	44.4	31.0
	Female	65–74	8.6	7.7	39.6	29.7	30.8	19.6
		75–84	11.9	17.0	43.4	64.3	41.8	28.0
		85+	13.7	15.8	54.4	73.7	52.1	38.7
		Total	12.2	15.9	48.3	67.7	46.2	32.1
	Total		12.5	16.3	50.2	67.7	45.9	31.9
Total			15.1	18.8	50.1	66.1	47.1	33.9

CI trigger is defined as a score in the range 0–23 on the MMSE, senility, or Alzheimer's disease.
Source: Author's calculations based on the 1999 National Long-Term Care Survey.

Table 14 Average hours of paid help per week among community residents reporting paid personal assistance within the prior week due to a disability or health problem; by HIPAA triggers by marital status, sex, and age, United States 1999, age 65 and above

Married	Sex	Age	HIPAA trigger					Total
			None	CI trigger only	ADL trigger only	ADL & CI trigger	Any trigger	
Yes	Male	65–74	–	6.5	31.8	2.5	20.9	20.9
		75–84	6.3	7.4	25.9	16.0	19.6	17.1
		85+	10.7	40.0	30.0	10.4	20.8	16.9
		Total	8.7	11.3	28.0	12.9	20.1	17.5
	Female	65–74	3.6	3.0	12.1	7.7	10.7	9.0
		75–84	8.7	7.7	20.0	23.5	20.2	15.3
		85+	15.5	2.0	10.8	36.0	20.0	19.3
		Total	8.2	5.6	15.0	23.6	17.2	14.2
	Total		8.4	9.1	21.7	17.7	18.8	15.9
No	Male	65–74	5.8	12.2	40.5	67.0	37.3	27.4
		75–84	8.3	15.3	54.1	2.5	33.8	24.2
		85+	7.2	8.8	43.1	19.0	32.4	21.2
		Total	7.5	13.1	47.8	34.9	33.9	23.4
	Female	65–74	6.5	14.7	21.2	25.8	21.4	15.4
		75–84	9.7	8.3	24.5	63.3	34.5	23.4
		85+	11.4	8.2	48.3	55.0	44.5	35.5
		Total	10.0	8.6	35.3	56.4	38.9	28.5
	Total		9.5	9.9	38.1	54.7	37.9	27.5
Total			9.3	9.8	33.4	45.3	33.2	24.9

CI trigger is defined as a score in the range 0–23 on the MMSE, senility, or Alzheimer's disease.
Source: Author's calculations based on the 1999 National Long Term Care Survey.

unmarried females had the highest average (39 h) and married females the lowest (17 h).

The weekly hours of paid help were similar or higher for persons who met both the ADL and CI Triggers: Married persons had a similar average of 18 paid h and unmarried persons a higher average of 55 paid h (combined average was 45 paid h).

Among those meeting only the ADL Trigger, married persons had an average of 22 paid h and unmarried persons an average of 38 paid h (combined average was 33 paid h). Among those meeting only the CI Trigger, married persons had an average of 9 paid h and unmarried persons an average of 10 paid h (combined average was 10 paid h).

Disability Declines

One of the most significant findings from the NLTCS was the discovery (Manton et al., 1993, 1997) and confirmation (Manton and Gu, 2001; Freedman et al., 2002, 2004) that LTC disability rates among the U.S. elderly were declining at a rate faster than the 0.6% per year expected based on the century-long trends established by Fogel and Costa (1997) and Costa (2000, 2002).

Stallard et al. (2004) used longitudinal weights to establish that the general decline in disability also applied to the more severe form represented by the HIPAA ADL Trigger. Longitudinal weights were used because concerns had been raised about the reliability of the standard cross-sectional weighting procedures in the NLTCS (Freedman et al., 2004).

The standard cross-sectional weighting procedures used the CDS Screener Cross-Sectional Weights for each indicated year, with adjustment for noncomplete institutional interviews. The longitudinal weights were defined as the cross-sectional weights assigned to the NLTCS respondents in 1984 or, if not then, the first cross-sectional weights assigned to the respondents as they aged in at some later date. The longitudinal weights did not include adjustments for non-response, in part because the response rates to the survey were very high (about 95%), and in part to minimize the number of assumptions used in their construction. However, the longitudinal weights included a one-time adjustment for deletions of certain persons aged 70–74 at their second survey, which reverted to the original longitudinal weights when these persons were reinstated beginning at their third survey. All of these deleted persons screened out at their first survey when they were aged 65–69. The surveys affected by these deletions were conducted in 1989, 1994, and 1999. The deletions were made because the vast majority of these persons were free of disabilities and the limited resources had to be directed toward the disabled.

Tables 15 and 16 display separately by sex the age-specific and age-standardized disability prevalence rates and their changes based on the HIPAA ADL Trigger using the standard cross-sectional weights for 1984 and 1999 and the longitudinal weights for 1999.

Table 15 Percent of population meeting HIPAA ADL trigger under cross-sectional and longitudinal weighting, United States 1984 and 1999, age 65 and above, males

	Cross-sectional weights			Longitudinal weights	
	Year			Year	
Age	1984	1999	Annual rate of decline; 15 year	1999	Annual rate of decline; 15 year
65–69	3.12	2.17	2.39%	2.17	2.39%
70–74	5.50	3.76	2.51%	3.76	2.50%
75–79	8.57	5.29	3.16%	5.24	3.22%
80–84	13.48	10.73	1.51%	11.21	1.22%
85–89	21.88	18.40	1.15%	17.87	1.34%
90–94	37.31	23.87	2.93%	25.10	2.61%
95–99	53.20	35.56	2.65%	31.61	3.41%
Age standardized rate	7.48	5.32	2.24%	5.35	2.21%

Results were age-standardized to the 1984 NLTCS weighted male population.
Source: Author's calculations based on the 1984 and 1999 NLTCS.

Table 16 Percent of population meeting HIPAA ADL trigger under cross-sectional and longitudinal weighting, United States 1984 and 1999, age 65 and above, females

	Cross-sectional weights			Longitudinal weights	
	Year			Year	
Age	1984	1999	Annual rate of decline; 15 year	1999	Annual rate of decline; 15 year
65–69	3.49	2.56	2.04%	2.56	2.04%
70–74	4.91	4.28	0.91%	4.41	0.71%
75–79	9.00	7.07	1.59%	7.05	1.62%
80–84	17.25	13.08	1.83%	13.42	1.66%
85–89	30.15	24.09	1.49%	24.69	1.32%
90–94	49.78	42.05	1.12%	43.52	0.89%
95–99	69.32	54.31	1.61%	56.75	1.33%
Age standardized rate	10.95	8.74	1.49%	8.94	1.35%

Results were age-standardized to the 1984 NLTCS weighted female population.
Source: Author's calculations based on the 1984 and 1999 NLTCS.

For both sets of weights, for all ages, and for both sexes, the prevalence rates for persons meeting the HIPAA ADL Trigger declined at rates faster than the expected rate of 0.6% per year. The age-standardized rates declined at a rate of 2.2% per year for males (for both sets of weights) and 1.4% or 1.5% per year for females (longitudinal vs. cross-sectional weights).

Significant areas of research involve the development and fielding of improved instruments for measurement of LTC disability and the analysis of existing data to enhance our understanding of the causes and public health implications of the declines.

Acknowledgments

The research in this article was supported by grants from the National Institute on Aging (Grants No. P01-AG17937 and U01-AG07198).

See also: Long Term Care in Health Services; Long Term Care, Organization and Financing.

Citations

Actuarial Standards Board (1999) *Long-Term Care Insurance.* Actuarial Standard of Practice No. 18. Washington DC: Actuarial Standards Board.

Blackwell DL and Tonthat L (2003) *Summary Health Statistics for the US Population: National Health Interview Survey, 1999. Vital and Health Statistics Series 10, No. 211.* Hyattsville, MD: National Center for Health Statistics.

Coronel S (2004) *Long-Term Care Insurance in 2002.* Washington DC: America's Health Insurance Plans.

Costa DL (2000) Understanding the twentieth-century decline in chronic conditions among older men. *Demography* 37(1): 53–72.

Costa DL (2002) Changing chronic disease rates and long-term declines in functional limitations among older men. *Demography* 39(1): 119–137.

Fogel RW and Costa DL (1997) A theory of technophysio evolution, with some implications for forecasting population, health care costs, and pension costs. *Demography* 34(1): 49–66.

Folstein MF, Folstein SE, and McHugh PR (1975) Mini-mental state: A practical method for grading the cognitive state of patients for the clinician. *Journal of Psychiatric Research* 12: 189–198.

Freedman VA, Martin LG, and Schoeni RF (2002) Recent trends in disability and functioning among older adults in the United States. *Journal of the American Medical Association* 288(24): 3137–3146.

Freedman VA, Crimmins E, Schoeni RF, et al. (2004) Resolving inconsistencies in old-age disability trends: Report from a technical working group. *Demography* 41(3): 417–441.

Internal Revenue Service (1977) *IRS Notice 97–31, Bulletin No. 1997–21, Internal Revenue Service,* May 27, 1977. pp. 5–8.

Kinosian B (2006) *The Department of Veterans Affairs Long-Term Care Planning Model and the National Long-Term Care Survey.* Philadelphia, PA: Department of Veterans Affairs.

Manton KG and Gu X (2001) Changes in the prevalence of chronic disability in the United States black and nonblack population above age 65 from 1982 to 1999. *Proceedings of the National Academy of Sciences USA* 98(11): 6354–6359.

Manton KG, Corder LS, and Stallard E (1993) Estimates of change in chronic disability and institutional incidence and prevalence rates in the US elderly population from the 1982, 1984, and 1989 National Long Term Care Survey. *Journal of Gerontology: Social Sciences* 48(4): S153–S166.

Manton KG, Corder LS, and Stallard E (1997) Chronic disability trends in elderly United States populations 1982–1994. *Proceedings of the National Academy of Sciences USA* 94: 2593–2598.

Perneczky R, Wagenpfeil S, Komossa T, Grimmer T, Diehl J, and Kurz A (2006) Mapping scores onto stages: Mini-Mental State Examination and Clinical Dementia Rating. *American Journal of Geriatric Psychiatry* 14(2): 139–144.

Pfeiffer E (1975) A short portable mental status questionnaire for the assessment of organic brain deficit in elderly patients. *Journal of the American Geriatrics Society* 23: 433–441.

Rogers S and Komisar H (2003) *Who Needs Long-Term Care.* Georgetown University Long-Term Care Financing Project. Washington DC: Georgetown University.

Stallard E and Yee RK (2000) *Non-Insured Home and Community-Based Long-Term Care Incidence and Continuance Tables. Actuarial Report.* Schaumburg, IL: Long-Term Care Experience Committee Society of Actuaries.

Stallard E, Wolf RM, and Weltz SA (2004) Morbidity improvement and its impact on LTC insurance pricing and valuation. *The Record* 30(1): Session #107PD, Society of Actuaries.

Wiener JM, Hanley RJ, Clark RJ, and Van Nostrand JF (1990) Measuring the activities of daily living: Comparisons across national surveys. *Journal of Gerontology: Social Sciences* 45(6): 229–237.

Wolf DA, Hunt K, and Knickman J (2005) Perspectives on the recent decline in disability at older ages. *The Milbank Quarterly* 83(3): 365–395.

Patient Empowerment in Health Care

J F P Bridges, Johns Hopkins Bloomberg School of Public Health, Baltimore, MD, USA
S Loukanova, University of Heidelberg, Heidelberg, Germany
P Carrera, Management Center Innsbruck, Innsbruck, Austria

© 2008 Elsevier Inc. All rights reserved.

Introduction

Empowerment is a term widely applied today in many domains of our lives. As such, it has been the focus of scholarship in various academic disciplines including psychology, sociology, education, economics, and community/organizational development. In recent years, the concept of empowerment has been the subject of great interest in the health-care context, especially given the many power imbalances that exist in medicine. While physicians have traditionally held considerable power – both over the patient in the consultation room and over other health-care workers in health-care facilities – recent trends toward centralized decision making and cost-containment have disrupted the traditional, physician-based power structures, leading to a situation in which they too now seek power.

Given both the traditional and modern power imbalances, for a health-care system to function correctly, both clinicians and patients need to be empowered and, more importantly, need to interact in an environment of mutual respect and partnership. This implies that health-care providers maintain sufficient power to fulfill their professional obligations to multiple constituencies, including the patients and communities they serve. With this power comes responsibility, as providers must share this knowledge while maintaining patient autonomy. Likewise, patients, their advocates/support networks, and families need power to realize their preferences and health-related needs and to fulfill their responsibilities both within and transcending the traditional doctor/patient dyad.

Empowerment Principles in Health-Care Literature

A recent review of the English language medical literature between 1980 and 2005, summarized in **Figure 1**, found a range of applications of empowerment principles in health care (Loukanova and Bridges, 2008). First, following more general social and political empowerment movements, 26% of all English language articles in the medical literature on empowerment have focused on

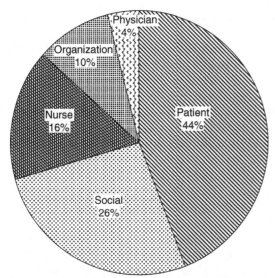

Figure 1 Focus on empowerment in medical literature (1980–2005). Proportion of empowerment articles published between 1980 and 2005 focusing on specific populations or entities. Adapted from Loukanova S and Bridges J (2008) Empowerment in medicine: An analysis of publication trends 1980–2005. *Central European Journal of Medicine* 3(1): 105–110.

issues of social empowerment, which relate to issues such as discrimination and health disparities. Second, research concerning nurse empowerment has been a major topic in health care, accounting for 16% of the literature. This body of work focuses on expanding nursing education, developing leadership and management skills, and fostering greater professional autonomy and job satisfaction. It also relates to the imbalances in professional power in the health-care workplace. Third, studies concerning the empowerment of organizations accounted for 10% of the literature. These papers have addressed issues such as improving staff performance, organizational culture, and the overall quality of the organization. Interestingly, there was very little research concerning the empowerment of physicians (only 4% of the literature). These articles focused on physicians' need for power to fulfill and manage their professional responsibilities to achieve outcomes of improved work efficiency, patient satisfaction, and physician self-governance.

The most prominent topic in the literature on empowerment in health focused on patient empowerment, accounting for 44%, and while we touch briefly on other types of empowerment in this article, we focus primarily on issues related to patient empowerment. The promotion of patient empowerment is dependent upon changing *both* patients and the health-care system. While patient empowerment can be established by introducing more choice for patients it also requires a system that is more patient centered to facilitate such choice.

Empowerment as an Idea

At the core of the concept of empowerment is the idea of physical or legal power. The word power comes from the Latin word *potere*, which means 'to be able' or to have the ability to choose. The verb empower means 'to give authority or power to; to authorize or give strength and confidence to.' In terms of its general use, Webster's dictionary defines power from a different perspective, citing the 'ability to act or produce an effect.' The concept of empowerment, however one defines it, seems to transcend its dictionary definition, representing a complex concept with a long and illustrious history. From an economic perspective, the roots of empowerment can be found during the Industrial Revolution in the late eighteenth century. The concentration of wealth in the ownership class was thrown into sharp relief by the effects of rapid industrialization and its effect on the class system. Empowerment evolved from the notion of increasing worker motivation and improving managerial leadership to the processes of giving subordinates greater resources and discretion today. Empowerment in the workplace is underpinned by Kanter's structural theory of organizational behavior (1993), which states that the empowerment of staff is important to overall work effectiveness and job satisfaction.

In the twentieth century, empowerment became associated with the struggle of those who held the least power in society. This was especially true for minority groups, who were discriminated against on the basis of their religion, gender, or race, perhaps best illustrated by the Civil Rights movement in the United States. Since the 1970s, empowerment has also served as the basis for defending community interests and promoting the mutual participation relationship between doctors and patients in the context of the consumer movement. And today, empowerment has a broader meaning, which focuses on types of self-realization and mobilizing the self-help efforts of people, rather than simply providing them with social welfare.

Empowerment in Medicine and Health

For most in medicine the thought of power is often focused on issues of control and domination. Focusing only on these aspects of power, however, limits our understanding of empowerment as it relates to any application in society. That said, the modern interpretation of power is extremely varied, and has to be considered in light of its use in technology, physics, mathematics, statistics, religion, politics, feminism, civil rights, psychology, disability, and even medicine. Taking this into account, the power element of empowerment has the potential for extremely broad interpretations, and as such could be applied to a broad range of stakeholders in health care. Early empowerment movements in health focused on services for and attitudes toward people with disabilities and mental illness, incorporating both community action and national/state legislation aimed at preventing discrimination. In more recent years, empowerment has hit the mainstream – being the focus of national attention and debate for a broader patient population.

Zimmerman (1990, 1995) and Rappaport (1984, 1987) are two of the leading researchers in the development of empowerment theory in health care. Zimmerman (1990) conceptualized empowerment at three different levels: (1) psychological empowerment is empowerment at the individual level of analysis; (2) organizational empowerment represents improved effectiveness resulting from organizations successfully competing for resources, networking with other organizations, or expanding their influence; and (3) empowerment, at the community level, refers to individuals working together in an organized fashion to improve their lives collectively and create links among community organizations and agencies that help maintain quality of life. Zimmerman (1995) expanded on his theory by distinguishing between processes and outcomes. Empowering processes refer to how people, organizations, and communities become empowered, whereas empowered outcomes refer to the consequences of those processes. He argues that empowerment can take many different forms and is dependent on the context for which it is being defined.

Rappaport (1984) takes a more pragmatic approach, noting that empowerment is easier to define in its absence – that is, through the eyes of the unempowered. Rappaport argues that it is simpler to identify the powerless, and significantly more difficult to define empowerment positively. He argues that the empowerment concept provides a useful, general guide for developing preventive interventions in which the participants feel they have an important stake. He also argues that empowerment should be adopted as a guiding principle for community psychology (Rappaport, 1987).

Despite the challenges in defining empowerment in positive terms, it does have a tremendously positive connotation, belonging to a class of similar positive constructs that have emerged in the past 20 years (e.g., patient activation, self-efficacy, shared decision making, patient autonomy). Empowerment has been employed universally in the medical literature as a positive construct independent of the area of its application. Interest in empowerment in medicine now transcends its initial application in the psychology literature (Rappaport, 1984) to includes issues of organizational and clinical management (Loukanova et al., 2007). Empowerment has become an important concept in understanding individual-, organization-, and community-level development in health care, although a widely accepted definition of empowerment still remains elusive (Gibson, 1991).

Patient Empowerment

Medicine's tradition of physician paternalism, in which physicians control much of the information and decision making, is currently giving way to one in which patients play a significant role in medical decision making in particular and their own health care in general. Concurrent with this trend have been continued calls for medicine to embrace patient-centered care and to better inform the patient, pay more attention to patient-reported outcomes including patient preferences, and to focus more on patient satisfaction. In both academic and policy circles there has also be a great deal of interest in patient empowerment, which can be considered an umbrella term, encapsulating a vast array of processes and outcomes.

Exact definitions of patient empowerment vary, depending on the disciplinary backgrounds of scholars as well the target populations of interest. In the context of nursing practice and education, Gibson defines empowerment "as a social process of recognizing, promoting and enhancing people's abilities to meet their own personal needs, solve their own problems and mobilize the necessary resources to feel in control of their own lives" (1991: 359). In their research with people with mental illness, Linhorst et al. define patient empowerment as "having decision-making power, a range of options from which to choose, and access to information" (2002: 472). According to Chamberlin (1997: 43), the key elements of empowerment in mental health are "access to information, ability to make choices, assertiveness and self-esteem." In relation to health information, empowerment means that patients are able to take control of their own health care and to make informed decisions. In parallel literature, the term activated patient has also been used to refer to patients who actively participate in their health care through knowledge of disease and treatment options and acquisition of skills to manage their health status (Hibbard et al., 2004).

Types of Patient Empowerment

The patient empowerment literature has focused on society in various ways, with subliteratures centered around individuals, families, or communities. Articles on individual patient empowerment focus on the relationship between the individual who receives medical attention and the health-care system, while articles on family empowerment take a broader perspective of care, involving other caregivers such as parents or spouses. Community empowerment encompasses a group of people living in the same locality, sharing a common disease, sharing ethnic or cultural characteristics, and taking action to improve their lives and to achieve greater equality of power (**Figure 2**).

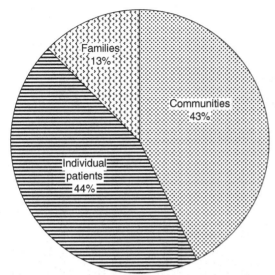

Figure 2 Focus of patient empowerment articles (1980–2005) Of the published articles in the medical literature focusing on patient empowerment, 44% focused on individual patients, 43% on communities, and 14% on families. Adapted from Loukanova S, Molnar R, and Bridges J (2007) Promoting patient empowerment in the health care system: Highlighting the need for patient-centered drug policy. *Expert Review of PharmacoEconomics and Outcomes Research* 7(3): 281–289.

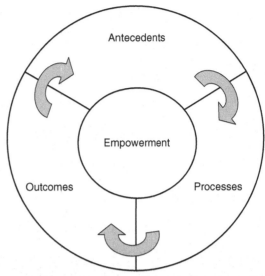

Figure 3 Empowerment as a self-perpetuating system. Patient empowerment is a system that involves important antecedents, processes, and outcomes. Adapted from Loukanova S, Molnar R, and Bridges J (2007) Promoting patient empowerment in the health care system: Highlighting the need for patient-centered drug policy. *Expert Review of PharmacoEconomics and Outcomes Research* 7(3): 281–289.

Models of Empowerment

Existing conceptual models in the literature involve issues such as community empowerment (Menon, 2002), nursing empowerment (Gibson *et al.*, 1991), or family empowerment. Population or disease-specific models have been published in the area of mental illness, brain damage (Man *et al.*, 2003), trauma patients (Fallot *et al.*, 2002), and diabetes (Anderson *et al.*, 2000). In a recent review of the literature, Loukanova *et al.* (2007) presented a conceptual model of empowerment for application to a general patient population. Here, empowerment is understood as a continually evolving process based on antecedents, or the necessary elements that allow patients to start the empowerment process; processes that emphasize the interaction between patients and the health-care system; and outcomes for the individual patient. This model tries to identify what is common about the patient empowerment process across different patient groups. It is presented (**Figure 3**) as a cycle, based on the type of relationships between the elements and the concept of a continuum with which this process is characterized.

Antecedents to empowerment include knowledge, health literacy, patient initiative, and advocacy and access to services. Important processes of empowerment are information sharing, doctor-patient communication, choice, and shared decision making. Finally, patient empowerment aims not only to improve health outcomes, but to generate patient-centered care that will affect patient satisfaction, self-efficacy, and adherence.

Measuring Empowerment

There are a number of instruments presented in the literature that attempt to measure patient empowerment, but they often focus on specific populations or diseases, rather than the general population. Examples include the Family Empowerment Questionnaire (Man *et al.*, 2003); the consumer-constructed scale in mental health services (Rogers *et al.*, 1997); Diabetes Empowerment Scale (Anderson *et al.*, 2000); Patient Activation Measurement (Hibbard *et al.*, 2004), and the Therapeutic Alliance Scale (Kim *et al.*, 2001) (**Table 1**). More research is needed to define in general the characteristics of the empowerment process that can serve as a basis for the development of a measure of patient empowerment in the general population.

A Holistic Model of Empowerment

Parallel to this recent rise in empowerment, a number of health-care systems have sought to become more patient-oriented. In the United States, a backlash against managed care and the growing number of uninsured and underinsured individuals with limited access to health care has in part precipitated calls for a more consumer-directed health-care system. In Europe, where there has been a long history of paternalism extending to medicine and where central agencies ration health care, there has also been an attempt to involve patients in medical decision making and introduce treatment options.

Table 1 Examples of validated measures of patient empowerment

Scale (Author)	Purpose	Validating study	Domains and items	Applications
The Diabetes Empowerment Scale (DES) (Anderson et al., 2000) and Short form of the DES (the DES-SF) (Anderson et al., 2003)	A measure of diabetes-related, psychosocial self-efficacy.	(DES) Patients with type 1 and type 2 diabetes (n = 375) (DES-SF) Patients with type 1 and type 2 diabetes (n = 229)	28-item DES with 3 subscales, derived from that behavior change model: Managing the psychosocial aspects of diabetes with 9 items; assessing dissatisfaction and readiness to change with 9 items; setting and achieving diabetes goals with 10 items. DES-SF is 8-item short form of the DES.	Shiu et al., 2005; Via et al., 1999; Glasgow et al., 2005
The Patient Activation Measure (PAM) (Hibbard et al., 2004) and Short Form of the Patient Activation Measure (Hibbard et al., 2005)	Patient knowledge, skill, and confidence for self-management.	A telephone survey of 1515 randomly selected adults in the United States, aged 45 years and older. A 48% response rate was achieved.	22-item measure that assesses patient knowledge, skill, and confidence for self-management. Stage 1 – believing the patient has an active role; stage 2 – having the confidence and knowledge to take action; stage 3 – taking action. The measure was developed using Rasch analyses and is an interval level, Guttman-like measure. The short form of PAM is 13-item measure.	(Hibbard et al., 2005)
Consumer-constructed scale to measure empowerment (Rogers et al., 1997)	Empowerment of consumers in mental health services	271 users of mental health services, members of 6 self-help programs in 6 states.	28-item questionnaire with 5 subscales measuring self-efficacy, self-esteem, power-powerlessness, community activism, righteous anger, and optimism-control over the future.	Hansson et al., 2005; Wowra et al., 1999; Corrigan et al., 1999; Geller et al., 1998
Patient empowerment scale (PES) in hospital environments catering to older people (Faulkner, 2001)	Identifying hospital environments that place patients at risk of becoming dependent, or which facilitate increasing independence.	Older hospitalized people (n = 102) from the elderly rehabilitation, acute surgery, and acute medicine	40 questions in a questionnaire with 2 types of items: 20 items coded E are empowering and 20 items coding D are disempowering acts.	Faulkner et al., 2006; Hage et al., 2005
Family Empowerment Questionnaire in brain injury (Man, 1998)	Empowerment among families with a member who has had a traumatic brain injury	Explorative factor analysis of responses of 211 families that included a brain damaged member	52-item Family Empowerment Questionnaire with 4 factors: skill, knowledge, support, and aspiration.	Man, 1999;
Empowerment questionnaire for people with brain damage (Man, 2001)	Empowerment of people with brain damage	112 people with brain damage	A 42-item questionnaire with 4 interpretable factors: support (13 items), skill (14 items), aspiration (9 items), and knowledge (6 items).	Man et al., 2003 Man et al., 2003
Treatment-related empowerment scale (TES) (Webb et al., 2001)	Patients' degree of control over the selection and use of drug therapy.	Anonymous survey of 43 patients with advanced HIV infection	10-item TES was specifically constructed to address components of communication, treatment choice, decision making, and satisfaction.	Man et al., 2004 Horne et al., 2004

In this section, we present a holistic model of empowerment that focuses on both patient and provider (or system) aspects of empowerment. In this model, patient empowerment is understood as a joint process whereby patients and providers work in partnership to enhance patients' involvement in their health and health care. This more complex system of empowerment brings together separate literatures on patient and provider empowerment, offering a more comprehensive account of empowerment. More importantly, the model highlights the role that the health-care system plays in patient empowerment. In this regard, patient empowerment is affected by all stakeholders of the health-care system including the state in its regulatory, financing, and purchaser role(s), and the profit and nonprofit sectors in financing, purchaser, and organizing roles. This model (**Figure 4**) also highlights some of the outcomes related to the fostering and promotion of empowerment for patients and providers.

Processes of Empowerment in Health Care

With all that has been written about empowerment in health care, little attention has been paid to how empowerment influences or impacts the provision of care. Based on a review of the literature, there are four overlapping themes in the literature that can be considered key processes involved in the empowerment of the patient, namely: (1) information sharing, (2) doctor-patient communication, (3) shared decision making, and (4) patient self-care.

(1) Information sharing

One of the principal processes of empowerment is information sharing, whether it is among patients, between the patient and physician, or with patients communicating with some external agency/advocate. Traditionally, information sharing efforts related to empowerment were based on grassroots and community programs, however, this has been affected dramatically by national public health campaigns (especially those using mass media), direct-to-consumer advertising, and by email and the Internet. While such broad-brush mechanisms prove to be a cost-effective method for information sharing, small-scale interventions and advocacy continue to play an important role in empowerment. Furthermore, mass media approaches to information sharing lack intimacy, partnership, and follow-up support that are synonymous with grassroots efforts.

For many, the easy availability of information has played an important role in transforming the doctor-patient relationship, while for others, it is a disruptive, potentially unempowering force. This bipolar view of information is best exemplified by the heated debate over direct-to-consumer advertising for pharmaceuticals (Gilbody et al., 2005), but it applies to any number of public health efforts that aim at changing patient behavior. It is certain that with better patient information comes patient responsibility, a responsibility that can be disruptive for many, leading some to classify information sharing as an antecedent to empowerment, rather than an activity of empowerment. Patient empowerment requires that patients are not just recipients of information – from only industry, providers, and government stakeholders communicating with the patient – but agents who can generate and

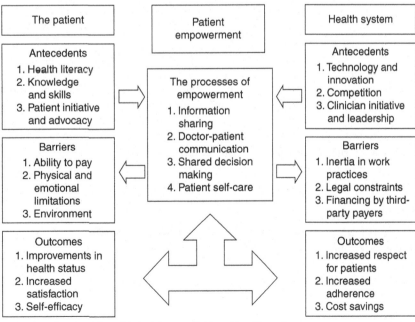

Figure 4 Patient empowerment as a partnership between patient and health system.

process information. For true patient empowerment, patients need to inform the health-care system about their own situation – both in terms of their health and what they would like out of health care. For example, new technologies, such as home-based monitoring devices, aim to facilitate this empowering process Patients are able to possess real-time knowledge about their (chronic) conditions, which can then facilitate more balanced communication between them and their physicians.

Patients can also possess valuable information in other ways. Self-help groups offer a supportive mechanism for which individuals with similar needs or experiences can be both student and teacher. Also, disease-specific patient associations serve as a valuable meeting place for patients to share information. In the United States, Medicare and Medicaid programs have a specific objective of nforming patients about their health-care opportunities – specifically aimed at promoting quality and price transparency.

(2) Doctor–patient communication

Focusing on the patient and the doctor, there has been an increasing emphasis on the transformation of the brief patient-doctor encounter into a lasting relationship with the mutual participation of both the patient and physician as the foremost goal. The active involvement of the patient is argued as a means by which problems inherent in health care (including information asymmetry between patient and physician and uncertainty) can be solved through honest and reasonable disclosure. As we move into an era of chronic illness, there is a growing need for better communication between doctor and patient. This interaction is impeded by time and resource constraints, language and cultural barriers, and by the notion (held by some patients and providers) that doctor knows best. While this latter notion has been reinforced by the professionalization of medicine over the past 100 years and the subsequent belief in informational asymmetries, it is also grounded in more ancient archetypes including tribal and religious convictions of the absolute power of the healer/redeemer (i.e., he or she who can give life also has the power to take it away).

Doctor-patient communication can serve both clinical and human needs. By necessity, such communication can be used to understand symptoms and patient histories, but more recently communication is used to understand the patient's needs and to discuss the optimal treatment path – including introducing the patient to any self-care tasks that they must undertake. On the human side, doctor-patient communication builds rapport and trust, an environment of empathy, and leads to more satisfaction for all parties involved (although a mismatch of patient and physician communication styles might not lead to rewarding communication). Thus, doctor-patient communication is not only vital to informed choice, but it leads to both positive health and nonhealth outcomes for the patient (Pignone et al., 2005).

(3) Shared decision making

Given the level of complexity of decision making in modern medicine and the differences between different patients (whether they be caused by variation in disease staging, genetics, lifestyles, or preferences), a shared decision-making framework is becoming increasingly necessary in medicine and a vital step in the empowerment of patients. Here we use shared decision making as an umbrella term to cover the principle of joint, doctor-patient decision making (in the literal sense) and policies, programs, and decision aides that facilitate a thoughtful discussion of health-care options between physician and patient. Given that involvement of the patients in decision making not only has important consequences for their own care (and how he or she feels about it), but also impacts the effectiveness of public health efforts in screening, treatment, disease-control programs, and (potentially) medical costs, a number of agencies now promote active, shared decision making. Surprisingly, there are many who believe that individual patients do not want to be involved in the decision-making process – often sighting ignorance, fear, or cultural barriers. Others believe that if prompted and assisted by an external advocate, these potentially unwilling patients can quickly learn and adopt shared decision making. To encourage such patients to speak up in the medical decision-making process, a number of agencies (both in the profit and not-for-profit sector) offer information about treatment options and decision aides in a range of conditions. A leader in this area is the Ottawa Health Research Institute which has developed numerous 'patient decision aids' to help patients and their health practitioners make tough health-care decisions (O'Connor et al., 1999). These decision tools prepare patients to discuss their health care with physicians by informing them about the options and possible consequences, creating realistic expectations, or providing balanced examples of others' experiences with decision making. Many patient groups now promote shared decision making, often using virtual support groups and storyboards/blogs to share patient experiences. These mechanisms foster doctor–patient communication by enlightening the patient to the various care paths and outcomes that other patients in their shoes have experienced.

(4) Patient self-care

One of the elements that best defines an empowered patient is patient self-care or self-management. Again, this encompasses a range of activities from patients triaging themselves to administering end-of-life pain management. It may involve preventative or behavioral change, or thorough self-management of medication for chronic diseases. Patient self-care may not necessarily place the patient in the driver's seat, but it does make them an important and valued member of the health-care team (as opposed to a passive player who is cared for or operated on). For some, this degree of patient involvement is unusual and infeasible given the lack of knowledge about health care, however, for the vast majority of cases, the patient is the initiator of care (e.g., 'something is wrong and I have to see the doctor'). Also, for chronic illnesses and other health-care issues that require care over long periods of time or across multiple providers, the patient often becomes the one constant in the health-care treatment equation. Movements toward patient self-care came to the forefront in areas such as mental health and care for people with disabilities, moving patients from institutional to community care and independent living. As lengths of stay have dropped, particularly in the United States after the adoption of prospective payments, additional care is provided in the patient's own home (assisted by home health-care services), requiring increased patient self-care. In Europe and Japan, patient self-care is also being promoted in care for the elderly to avoid the prohibitive costs of institutionalized aged care.

Patient self-care promotes personal initiative and responsibility for one's health, and helps patients make therapeutic choices that are more relevant to their own circumstances and preferences. This said, the ultimate goal of patient care is not just to improve the quality of life, but to increase the effectiveness of care. Existing patient self-management programs are often well monitored and supported by the health-care system, which needs to provide the necessary information, skills, and techniques for patients to be competent in the provision of their self-care. Traditional programs target consumers at risk of declining health or costly medical services through the application of evidence-based care, self-care support, multidisciplinary care coordination, and community collaboration. Self-care is a key to effectiveness and efficiency in the care of chronic disease, like diabetes, asthma, and mental diseases, which can be delivered directly by health-care providers, by specialized disease management organizations, or even by patients and patients' groups.

Patients' Role in Empowerment

As seen in **Figure 4**, the processes of empowerment are affected by both the patient and health-care system. Focusing first on the patient, a number of antecedents and barriers have been identified that support/limit patients' involvement in the empowerment process. A number of patient outcomes of empowerment have also been identified in the literature.

Patient antecedents

From the patient's perspective, there are several antecedents to empowerment, including health literacy, knowledge and skills, and patient initiative and advocacy. Patients must have a degree of health literacy to be active participants in health-care delivery and decision making. Health literacy affects the ability of the patient to comprehend health-care providers and to understand the diagnosis, treatment, and expected outcomes. Patients also need a basic knowledge of health and health care, and the necessary cognitive skills and time to participate when necessary. The final key to patient empowerment is patient initiative: the ability and motivation to become involved in decision making or to marshal the necessary advocacy resources to precipitate change.

Patient barriers

There are also several barriers that patients face in the road to empowerment, including ability to pay, physical and emotional limitations, and environment. Inability to pay for, or a lack of access to, health-care services is a key destabilizing force in the empowerment process. Patients may be further limited by their mental and health status and by the social environment in which they are situated. Addressing the barriers to empowerment at the individual level can be arguably more complicated, since these barriers concern attitudes and values, which are also often related to the social environment. For example, individuals have different attitudes regarding their willingness to participate in the medical decision-making process. One possible barrier to patient empowerment is that, a priori, patients might feel burdened by the process of decision making for the treatment of their health problems and may prefer to delegate all the decisions to their physician, although such decisions might not fit their needs, preferences, and values. Environment, or what is often referred to in the health systems literature as 'place,' also can act as a barrier to becoming empowered. For example, patients in rural or poor, inner-city areas may not only face access barriers to health care, but also have decreased access to education and advocacy groups. Access to both information and services is complicated, and hence often neglected, for people with disabilities.

Patient outcomes

A range of outcomes of empowerment have been noted in the literature including improvements in health status, increased satisfaction, and self-efficacy. Empowerment has been studied in a number of clinical areas leading to a solid literature linking patient empowerment to better health outcomes, such as for chronic conditions, asthma, and diabetes. Empowerment leads to patient satisfaction given that an empowered patient will have more say in their health care and (more importantly) be aware of the complexities involved in determining the optimal treatment. Some longitudinal studies have also demonstrated the impact of education or self-management training on self-efficacy, which is among the most important outcomes of empowerment. Self-care in particular is an important way in which the patient, instead of the physician, takes control over his or her health, lifestyle changes, and care-seeking behavior, understanding when medical attention is necessary.

The Health-Care System and Patient Empowerment

It is unclear if, left to their own devices, the providers who run health systems would aim to promote or restrict patient empowerment. While all health-care systems strive for the good of their constituents, it has been recognized that paternalism has dominated the practice of medicine (i.e., physicians 'care for' patients rather than provide clients a service). While a number of health systems have attempted to promote consumer rights and patient-centered medicine, these are potentially a reaction to external pressures from patient groups calling for patients' rights, as well as financial pressures from increased health-care consumerism, health tourism, and competition between providers. Again antecedents and barriers that support/limit the health-care system's role in patient empowerment have been identified in the literature, as well as potential outcomes of patient empowerment on the health-care system.

Health system antecedents

Regardless of how paternalistic or patient-centered health-care systems may set out to be, there are a number of antecedents that promote an atmosphere of patient empowerment within the health-care system: technology and innovation, competition, and clinician initiative and leadership. Arguably, technological change has done more to empower patients in the past 30 years than any other factor. Not only do we have new treatments, and even cures, for many diseases, but through innovation patients now need to spend less time in the hospital, have better access to information (especially through the Internet), and play an increased role in their own care. Competition drives innovation, whether it is promoted by way of professional, academic, or financial motives. By attempting to reach a larger customer base, physicians, hospitals, insurers, and industry have to provide products and services that patients deem beneficial. Finally, through the leadership of clinicians (especially nurses, social workers, and a limited number of physicians), health-care systems are changing to become more patient friendly. For example, the Institute of Medicine has been a major promoter of patient-centered care in the United States, and, at the micro and meso levels, physicians, nurses, and other health-care professionals have, and will continue to play, an important role in the empowerment of patients. While patient-centered care is not new, some of the interest in patient-centered care, especially in the United States, can be seen as a backlash to the 'financial-centered care' approaches of managed care or reaction against health-care rationing in countries with national health systems with *finite* resources.

Health system barriers

From a social justice perspective, health care is widely considered as a special good. Health care is also a complex good in that there is a great deal of uncertainty surrounding it. Limited resources for health care and substantial variations in care quality have led to government involvement in the financing and delivery of health care to ration and redistribute health care equitably. Rationing is often based on egalitarian principles, so that most people can afford health care as a means to function in society, or as a right. However, this perspective is often manifested as a form of paternalism instead of a respect for individual patient values and preferences. The historical development behind public provision, regulation, and financing of health care has often resulted in systems that impose barriers for patient empowerment in the health-care system such as inertia in work practices (especially in government bureaucracy), legal constraints, and financing by third-party payers.

Health care in any country is delivered (and in certain cases, financed) by a nexus of autonomous and semiautonomous agencies, spanning a range a professional and even cultural barriers, and thus pervaded by inertia. This is complicated by the traditional approach to medicine predominantly based on expert opinion and clinical judgment; thus care practices established over time have strongly influenced regulations, the role of professional societies, and governing agencies. Such an entrenchment of institutions/work practices – understood here as the customary ways, working rules, and legal regulations that shape and pattern behavior – in turn provides a context that explains the political and legal constraints to empowerment. For example, health reforms in many countries have encountered resistance to changes in medicine – a type of stickiness or path dependence – resulting in incremental reforms dominating the landscape of health policy making. Reliance on third-party payers or insurers can similarly inhibit empowerment as manifested by the development and spread of managed care financing approaches that insulate patients from decisions about health-care purchases. These three types of barriers may impede patient empowerment and perpetuate the current paternalist culture in medicine.

In the name of cost efficiency, choices are made on behalf of the patient. Choices available to the patient are purposely restricted both in terms of the range of providers available and the level of health care that can be consumed. The development of health technology assessment agencies aimed at promoting cost effectiveness, efficiency, and value of health care similarly have the potential to perpetuate medical paternalism and ignore the values of the patient through technically oriented evaluations and assessments, especially if they are restricted to the financial need of payers. In recognition, there is currently a movement to make these systems of evaluation more patient-centered, by explicitly assessing patient satisfaction with care and patients' involvement in care, eliciting patient preferences about care and desired health outcomes to support shared and informed decision making, so that a dialogue is opened up between the health-care system and patients, expanding patient choice and patient involvement.

Health system outcomes

The benefits of patient empowerment are not limited to the patient, but can affect health-care providers and the health-care system in positive ways, especially through increased respect for patients, increased adherence, and cost savings. As mentioned earlier, the active involvement of the patient has important consequences not just at the micro level (the patient's own health) but at the macro level as well in terms of successful public health efforts to improve health and achieve cost savings from effective programs. A major outcome of patient empowerment in the health system will relate to how patients are viewed. If patients are perceived as co-equals with health-care providers, then they will be treated in a manner that respects their unique needs, individual priorities, and personal well-being. Recognizing the individuality of every patient may lead to greater support from patients in their treatment plan – a mutually agreed to regimen. This may represent an ideal model of care given the high prevalence of poor treatment adherence, limiting ability to achieve therapeutic goals as well as the efficient use of resources. Cost savings can be generated from a decrease in the duplication and misuse of services, a reduction in hospitalization rates in favor of outpatient services, and an increase in the use of efficacious and acceptable medical regimens.

Conclusions

While many of the processes supporting patient empowerment have been occurring through patient advocacy, facilitated though professional encouragement by some key clinicians, the path to widespread patient empowerment will require significant health system reforms. These system reforms need to institutionalize empowerment concepts, approaches, and processes, as well as to correct power imbalances in the system. Such reforms will need to challenge existing power structures, especially the dominance of the physician. Further, such reforms will challenge existing systems of health-care financing, particularly the paternalistic national, social solidarity systems that emerged over the twentieth century. Health-care reforms will also be needed to transfer a greater degree of control to patients over their own health care. These include giving insured individuals greater choice in selecting treatments, level of premium payments, and user-fees. An example worth noting in this regard is Switzerland, which is regarded as a model of consumer-driven health care (CDHC). Switzerland reformed what was essentially a mosaic of 26 unique health-care systems into one health-care system through the Health Insurance Law, which took effect in 1996. From voluntary coverage, the reform made compulsory the purchase of health insurance coverage by households and redefined solidarity in the context of calculated premiums and premium subsidies. From risk-related premiums prior to 1996, premiums are community-rated while subsidies of health insurance premiums are means-tested.

Another example can be found in the Netherlands, which replaced its system of compulsory health funds and private health-care insurance with a single statutory regime anchored in individual choice and responsibility beginning in 2006. Under the new system, every resident has the choice of insurer and policy, including a replacement scheme in the form of a health savings account for conscientious objectors (i.e., people who are opposed to insurance in principle). Like Switzerland, individuals in the Netherlands are free to choose the level of out-of-pocket costs that they are willing and/or able to bear.

In the United States, there has been considerable discussion in recent years about the potential empowering effects of consumer-directed health care (CDHC) – a type of health insurance that combines high deductibles (expenditures, set at some predetermined level, that a patient or family has to pay out of pocket before the insurer will contribute to costs) and, in certain situations, a savings account option. So, the majority of patients are essentially paying out of pocket, because most annual expenditures, barring any catastrophic events, do not exceed the deductible level. With regard to the savings option, similar to a health savings account (HSA), insurance providers offer incentives not to spend the money, including rollover and the ability to 'cash in' the savings. A limited number of other countries have explored consumer-directed, health-financing options; Singapore is a notable example, as it is the first country to institutionalize HSAs. While there has been a great deal of rhetoric concerning the potential empowering nature of CDHC and HSAs, there is a lack of strong evidence as to the mechanism by which they do contribute, if any, to patient empowerment. In the United States, CDHC is often justified on the basis of cost savings (especially to the employer) and as a mechanism to cover uninsured persons who might not be able to afford the high cost of 'first dollar' (high deductible) health insurance. This said, these financing mechanisms have a great deal of potential to increase patient empowerment.

As health-care systems move in the right direction of involving patients as key stakeholders, there is hope that the patient will no longer be seen as a mere recipient of care. And, as health-care systems seek to become more responsive to the needs and preferences of patients, patients will become even more educated and involved in their own health care – in terms of better communication with their physician, being more selective of their insurer or provider, and being even more vocal in the health-care policy arena. The process of patient empowerment is changing the symbiotic roles of patients and providers in the health-care system, as is the responsiveness of the health-care system so as to create a partnership with the patient.

Citations

Anderson R, Funnel M, Fitzgerald J, and Marrero D (2000) The diabetes empowerment scale. *Diabetes Care* 23(6): 739–743.

Chamberlin J (1997) A working definition of empowerment. *Psychiatric Rehabilitation Journal* 20(4): 43–46.

Fallot RD and Harris M (2002) The Trauma Recovery and Empowerment Model (TREM): Conceptual and practical issues in a group intervention for women. *Community Mental Health Journal* 38: 475–485.

Gibson CH (1991) A concept analysis of empowerment. *Journal of Advanced Nursing* 16: 354–361.

Gilbody S, Wilson P, and Watt I (2005) Benefits and harms of direct to consumer advertising: A systematic review. *Quality and Safety in Health Care* 14(4): 246–250.

Hibbard JH, Stockard J, Mahoney ER, and Tusler M (2004) Development of the Patient Activation Measure (PAM): Conceptualizing and measuring activation in patients and consumers. *Health Services Research* 39: 1005–1026.

Kanter RM (1993) *Men and Women of the Corporation*, 2nd edn. New York: Basic Books.

Kim SC, Boren D, and Solem SL (2001) The Kim Alliance Scale. Development and preliminary testing. *Clinical Nursing Research* 10(3): 314–331.

Linhorst DM, Hamilton G, Young E, and Eckert A (2002) Opportunities and barriers to empowering people with severe mental illness through participation in treatment planning. *Social Work* 47(4): 425–434.

Loukanova S, Molnar R, and Bridges J (2007) Promoting patient empowerment in the health care system: Highlighting the need for patient-centered drug policy. *Expert Review of PharmacoEconomics and Outcomes Research* 7(3): 281–289.

Loukanova S and Bridges J (2008) Empowerment in medicine: An analysis of publication trends 1980–2005. *Central European Journal of Medicine* 3(1): 105–110.

Man DW, Lam CS, and Bard CC (2003) Development and application of the Family Empowerment questionnaire in brain injury. *Brain Injury* 17(5): 437–450.

Menon ST (2002) Toward a model of psychological health empowerment: Implications for health care in multicultural communities. *Nurse Education Today* 22: 28–39.

O'Connor AM, Rostom A, Fiset V, et al. (1999) Decision aids for patients facing health treatment or screening decisions: A Cochrane systematic review. *British Medical Journal* 319: 731–734.

Pignone M, DeWalt DA, Sheridan S, Berkman N, and Lohr KN (2005) Interventions to improve health outcomes for patients with low literacy. A systematic review. *Journal of General Internal Medicine* 20(2): 185–192.

Rappaport J (1984) Studies in empowerment: Introduction to the issue. *Prevention in Human Services* 3: 1–7.

Rappaport J (1987) Terms of empowerment/exemplars of prevention: Toward a theory for community psychology. *American Journal of Community Psychology* 15: 121–148.

Rogers ES, Chamberlin J, Ellison ML, and Crean T (1997) A consumer-constructed scale to measure empowerment among users of mental health services. *Psychiatric Services* 48: 1042–1047.

Zimmerman MA (1990) Taking aim on empowerment research: On the distinction between individual and psychological conceptions. *American Journal of Community Psychology* 18(1): 169–177.

Zimmerman MA (1995) Psychological empowerment: Issues and illustrations. *American Journal of Community Psychology* 23(5): 581–599.

Further Reading

Acquadro C, Berzon R, Dubois D, et al., PRO Group (2003) Incorporating the patient's perspective into drug development and communication: An ad hoc task force report of the patient-reported outcomes (PRO) harmonization group meeting at the Food and Drug Administration, February 16, 2001. *Value in Health* 6(5): 522–531.

Anderson RM and Funnel MM (2005) Patient empowerment: reflections on the challenge of fostering the adoption of a new paradigm. *Patient Education and Counseling* 57: 153–157.

Arnstein SRA (1969) Ladder of citizen participation. *Journal of the American Institute of Planners* 35(4): 216–224.

Bastian H (1998) Speaking up for ourselves. The evolution of consumer advocacy in health care. *International Journal of Technology Assessment in Health Care* 14(1): 3–23.

Bridges J (2003) Stated preference methods in health care evaluation: An emerging methodological paradigm in health economics. *Applied Health Economics and Health Policy* 2(4): 213–214.

Bridges J and Jones C (2007) Patient based health technology assessment: A vision of what might one day be possible. *International Journal of Technology Assessment in Health Care* 23(1): 30–35.

Gagnon M, Hibert R, Dube M, and Dubois MF (2006) Development and validation of an instrument measuring individual empowerment in relation to personal health care: The Health Care Empowerment Questionnaire (HCEQ). *American Journal of Health Promotion* 20(6): 429–435.

Glasgow RE, Wagner EH, Schaefer J, Mahoney LD, Reid RJ, and Greene SM (2005) Development and validation of the Patient Assessment of Chronic Illness Care (PACIC). *Medical Care* 43(5): 436–444.

Tomes N (2006) The patient as a policy factor: A historical case study of the involvement of the consumer/survivor movement in mental health. *Health Affairs (Millwood)* 25(1): 720–729.

Relevant Websites

http://www.aachonline.org – American Academy on Communication in Healthcare.

http://www.consumersinternational.org – Consumers International.

http://www.each.nl – European Association for Communication in Health Care.

http://www.eurordis.org – European Organization for Rare Diseases.

http://www.eu-patient.eu – European Patients Forum.

http://www.gesundheitsinformation.de – Gesundheits information, Institut für Qualität und Wirtschaftlichkeit im Gesundheitswesen (IQWiG) (German).

http://www.informedhealthonline.org – Informed Health Online (English).

http://www.patientsorganizations.org – International Alliance of Patients' Organizations.

http://www.npsf.org – National Patient Safety Foundation.

http://decisionaid.ohri.ca – Patient Decision Aids, Ottawa Health Research Institute.

http://www.pickerinstitute.org – Picker Institute.

http://thepatient.adisonline.com – *The Patient: Patient-Centered Outcomes Research Journal*.

Community Health Workers

S B Rifkin, London School of Economics and Political Science, London, UK

© 2008 Elsevier Inc. All rights reserved.

History and Background

Community health worker (CHW) is an umbrella term to describe a lay person who lives and/or works closely with local communities and who provides basic health care, including health education. Community health workers emerged as part of the health workforce during the twentieth century as a result of the changing environment. New discoveries in causes of disease during the nineteenth century began to translate into public health interventions (such as the provision of clean water and disposal of human waste) during the twentieth century. As a result, prevention was seen to be equally important as cure, and involving local communities in public health actions became increasingly necessary. This new situation gave rise to two developments that underpinned the role of the CHW at the end of the century. The first, resulting from the lack of human resources to deliver the new interventions, particularly in the less developed (and often postcolonial) world, was the involvement of local lay people in health-care delivery. The second, promoted in a classic text on health care in the developing world edited by Maurice King in 1966 (King, 1966), was the advocacy of involving local communities through their leaders in planning, executing, and managing health prevention activities focusing on health education for behavioral changes and health actions for sanitation.

As a result of this new situation, health professionals began to use lay people in the community to deliver health care. In China, in the 1920s, a Rockefeller Foundation pilot program in Ding Xian trained farmers to record births and deaths, vaccinate for smallpox and other diseases, give first aid, give health education talks, and maintain clean wells. In other countries in the developing world, locals were trained for control of infectious diseases such as diarrhea and malaria. In rural Africa, doctors would train locals to help with surgery. In the United States, health guides were trained to link the health services with black communities.

Experiences of local community involvement in health provided evidence and inspiration for the World Health Assembly's 1978 meeting in Alma Ata. At that meeting, the policy of primary health care (PHC) was proposed and accepted by all member states. PHC, reflecting concerns for social justice, highlighted the values of equity, community participation, prevention, multisectoral collaboration, and appropriate technology to rapid health improvements (WHO, 1978). It has been argued that a health-care model (often described outside the political context of the Chinese revolution) developed in the People's Republic of China gave proof of reasons to pursue these principles. The most highly profiled contribution was a community health worker, seen to be a replication of China's 'barefoot doctor.' Supporting solutions to few human resources for health care and promoting the political context of a mass people's revolution, a 'barefoot doctor' was a local person trained to give basic health care but also to become an 'agent of change,' promoting broader engagement of community people in decision making and responsibility. Although most often taken outside the political context in which it developed, the 'barefoot doctor' concept became the focus of debates about the role of the community in health care.

In the Alma Ata aftermath, there was a flurry of documents and activities pursuing CHW programs. Many governments, reacting to the lack of more concrete proposals to implement PHC, focused on launching CHW programs to prove their commitment to the new strategy. A tendency arose to identify PHC as CHWs (Mburu, 1994).

More critical than the limited interpretation of PHC, however, was the development and implementation of the programs themselves. The debates focused around two sets of issues. The first was the technical issues, including training, tasks, competencies, payment (or volunteer), support and supervision, and sustainability. The second group of issues revolved around the CHW as an 'agent of change,' highlighting issues around power and control. These issues, best articulated in an article by David Werner (1977) included whether CHWs were empowered or oppressed as a result of the existing socio-economic-political structures, bureaucracies, and health professionals; whether CHWs were valued by community people; whether CHWs used their positions to gain material rewards for themselves; and whether CHWs promoted the medicalization of health by overprescribing medicines.

The decade following the Alma Ata Declaration saw a proliferation of both governments and nongovernmental organizations (NGOs) initiating and supporting CHW programs, both in developing and developed countries. By the end of the 1980s, researchers had collected data to examine the above issues in some detail. The experiences of several smaller NGOs in impoverished rural areas recorded success stories. Several of them, such as Jamkhed in India, gave proof of how CHWs could extend medical care and create opportunities for community participation and empowerment. In 1959, Maybelle and Raj Arole graduated from Vellore Medical College in India and began their rural service, which led them to commit their lives to the rural poor. By 1970, their experience inspired them to set up a program in one of the poorest and most remote places in India. Using curative services as a community entry point, they began to gain the trust and confidence of the local people. Responding to the most immediate need – no water – the doctors worked with local people to build wells, siting them in the lowest-caste areas so caste taboos would begin to break. In 1974, members of farmers' clubs attached to the hospital carried out a health survey. As a result of this exercise, the farmers' club demanded that women be trained as village health workers. These workers served community people and began to develop community funds helping those who lacked resources. They did follow-up on mothers to ensure antenatal care and vaccination of newborns, gave health education, and carried out 'village clean-up' drives. The program spread throughout the district. By 1990, Jamkhed was providing training for other CHWs, both Indian and foreign (**Figure 1**) (Arole and Arole, 2002).

Other NGO experiences, such as the White Mountain Apache program in eastern Arizona, USA, gave evidence of success in attacking rural poverty and poor health in areas of deprivation in comparatively rich industrial nations (Taylor-Ide and Taylor, 2002).

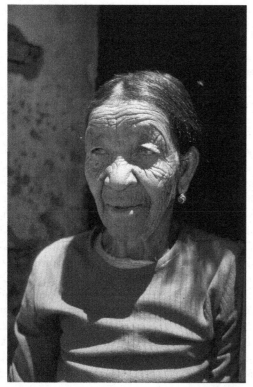

Figure 1 The face of a CHW — kind, caring, compassionate, and experienced. Photo courtesy by Pitt Reitmaier.

However, data from large government programs recorded more difficulties. Examining government programs in *Community Health Workers in National Programmes? Just Another Pair of Hands?*, Walt (1990) and her colleagues investigated three programs (in Botswana, Colombia, and Sri Lanka). They concluded that needs for local health care, the demands of government bureaucracy, and the lack of money and support by professionals for wider community development (change agent) roles meant that the CHW was essentially a low-cost health worker extending government services. The vision of a community person able both to extend health services and to facilitate greater choice and potential for individual health and material improvement proved difficult to realize.

The period from the 1990s until the early 2000s saw interest in CHWs begin to wane. Several national programs disappeared. PHC and CHW programs in particular proved to be much more costly than previously considered. Concerns about cost-effectiveness overtook the Alma Ata vision of a more just, equitable, and people-oriented health system. The political environment that supported more social welfare concerns and broad government benefits gave way, after the collapse of the Soviet Union, to a more market-oriented political and economic system. This new environment had several consequences for CHW programs. On the one hand, the new role of government to oversee rather than to provide health care meant much less money for government health delivery programs. On the other hand, decentralization and reduced state support for care provision stimulated communities to become more involved in health care at the local level.

In the new millennium, with growing emphasis by international organizations including the World Bank, which provides the greatest amount of funding to the UN, and other Bretton Woods institutions for poverty alleviation, the CHW has again attracted interest. The agendas of many international organizations and bilateral donors began to focus on equity and empowerment as the way of improving and sustaining the lives of the poor. As a result, promotion of community-based activities as a means to break cycles of poverty regained ground. In health, for example, India has initiated a Rural Health Mission in 2005, calling again for the support of an expanded female CHW cadre responsible for building awareness around village health rights, giving first-level health care with appropriate referrals, and supporting family welfare programs (GOI, 2005). Interest also has been stimulated in training local people to fill large gaps created by migration of trained health staff to more lucrative jobs in industrialized countries (Haines et al., 2007). For example, the United Nations Millennium Project in 2005 called for a massive increase in human resources to meet the UN Millennium Development Goals.

This overview of the development of CHWs suggests the importance, value, success, and/or failure of CHW program can be analyzed by examining five issues.

Issue One: Who is a CHW?

The CHW is a local resident who learns health knowledge and skills, particularly in the area of preventive work and health education, and serves the local community people. This person (usually female) should be accountable to the community for her work. She should be supported by the health system, but not part of it, and should be trained for meeting community needs with shorter courses than professionals (Kahassay et al., 1998).

This wide definition covers both men and women without defining educational qualifications. This definition covers uneducated women who learn to perform tubectomies with highly successful outcomes in a rural health program in Bangladesh. This definition also includes people trained to extend clinical and preventive services that focus on a single disease such as malaria. It includes local high school graduates in New York City, trained to encourage behavioral change to prevent hypertension-related disease (Walt et al., 1990). However, traditional healers who are part of local communities are not covered by this definition unless they are specifically trained as part of a CHW program. CHWs are not part of the formal health system, but rather an important support for the system at the grassroots level.

There has been some discussion as to whether a standard definition of CHW is critical to their development. It has been suggested that without such a definition, the tasks to be carried out and quality of service cannot be assured. However, the range of experiences of CHW programs is wide and varied. CHWs record results both positive and negative that reflect the culture and environment in which they operate. The reality of CHW programs rather suggests that flexibility is more important than standardization, because it allows programs to meet needs defined by the community that each CHW serves.

Kaseje and Sempebwa (1987) give an example of community health workers in Saradidi, Kenya. This program sought to provide outreach to villages covering about 43 000 people in 56 villages. As a beginning 126 CHWs were trained. Each CHW served 10 households that had about an average of 4 persons per household. The CHWs were chosen and supported by the community in which they lived. They were not required to be literate or to have a formal education. About 98% were women between 25–39 years old. They spent about 5–10 days in the program each month spending about 2 hours with each household they visited. Although barriers were identified barriers such as lack of pay, lack of transport, weak village support committees, and lack of medicines, only 4 of the 126 CHWs dropped out of the program after 4 years. The reasons for remaining included: receiving continuous training; their commitment to serving the village; their view that they were contributing to the health of the community; the pay they occasionally received; and their own personal development.

Experience shows that the CHWs are people who work with local communities carrying out tasks that range from extending clinical services to mobilizing at-risk individuals or all community members to undertake preventive activities. While small NGO programs have explored and promoted programs in which CHWs became involved in wider community development work and empowerment activities, it appears their immediate value to health improvements is as an extension of a resource-constrained health service.

However, demands continue for addressing the role of CHW as an agent of change.

Issue Two: Can CHWs Be Both Service Extenders and Facilitators for Community Improvement?

CHWs within the PHC framework were conceived to be both service providers and agents of change. The Alma Ata Declaration posed a challenge for this vision to be realized. PHC broadened the definition of good health to include addressing root causes of poor health in the existing social, economic, and political environment. The view recognized that health improvements were not simply the result of health service provision.

The experiences of poverty and community over the last 30 years gives evidence that to be effective CHWs need to play both roles. They must respond to the community needs of health provision but also support community people to make changes to improve their lives. A study by Bhattacharyya et al. (2001) reviewing incentives for CHWs well illustrates this point.

The study reviewed the experiences of a number of CHW programs. The main conclusion was that the effectiveness of CHWs depends primarily on their relationship to the community. They noted that it was vital to involve the community in all aspects of the program. For this reason, CHWs must play a role as a facilitator in order to function as a health service provider. One example is that community people use CHWs for health care when trust and credibility has been established between provider and patient. Another example is to meet the high demands for health care; when the CHWs have worked closely with other community organizations such as religious groups or women's groups and shared concerns and objectives, these groups can lighten the load by taking on health education activities.

An equally important aspect of facilitation is the process that supports empowerment. This process has been critical, particularly for women, who are the majority of CHWs around the world. The CHW profits from this process, in the first instance, by learning new skills and knowledge and gaining confidence through working with colleagues and trainers in the program. She helps to empower the people she serves by giving them the benefits from her own experience and serving as a role model. This role is particularly evident in countries where women's movements and opportunities are limited. The female CHW is allowed to go to meetings with other CHWs to promote her work and also take knowledge and skills to other women who are fairly isolated in their homes. For women in particular, the facilitation role is as important as the health provider role. It enables both the CHW and those she serves to find ways of improving their lives and their health.

Sheikh et al. (2007) give an example of women health volunteers in Tabriz City, Iran that illustrates this point. In the city of Tabriz, a cadre of Women Health Volunteers (WHV) was created in 1994 to provide health center outreach to urban women. In the early years, this program focused on collecting vital statistics from and giving health education (mainly family planning information) to the 50 families to whom each WHV was assigned. In 2005, a pilot program was designed to shift the emphasis of work from information provision to opportunities for empowerment. A group of WHV were trained in participatory methods then used these visualization of mapping and priority matrices to do a participatory needs assessment with volunteers from their assigned cohorts. The needs assessment revitalized the WHV and engaged the local women actively in health promotion activities. In one case, the neighborhood women identified priority as 'reclaiming' the local park from drug addicts who prevent them from using it. With the help of one of the WHV an exercise hour was organized each morning where 40–50 local women would walk together in the park for one hour. The sight of a large number of women dressed in traditional chador (a black material covering women from head to foot) frightened addicts from the park. The group continued to walk and to organize other activities such as health education classes for women over 50 and meetings with young men at the local mosques to discuss the problem of drug addiction (**Figure 2**).

The role of a community worker as change agent and a focal point for the process of empowerment has been particularly difficult in the field of health. In large part, the reason is because health professionals define most causes of health improvements as 'interventions.' Such a framework demands standard indicators for outcome and impact. It does not give flexibility to assess individual experiences or examine community work as a process. It restricts the understanding about how this process links to

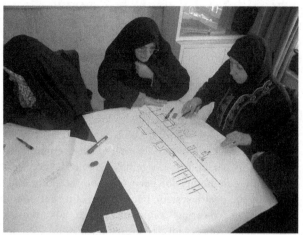

Figure 2 CHWs—mapping community health problems in Iran. Photo by SB Rifkin.

attitudes, beliefs, and behaviors of people and how the CHWs promote positive change in these areas (Rifkin, 1966). This aspect of the contribution of CHWs calls for a new framework and more research.

Issue Three: What Training and Support Does the CHW Need?

CHW programs developed in response to specific situations. Because there was no standard definition of the term, there has been no standard program of training. Most training programs are focused on teaching CHWs to respond to local health problems. CHWs are most often trained in the place where they live. This situation allows the training to be responsive to other demands on the trainee's time. Lankester and his colleagues (1992) describe a model that has been adapted by many other CHW programs. It suggests that the training program begins by teaching CHWs for a period of one week to three months. After this period, training continues once a week or every two weeks until the participants cover the material that has been designed for their program. Training can also be done intermittently, teaching one or two days per week. However, this obviously takes more time and risks the problem of the community losing interest.

CHW training programs focus, for the most part, on health and disease problems and solutions. Topics covered are commonly: care of children under 5 years old, care of pregnant mothers, prevention and treatment of common diseases in the location of the community, first aid, and environmental health, as well as more general topics such as record-keeping, methods of communication, and building partnerships with those concerned with health in the community. Programs in which the aspects of agents of change are important emphasize communication and, at present, participatory approaches to health promotion (**Figure 3**).

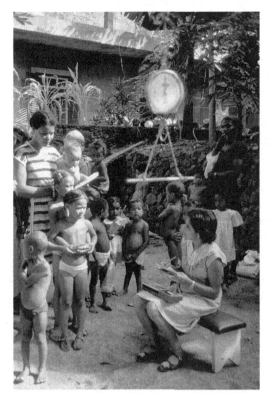

Figure 3 A CHW weighing children to check if they are malnourished. Photo courtesy of Pitt Reitmaier.

Topics on community facilitation have gained more emphasis with the recognition of the threat of the HIV/AIDS epidemic. CHW programs expanded in communities where this disease is rampant. CHWs supervise the use of antiretroviral therapy, encourage people to take up services, and reach out to vulnerable groups to involve them in prevention, care, and treatment. However, WHO promotes a wider role for workers in this area. In the *World Health Report* (2004), WHO argues that CHWs should not merely be seen as a source of cheap health-care delivery. Rather, they can and should be a part of the broader strategy to help community people gain more control over their own health and their own lives. HIV/AIDS has helped to bring the idea of CHWs as agents of change back on the agenda, and WHO has sought to integrate this training in the programs to address issues around the control of this disease.

Support for CHWs and their work depends on three pillars: the community, the health system, and internal program incentives. Support from the community is perhaps the most critical. Without this support, the CHW cannot operate. A major contribution to gaining this support has been to ask the community to choose its own workers. Although this process can and has been abused, it is the only one that has the potential to create a sense of ownership and accountability between CHWs and the people they are to serve. Small-scale programs have tried to strengthen this bond by forming community health committees to provide a direct link between the CHW and community representatives. However, these committees appear not to have been as successful as the individual relationships the CHW forms.

Support from the existing health system is critical for cementing the relationship between the community and the CHW. Components of this support include the health service structure (hospitals, health centers, and health posts); the health service management (the heads of all local health units); and, in the presently promoted decentralization policies in an expanding number of countries, the district and lower government units as well as civil society (members of groups outside the health system such as women's groups, labor groups, etc.). These components support CHWs by providing referral units for care, providing supervision of their work, giving them recognition for their contributions, and building local-level partnerships so their work can be carried out effectively. Where these systems are unstable, where the infrastructure and/or management capacity is weak or nonexistent, and where funds and/or commitment are lacking, CHWs struggle to provide effective and valued contributions (Kahssay *et al.*, 1998).

CHWs want to know what incentives the program provides for them as individuals. Receiving payment is the most obvious. There are no standard remuneration schemes for CHWs. Programs vary from giving a small standard payment each month to having people work as volunteers without any money. CHWs do sometimes get nonmonetary contributions from community people. However, a study by Bhattacharyya *et al.* (2001) gives evidence that money is not the sole incentive. CHWs are supported by recognition of their work, by gaining new skills, by gaining status in the community, by getting preferential treatment, and by having flexible hours and clear roles. The study highlights that the main incentive is the commitment of the CHW to contribute to improving health in his or her own community. Where this commitment is not recognized and supported, programs have high dropout rates or may close.

Issue Four: Are CHW Programs Effective?

The promotion of CHWs in the 1970s and in the wake of the Alma Ata Declaration was based on the failure of clinical care to meet the need of the majority of people, particularly the rural and the poor. Clinical care was limited to institutional curative care. It did not reach those far from clinics, nor did it address integrating other aspects of care, such as prevention and health promotion activities needed to insure good health. The introduction of CHWs was an attempt to overcome these barriers. What is the evidence that these programs have met these expectations?

A study undertaken by Witmer and colleagues (1995) summarized the evidence of CHW contributions to the delivery of primary and preventive care in the United States. The studies showed that, working with underserved populations, CHWs facilitate health care through outreach, prevention, and health-promotion services. They also have been effective in maternal and child health programs through health education and improved service access. They helped people in the community keep health service appointments and follow their medication regimens. They proved to be an effective link with mental health services and with services to those vulnerable to HIV/AIDS. Beyond service provision, CHWs have informed healthcare providers about community needs for the communities with which they work, CHWs promote consumer protection and advocacy. CHW programs also contribute to the empowerment of the CHW by allowing low-skilled unemployed workers and welfare recipients to seek new jobs and career advancement (**Figure 4**).

In the area of disease control and prevention programs, there also is evidence of some success. Data from Latin America shows that CHWs have been key to full immunization coverage in urban areas of Mexico and rural Ecuador (Walker and Jan, 2005). Their flexibility for service delivery and their ability to target each separate household was key to this success. A review of CHWs in Africa assessed their contribution to disease control programs, particularly to malaria and TB with the administration of directly observed treatment, short course (DOTs) (Lehmann *et al.*, 2004). HIV/AIDS is another area in which using CHWs as service providers has recorded positive results. These programs have also often expanded the role to emphasize CHWs as change agents as described above. In Haiti, for example, a small NGO called Zanmi Lasante uses CHWs (called 'accompagnateurs') to supervise antiretroviral therapy and provide community outreach, including case identification in marginalized populations. A study showed that the CHWs properly identified at-risk people at the community level and facilitated uptake of services. These encouraging results will be used to argue for a standardized training for all CHWs in both biological and social realms (Mukherjee, 2007).

In a review of the evidence, Berman and his colleagues (1987) concluded that in small-scale, well-managed programs, CHWs had the potential to overcome problems of health-care delivery due to limited human resources. There is much less evidence that this potential has been equally recognized in large-scale government programs. Many governments reduced or discontinued their CHW programs in the 1980s due to the pressures of financial constraints and health system reforms. However, in Pakistan, where a program training CHWs (called 'lady health workers') was created in the 1990s, some positive gains have been seen (Douthwaite and Ward, 2005). The tasks of the lady health workers focused on promotion of health for women of reproductive age. In addition to making contraception services available in the home, they promoted childhood vaccinations, monitored children's growth, gave first aid, made referrals for more serious cases, and gave health education. Evidence shows that in the first years of the program, contraceptive uptake grew from 12% to 28%.

However, experience also suggests there are major barriers that result in CHW programs not reaching expectations. The following are some of the more frequent:

1. CHWs' roles are fragmented. They are asked to deliver services and facilitate community change. In terms of

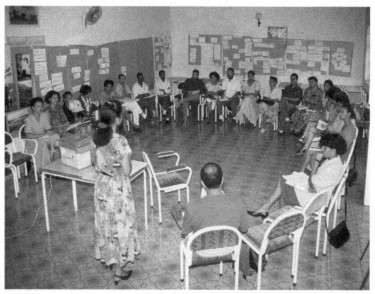

Figure 4 CHW providing health education for a group of community people. Photo courtesy of Pitt Reitmaier.

the former, the demands of the health service and of the community means that they must have knowledge about a very wide range of topics. As a result, they often do not have basic knowledge about topics that are the most relevant at the moment. In terms of the latter, they do not receive support from professionals. Often, health professionals do not have skills and attitudes to promote wider community development roles.
2. Their training is not standardized. Thus, some CHWs might know quite a bit about a topic while others may know very little. Available training material has not been disseminated, used, or adapted. There is no system to check information or integrate new information into training and in-service programs.
3. Supervision from formal health staff and monitoring and evaluation of CHW work is often weak. Supervision is erratic or often not done. Lack of monitoring and evaluation means programs cannot correct faults.
4. Incentives are not supportive of their work. Payment is not standard. There are few opportunities to learn new skills and knowledge. CHWs are often treated as low or nonpaid labor and see themselves as being exploited.
5. CHWs do not integrate with other health providers. They do not receive support for their work from other health-care organizations in the community. Their links to the formal health-care system are weak, so they do not get support from government institutions. They often are seen as rivals for work from private providers or traditional healers.

The above barriers also help to explain why the role of a change agent is difficult to assess. It is not only because there are no adequate frameworks at present to assess the effects of community interactions with CHWs but also because there are difficulties in formulating these interactions in a standard model. These difficulties reflect both the problems of describing what a supportive environment is as well as describing replicable relationships between CHWs and community people. As a result, studies that assess the influence of the CHW on empowerment of communities are either anecdotal or combined with program descriptions of the entire range of CHW work, which mainly focuses on health-care provision.

Issue Five: Are CHW Programs Sustainable?

With examples of positive program results and increasing interest in developing CHWs as a supplement to increased demand for but reduction in supply of health service providers, programs are likely to expand. What is known about their sustainability?

In the present environment of neoliberal economics and health system reform, sustainability is most often discussed in the context of cost-effectiveness. In other words, what is the return on investment in any specific intervention? Some of the early thinking about CHWs suggested that there was very little cost, so this criterion was not often considered. However, it very soon became apparent that even with free voluntary labor, primary health-care programs and CHW programs generated considerable expenditures. CHW programs needed trainers, training materials, upgraded training sessions and materials, medicines, often transport, and supervision and support from health professionals. Such expenditures had to be traded off against other types of interventions and use of human resources. Thus, CHW programs were quickly absorbed into this framework for the assessment of value for money.

The criteria for biomedical interventions are fairly easy to determine. Costs and expected outcomes are readily identifiable. In the case of making the same analysis for CHWs, there are several constraints. In their article, Walker and Jan (2005) discuss in detail some of these problems. They note that objectives of CHW programs can be classified into three categories: health gains, individual nonhealth benefits (looking at benefits to individuals resulting from the process of care and the information given in the cultural context and in autonomy given to patients in treatment), and social nonhealth gains (the changes that take place in the wider community because of the existence of the program). Particularly the last two criteria are obviously not amenable to a single standard indicator.

Despite these recognized constraints, there have been attempts to examine whether investment in CHWs gives enough benefit to continue to fund them. A study by Islam *et al.* (2002) published in the *Bulletin of the World Health Organization* reports research that compared the cost of a TB control program run by an NGO, Bangladesh Rural Advancement Committee (BRAC), with a program run by the government that did not use CHWs in the same area. In the government area, 185 patients who were identified as positive cases and were treated by DOTS provided at health units had an 82% cure rate. In the BRAC areas, a total of 186 patients used CHWs to deliver DOTS with an 84% cure rate. The government program cost US$96 per patient while BRAC's program cost US$64 per patient. Thus, the BRAC program was found to be more cost-effective than that of the government.

In an earlier study, Berman and colleagues (1987), while acknowledging the difficulties of using cost-effectiveness, nevertheless reviewed a number of programs in this context. This article served as a basis for other evaluations of programs. After reviewing six large-scale CHW programs and several small-scale programs, the authors concluded: (1) in the programs under review, CHWs reached more people than programs that were clinic-based, (2) after a review of the costs, CHW programs in general had a lower cost than clinic-based programs, (3) CHWs had the potential of delivering effective interventions that addressed the health problems causing major mortality in the population, but (4) the quality of care was poor due to failures in training, supervision, and logistics, and (5) to date there was no evidence of a large-scale impact on health . Their review suggested that in the 10-year period following Alma Ata, CHW programs had both low cost and low effectiveness. What the programs needed to improve was the combination of more adequate support, and that implied more resources.

Whether more support and more money will be forthcoming depends. Haines and his colleagues (2007) suggest it depends on four factors. The first is the national socio-economic and political environment in the countries where CHWs operate. Influences here include the political will, the level of poverty, the existence and support for participatory structures and governance, and the level of corruption.

The second factor is the community. Whether programs will be sustained and grow depends not only on cultural factors but, equally important, on community leadership and location of the community. It depends on the health situation and health beliefs. More critically, it depends on community support and the commitment of CHWs to work in the community. The situations that influence this factor have been discussed previously, concerning barriers to CHWs being effective. In addition, it depends on how issues of community mobilization and empowerment are addressed. CHW programs that succeed are 'owned' by the community – the community is not merely mobilized to support the program.

The third factor is the health system. The links and support of health system infrastructure and professional health staff, as seen above, are key to program sustainability. Where there is unclear communication, lack of interest from and/or competition with health staff, lack of recognition and value for CHWs, and no perception of future developments for CHWs, programs are weak or fail.

The fourth factor is the international environment. What determines support for CHW programs is, first, the support, particularly in financing, from the international and bilateral donor agencies. Particularly in low-income countries, where there is a great need for more human resources (often the result of migration of local health staff) to deliver low-cost and effective interventions, donor aid is needed to support these programs. Donor support depends on evidence that the community values the role of CHWs in service delivery and that CHWs' work contributes to empowerment of themselves and community people. The international environment also contributes to more technical developments affecting CHW work. These developments include both biomedical research for new cost-effective interventions and technical assistance to improve the delivery of interventions at the community level.

Community Health Workers: The Way Forward?

This review of CHWs has described and analyzed the role of CHWs in both health-care delivery and in becoming catalysts for changing attitudes, beliefs, and behaviors of people at the community level. It reviewed the history of the theory and practice of CHW programs. It highlighted how the role of the CHW has reflected advances in medicine, particularly in public health, as well as the international and local social, political, and economic environment. It summarized the experiences of CHW work. The remaining question is: What is the way forward?

In the immediate future, the value of the CHW is seen mainly as an additional resource for meeting increasing demands from overstretched health professionals in all parts of the world. There is also recognition of the value of CHWs in supporting empowerment among themselves and local people to break the cycle of poverty. This situation provides the possibility for poor people who have the potential to contribute to health care, mainly women, to gain skills and knowledge to improve their own health and their own lives. It also provides opportunities for others in the community to get the same opportunities. For these reasons, it can be argued that CHW programs continue to be relevant and will gain new and critical support.

In the longer term, the determinants of the future of medicine and society will also determine the role of the CHW. While it is predictable that biomedical advances will need people to deliver these interventions and to promote changes in the community to make the interventions effective, it is less predictable that CHWs will be able to play an important role. One reason is that the political environment that promoted social justice in health now emphasizes a market economy with incentives for individual community gains. Another reason, in part a response to these new values, is that communities where CHWs functioned best (tightly bound communities with a history of mutual support, most often poor and fairly isolated) are beginning to break down. The young, wanting to take advantage of this new environment, leave rural areas for the big cities. In rapidly growing urban areas, communities are much less structured, competition is fierce, and there is less support for individuals. This situation poses new challenges for community workers in all fields of development.

In the field of health, the role of the CHW will depend on answers to a number of questions. These include, for example: What are the incentives for those who get training and opportunities to remain in their own communities and help those less well off? How can those who move out and gain better living conditions help support those who remain at home? More questions and more answers will determine the future of the CHW.

In conclusion, this review gives evidence of the contribution CHWs have made to health improvements at the community level in the twentieth and early twenty-first centuries. Although hard to quantify and generalize, this support has a wide range of evidence to suggest an impact on health improvements. However, in a rapidly changing world, it is difficult to make predictions about how this important role will develop and whether and how it will remain relevant. CHWs were a creation of the changes in understanding about how health improves. Their future rests in the continual exploration of this topic and, as in the past, in the political, social, and economic environment that creates the response to this change.

See also: Health Issues of the UN Millennium Development Goals.

Citations

Arole M and Arole R (2002) Jamkhed, India: The evolution of a world training center. In: Taylor-Ide D and Taylor C (eds.) *Just and Lasting Change: When Communities Own Their Future.* Baltimore, MD: Johns Hopkins University Press.

Berman P, Gwatkin D, and Burger S (1987) Community-based health workers: Head start or false start towards health for all? *Social Science and Medicine* 25: 443–459.

Bhattacharyya K, Winch P, LeBan K, and Tien M (2001) *The Community Health Worker: Incentives and Disincentives; How They Affect Motivation, Retention and Sustainability.* Arlington, VA: Basic Support for Institutionalizing Child Survival Project (BASICS II) for the United States Agency for International Development.

Douthwaite M and Ward P (2005) Increasing contraceptive use in rural Pakistan: An evaluation of the lady health worker programme. *Health Policy and Planning* 2: 117–123.

GOI (Government of India) (2005) *Rural Health Mission.* New Delhi, India: Government of India.

Haines A, Sanders D, Lehmann U, et al. (2007) Achieving child survival goals: Potential contribution of community health workers. *Lancet* 369(9579): 2121–2131.

Islam A, Wakai S, Ishikawa N, Chowdhury AMR, and Vaughan J (2002) Cost effectiveness of community health workers in tuberculosis control in Bangladesh. *Bulletin of the World Health Organization* 80(6): 445–450.

Kahssay HM, Taylor ME, and Berman P (1998) *Community Health Workers: The Way Forward.* Geneva, Switzerland: World Health Organization.

Kaseje DC and Sempebwa EK (1987) Characteristics and functions of community health workers in Saradidi, Kenya. *Annuals of Tropical Medicine and Parasitiology* 81(supplement 1): 56–66.

King M (ed.) (1996) *Medical Care in Developing Countries.* Nairobi, Kenya: Oxford University Press.

Lankester T (2000) *Setting up Community Health Programmes: A Practical Manual for Use in Developing Countries.* London: Macmillian.

Lehmann U, Friedman J, and Sanders A (2004) A joint learning initiative: human resources for health and development: review of the utilization and effectiveness of community-based health workers in Africa. *JLI Working Paper* 4–1.

Mburu FM (1994) Whither community health workers in the age of structural adjustment? *Social Science and Medicine* 39(7): 883.

Mukherjee JS (2007) Community health workers as a cornerstone for integrating HIV and primary health care. *AIDS Care* 19(Suppl.1): S73–S82.

Rifkin SB (1996) Paradigms lost: toward a new understanding of community participation in health programmes. *Acta Tropica* 61: 79–92.

Sheikh M, Tarin E, Behdjat H, and Rifkin SB (2007) *From informers to transformers: a new role for Women Health Volunteers in Tabriz City, Iran.* Presented to 5th European Congress on Tropical Medicine and International Health, Amsterdam.

Taylor-Ide D and Taylor C (2002) *Just and Lasting Change: When Communities Own their Future.* Baltimore, MD: The John Hopkins University Press.

Walker D and Jan S (2005) How do we determine whether community health workers are cost-effective? Some core methodological issues. *Journal of Community Health* 30(3): 221–229.

Walt G (ed.) (1990) *Community Health Workers in National Programmes: Just Another Pair of Hands?* Milton Keynes, UK: The Open University Press.

Werner D (1977) *The Village Health Worker: Lackey or Liberator?* http://www.healthwrights.org/articles/lackey_or_liberator.htm (accessed November 2007).

Witmer A, Seifter W, Finocchio L, et al. (1995) Community health workers: integral members of the health care work force. *American Journal of Public Health* 85: 1055–1058.

World Health Organization (1978) *Primary Health Care.* Geneva, Switzerland: WHO.

World Health Organization (2004) *The World Health Report: Changing History.* Geneva, Switzerland: WHO.

Further Reading

Abbatt F (2005) *Scaling Up Health and Education Workers: Community Health Workers; Literature Review.* London: DFID Health Systems Resource Centre. www.dfidhealthrc.org/publications/health_service_delivery/05HRScalingUp03.pdf (accessed November 2007).

Binka FN, Nazzar A, and Phillips JF (1995) The Navrongo community health and family planning project. *Studies in Family Planning* 26(3): 121–139.

Frankel S (1992) *The Community Health Worker: Effective Programmes for Developing Countries.* Oxford, UK: Oxford University Press.

Gilson L, Walt G, Heggenhougen K, et al. (1989) National community health worker programs: How can they be strengthened? *Journal of Public Health Policy* 10(4): 518–532.

Lewin SA, Dick J, Pond P, et al. (2005) Lay health workers in primary and community health care. *Cochrane Database of Systematic Reviews* 1: CD004015.

Love MB, Gardner K, and Legion V (1997) Community health workers: Who they are and what they do. *Health Education and Behaviour* 24(4): 510–522.

Niettaamaki L, Koskela K, Puska P, and McAlister AL (1980) The role of lay workers in community health education: Experiences of the North Karelia project. *Scandinavia Journal of Social Medicine* 8(1): 1–7.

Werner D (1983) *Where There Is No Doctor: A Village Health Care Handbook.* London: Macmillan.

World Health Organization (2007) *Community Health Workers: What Do We Know About Them? The State of Evidence on Programmes, Activities, Costs and Impact on Health Outcomes of Using Community Health Workers.* Geneva, Switzerland: WHO. www.who.int/entity/hrh/documents/community_health_workers_brief.pdf (accessed November 2007).

Relevant Websites

http://www.brac.net – Bangladesh Rural Advancement Committee.
http://www.healthlink.org.uk – Healthlink Worldwide.
http://www.hesperian.org – Hesperian Foundation.
http://www.hreoc.gov.au/HUMAN_RIGHTS/rural_health/nyirrpi_grandmothers.html – Human Rights and Equal Opportunity Commission, Rural Health Examples.
http://www.pih.org/home.html – Partners in Health.
http://bhpr.hrsa.gov/healthworkforce/chw/5.htm – US Department of Health and Human Services, Community Health Workers National Workforce Study, Chapter 5.
http://www.who.int – World Health Organization (WHO).

KEY FEATURES OF HEALTH SYSTEMS AROUND THE WORLD

National Health Systems: Overview

N Goodwin, King's Fund, London, UK

© 2008 Elsevier Inc. All rights reserved.

Introduction: What is a National Health System?

There is no single definition of what might comprise a 'national' health system. According to the World Health Organization (WHO, 2000), for example, it comprises "all activities whose primary purpose is to restore and maintain health ... improving the health of the population they serve, responding to people's expectations, and providing financial protection against the costs of ill-health" (WHO 2000: 5–8). The activities (health actions, according to WHO) of a national health system are thus characterized by the expressed intent of those within it to improve health. The definition is a useful one in that it recognizes that any health system is a combination of resources, organizations, and financing and management arrangements that ultimately culminate in the delivery of health services to a population. Therefore, every country can be said to have some form of national health-care system, regardless of how unstructured or unsystematic its operation.

Building an effective and affordable national health system is a major preoccupation of governments around the world as they attempt to bring together – whether by contractual incentives or through publicly delivered services – the necessary components that are needed to improve health status and provide accessible and responsive services to the needs of individuals, families, and communities. A major difference, therefore, between a health system and a 'national' health system is the involvement of the state (governments and legislative bodies). Consequently, the nature of a national health system is characterized as much by predominant political motivations as it is by the opportunities and/or limitations imposed by the availability of financial and human resources.

As Maxwell (1992) discusses in his six dimensions of quality (**Table 1**), the principles of all national health-care systems are broadly the same yet the combination of these principles can lead to competition, both politically and financially, depending on which principles are regarded as more or less important. If one was to think of a national health system as an automobile, for example, there are trade-offs to be had between choosing a model that is eco-friendly and economical with one that has a high-performance engine and a higher specification of internal comfort. What aspects of care make a national health-care system more or less effective can, therefore, depend on individual circumstances or point of view. It is because of this that national health systems can be seen to have varying degrees of success in living up to these different principles and are so readily influenced by political objectives.

The Functions of a National Health-care System

The basic structure of a national health system can perhaps best be illustrated in **Figure 1**. It reveals that all national health systems are split into four principal functions: financing, purchasing (or resource allocation), service provision, and stewardship. Within each principal function are a number of important subfunctions. For instance, the financing element to a national health-care system requires not only the ability to collect revenue but also a process of managing that revenue collection through, typically, the pooling of resources to ensure that the risk of having to pay for health care is shared across a population rather than by each contributor individually. Similarly, the provision of services can be usefully split between personal services (services that people receive from a health agent, such as a doctor or dentist) and nonpersonal services (programs manifested in public health measures to promote healthy lifestyles or public works that improve water quality and reduce the prevalence of disease). Stewardship, which is represented as a theme working across the three main delivery elements of the system, represents the important process of managing and/or regulating the national health system. This is an important aspect because it is the responsibility of the system to protect the people by ensuring their money is used wisely. Stewardship of the system, through regulation and governance of activities, can also promote efficiency and quality in care delivery practice and may also help to engender a sense of national citizenship. These four principal functions of national health systems are performed very differently internationally. The following sections will illustrate these variances using case examples.

Formal Care and Lay Care

Before embarking on an analysis of the different functions of a national health system, it is important to make a quick distinction between formal and lay (or informal) care. When considering the components that make up a national health-care system, it is tempting to think immediately of doctors and nurses, of surgeries and hospitals, or of educational and health promotional interventions. However, it is a fact that the majority of health care (over 80%) is administered by one's self (self-care), family members, friends, and 'lay carers.' This is true regardless of a country's level of development. Hence, while a national health system encompasses a wide range of activities with a health improvement goal, the major part of care is provided in the informal setting and is unpaid.

In the United Kingdom, for example, about one-eighth of adults act as 'health carers' to some extent (not including routine parenting such as care for a sick child). Whereas much of this is social care (feeding, washing, dressing, and providing emotional support) the system has begun to invest in 'expert carers' that, for instance, enable more lay people to provide care advice, dress wounds, or give intravenous drugs. That the services provided by lay carers in the UK crosses the boundary with formal care provides recognition that there is a significant gray area in distinguishing between the formal (within the system) and the informal (out of the system).

Financing Health Care

Financing a health-care system is critical to its sustainability and key challenges are faced in ensuring that the necessary organizational and institutional arrangements are in place to raise revenue from which to reward and motivate health-care providers. There are two principal functions to financing: (1) revenue collection, the process by which a national health system receives money, and (2) pooling resources, the process by which this revenue is managed to ensure that individual contributors are not exposed to the high costs of having to pay for health care through risk sharing with other members of the pool. According to the World Health Organization (2000), differences in how these functions are administered impact directly on the relative performance of national health-care systems, yet the mechanisms through which financing systems operate can vary dramatically between nations.

In an excellent analysis of the advantages and disadvantages of different funding options, Mossialos *et al.* (2002) show that revenue can be collected from a range of sources, through varying collection mechanisms, and by different collection agents. Examples of funding sources, contribution mechanisms, and collection agents (and their various combinations) can be seen in **Figure 2**. This reveals that the sources of funds – or who pays for health services – can vary from individuals, households, employees, and employers (firms and corporate bodies) to loans, grants, and donations from foreign governments, nongovernmental organizations (NGOs), and charities. In most national health systems, however, funds derive primarily from the population (by individuals and/or those that employ them).

Methods of Revenue Collection

As **Figure 2** shows, there are many different approaches to collecting revenue including taxation, social health insurance, private health insurance, out-of-pocket payments, and loans and donations. National health systems are often defined by their dominant revenue collection. Thus, health systems in France and Germany are known as social health insurance systems because it is that method that generates the principal source of funding. In a similar way, countries such as the United Kingdom or Sweden are often referred to as tax-based systems while in the United States it is private health insurance within a business model of health-care provision that predominates.

In many low-income countries, however, economic hardship means that their ability to collect prepayments by way of social health insurance or tax revenues is

Table 1 Maxwell's (1992) six dimensions of quality in a health-care system

1. Access to services
2. Relevance to need (for the whole population)
3. Effectiveness (for individual patients)
4. Equity (fairness)
5. Social acceptability
6. Efficiency and economy

Adapted from Maxwell R (1992) Dimensions of quality revisited: From thought to action. *Quality in Health Care* 1(3): 171–177.

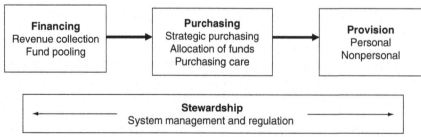

Figure 1 The basic structure of a national health system.

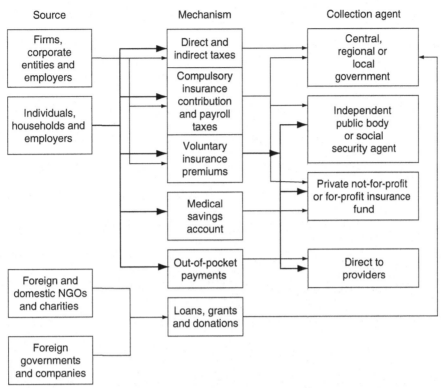

Figure 2 Examples of funding sources, contribution mechanisms, and collection agents within a health system. Adapted from Mossialos E, Dixon A, Figueras J, and Kutzin J (2002) *Funding Health Care: Options for Europe.* Buckingham, UK: Open University Press.

limited, so their systems rely on out-of-pocket charges and donor contributions. Indeed, in lower-income countries around the world, revenue collection methods tend to be less able to finance care through forms of prepayment. For example, in Latin America, most countries employ a mixed model of social health insurance, private health insurance, and taxation for public health services with a higher percentage of out-of-pocket expenditure. In sub-Saharan Africa, out-of-pocket payments are the principal source of revenue, exposing individuals to the risks associated with meeting health-care costs that prepayment schemes that pool funds for a defined population do not.

Taxation

Taxation methods of raising revenue for health systems can vary a great deal. For example, taxes may be raised for general purposes (the proportion allotted to health care to be determined later) or hypothecated such that a certain proportion is earmarked for health purposes. The potential advantage of the latter is that it directly links tax and spending, making it more transparent to the public where tax money is spent. A key disadvantage, however, is that it reduces the ability to be flexible in the prioritization of government tax revenue and limits the range of tax sources that governments may use to obtain health funding. Taxation may also be 'direct' – for example, levied on individuals through an income tax or on businesses by a company tax – or 'indirect' such as taxes on goods and services that people buy, import, and export. Whereas direct taxes have the advantage over indirect taxes in their ability to be progressive (high-income earners pay relatively more yet health benefits are available to all) rather than regressive (fixed amounts, e.g., for a vehicle license), certain direct taxes can have the benefit of influencing consumer behaviors. Taxing goods such as tobacco or alcohol may deter consumption of goods regarded to do harm to health and so help improve health itself. Taxes that go to health care are often also raised locally as well as nationally – an approach that is argued to improve accountability and responsiveness to local people because the system provides more transparency since health-care expenditure in a local tax system is usually the largest percentage of what a local authority spends (e.g., up to 70% in Sweden). However, in systems without adequate redistributive mechanisms of tax income between rich and poor localities, inequalities in health-care provision inevitably arise.

A good example of a national health system that is predominantly funded through taxation is Sweden (**Figure 3**). In Sweden, there are three independent

National Health Systems: Overview

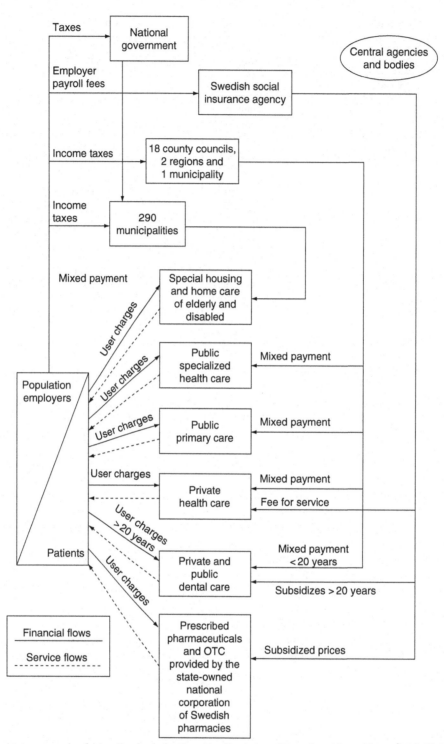

Figure 3 Sweden as an example of a taxation-based national health system. Reproduced from Glenngård A, Hjalte F, Svensson M, Anell A, and Bankauskaite V (2005) *Health systems in transition: Sweden,* p. 2. Copenhagen: WHO Regional Office for Europe on behalf of the European Observatory on Health.

government levels involved in health care: the national government, the county councils, and the municipalities. All three levels play an important role in the welfare system and are represented by directly elected bodies that have the right to levy taxes on the population to finance their activities. Overall goals and policies are set at a national level by the Ministry of Health and Social Affairs, while both the financing and provision of healthcare services are primarily the responsibility of the county councils. According to Sweden's three basic principles for public health and medical care – the principle of human dignity, the principle of need and solidarity, and the principle of cost-effectiveness – care should be provided on equal terms, according to need, and it should be managed democratically and financed on the basis of solidarity (Glenngård et al., 2005).

Social Health Insurance

Social health insurance is a system of contributions (usually compulsory) shared between employee and employer who pay a percentage of income to a government-sanctioned insurance fund. Like taxation-based funding, a key advantage is the process of prepayment into a large risk pool (discussed later), and like taxation-based funding, there is tremendous variance in the methodologies employed internationally to collect the insurance payments. Hence, in Germany, 'sickness funds' are created both by geographical locality and by occupational group, while in France and the Netherlands, the system is organized through smaller independent funds that provide the population with choices on the types and levels of care coverage they would prefer. Single national insurance funds are also common, such as those that existed in Croatia and Slovakia.

Social health insurance systems are often regarded as preferential to taxation models of funding since budgetary and spending decisions are ring-fenced (that is, funds are reserved specifically for expenditure on health care). In theory, this protects health-care funding from political interference. Moreover, a key element to such systems is the development of social solidarity since the system guarantees the entitlement to individuals of a set level of health-care coverage at a cost that is highly visible to them. However, as Goodwin et al. (2006) note, the system is not without its disadvantages. For instance, since eligibility is based on employment, there is the potential for restricted access to the elderly and unemployed. Also coverage tends to focus primarily on personal health care, rather than on the nonpersonal elements of a health system that emphasize public health interventions. Significantly, as costs of health systems in all Western countries rise, social health insurance is less able to adapt to the rising costs of provision. Indeed, as the example of the French health-care system shows (**Figure 4**), social health insurance systems often include significant elements of taxation-based subsidies, additional voluntary insurance, and various user charges that help to bridge the gap between revenues collected and expenditure.

The French health-care system (see **Figure 4**) was inspired by the Bismarckian (German health system founded by Bismarck) model, with health insurance funds under the supervision of the state. It relies on a combination of public and private supply, even in the hospital sector. Patients benefit from easy access to care (freedom of choice, direct access to the specialists) and an abundant supply of self-employed doctors, in particular. Complementary voluntary health insurance to cover the cost of statutory copayments is widespread (Sandier et al., 2004). The financial sustainability of the French health-care system is a perpetual source of concern, particularly due to the fact that actual expenditure consistently exceeds the targets set. Until now, the high cost of the health-care system has been accompanied by high levels of access to health care, but the demographic change expected within the health professions may lead to an increase in explicit rationing in future years. Nonetheless, the French health-care system was ranked the best in the world in the World Health Report 2000 for its effective combination of responsiveness to demands and social equality (WHO, 2000).

Private Health Insurance

Unless you live in the United States, private health insurance is usually of a second order of significance in the funding of your national health system. In low-income countries, for example, private insurance accounts for less than 2% of total health expenditure whereas in high-income countries it rarely exceeds 15%. Private health insurance is obviously least affordable to those on the lowest incomes yet is not necessarily the domain of the most affluent. For example, in both social health insurance and tax-based national health systems, private health insurers are often used by individuals to fill gaps in service coverage that are otherwise excluded from the nationally funded system. This form of private insurance is thus complementary to existing entitlements and is sometimes known colloquially as a top-up policy.

There are two other main forms of private health insurance: supplementary and substitutive. Supplementary insurance takes the form of an additional payment to receive enhanced benefits in addition to those offered through a social health insurance scheme. Hence, it may allow for quicker access to care, can be located in more comfortable surroundings, or be exempt from the costs of copayments such as those levied on drugs or inpatient stays. As **Table 2** shows, more than 90% of individuals in the French health system take out supplementary private insurance to protect against the high level of copayments involved in accessing the nationally funded system.

Substitutive private insurance, as the name implies, is an alternative to social health insurance and is taken up by those who may be excluded from public cover. In Germany and the Netherlands, for instance, employees earning above a certain income are excluded from care provided by the social insurance scheme (though not exempt from making payments) and are required to take out 'compulsory voluntary' insurance to get the care they

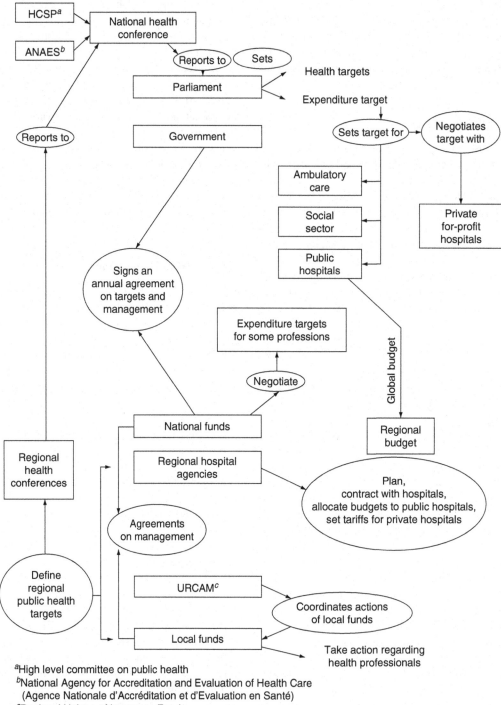

Figure 4 France as an example of a social health insurance-based national health system. Reproduced from Sandier S, Paris V, Polton D (2004) Health care systems in transition: France, p. 21. Copenhagen, Denmark: WHO Regional Office for Europe on behalf of the European Observatory on Health Systems and Policies.

require. Depending on their level of income and personal choice, individuals may opt back into the national system of social insurance health coverage or seek a private insurance agent. As **Table 2** shows, supplementary, substitutive, and complementary private health insurance tends to be prevalent in certain types of national health systems.

The United States remains the only Western healthcare system whose primary source of funding comes

Table 2 Forms of private health insurance in taxation and social insurance-based health systems

Country	Main source of funding for health system	% population covered by health system	% population with private insurance	Type of private insurance
Denmark	Taxation	100%	28%	Complementary
France	Social health insurance	100%	>90%	Supplementary
Germany	Social health insurance	88%	9%	Substitutive
Netherlands	Social health insurance	64%	29%	Substitutive
Sweden	Taxation	100%	1.5%	Supplementary
UK	Taxation	100%	11.5%	Supplementary

Reproduced from Organisation for Economic Co-operation and Development (OECD) (2004) Towards high performing health systems: Summary report. Paris: OECD.

through private health insurance. It is also the only country among the most developed nations without universal health-care coverage. Often referred to as a business model, the health system in the United States comprises a complex array of competing company-based and private for-profit and not-for-profit health insurance agencies offering a range of care plans to consumers and/or their employers. Providers of care, often working in large group practices and/or associations, contract with insurance agents (sometimes exclusively) and are generally paid on a fee-for-service basis. Cost inflation in the U.S. health system – influenced by the predominance of fee-for-service provision, investment in medical technologies, the high cost of medical malpractice claims, and high consumer demands – has resulted in the most expensive health-care system in the world (16% of GDP in 2004). Such rising costs have led to a growing number of citizens who are underinsured or without any health insurance coverage, despite a significant tax-funded component manifest in Medicare (for the elderly) and Medicaid (for the poor and disabled). To counteract these system failures, local managed care systems run by health maintenance organizations (HMOs) developed in the 1980s to provide enrollees with comprehensive care packages through an exclusive and integrated network of providers. However, antitrust legislation and consumer demands for lower-priced health plans have all but led to the demise of the HMO movement.

Out-of-Pocket Payments

Unlike in the previous three prepayment models, where it is possible to pool funds and spread risks among a population, a health system in which people must pay out of their own pockets for a substantial part of the costs of health services clearly restricts access to the more expensive forms of care. In most low-income countries, where prepayment systems are unavailable, out-of-pocket payments are often the only way to raise revenue and cover costs – leaving those who cannot afford treatment at higher health risks. Community financing is a method often promoted in such countries in an attempt to create pools of funds and reduce risks. For example, the Bamako Initiative – promoted in many parts of Africa since 1987 – helps provide local access to essential primary care services by decentralizing revenue collection and decision making to local communities. The basis of this approach to health system funding is to levy a small out-of-pocket charge when a drug or basic care is provided and then invest this in a fund from which local people prioritize investment into their community's health needs. The approach has been moderately successful and has led to relative improvements in coverage, affordability, and use of care in many parts of Africa (McPake et al., 1993).

In high-income countries, where prepayment models exist, copayments and user charges are often employed as a form of both income generation and also demand management by health system architects faced with the prospect of rising health expenditures resultant from growing consumer needs and demands. Depending on the level at which these user charges are set, and on the use of exemption strategies for at-risk populations, such fees have been criticized for dissuading the poor from using services. They also do not appear to raise revenue to enable sustainable improvements to care and are inequitable.

Loans, Grants, and Donations

External aid is a substantial source of funding for the health sector in many low-income countries where it can account for as much as 90% of the overall health budget. Aid is most often provided by bilateral agencies (donors from a particular country) such as USAID (United States), DANIDA (Denmark), and DFID (UK). Multilateral agencies (pooled donor resources between countries) are also prevalent and include organizations like the World Bank and the United Nations Development Fund (UNDF). Aid from such organizations is often provided as loans or grants to which a set of conditions concerning their use is established by donors; in most cases, these are linked to specific projects that are developed and delivered separately between donors and national governments. While many projects have been successful, project-based approaches have been seen to lead to fragmentation and duplication of effort and/or time and effort from national governments in responding to the priorities of donors rather than concentrating on wider health sector programs. Moreover, grants do not necessarily lead to greater expenditure in the health sector as governments may view the funding as a substitute for their own expenditure, or as an opportunity to channel resources toward other priorities. Loans, grants, and donations, if not managed carefully, may thus do more harm than good. Aware of this, many donors and governments are beginning to embrace longer-term and strategic support programs; such sector-wide approaches have been seen to be successful in countries such as Bangladesh, Ghana, and Pakistan.

Pooling Resources

Fund pooling is the sharing of risk between contributors. The ability to prepay for care services and to pool funds has significant advantages for a national health system because it enables the equalization of contributions among members, regardless of their risk of needing to use services. Moreover, the approach has the benefit of economies of scale, thus allowing for cross-subsidization. **Table 3** gives examples of how different countries can approach risk pooling, for example, from the development of social insurance funds (sometimes called sickness funds) to smaller community-based pools. As the examples imply, a range of agents might be involved in the pooling process from which a larger central pool is developed or, conversely, pooling might be devolved on the basis of risk-adjusted allocations to regional or local agencies who are then enfranchised to address local health-care needs and priorities.

Larger risk pools are obviously better than small ones because they can increase the overall availability of funds to improve and develop health services, enable economies of scale in administration, and reduce the levels of contribution to protect individuals against uncertain need. From **Table 3**, it might be predicted that Colombia's fragmented system of small organizations would damage the performance of the health system in these three areas. Evidence from Argentina pre-1996, in which there were more than 300 small pooling organizations in the system – most with fewer than 50 000 members – would support this proposition. The many small pools of funds meant that available health-care packages were very limited (especially in poor areas where low wages limited contribution levels). In West Africa, community financing initiatives to raise local pools of funding to plan and deliver drugs and care to local people have in many cases provided some protection from the risks of out-of-pocket payments, but the low level of pooled resources means such approaches are beset with problems of financial sustainability (Goodwin et al., 2006).

The key lesson to be learned from this section is that the ability of a national health system to prepay for health care, and to develop large resource pools to cross-subsidize care between high- and low-risk people, is fundamental to a national health system's sustainability and operational effectiveness. It should be noted that it is not the number of pools that is the issue, but their size relative to population health-care needs.

Purchasing Health Services

The management of purchasing is essential in ensuring that providers of services meet the goals of a national health system. As Goodwin et al. (2006) discuss, purchasers of health services face three fundamental challenges: which packages of care to buy, from whom to buy them, and how to buy them. Size is important for purchasing organizations because larger purchasers not only have

Table 3 National examples of approaches to spreading risk and subsidizing the poor

Country	System	Spreading risk	Subsidizing the poor
Colombia	Large number of small multiple pools	Competing social security	Organizations, municipal health
Netherlands	Multiple pools; mostly private competing social insurance funds	Intrapool via nonrisk-related contribution and interpool via central risk equalization fund	Via risk equalization fund, excluding the rich
Republic of Korea	National health insurance (covers 30% of total expenditure of any member) and Ministry of Health	Intrapool via nonrisk-related contributions. Explicit single benefits package for all members	Salary-related contribution plus supply-side subsidy from Ministry of Health. Public subsidy for insurance to the poor and to farmers
Zambia	Single formal pool held by Central Board of Health	Single benefit package for all financed by general taxes	Intrapool via general taxation. Supply-side subsidy via the Ministry of Health

Reproduced from World Health Organization (WHO) (2000) The World Health Report 2000. Health systems: Improving performance. Geneva: WHO.

administrative advantages in terms of economies of scale, but also have more bargaining capacity over both price and quality.

Which Packages of Care to Buy: The Role of Strategic Purchasing

Strategic purchasing requires a continuous search for the best interventions and care packages to purchase. This can be seen to occur at two levels in national health systems – first, at a societal and political level, the extent of health-care coverage and the goals of the system (related to the section entitled 'Stewardship' later in this article); and second, the identification of those services and interventions that will meet these goals best. The latter implies responsibility for allocating resources and/or creating incentives and negotiating with providers.

Many countries, especially low-income countries, cannot afford to provide comprehensive health-care benefits for the entire population and face major imbalances in resource allocation – for example, between rural and urban regions, and between rich and poor communities. Defining priorities to achieve maximum health gain for the money that is available to purchase services becomes a key task. Many countries address this through a policy of essential care packages (ECPs) aimed at purchasing services with the greatest potential of reducing the burden of disease. The policy of ECPs has been promoted internationally as the most effective way of channeling scarce resources into interventions with the highest health impact.

How Health Systems Purchase Services

The mechanism through which care is bought – that is, how to purchase services – is crucial because the method of payment establishes different kinds of incentives that providers will react to and the subsequent cost and quality of the services they provide. As Goodwin *et al.* (2006) describe, there are three main methods by which health systems purchase services:

1. Full retrospective reimbursement for all expenses incurred, manifest in fee-for-service payments;
2. Reimbursement for all activity based on a fixed schedule of fees using a tariff, based on a system of health- or diagnostic-related groups (HRGs and DRGs); and
3. Prospective funding based on the expected future expenditure using a fixed budget, manifest in salaried employment, directly managed and/or devolved budgets, and capitation.

Retrospective reimbursement is a payment scheme whose level is determined only after services have been provided. It may involve *per diem* payments, a cost-per-case, or a direct service payment. To health systems, the main problem with this model of purchasing is the inability to control provider costs effectively due to weak forms of audit and control of activity. In the United States, for example, the cost of Medicare and Medicaid services (tax-based funding for the old and poor) that began in the 1960s could not be maintained beyond 1983 because federal government income did not provide enough revenue to cover costs. It was known as the blank-check era since providers received payment for all care deemed 'customary, usual, and reasonable.' As the number of people on Medicare rapidly climbed and costs spiraled the system was replaced with DRG-based funding; a similar policy shift occurred in Germany's social insurance system in the early 1990s.

Prospective payment requires a tariff to be set to charges agreed in advance with providers, the most common being the DRG. DRGs categorize patients based on their primary and secondary diagnoses, primary and secondary procedures, age, and length of stay. The categories establish a uniform cost, enabling funders to set a maximum amount payable for a suite of care to a patient. Under this system, providers are given the incentive to keep their costs down as they would experience a profit (or surplus) if their costs are below the tariff in the DRG category. National health systems, therefore, benefit from more efficient providers and provider competition based on quality rather than cost. Such as system, called payment by results, has recently been established in the English National Health Service (NHS) to replace traditional capitation-based funding.

Prospective funding is a system that many national health-care systems have in place. Under this system, a global budget for health-care spending is often set within which envelope care can be purchased. Funding agencies acting on behalf of governments then allocate a fixed proportion of that budget to providers. The method of allocation can vary, for example, from political negotiation (a settlement), to provider competition (a bid), or by way of historic precedent and activity. Most countries use more sophisticated combinations of the three, for example, devolving resources to local purchasing agencies based on the needs of local populations based on their demographic profiles (capitation). This approach is favored in most high-income countries of Europe where a fair share of resources through capitation-based formulae is generally mixed with historic local expenditures and political negotiations. Variations to the approach are, therefore, commonplace. For example, budgets in Italy are renegotiated retrospectively; local taxes are raised in Sweden to supplement the national allocation; care is rationed in Norway through waiting lists or entitlement changes; and in most countries, such as Finland, copayments are levied to raise revenue and manage demand.

Types of provider payment mechanisms, therefore, produce different system incentives (**Table 4**). Fee-for-service and prospective payment mechanisms provide strong incentives to meet consumer demands and deliver timely services, but are weaker in containing costs and do not necessarily invest in services that prevent health problems. France is a classic example, and the rising costs of the system has led the French to reconsider its strategic priorities including limiting entitlements, increasing the use of copayments, and introducing capitation payments as a way of controlling costs. By contrast, the English NHS, historically highly cost-effective in service delivery terms due to its capitation-based system and primary care-led system of gatekeeping, has encouraged the move to a DRG-style system of funding to encourage providers to become more responsive to patient demands and so reduce waiting lists and improve access. National health systems, therefore, need to combine payment mechanisms if they are to achieve all their objectives. The French and English diversions away from their historical positions show how countries have attempted to change provider behavior to meet system needs – choice and responsiveness (in England) and cost containment (in France).

In national health systems, purchasing needs to be actively managed since the process of making strategic investment priorities can impact on equity and efficiency in provision. The performance of a health system is likely to fall short of its potential if resources are not allocated and spent wisely to gain the best mix of responses from providers that help to satisfy needs and improve care quality.

Providing Health Care

Referring back to **Figure 1**, health-care provision can usefully be split between personal and nonpersonal services. Personal services are those that people receive from a health agent, such as a doctor or dentist, while nonpersonal services are manifest in wider health promotion and disease prevention activities such as public health programs to promote healthy lifestyles or improve local environmental health.

The provision of personal health-care services within a national health system has most often been categorized through a threefold classification – primary, secondary, and tertiary care (**Figure 5**). Primary care is regarded as the first level of contact between individuals, the family, and/or communities with the health system itself. The purpose of primary care services is to bring basic health care as close as possible to where people live and work. Primary care can be delivered by way of a wide range of community-based health professionals, such as family physicians, pharmacists, therapists, and dentists. Primary care forms an integral part of most country's health systems and, as this article will show later, having an effective system of primary care providers is of crucial importance to overall national health system effectiveness. Secondary care, often referred to as the acute sector due to its predominant basis in hospital institutions, can be described as

Table 4 Provider payment mechanisms and provider behavior

	Ability to prevent health problems	Delivering services	Responsiveness to expectations	Containing costs
Salaried/global budget	++	––	+/–	+++
Capitation	+++	––	++	+++
Diagnostic related payment	+/–	++	++	+/–
Fee-for-service	+/–	+++	+++	–––

+++: very positive effect; ++: positive effect; +/–: little effect; ––: negative effect; –––: very negative effect. Reproduced from World Health Organization (WHO) (2000) The World Health Report 2000. Health systems: Improving performance. Geneva: WHO.

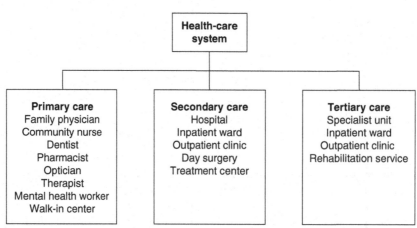

Figure 5 Sectors of 'personal' health care within a national health system.

the episodic treatment provided for an illness or health problem and is primarily curative in nature. Often, secondary care services are accessed through referrals from family physicians and/or through direct access for accident and emergency care. Tertiary care takes the form of more specialized care often within a specialist center serving a larger population or even the whole country.

Across a national health system, the number of patient contacts and episodes decreases as one moves from informal lay care to primary, secondary, and tertiary sectors. Despite the reduced number of patients accessing care in each sector, the proportion of costs of health services provision to the system as a whole tends to rise exponentially. This can be seen in **Figure 6**. However, making generalizations about the structure of health-care provision using the general classifications discussed previously is invidious. In reality, the boundaries between care sectors are often ambiguous and blurred since care can shift seamlessly from one sector to another.

Care Pathways and Disease Management: The Emergence of New Health System Models

There is a constant pressure to address increasing health-care costs in most national health systems by attempting to develop more efficient and appropriate care practices. For example, many national health-care systems have taken the opportunity to redesign and streamline the care process to reduce the number of contacts with the different parts of the system, minimize the numbers of handovers and referrals between providers, and so make more appropriate (and cost-effective) the use of each sector. Purchasing and/or commissioning care delivery across a redesigned care pathway has been claimed to be more efficient in terms of resource use, enabling patients quicker access to treatment and maximizing long-term health outcomes.

An alternative, often linked, approach is based on the greater ability of the system to promote good health and/or enable the management of illness without recourse to the need for the more expensive forms of care. Indeed, most countries, whether high or low income, seek to promote health and manage illness outside of institutionalized structures. As a consequence, patients are increasingly being prescribed integrated care packages across the previous dimensions of care (such as a disease management program) and/or investment is made in the capacity of primary care providers, and indeed of people themselves ('self-care') to promote good health and provide effective and early interventions that limit the need for people to access the more expensive forms of care.

Disease management as the basis for a health systems design is a concept developed in the United States during the 1990s and has been a growing phenomenon in health systems around the world, although its specific forms strongly depend on the health-care system in which it is applied. A number of definitions for this model of care exist, but roughly it encompasses a systematic, population-based approach to tackling specific diseases and health problems by developing programs of care to advance health system quality, efficacy, and health outcomes. In the United States, disease management programs mainly focus on reduction of costs by targeting short-term interventions to patients currently in relatively good health yet at high risk of using secondary and tertiary care in the near future. In Europe the use of disease management mechanisms is accelerating. For example, in Spain, Insalud (the Spanish National Health Service) has contracted out disease management programs for heart failure and diabetes in Barcelona and Madrid. In Germany, national government has by law introduced disease management programs as a lever to break up the traditional authority of physicians while seeking to reduce rising long-term costs.

Figure 7, adapted from the 'Kaiser Triangle' disease management model of the U.S. managed care organization Kaiser Permanente and later adopted by the Department of Health in England (Department of Health, 2004), describes the type of health-care system that should be provided to people suffering from, or at high risk for, chronic disease. Unlike the care triangle described in **Figure 6**, the health system model is not based on institutional sectors (i.e., primary, secondary, and tertiary care), but on different approaches to manage patients' needs. At the top of **Figure 7** lies case management (the top 5% of people with chronic disease) for people with advanced and acute conditions who require intensive and actively managed care by professionals. At the second level – disease management (the next 15% of cases) – proactive case management by multiprofessional and integrated teams is required, perhaps following specified pathways of care, but including a high degree (about 50%) of support to self-care. For the majority of patients (about 80%), chronic disease remains a condition (or a

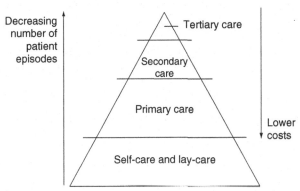

Figure 6 Relationship between health-care expenditure and levels of care.

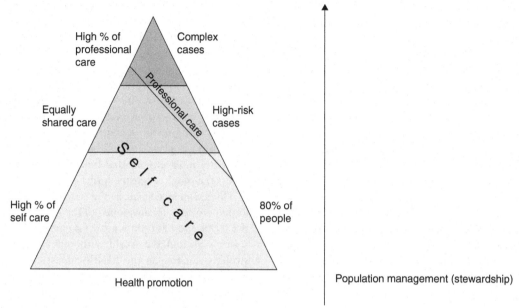

Figure 7 A health-care system model based on the management of chronic diseases and long-term conditions. Adapted from Department of Health (2004) *Improving Chronic Disease Management*. London: Department of Health.

risk) that does not require active professional intervention but can, through the right support, be addressed by engaging patients to be active in the self-management of their conditions and so prevent any deterioration. Given the numbers of people in this part of the triangle (about 80% of cases, or 48% of the whole population) one can see that effective self-care strategies are crucial to the overall effective support for people with long-term conditions (i.e., reducing the numbers of people subsequently moving up the triangle) (Department of Health, 2004).

Figure 7 also shows that for such a health-care system based on disease management to be effective, it requires a significant degree of management to ensure that local services to a defined population are tailored to meeting needs. As the model implies, it is the purchasers' responsibility to ensure that strategies are in place for high-risk groups to help prevent the onset of chronic disease, and to enable self-management for those living with such conditions. The range of self-care support tools that purchasers might seek to encourage, therefore, lies both within and out of the personal health sectors and includes: patient education, self-skills training, self-diagnostic and self-monitoring tools, home adaptations, and peer support networks. As national health systems develop in high-income countries, the needs of an aging population and the rising burden of chronic disease and long-term care needs have begun to shift how care is provided from an acute sector paradigm (based on episodic care in hospital institutions) to one based on disease management (based in primary and community care sectors and blurring the boundary between the formal and informal care sectors).

Public Health

Until the 1970s it was commonly assumed that improvements in health experienced in most countries during the last century occurred as a consequence of advances in medical care. However, the evidence collated in the key work by Wilkinson and Marmot (2003) has shown that the most important factors to improve the health of people, patients, and populations lies primarily outside the formalized system of health care. This led the authors to a key observation that the amount of money spent on health care (in terms of percentage of GDP) is not in itself a direct and causal contributor to a nation's health profile.

Many health-care systems internationally have made fundamental changes to the management and delivery of care in attempts to reduce inequalities in both health status and access to services following the realization that the role of a national health system must extend beyond the formalized systems of medical care to address the wider public health agenda through services and strategies aimed at improving well-being. At present, there is a struggle taking place in many health systems around the world to rebalance their policies and practices. Whereas there is a recurring policy theme internationally in the importance of developing a more proactive public health-based system, the necessary restructuring and reengineering of existing ways of purchasing and providing care services to achieve this implies radical system change (**Table 5**). For example, the core features of a public health system would require the provision of comprehensive public health programs for populations

Table 5 Characteristics of a proactive public health system

Public health at the center of decision making
Public health at the cultural heart of care organizations
Finance, purchasing, and provider strategies integrated to assist health improvement
Ring-fenced resources for public health
Interventions at the earliest opportunity to address avoidable deaths
Preventative initiatives to promote good health and well-being
Responsibility to the citizen by helping fulfill their economic potential to improve health
Primary care organizations to manage patients and prevent ill health
Workforce development and training tailored to meet health improvement agenda

to improve and protect health, public health interventions that are integrated into the daily work of professionals in primary care, and the creation of multidisciplinary public health teams working in community-based managed care networks.

Stewardship

In the view of international agencies that have examined the relative performance of national health systems, it is clear that more effective health-care systems are those which are carefully and responsibly managed (WHO, 2000; OECD, 2004; Davis *et al.*, 2007). Stewardship of a nation's health system is important because it is people who entrust themselves (and their money) to a health service and so, in return, it becomes the responsibility of the system to protect the population by ensuring resources are used wisely. Most organizations cannot be left to themselves to deliver effective and excellent services, and improve quality, safety, and efficiency, so in most national health systems the government must fulfill the task of stewardship – whether through direct regulation of nationally funded providers or by way of the use of independent regulators in a mixed economy of public and private providers.

Stewardship of a health system through forms of regulation and governance can have three main objectives. First, policy makers may wish to stimulate capacity and productivity through entrepreneurial opportunities by encouraging competitive behavior. This might include permitting hospitals to retain operating surpluses, moving payment systems from fixed budgets to fee-for-service, or allowing hospitals to set their own fees. Second, regulators might wish to protect the system from the more negative aspects of competition through activities such as reducing adverse selection by health-care payers and providers, requiring insurance providers to accept all applicants, or setting minimum quality standards through licensing or accreditation. Third, regulation can concentrate on safeguarding social objectives, such as stipulating minimum waiting times or opening hours, setting uniform prices (tariffs), providing treatment guidelines and protocols, and undertaking quality assurance audits.

Many Western countries have introduced regulatory reforms to alter system behaviors. As a result, there has been a general increase in the number of regulatory bodies and activities at state and local levels in health care. For example, in the English NHS, a statutory duty to assess the performance of health-care organizations and publish performance ratings was established in 2004 by way of the Health Care Commission. The purpose of the approach was to ensure that providers – now enjoying greater entrepreneurial freedom and autonomy from the state – were still meeting core government standards of quality, safety, cleanliness, and waiting times (i.e., safeguarding social objectives). Such 'steer and channel' regulation is likely to play an important role in the short and medium term in many countries that are simultaneously encouraging competition but through rules consistent with core social objectives. Hence, well-designed regulatory mechanisms can stimulate needed entrepreneurialism while simultaneously safeguarding social objectives – the essence of stewardship.

The nature of stewardship has an important role to play in defining the characteristics of national health-care systems. Political leadership and legislation practice together defines the principles and conceptual frameworks around which health system financing, purchasing, and delivery operate. For example, in England, the core principles of a tax-funded NHS that is free at the point of delivery to all citizens according to need has remained unchallenged despite far-reaching reforms that have injected private-sector capital and management practices into the system. In France, the principle of *la medicine liberale* remains culturally important to citizens who value freedom of access to specialists within a socially equitable social health insurance-based system. As the WHO (2004) commented, leadership by the state – its vision, direction, and relationship with citizens – tends to define the overall strategic framework in which the component parts of a national health system operate.

What Factors Constitute a More Effective Health-Care System?

In Alan Gillies' (2004) book that examined this question it was suggested that individuals wanted three fundamental things from their national health-care system: first, they wanted to be kept as healthy as possible; second, when this is not possible, they want to be treated and made better as soon as possible; and third, they want care provided at a minimum (or best value) cost consistent with the first two goals. Hence, Gillies argued that the best health-care systems were those that enabled the greatest possible health improvement and health-care provision within the funding available. In common with international studies examining the factors associated with better health-care systems (OECD, 2004; WHO, 2000; Davis et al., 2007) these observations reveal that it is not the level of spending that counts – as there is no single most appropriate level – but how that spending is used that matters.

Responsiveness and choice have become important criteria in the more affluent nations as they seek to meet personal demands for health care (as opposed to national needs) through patient-led care. However, as Gillies argues, the priorities that have become prevalent in Western countries are for most parts of the world an unrealistic dream. Hence, he argues that it should never be forgotten that the basic responsibility of a national health system is to deliver the basics. Reflecting back to Maxwell's (1992) basic quality measures that define the purpose of national health systems (see **Table 1**), and the realization that no single principle is necessarily more important than another, how might it be possible to objectively measure, on a comparative basis between nations, which type of national health system performs better than another?

The question is problematic because data that may be used to make effective comparisons between countries are fraught with difficulties. For example, comparisons are often made between national health systems based on their respective health expenditure relative to their nation's wealth (as characterized by the percentage of GDP allocated to financing health care). However, understanding what can be, or is actually, purchased with this funding varies markedly in real terms (purchasing power) or in terms of the coverage and entitlement to care for all citizens. Moreover, meaningful health outcome comparisons can be argued to be confounded by contextual variances in the demographic, geographical, and socioeconomic profiles of different countries. As a result, comparisons have tended to use high-level indicators of performance between countries – such as levels of infant mortality or life expectancy at birth – all factors that we know are influenced more by factors outside the influence of formal health system interventions (Wilkinson and Marmot, 2003).

Perhaps the most famous comparative study is contained in the World Health Report 2000, which compares the health systems of 191 countries based on a ranking of eight key system measures, leading with a composite measure of these systems for overall health system performance (WHO, 2000). More recently, the Commonwealth Fund's comparative analysis of six national health-care systems has added to the debate (Davis et al., 2007). What both uncover is that systems without universal health coverage and/or fragmented rather than coordinated care delivery fare worse in comparison to those that do, regardless of the amount of money spent on health care. For example, the United States (the most expensive health system) was ranked 37th in the World Health Report 2000 and last out of the six nation summary scores (Australia, Canada, Germany, New Zealand, UK, and the United States) in the Commonwealth Fund's assessment (**Table 6**).

The OECD's (2004) study of 29 industrialized nations suggested that the following key factors were associated with high-performing health-care systems:

Table 6 Six nation summary scores on health system performance, Commonwealth Fund (2007)

	AUS	CAN	GER	NZ	UK	US
Overall ranking	3.5	5	2	3.5	1	6
Quality care	4	6	2.5	2.5	1	5
Right care	5	6	3	4	2	1
Safe care	4	5	1	3	2	6
Coordinated care	3	6	4	2	1	5
Patient-centered care	3	6	2	1	4	5
Access	3	5	1	2	4	6
Efficiency	4	5	3	2	1	6
Equity	2	5	4	3	1	6
Healthy lives	1	3	2	4.5	4.5	6
Health expenditures per capita*	$2876	$3165	$3005	$2083	$2546	$6102

Note: 1=highest ranking, 6=lowest ranking.
*Health expenditures data are from 2004 except Australia and Germany (2003).
Health expenditures per capita figures are adjusted for differences in cost of living. Source: OECD, 2004.
Source: Calculated by The Commonwealth Fund based on the Commonwealth Fund 2004 International Health Policy Survey, the Commonwealth Fund 2005 International Health Policy Survey of Sicker Adults, the 2006 Commonwealth Fund International Health Policy Survey of Primary Care Physicians, and the Commonwealth Fund Commission on a High Performance Health System National Scorecard.
Source: Davis K, Schoen C, Schoenbaum S, Doty M, Holmgren A, Kriss J, and Shea K (2007) *Mirror, Mirror on the Wall: An International Update on the Comparative Performance of American Health Care*. New York: The Commonwealth Fund.

- a sustainable and robust financing system;
- care that is provided to all the population and care that is coordinated so recipients are looked after 'from cradle to grave';
- a focus on prevention of ill health and the promotion of public health;
- an effective monitoring and regulation system; and
- strategic planning to ensure resources for health care are being put to good use, for example, harnessing the potential of advances in information technology.

Each of these reports can rightly be criticized for the methodological inadequacies in their assessments. Yet, each serves to highlight two central issues we know about the effectiveness of national health systems: first, that achieving good health outcomes in a national health system is more about how the system is designed and not necessarily related to how much is spent; and second, that different health-care systems are simultaneously trading off the achievement of different measures of system quality (e.g., in terms of access, efficiency, equity, and responsiveness).

Regardless of funding type, there is also evidence to suggest that more effective health-care systems have a stronger orientation to health promotion, disease prevention, and the provision of accessible and universal primary and community care-based services. The benefits of such a strong primary care-based component to a health system have been identified through influential analysts such as Barbara Starfield. By ranking the primary care orientation of 12 Western industrialized nations, she concluded that countries with a strong primary care base to their healthcare system achieved better outcomes, and at lower cost, than countries in which the primary care base was weaker (Starfield, 1998). In Starfield's analysis, features that were consistently associated with good or excellent primary care included the comprehensiveness and family orientation of primary care practices, within a wider system in which governments regulated the distribution of healthcare resources by way of taxation or national insurance. Given that the burden of disease is shifting to the long-term chronically ill, national health systems must adapt to meet this challenge – a task requiring a move away from episodic care undertaken in specialist hospital institutions to long-term care management and coordination undertaken in the community. The importance of a primary care orientation to health system design with a strong public health component has never been more relevant.

Conclusions

In almost all Western countries, health-care systems are in a state of radical transformation as they simultaneously attempt to meet the demands of empowered consumers, incorporate evidence-based modes of working, apply disease management principles, and contain costs. The tensions implicit in these changes mean that the relationship between governments, insurance funds, health-care providers, medical professionals, and the public is in constant need of effective stewardship if the espoused goals of a national health system are to be achieved. Such stewardship requires effective regulation of activities to connect together the constituent parts of a national health system and enable, for example, the reconfiguration of personal and nonpersonal services to meet future health-care needs through a shift from a preoccupation with downstream care services to an upstream focus on the health of communities. However, achieving such ideals will be influenced by the two key features controlling the overall nature of a national health system: the involvement of the state (the ability of governments and legislative bodies to respond to system needs) and the limitations imposed by political and resource pressures.

See also: Health System Organization Models (Including Targets and Goals for Health Systems); Urban Health Systems: Overview.

Citations

Davis K, Schoen C, Schoenbaum S, et al. (2007) *Mirror, Mirror on the Wall: An International Update on the Comparative Performance of American Health Care.* New York: The Commonwealth Fund.

Department of Health (2004) *Improving Chronic Disease Management.* London: Department of Health.

Gillies A (2003) *What Makes a Good Healthcare System?* Abingdon, UK: Radcliffe Medical Press.

Glenngård A, Hjalte F, Svensson M, Anell A, and Bankauskaite V (2005) *Health Systems in Transition: Sweden.* Copenhagen, Denmark: WHO Regional Office for Europe on behalf of the European Observatory on Health.

Goodwin N, Gruen R, and Iles V (2006) *Managing Health Services.* Maidenhead, UK: Open University Press.

Maxwell R (1992) Dimensions of quality revisited: From thought to action. *Quality in Health Care* 1(3): 171–177.

McPake B, Hanson K, and Mills A (1993) Community financing of health care in Africa: An evaluation of the Bamako Initiative. *Social Science and Medicine* 36(11): 1383–1395.

Mossialos E, Dixon A, Figueras J, and Kutzin J (2002) *Funding Health Care: Options for Europe.* Buckingham, UK: Open University Press.

Organisation for Economic Co-operation and Development (OECD) (2004) *Towards High Performing Health Systems: Summary Report.* Paris, France: OECD.

Sandier S, Paris V, and Polton D (2004) *Health Care Systems in Transition: France.* Copenhagen, Denmark: WHO Regional Office for Europe on behalf of the European Observatory on Health Systems and Policies.

Starfield B (1998) *Primary Care: Balancing Health Needs, Services and Technology.* Oxford, UK: Oxford University Press.

Wilkinson R and Marmot M (eds.) (2003) *Social Determinants of Health: The Solid Facts,* 2nd edn. Geneva, Switzerland: World Health Organization.

World Health Organization (2000) The World Health Report 2000. *Health Systems: Improving Performance*. Geneva, Switzerland: World Health Organization.
World Health Organization (2004) The World Health Report 2004. *Changing History*. Geneva, Switzerland: World Health Organization.

Further Reading

Hunte D (ed.) (2007) *Managing for Health*. London: Routledge.
Schrijvers G (ed.) (2005) *Disease Management in the Dutch Context*. Netherlands: ZuidamUithof Drukkerijen.
Smith J and Goodwin N (2006) *Towards Managed Primary Care: The Role and Experience of Primary Care Organizations*. Aldershot, UK: Ashgate.
Walshe K and Smith J (eds.) (2006) *Healthcare Management*. Maidenhead, UK: Open University Press.

Relevant Websites

http://hospitalconnect.com/aha/about – American Hospital Association.
http://www.dh.gov.uk – Department of Health, England.
http://www.ehma.org – European Health Management Association.
http://www.euro.who.int/observatory – European Observatory on Health Systems and Policies.
http://www.epha.org – European Public Health Alliance (EPHA).
http://www.healthcarecommission.org.uk/homepage – Healthcare Commission.
http://www.dmalliance.org – International Disease Management Alliance (IDMA).
http://www.ijic.org – International Journal of Integrated Care (IJIC).
http://www.oecd.org – Organisation for Economic Co-operation and Development (OECD).
http://who.int – World Health Organization (WHO).

Urban Health Systems: Overview

D C Ompad, Center for Urban Epidemiologic Studies, New York Academy of Medicine, New York, NY, USA
S Galea, University of Michigan School of Public Health, Ann Arbor, MI, USA
D Vlahov, Mailman School of Public Health, Columbia University, New York, NY, USA

© 2008 Elsevier Inc. All rights reserved.

Introduction

Demographic trends suggest that there is an urgent need to consider the health of urban populations. Cities are becoming the predominant mode of living for the world's population. According to the United Nations (UN), approximately 29% of the world's population lived in urban areas in 1950. By 2000, 47% lived in urban areas and the UN projects that approximately 61% of the world's population will live in cities by 2030. Overall, the world's urban population is expected to grow from 2.86 billion in 2000 to 4.94 billion in 2030. As the world's urban population grows, so does the number of urban centers. The number of cities with populations of 500 000 or greater grew from 447 in 1975 to 804 in 2000. In 1975 there were four megacities with populations of ten million or more worldwide; by 2000 there were 18, and 22 are projected by 2015. As illustrated by **Figure 1**, most cities are in middle- to low-income countries; in 2000 middle- to low-income countries contained 72% of the world's cities. During the second session of the World Urban Forum in 2004, world leaders and mayors warned that rapid urbanization is going to be one of the most important issues in this millennium.

A Brief History of Urban Health

Cities and their impact on health have been a concern for millennia. City architects as early as the fourth century BCE designed cities to maximize exposure to the sun in winter, minimize solar exposure in the summer, and take advantage of mountain and sea breezes (Semenza, 2005). More familiar, recurrent plague epidemics in European cities between the fourteenth and sixteenth centuries, and pestilence within slums early in the Industrial Age became a major concern for urban dwellers such that authorities were required to develop and maintain knowledge for dealing with the epidemics.

For centuries, researchers and scholars have considered the study of how cities may shape health an important area of inquiry. Some of the early epidemiological studies and interventions were centered on urban populations. John Graunt, considered by many to be the first epidemiologist, published *Natural and Political Observations Mentioned in a Following Index, and Made upon the Bills of Mortality* in 1662. In it, he presented the first life tables, as well documenting increases in urban populations due to immigration. Almost two centuries later, John Snow, in what might be considered a prototypical urban health intervention, removed the Broad Street pump handle after observing differential attack rates for cholera in London.

Until relatively recently, in the academic literature, urban living and its related exposures were considered mainly in terms of their detrimental effects. This urban health 'penalty' perspective, described by Andrulis and others, focused attention on poor health outcomes in an inner-city environment and disparities in the burden of morbidity and mortality, as well as disparities in

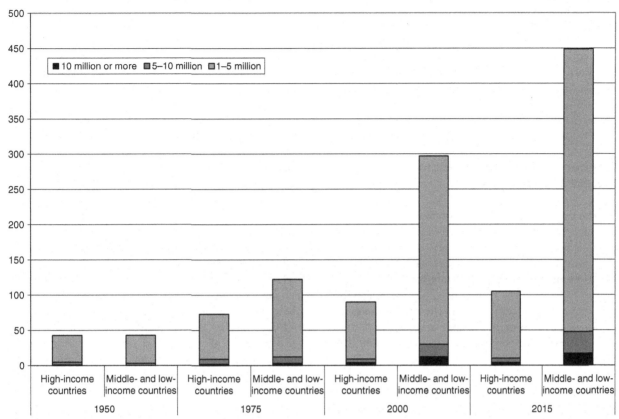

Figure 1 Number of cities with 1 million or more residents. Adapted from United Nations, Department of Economic and Social Affairs, Population Division World urbanization prospects: World urbanization prospects: The 2003 revision, data tables and highlights. http://www.un.org/esa/population/publications/wup2003/2003wupu.

health-care access, among specific subgroups. Recent work, however, has shown that urban living may be health promoting and may confer an urban health 'advantage.' Urban areas can provide access to cultural events, educational opportunities, cutting-edge medical facilities, and a plethora of health and social services. Moving forward, academic interest in urban health will likely balance the features of the urban environment that both promote and harm population health.

Defining Urban Areas

There is little consensus about the definition of urban and what constitutes a city across national and international entities and disciplines. The U.S. Bureau of the Census defines an urbanized area as "a place and the adjacent densely settled surrounding territory that together comprise a minimum population of 50,000 people," where the "densely settled surrounding territory" is defined as "one or more contiguous block having a population density of at least 1,000 people per square mile." The Census bureau thus provides a dichotomy whereby territory, population, and housing units within specific size and density parameters are designated urban and those that are outside those parameters are nonurban. However, there are inherent limitations to these definitions: urban areas exist in contrast to rural or simply in contrast to nonurban areas. In the twenty-first century, few cities exist in extreme isolation such that what is not defined as city is rural (e.g., Las Vegas). Most cities (e.g., New York City, London, Bangkok, etc.) are actually far-reaching densely populated areas, containing peri-urban and suburban areas, which continue relatively uninterrupted for miles beyond the municipal city boundaries and the city center. Alternative definitions have been developed and rates of disease, risk, and protective behaviors vary between definitions.

The definition of urban also varies widely between countries. Among 228 countries on which the UN had data for in 2000, almost half (100) include size and density as criteria, 96 include administrative definitions of urban (e.g., living in the capital city), 33 include functional characteristics (e.g., economic activity, available services, etc.), 24 have no definition of urban, and 12 define all (e.g., Anguilla, Bermuda, the Cayman Islands, Gibraltar, the Holy See, Hong Kong, Monaco, Nauru, Singapore) or none (e.g., Pitcairn Island, Tokelau, and Wallis and Futuna Islands) of their population as urban. Official statistics (e.g., UN statistics detailed previously) rely on country-specific designations and as such vary widely. In specific instances, definitions of urban in adjacent countries vary tremendously (e.g., Cambodia vs. Vietnam). Furthermore, definitions of urban have changed over time in different ways in different countries. Therefore, global statistics are subject to country-level differences in the definition of urban that may be based on population density or specific urban features (e.g., proportion of agricultural workers, municipal services).

Conceptualizing Urban Exposure as a Determinant of Health

We can conceptualize urban exposure in three main ways: urbanicity, urbanization, and the urban environment. 'Urbanicity' focuses on characterizing the presence of conditions at a particular point in time (i.e., prevalence) that are particular to urban areas or present in urban areas to a much greater or lesser extent than in nonurban areas. The focus on urbanicity is important to public health assessments on prioritizing current needs and approaches.

Urbanization is more dynamic in that it refers to the change in size, density, and heterogeneity of cities and provides a perspective for public health planning. Factors such as population mobility, segregation, and industrialization frequently accompany urbanization. More simply stated, urbanization is the process that involves the emergence and growth of cities. Thus the process of urbanization is not dependent on definition of urban *per se*, but rather on the dynamics of agglomeration of individuals. Although the pace of urbanization is independent of the base size of the population, the population size/density of surrounding areas may shape the pace of urbanization. For example, urbanization may include the establishment (or destruction) of new buildings or neighborhoods, development (or removal) of transportation routes, and the in-migration and out-migration of people, changing the racial/ethnic composition of cities. The process of urbanization gives rise to unique features of urban areas that merit separate study. How the dynamics of urbanization affect health can be considered with examples. An influx of impoverished peoples to a city (e.g., immigration driven by food or work shortages in nonurban or other urban areas) in search of jobs and services may tax available infrastructure including transportation, housing, food, water, sewage, jobs, and health care. Overtaxed sanitary systems may directly lead to rapid spread of disease as has been the case many times in North America during the past century and as continues to be the case in the developing world today. Also, the population strain on available jobs may result on devaluation of hourly wage rates, higher unemployment, and changing socioeconomic status for persons previously living in a given city. This lowering of socioeconomic status can result in more limited access to health care and to poorer health. Therefore, characteristics of urbanization, including the intensity, rate, and duration of these changes, and the response to these changes, all may have health effects on urban residents. Common mechanisms may exist through which urbanization affects health independent of the size of the city in question.

The urban context or environment can be defined as the specific characteristics or features of cities that influence health. Consider the urban environment as three distinct concepts: the social environment, the physical environment, and the urban resource infrastructure. The social urban environment comprises contextual factors that include social norms and attitudes, disadvantage (e.g., neighborhood socioeconomic status), and social capital (e.g., social trust, social institutions, etc.). The urban physical environment refers to the built environment, pollution, access to green space, transportation systems, and the geological and climate conditions of the area the city occupies. Features of the urban resource infrastructure that influence health may include factors such as the availability of health and social services, and municipal institutions (e.g., law enforcement). Features of the urban environment – the social and physical environment, as well as the infrastructural resources – all in turn are influenced by municipal, national, and global forces and trends.

Types of Studies to Investigate Issues of Health in Urban Populations

Urban Versus Rural

Urban versus rural studies typically contrast urban areas with rural areas in the same country or consider morbidity and mortality in urban versus nonurban areas. Essentially, these studies seek to determine whether morbidity and mortality due to a specific health outcome is different in specific urban areas as compared to specific nonurban areas.

Urban versus rural (or nonurban) comparisons are useful in drawing attention to particular health outcomes that may be more or less prevalent in urban areas and merit further investigation to examine the specific features of the urban (or rural) environment that are associated with that outcome. Recognizing that urban–rural comparisons are too blunt, more recent work has refined distinctions such as urban core, urban adjacent, urban nonadjacent, and rural. However, such studies are limited in their ability to identify what those factors may be and what the pathways are through which they affect the health of urban dwellers. Features of cities change over time and some factors may not be conserved between cities (e.g., racial/ethnic distribution). It is unsurprising then that different urban–rural comparisons have provided conflicting evidence about the relative burden of disease in urban and nonurban areas. At best, these studies reveal gross estimates of the magnitude and scope of health measures in broad areas by geographical areas typically defined by size and population density.

Interurban

Interurban studies typically compare health outcomes between two or more urban areas between or within countries. Such studies can simply identify differences between cities or they can begin to examine specific features of cities that influence health. Examples of the former are numerous. For example, Vermeiren and colleagues (2003) have compared mental health outcomes among adolescents in New Haven (United States), Arkhangelsk (Russia), and Antwerp (Belgium), providing insights about cross-cultural, cross-urban similarities and differences in antisocial behavior, depression, substance use, and suicide. A study of Puerto Rican injection drug users in New York City (United States) and Bayamón (Puerto Rico) revealed several differences between the two ethnically similar populations; injection drug users in Puerto Rico injected more frequently (Colon et al., 2001) and had higher rates of needle sharing as compared to their New York counterparts (Deren et al., 2001). The authors pointed to similarities in drug purity (Colon et al., 2001) and differences in the onset of the crack epidemic (Deren et al., 2001) as city-level factors that influenced injector risk behaviors. When using the city as the unit of analytic interest, one implicitly assumes that city-level exposures are equally important for all residents. Studying differences in drug use risk behaviors among two cities does not permit analysis of differences in behaviors within cities because of location of residence, intraurban variability in barriers to safer behaviors, or variations in access to key services (e.g., drug treatment, needle exchange) provided to different urban residents. However, interurban studies such as the examples mentioned here can help guide municipal and state policy makers when making decisions on service provision throughout a city.

Intraurban

Intraurban studies typically compare health outcomes within cities and are becoming widely used to investigate specific features of the urban environment. These studies often focus on neighborhoods, specific geographic areas within a city that are generally administrative groupings (e.g., census tracts in Canada, subareas or suburbs in South Africa). However, it is important to note that these areas may not represent residents' perceptions of their neighborhoods. The Project for Human Development in Chicago Neighborhoods (PHDCN), which identified collective efficacy as a determinant of violence in urban neighborhoods (Sampson et al., 1997), is an example of such a study and has demonstrated their potential to guide specific interventions to improve urban health. As a result of findings from the PHDCN, public health interventions have been developed that attempt to increase collective efficacy and social capital in particular urban neighborhoods.

Intraurban studies may contribute important insights into the relations between specific urban features and health outcomes. However, it may be difficult to generalize from one city to another. For instance, the relation between collective efficacy and violence may be modified by different levels of policing or differential access to illicit substances within a given city. Furthermore, it is important to consider that neighborhood residence is a function of geographical location and other types of social ties that are facilitated or necessitated by the urban environment.

Defining and Quantifying Urban Exposures

Social Environment

The urban social environment includes features such as social norms and attitudes, income distribution, and social capital. Although we summarize some key aspects of the social environment, the list provided here is by no means exhaustive. (For a more comprehensive consideration of the urban social environment, see the section titled 'Further reading.')

Social norms are patterns of behaviors that are considered accepted and expected by a given society. From the perspective of urban health, societal and cultural norms are important considerations when thinking about the behavior of urban dwellers and may exist on several levels. For example, Frye et al. (2006) considered the role of social norms in shaping behaviors among men who have sex with men (MSM) in urban communities. They posited that MSM may be influenced by the social norms of the gay community, with its unique physical and social structures and cultural characteristics as well as smaller subpopulations within the gay community. These communities may not be limited to one geographic location, however. Thus, MSM may also be influenced by the norms operating within their geographical neighborhood, which may have norms that operate in conjunction with, or opposition to, the prevailing norms of the broader gay community.

Income inequality is the relative distribution of income within a city or neighborhood, and is typically operationalized with the Gini coefficient. Income inequality has been associated with several health outcomes, including self-rated health, cardiovascular mortality, and consequences of illicit drug use. Income inequality is thought to operate through material and psychosocial pathways to shape population health independently of absolute income. For example, Subramanian et al. (2003) reported a significant association between self-rated health and community-level income inequality among adults in Chile, even after adjusting for absolute household and community income.

According to Berkman and Kawachi in *Social Epidemiology* (2000), social cohesion is the connectedness among groups and includes elements such as strong social bonds and a lack of conflict within the community. Social capital is thought to provide resources for collective action. There is evidence that the absence of social capital is associated with negative health outcomes such as increases in mortality, poor self-rated perception of health, higher crime rates, and violence.

Physical Environment

The urban physical environment refers to the built environment (e.g., green space, housing stock, transportation networks, etc.), pollution, noise, traffic congestion, and the geological and climate conditions of the area the city occupies. The built environment refers to "housing form, roads and footpaths, transport networks, shops, markets, parks and other public amenities, and the disposition of public space" (Weich *et al.*, 2001). Recent studies have suggested that poor-quality built environments are associated with depression, drug overdose, and physical activity. Examination of the association of built environment and health overall is a relatively recent area of inquiry (for a more thorough treatment of health and the built environment, see the September 2003 issues of the *Journal of Urban Health* 80(3): 359–519 and the *American Journal of Public Health* 93(9): 1376–1598).

Green space (e.g., parks, esplanades, community gardens, etc.) has the potential to significantly contribute to the health of urban dwellers. Living in areas with walkable green spaces has been associated with increased longevity among elderly urban residents in Japan, independent of their age, sex, marital status, baseline functional status, and socioeconomic status (Takano *et al.*, 2002).

Urban transportation systems include mass transit systems (i.e., subways, light rail, and buses) as well as streets and roads. According to the Light Rail Transit Association, there are 135 subways currently operating in 67 countries worldwide. Urban transportation systems on one hand are key in the economic livelihoods of city residents as well as cities as a whole. Yet on the other, there are significant health considerations for mass transit and roadways including security and violence, noise, and exposure to pollutants. These exposures are relevant not only for transit workers, but also for transit riders.

Pollution is one of the well-studied aspects of the urban physical environment. Urban dwellers are exposed to both outdoor and indoor pollutants that include heavy metals, asbestos, and a variety of volatile hydrocarbons. For example, one study in Bangkok (Thailand) reported high levels of benzene and polycyclic aromatic hydrocarbons among street vendors and school children sampled from traffic-congested areas as compared to monks and nuns sampled from nearby temples (Ruchirawat *et al.*, 2005).

Urban Resource Infrastructure

The urban resource infrastructure can have both positive and negative effects on health. The urban infrastructure may include more explicit health-related resources such as health and social services as well as municipal structures (e.g., law enforcement), which are shaped by national and international policies (e.g., legislation and cross-border agreements).

The relation between availability of health and social services and urban living is complicated and varies between and within cities and countries. In wealthy countries, cities are often characterized by a catalog of health and social services. Even the poorest urban neighborhood often has dozens of social agencies, both governmental and nongovernmental, each with a distinct mission and providing different services. Many of the health successes in urban areas in the last two decades, including reductions in HIV transmission, teen pregnancy rates, tuberculosis control, and new cases of childhood lead poisoning, have depended in part on the efforts of these groups. For example, social and health services are frequently more available in cities than they are in nonurban areas, which may contribute to better health and well-being among urban residents. Despite wider availability of social and health services in cities, many cities are experiencing remarkable disparities in wealth between relatively proximate neighborhoods, which are often associated with disparities in the availability and quality of care. Low-income urban residents face significant obstacles in finding health care both in wealthy and less-wealthy countries.

Municipal, National, and Global Forces and Trends

Municipal, national, and global forces and trends can have a far-reaching impact on both urban living and urbanization. Legislation and governmental policies can have substantial influence on the health of urban dwellers. Historically, municipal regulations regarding sanitation in the nineteenth and twentieth centuries facilitated vast improvements in population health and led to the formation of national groups dedicated to improving population health like the American Public Health Association. A contemporary example of the power of legislation to influence health has been ongoing in the state of New York (United States) since the early 1970s. In 1973 the New York state legislature, with the encouragement of then Governor Nelson Rockefeller, enacted some of the most stringent state drug laws in the United States. Characterized by mandatory minimum sentences, the Rockefeller Drug Laws have led to the incarceration of over 100 000 drug users since their implementation. Those incarcerated under the Rockefeller Drug Laws overwhelmingly are New York City residents (78%) and black or Hispanic (94%). Assuming that each year incarcerated was a year of life lost, Drucker estimated the potential years of life lost as a result of the Rockefeller Drug Laws to be equivalent to 8667 deaths (Drucker, 2002).

Regional and global trends can affect not only urban living, but also the rate and process of urbanization or de-urbanization. Changes in immigration policies or policy enforcement can impact urban dwellers in a variety of ways including, but not limited to, changes in access to key health and social services for some subpopulations, changes in community policing practices and changes in social cohesion and levels of discrimination. Terrorist attacks in urban centers (e.g., Baghdad, Jerusalem, London, Madrid, New York) are associated not only with morbidity and mortality among those directly affected by the event, but also significant psychological distress for other residents of the cities. Armed conflicts have resulted in mass displacement of individuals, some of whom have fled cities for other cities, regions or countries, or camps for displaced individuals (e.g., Darfur).

Methods for Studying Urban Health

The study of urban health requires the employment of analytic resources from diverse disciplines that can combine to produce an understanding of how features of the urban environment influence population health. We summarize the contribution of selected qualitative and quantitative methods to the study of urban health.

Qualitative Methods

Participant observation
Participant observation involves systematic observation of a phenomenon of interest while engaging as a participant in that setting. Participant observation offers opportunities for the researcher to develop an in-depth understanding of a particular social context through their experience as an actor within that context. Some of the classic studies of urban life were developed using participant observation, including William Foote Whytes's *Street Corner Society* (1943) and Carol Stack's *All Our Kin* (1977). A more recent example of participant observation in an urban community was Bourgois's (2003) study of crack cocaine sellers in East Harlem, New York City. This study highlighted the unstable, contingent, and constantly negotiated nature of city living within the context of a predominantly minority and economically disadvantaged neighborhood with open-air illicit drug markets.

In-depth interviews
In-depth interviews are designed to gather information about the experience, interpretations, understandings, and reactions to a particular phenomenon in a respondent's own words. Whereas quantitative interviews offer respondents a set of predetermined response categories from which to choose, qualitative interviews are usually open-ended and invite respondents to discuss the topic of interest in their own words. The structure of in-depth interviews is variable, ranging from a set of predetermined questions presented in a predetermined order to a set of topics to be covered in no particular order within the span of the interview. Often, the open-ended nature of the questions allows researchers to explore and elucidate areas that would not be captured in qualitative interviews. Similarly, analysis of in-depth interviews can be conducted in a manner that ranges from the application of predetermined categories to more inductive approaches in which the goal is to identify constructs and their relationships based on their presentation in the interviews.

Within urban contexts, in-depth interviews can be used productively to elicit residents' understandings of their environments and perceptions of the ways that those environments influence residents' health. Correspondingly, they can be used productively with urban residents, health providers, and key decision makers to develop mechanisms to improve social contexts and address health issues within urban environments. Sampling decisions should be shaped by the specific question of interest and may range from random sampling to specific selection of key informants (e.g., decision makers, longtime neighborhood residents).

Focus groups
Focus groups are interviews that are generally made up of small samples of individuals – generally between 6 and 12 per group – to discuss a topic or process of interest in detail. Focus groups are often used when the topic is one that is not highly sensitive and when a goal is to enable participants to interact with one another around the topic. Focus group interviews often rely upon interactions among group members on a topic provided by the researcher (who may take the role of facilitator). Participants discuss ideas, issues, insights, and experiences among themselves, commenting, criticizing, or elaborating on the views expressed by previous speakers.

As with in-depth interviews, focus groups can be relatively structured or unstructured. A facilitator knowledgeable about the topic of interest, skilled in group facilitation, and able to develop rapport with the focus group participants is essential to successful data collection. Analysis of focus group interviews may proceed using a deductive approach with categories determined *a priori* or with an inductive approach that seeks to develop themes and categories out of the focus group material itself.

Quantitative Methods

Ecological analyses
Ecological analyses consider associations using grouped or aggregated data for both exposure and outcomes. For example, ecological analyses can be used to consider

the association between HIV prevalence and legal repressiveness across cities (defined as hard drug arrests per capita, police employees per capita, and corrections expenditures per capita; Friedman et al., 2006). Such simple correlations can suggest city features that covary with measures of city-level health for further consideration. More sophisticated techniques (e.g., multilevel multivariate regression analyses) can consider how particular features are associated with particular outcomes while accounting for the contribution of other potentially important variables. Ecological analyses have historically been the primary method used in interurban comparisons. In urban health research, ecological studies have been used for generating hypotheses. For example, ecological studies demonstrating that relative income within cities was associated with asthma hospitalization rates in New York City generated theories about the role of race/ethnicity and the neighborhood environment on the occurrence of asthma in cities.

Although ecological analyses are potentially useful in identifying features of the urban environment that may be associated with health, there are several inherent limitations to inferences that may be drawn from ecological analyses about how these features may impact health on the individual level. Causal inferences at the individual level cannot be drawn from ecological studies. For example, the ecological observation that residential areas in Tshwane (South Africa) with high socioeconomic circumstances have higher suicide mortality rates does not necessarily imply that wealthier individuals are more likely to commit suicide (Burrows and Laflamme, 2005). Such an inference is frequently referred to as the ecological fallacy, and highlights the limited interpretations that should be drawn from ecological studies. Still, ecological analysis will continue to be an urban health research tool for hypothesis generation and will continue to suggest features of cities that may be associated with health outcomes. It is important to note that ecological studies are not limited to interurban comparisons but can equally generate hypotheses about features of intraurban units, such as neighborhoods or residential areas, which can shape population health.

Multilevel methods

Multilevel analyses integrate individual-level variables with group- and macro-level variables so that multiple levels of influence can be assessed simultaneously. Multilevel models have been available since the 1960s although they did not come into widespread use for more than two decades due to limitations of early models. Multilevel analyses allow researchers to consider how specific features of cities or of units within cities (e.g., neighborhoods) contribute to individual health independent of the contribution of other individual and contextual variables.

In its simplest application to urban health, a multilevel analysis uses data from individuals in multiple cities (or neighborhoods within a city) to consider whether city living independently explains interindividual variability in health status after controlling for other relevant individual characteristics. More useful to the study of urban health, however, is the consideration of how different characteristics of urban living at multiple levels may be associated with a particular health outcome. For example, multilevel analysis can test whether racial/ethnic segregation between neighborhoods is associated with individual access to preventative health care (e.g., influenza vaccination) while controlling for social ties at the neighborhood level and for individual race/ethnicity and other key variables. With multilevel analyses, researchers can evaluate the possibility that the effect of urban living on health is different within and between cities by introducing random slopes that allow for varying strengths of the associations between urban characteristics and health.

Conclusion

Urban health is the study of urban characteristics – including features of the social and physical environment and features of the urban resource infrastructure – that can influence health and disease in the urban context. Global demographic trends suggest urban living has become normative and thus there is an urgent need to consider how urban living may influence the health of populations. The study of urban health requires a multidisciplinary perspective that can consider different types of studies, including inter- and intraurban studies and urban–rural comparisons, and employs a multiplicity of methods including qualitative and quantitative methods. Epidemiologists, public health practitioners, urban planners, as well as social, behavioral, clinical, and environmental health scientists can contribute to the study of urban health in conjunction with the active participation of community residents, civic, business, faith-based, and political leaders. The International Society for Urban Health (see the section titled 'Relevant websites') is an organization devoted to furthering perspectives and approaches to improving health in cities and can serve as a resource for those interested in further reading about the study of urban health.

Citations

Berkman LF and Kawachi I (eds.) (2000) *Social Epidemiology*. New York: Oxford University Press.

Bourgois PI (2003) *In Search of Respect: Selling Crack in El Barrio*, 2nd edn. New York: Cambridge University Press.

Bureau of the Census (2002) Qualifying urban areas for Census 2000. Department of Commerce. Federal Register, vol 67, No. 84. May 1, 2002: 21962.

Burrows S and Laflamme L (2005) Living circumstances of suicide mortality in a South African city: An ecological study of differences across race groups and sexes. *Suicide and Life-Threatening Behaviour* 35: 592–603.

Colo HM, Robles RR, Deren S, et al. (2001) Between-city variation in frequency of injection among Puerto Rican injection drug users: East

Harlem, New York, and Bayamon, Puerto Rico. *Journal of Acquired Immune Deficiency Syndrome* 27: 405–413.

Deren S, Robles R, Andia J, Colon HM, Kang SY, and Perlis T (2001) Trends in HIV seroprevalence and needle sharing among Puerto Rican drug injectors in Puerto Rico and New York: 1992–1999. *Journal of Acquired Immune Deficiency Syndrome* 26: 164–169.

Drucker E (2002) Population impact of mass incarceration under New York's Rockefeller drug laws: an analysis of years of life lost. *Journal of Urban Health* 79: 434–435.

Friedman SR, Cooper HLF, Tempalski B, et al. (2006) Relationships of deterrence and law enforcement to drug-related harms among drug injectors in US metropolitan areas. *AIDS* 20: 93–99.

Frye V, Latka MH, Koblin B, et al. (2006) The urban environment and sexual risk behavior among men who have sex with men. *Journal of Urban Health* 83: 308–324.

Ruchirawat M, Navasumrit P, Settachan D, Tuntaviroon J, Buthbumrung N, and Sharma S (2005) Measurement of genotoxic air pollutant exposures in street vendors and school children in and near Bangkok. *Toxicology and Applied Pharmacology* 206: 207–214.

Sampson RJ, Raudenbush SW, and Earls F (1997) Neighborhoods and violent crime: A multilevel study of collective efficacy. *Science* 277: 918–924.

Semenza JC (2005) Building healthy cities: A focus on interventions. In: Galea S and Vlahov D (eds.) *Handbook of Urban Health: Populations, Methods and Practice*, pp. 459–478. New York: Springer.

Stack C (1977) *All Our Kin: Strategies for Survival in a Black Community.* New York: Harper and Row.

Subramanian SV, Delgado I, Jadue L, Vega J, and Kawachi I (2003) Income inequality and health: Multilevel analysis of Chilean communities. *Journal of Epidemiology and Community Health* 57: 844–848.

Takano T, Nakamura K, and Watanabe M (2002) Urban residential environments and senior citizens' longevity in megacity areas: The importance of walkable green spaces. *Journal of Epidemiology and Community Health* 56: 913–918.

Vermeiren R, Schwab-Stone M, Deboutte D, Leckman PE, and Ruchkin V (2003) Violence exposure and substance use in adolescents: Findings from three countries. *Pediatrics* 111: 535–540.

Weich S, Burton E, Blanchard M, Prince M, Sproston K, and Erens B (2001) Measuring the built environment: Validity of a site survey instrument for use in urban settings. *Health and Place* 7: 283–292.

Whyte WF (1943) *Street Corner Society: The Social Structure of an Italian Slum.* Chicago, IL: University of Chicago Press.

Further Reading

Andrulis DP (1997) The urban health penalty: New dimensions and directions in inner-city health care. *Inner City Health Care.* Philadelphia, PA: American College of Physicians. http://www.acponline.org/hpp/pospaper/andrulis.htm.

Bureau of the Census (2002) Qualifying urban areas for Census 2000. Department of Commerce. Federal Register, vol 67, No. 84. May 1, 2002: 21962.

Diez Roux AV (2001) Investigating neighborhood and area effects on health. *American Journal of Public Health* 91: 1783–1789.

Freudenberg N, Silver D, Carmona JM, Kass D, Lancaster B, and Speers M (2000) Health promotion in the city: A structured review of the literature on interventions to prevent heart disease, substance abuse, violence and HIV infection in US metropolitan areas, 1980–1995. *Journal of Urban Health* 77: 443–457.

Freudenberg N, Vlahov D, and Galea S (2005) Beyond urban penalty and urban sprawl: Back to living conditions as the focus of urban health. *Journal of Community Health* 30(1): 1–11.

Galea S and Vlahov D (eds.) (2005) *Handbook of Urban Health: Populations, Methods and Practice.* New York: Springer.

Harpham T and Tanner M (1995) *Urban Health in Developing Countries*, London: Earthscan.

Kawachi I and Berkman LF (eds.) (2003) *Neighborhoods and Health.* New York: Oxford University Press.

Leviton LC, Snell E, and McGinnis M (2000) Urban issues in health promotion strategies. *American Journal of Public Health* 90: 863–866.

Luke DA (2004) *Multilevel Modeling.* Thousand Oaks, CA: Sage.

Patton MQ (2001) *Qualitative Research and Evaluation Methods.* Newbury Park, CA: Sage.

Raudenbush SW and Bryk AS (2002) *Hierarchical Linear Models*, 2nd edn. Thousand Oaks, CA: Sage.

Vlahov D and Galea S (2002) Urbanization, urbanicity, and health. *Journal of Urban Health* 79(supplement 1): S1–S12.

Vlahov D, Galea S, and Freudenberg N (2005) The urban health "advantage." *Journal of Urban Health* 82: 1–4.

Relevant Websites

www.isuh.edu – International Society of Urban Health.

http://www.un.org/esa/desa – United Nations Department of Economic and Social Affairs.

http://www.unhabitat.org – United Nations Human Settlements Program.

http://www.who.int/social_determinants/knowledge_networks/settlements – Commission on Social Determinants of Health, Knowledge Network on Urban Settings.

http://www.who.or.jp – WHO Center for Health Development, Kobe, Japan.

Comparative Health Systems

H Wang, Yale University School of Public Health, New Haven, CT, USA

© 2008 Elsevier Inc. All rights reserved.

Introduction

A good health system is one of the most important elements in ensuring the health of a population in any modern society. Although all nations share the same goal of improving the health of a population in a cost-effective and equitable manner, health systems vary greatly from country to country. However, a perfect health system does not exist. In fact, nearly every nation is continuously undergoing certain health system reforms and system improvements. Governments are constantly striving for a high-quality, cost-effective, and universal health-care system.

Comparative health-care systems is a rapidly growing field that is being called on more and more frequently in health policy and health service research communities. This is particularly true in the current trend of globalization, wherein alternative ways to solve inherent problems in health systems and to improve the performance of health systems are being analyzed.

Experience from previous decades shows that the development of a health system is facilitated with international comparisons of other nations' health systems. First, the comparative nature of the analysis allows for a greater number of policy options to be identified, which will likely assist policy makers in the implementation of health strategies. Second, the comparative analysis of a health system can help people realize the consequences of various policy decisions: the successes that they might consider adopting and the failures that they should avoid. Finally, comparative analyses can act as benchmarks for in-depth evaluations of the performance of a health system.

Concept of Health System

Health systems have been conceptualized in various ways. Roemer (1991) defines a health system as "the combination of resources, organization, financing and management that culminate in the delivery of health services to the population." This definition emphasizes the input requirements of a health system. The World Health Organization's (2000) definition includes "all the activities whose primary purpose is to promote, restore or maintain health." Rather than emphasizing inputs such as resources, this definition focuses primarily on the outcome aspects of a health system. Irrespective of the definition, a health system should include the following two major components: The first component is the goal of a health system, that is, to address health and illness in society, and the second component is a set of mechanisms that transform health-related resources into health services in order to achieve the goal of a health system.

Although health systems vary across countries, all include similar structural components (see **Figure 1**): health-care providers, consumers of health-care services, health financing agencies, resources suppliers, and government/regulatory entities. Each component is directly linked to the other four components. For example, health providers provide health-care services to the consumers, receive payments from a financing agency to recover the cost of health services, obey the regulations imposed by the regulatory entity, and receive resources from resource suppliers.

The variations arise from the individuals that comprise the components, the manner in which the individuals function collectively, the importance of each component in the system, and the relationships among the components of a specific health system. For example, all health systems have health-care financing agencies. However, these agencies vary, from governments to private health insurance to

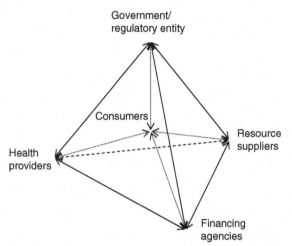

Figure 1 The common structure of health systems.

individual consumers themselves. In some health systems, governments are the major agencies for health financing; in other cases, out-of-pocket payments are the main sources of health financing; that is, the individual health-care consumer acts as the health financing agency. The relationships between health financing agencies and health-care providers are based on the contract arrangements of capitation or fee-for-services payments.

Methods in Comparative Health Systems

Methods to compare health systems have evolved into three types (Rodwin, 1995). The first type can be summarized as random observations in the early stage of comparative analysis. That is, "travelogues ... written by physicians from overseas tours" to express the variations of health systems without specific policy purposes. The second type can be summarized as purposeful learning of comparative analysis, which focuses primarily on the practical issues of improving the performance of a health system through health system reform. The third type can be summarized as a social science comparison of health systems. Comparative health system analysis involves a multidisciplinary approach and incorporates disciplines such as anthropology, sociology, political science, and economics. Furthermore, rigorous study design with elaborate hypotheses and sophisticated analytic methods are applied in comparative analysis.

In terms of study design, the majority of comparative analyses of health systems have been cross-sectional. In order to make the health systems as comparable as possible, countries with similar socioeconomic environments (serving as the control variable) are often selected for comparative analysis. Since an experimental study design is rarely feasible, quasi-experimental study designs have been used instead. However, this type of study is very expensive and is able to test multiple sites only within the same country.

Comparative analyses of health systems can be performed by a 'snapshot' approach to examine the overall performance of a health system or by an 'anatomical' approach to examine the effects of specific components on the outcomes or overall function of a health system. The snapshot approach commonly uses the following measures to compare health systems: total health-care expenditure, life expectancy or healthy life expectancy, or health system outcomes. These are then used to judge the overall performance of a health system. Although this approach is intuitive and easy to understand, it does not provide significant details for the policy learning purpose. The second approach incorporates a more in-depth analysis of each component of the health system in order to gain a greater understanding of how a specific system works. Certainly, these two approaches are not mutually exclusive. A snapshot approach is usually the first step of a more elaborate comparative analysis of a health system.

The framework of "structure, process, and outcome" (Aday, 1998) is often implicitly or explicitly applied in comparative health system analyses. Structure refers to the investment of health resources – including resources for the delivery of health services, as well as resources for the organizational structure of health services – and the health status of a population in a specific society. Process encompasses the delivery of health services, as well as the utilization of health services. Outcome can be dissected into two groups: intermediate outcomes and ultimate outcomes. Intermediate outcomes refer to the immediate outputs of health system performance such as quality, efficiency, and access to health services. Although these outputs are the consequences of health system performance, they are not necessarily the final goals from a societal perspective. The ultimate outcomes refer to health status, customer satisfaction, and financial risk protection (Roberts et al., 2004). According to a World Health Organization report, the goal of customer satisfaction is replaced by "increasing responsiveness to the legitimate demands of the population" (World Health Organization, 2000). In addition to the overall level of these indicators, the distribution of these indicators among various factors, such as socioeconomic status, race, ethnicity, and gender, is also of particular interest in health policy. Health equity with respect to health-care financing and health-care utilization has become an increasingly important goal in modern society. Commonly used indicators to measure ultimate and intermediate goals are listed in **Table 1**.

Variation of Health Systems and Their Performance

There are a variety of health systems. Field (1973) observed five types of health systems based on the evolutionary progress of industrialized nations: the private health system, the pluralistic health system, the national health insurance system, national health services, and socialized health services. Bambra (2005) grouped the health systems of OECD countries into three categories, liberal, conservative, and social democratic, on the basis of the degree of health-care decommodification. Lassey (1997) classified health systems into "most advanced," "somewhat advanced," and "less advanced" on the basis of technology use, resource availability, and health service accessibility.

Rather than classifying different types of health systems, this article uses the anatomic approach to examine the method by which each component of a health system functions and to assess the potential outcome indicators of a particular health system. This approach is likely to facilitate the translation of comparative results into policy recommendations.

Epidemiological Profiles of Populations or Patients

The centerpiece of a health system is its beneficiaries – that is, the population or patients. The health of a population varies greatly from country to country. Disparities in population health are often used to compare the performance of health systems. In addition, the health status of a population, determined by epidemiological profiles, is an important factor that influences the development of a health system in a specific society. For example, in a society with a high prevalence of communicable diseases, tax-based financing for disease prevention at population level, as well as emergency services for disease treatment, will be required. However, in a society characterized by chronic disease, community-based disease prevention and disease management are essential components of the health system. Therefore, health system development requires the population or patients to be the centerpiece. Health systems should reflect the health demands and needs of a specific society. Health systems should also evolve as the populations or the patients' health status changes.

Financing of Health Services

Financing is one of the most important components and functions of a health system. Health system financing varies depending on how resources are generated, pooled, and used. Health services can be financed in a variety of ways: from an individual who is self-insured, through an insurance agency, or through a government agency that provides health insurance to a specific group or the entire population.

There are three basic issues that policy makers must address in terms of health financing. The first is the amount of resources that a financing system can mobilize

Table 1 Ultimate and intermediate goal indicators of a health system

Categories	Key indicators / Levels	Distribution
Ultimate goals of health system		Indicators of equity, which refers to the difference of the outcomes among different groups of the population. The most commonly used indicators for assessing a health system include health equity, financial equity, and access equity
1. Health status	Life expectancy at birth	
	Infant mortality	
	Maternal mortality	
	Life expectancy at 65	
	Disability-adjusted life year (DALY)	
	Quality-adjusted life year (QALY)	
2. Financial risk protection or the share of financial burden	Health insurance coverage	
	Percentage of out-of-pocket payment of total health expenditure	
	Percentage of poverty due to illness	
3. Customer satisfaction or responsiveness to people's nonmedical expectations	Consumer-satisfaction survey indicators	
Intermediate goals of health system		
1. Efficiency	Cost per unit of outcome (health improvement)	
2. Quality	Appropriateness (overused, underused, or misused)	
3. Access	Utilization rates of health services	
	Physician/hospital beds per 1000 population	
4. Cost	Total health expenditure	
	Percentage of health expenditure in gross domestic product	

This table is based on information from Roberts MJ, Hsiao W, Berman P, and Reich MR (2004) *Getting Health Reform Right: A Guide to Improving Performance and Equity*. New York: Oxford University Press and World Health Organization (2000) *The World Health Report 2000: Health Systems: Improving Performance*. Geneva: WHO.

and then allocate to health services. The combination of multiple sources of financing is the total health expenditure in a specific society. The second issue is the type and amount of services that can be purchased. This refers to the benefit package design in response to the demand and/or needs for health services and resource constraints. The third issue involves the purchase of health services through the use of incentives in order to achieve the desired outcomes of a health system.

The level of health expenditures varies greatly from country to country. **Table 2** summarizes total health expenditure per capita, the health expenditure as a percentage of Gross Domestic Product, and sources of health financing in selected countries. There is no consensus on the appropriate amount that should be allocated to health financing. In many of the poorest countries, the level of spending is still insufficient to ensure equitable access to basic and essential health services and interventions. Thus, a major health policy issue in poor countries is ensuring adequate and equitable resource mobilization for health. On the other hand, in many of the richest countries, the level of spending is considered too high, and the concomitant benefits from these investments do not generate a reasonable return in terms of health gain. Consequently, a major policy issue in the wealthiest nations is controlling the cost of health services and ensuring their maximum efficiency.

Although there is ongoing debate over the appropriate amount of health-care spending per country, there is fairly common agreement on how health expenditures should be financed. For example, if out-of-pocket payments for health-care financing are too high, the financial risk protection of a health system will be low in a given society. **Table 3** summarizes financial risk protection and other selective effects of various health financing mechanisms.

Provider Payment Methods

Provider payment methods are a set of contracts made between health-care providers and financing agencies

Table 2 Total health expenditure and financing mechanisms

			Source of financing, % of total health expenditure			
Country	Total expenditure per capita (international dollar)	Total expenditure on health as % of GDP	Government expenditure	Private prepaid plans	Out-of-pocket	Other
Algeria	186	4.1	80.8	0.8	18.3	0.1
Argentina	1067	8.9	48.6	19.6	28.6	3.2
Australia	2874	9.5	67.5	7.8	22.0	2.7
Brazil	597	7.6	45.3	19.6	35.1	0.0
Canada	2989	9.9	69.9	12.7	14.9	2.4
China	278	5.6	36.2	3.7	55.9	4.2
Czech Republic	1302	7.5	90.0	0.3	8.4	1.4
Germany	3001	11.1	78.2	8.8	10.4	2.6
Japan	2244	7.9	81.0	0.3	17.1	1.6
Kenya	65	4.3	38.7	3.7	50.6	7.0
Mexico	582	15.2	44.6	36.5	13.5	5.4
Mozambique	45	4.7	61.7	0.2	14.9	23.2
Namibia	359	6.7	70.0	22.8	5.8	1.4
Republic of Korea	1074	5.6	49.4	2.1	41.9	6.6
Russia	551	5.6	59.0	2.7	29.2	9.1
Singapore	1156	4.5	36.1	0.0	62.0	1.9
Spain	1853	7.7	71.3	4.3	23.5	0.9
Sweden	2704	9.4	85.2	0.3	13.6	0.8
Switzerland	3776	11.5	58.5	9.0	31.5	1.0
United Kingdom	2389	8.0	85.7	3.3	11.0	0.0
United States	5711	15.2	44.6	36.5	13.5	5.4
Zimbabwe	132	7.9	35.9	13.5	36.3	14.3

Source: World Health Organization (2006) *The World Health Report*. Geneva: WHO.

Table 3 Source of health-care financing

Types	Financing mechanisms	Efficiency	Equity	Financial sustainability	Financial risk sharing	Service utilization
Out-of-pocket	Individuals	Low	Low	Low	Low	Low
Medical saving account	Individuals	Medium	Low	Medium	Low/medium	Low
Community financing	Premium contribution	Medium	Low	Medium	Medium	Medium
Private health insurance	Premium contribution	Medium	Low	Medium	High	High
Social insurance	Payroll and tax deduction	High	Medium	High	High	High
National health insurance	General tax	High	High	High	High	High

This table is created mainly based on World Bank (1999) *Teaching materials of the Flagship Program on Health Sector Reform and Sustainable Financing*. Washington DC: World Bank; Roberts MJ, Hsiao W, Berman P, and Reich MR (2004) *Getting Health Reform Right: A Guide to Improving Performance and Equity*. New York: Oxford University Press; and World Health Organization (2000) *The World Health Report 2000: Health Systems: Improving Performance*. Geneva: WHO.

with respect to compensation for provider health service delivery. Since different payment arrangements alter the financial risk-bearing status of providers, they impose differing financial incentives for providers and thus influence the performance of a health system. **Table 4** lists seven of the most commonly used provider payment methods, as well as their incentives for providers in terms of quantity, quality, and cost control. In practice, however, there are payment methods that combine different payment mechanisms into one payment arrangement. For example, salary plus bonus payments combine both fee-for-services and salary into one payment method in order to balance the incentives for quantity, quality, and cost of services.

Delivery of Health-Care Services

The delivery of health-care services can be divided into two components: the types of services delivered and by whom, that is, its ownership. The types of services vary

Table 4 Provider payment mechanisms

Payment methods	Unit of payment	Financial risk-bearing of providers	Financial incentives for providers		
			Quantity	Quality	Cost control
Fee-for-service	Per service item	No	High	High	Low
Salary	Monthly payment	No	Medium	Medium	High
Capitation	Per contracted patient/person	Yes	Low	Low/High	High
Daily payment	Per patient day	Partial	Low/High	Low/High	Medium
Case payment	Per case of different diagnosis	Partial	Low/High	Low/High	Medium
Line item budget	Budget line	No	Low	Low	Medium
Global budget	All services	Yes	Low	Low/High	High

This table is created mainly based on World Bank (1999) *Teaching materials of the Flagship Program on Health Sector Reform and Sustainable Financing*. Washington DC: World Bank; Roberts MJ, Hsiao W, Berman P, and Reich MR (2004) *Getting Health Reform Right: A Guide to Improving Performance and Equity*. New York: Oxford University Press; and World Health Organization (2000) *The World Health Report 2000: Health Systems: Improving Performance*. Geneva: WHO.

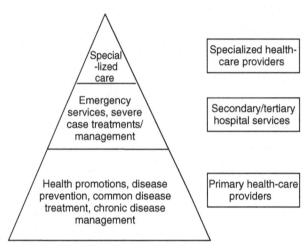

Figure 2 The structure of health services delivery.

from community-based health services for the majority of the population to hospital-based services for a select group of patients with severe health problems, to specialized health services for those patients who require specialized care (see **Figure 2**). In some health systems, providers are organized into a three-tier hierarchical system. Primary health-care providers often serve as gatekeepers of the health system; a referral system is often in place in order for patients to receive higher-level hospital and/or specialized care. In other systems, these three tiers may not be present. For example, a lack of resources may force informal health-care providers, such as traditional healers, birth attendants, and community health workers, to act as the primary health-care providers although they are not considered part of the formal health system. Another example is the direct entry of patients into tertiary and specialized health services. The referral system is bypassed in order to increase a patient's freedom of choice among health providers. These structural differences in the delivery of health services may have great impact on access, quality, and efficiency of health services.

The second component of health service delivery is ownership. Health-care providers may be part of a publicly owned or a privately owned system. Recently, a trend has been growing toward converting publicly owned delivery systems to public–private partnerships. Public–private partnerships are viewed as a 'win–win' arrangement, with various motivations and philosophies working together – albeit with different incentives – to contribute to the improvement of the health status of a population. **Table 5** lists the major characteristics of publicly and privately owned delivery systems, as well as the predicted outcomes of the performance of the delivery systems. In the public–private partnership, the public system can take advantage of the higher levels of efficiency and quality of a private system, while at the same time maintaining its equity and cost-control goals.

Regulation of a Health System

Regulations are rules or orders mandated by a government in order to improve the outcomes of a system through behavior change. Health regulation functions to (1) ensure the fairness of market exchange in a health system, (2) correct the market failure of a health system, and (3) ensure the equity of financing and delivery of health-care services.

Regulatory policy is incorporated into almost every aspect of a health system. From a functional perspective, regulations have the following four objectives: financial risk sharing; quality and safety; equity of health services; and cost-effectiveness, or value for money (**Table 6**).

Criticism of Comparative Analysis of Health Systems

Comparative health systems is a rapidly growing field that is being used more and more frequently in health policy and health service research communities. However,

Table 5 Health-care providers by ownership

Variables	Public	Private	Public–private partnership
Characteristics			
Incentives	Low	High	Medium
Financial risks	Low	High	Shared
Decision space	Centralized	Decentralized	Shared
Profit	No	Varies	Controlled
Performance			
Efficiency	Low	High	Medium
Quality	Medium	High	Cost-effective
Equity	High	Low	Medium
Responsiveness	Low	High	Medium
Cost control	High	Low	Medium

This table is created mainly based on World Bank (1999) *Teaching materials of the Flagship Program on Health Sector Reform and Sustainable Financing*. Washington DC: World Bank; and World Health Organization (2000) *The World Health Report 2000: Health Systems: Improving Performance*. Geneva: WHO.

Table 6 The objectives and options for regulation in health system

Objectives	Regulations
Financial risk sharing	Mandating enrollment for health insurance
	Setting community rate
	Providing open enrollment
	Ensuring minimum benefit package
Medical safety	Market entry license, including doctor's practice license, hospital licenses, drug manufacture license, etc.
	Practice guidelines and procedures
	Drug quality
Equity	Medical safety net
	Medical resource reallocation
Cost-effectiveness	Services prices control
	Profit/surplus regulation
	Capital investment

there are many criticisms, including questions about the usefulness of international comparisons, the simplicity of methods used in the analysis, and the value of international experiences as a means of health system improvement.

Although many comparative analyses attempt to conduct objective comparative analyses using similar frameworks and statistical indicators, the results of the comparison remain debatable. Often, the information is not reported in the same format, and statistics are calculated differently and use dissimilar definitions. This issue raises concern about the use of simple statistical comparisons as a method of comparative analysis. Comparative analyses should be made for countries with similar characteristics – serving as control factors – and with elaborate and careful interpretation.

Many health system comparative analyses attempt to establish a causal relationship between a health system and its outcomes. However, the majority of these analyses are based on cross-sectional data. Furthermore, the outcomes of a health system, particularly the health of a population, are influenced by many factors that exceed the boundaries of the health system. These factors are difficult to control in comparative analyses. Therefore, the results derived from comparative analyses must be interpreted with caution as they may not be valid or reliable results.

Health systems are deeply rooted in their country's historical, cultural, ethical, political, social, and economic development. The successes of one health system may not apply to another health system in a different society. For example, a community health financing scheme may work well in a society with a high degree of trust, reciprocity, and social networking but may not work well in a society with low social capital. Therefore, the transfer of knowledge should be done cautiously when adapting successful strategies.

In summary, there is great variation in terms of health systems and their levels of performance. Health systems are dynamic and evolve in response to changes in the epidemiological profiles of the population, improvements in medical technology, and people's knowledge of the health system. Although there is criticism regarding the methodology and results of comparative health system analyses, the field is growing rapidly and is being used more and more frequently in health policy and health service research communities. Comparative health system analyses are still considered useful learning tools for health system improvement, particularly in the current environment of globalization.

See also: Global Health Initiatives and Public Health Policy; Health Policy: Overview; Human Rights, Approach to Public Health Policy; Politics, and Public Health Policy Reform; Resource Allocation: International Perspectives on Resource Allocation; The State in Public Health, The Role of.

Citations

Aday LA, Begley CE, Lairson DR, and Slater CH (1998) *Evaluating the Healthcare System: Effectiveness, Efficiency, and Equity*. Chicago, IL: Health Administration Press.

Bambra C (2005) Worlds of welfare and the health-care discrepancy. *Social Policy & Society* 4: 31–41.

Field M (1973) The concept of health system at the macrosociological level. *Social Science and Medicine* 7: 763–785.

Lassey ML, Lassey WR, and Jinks MJ (1997) *Health Care Systems around the World*. Upper Saddle River, NJ: Prentice Hall.

Roberts MJ, Hsiao W, Berman P, and Reich MR (2004) *Getting Health Reform Right: A Guide to Improving Performance and Equity*. New York: Oxford University Press.

Rodwin VG (1995) Comparative health systems: A policy perspective. In: Kovner AR (ed.) *Jonas's Health Care Delivery in the United States*. New York: Springer.

Roemer M (1993) *National Health Systems of the World*. New York: Oxford University Press.

World Health Organization (2000) *The World Health Report 2000: Health Systems: Improving Performance*. Geneva, Switzerland: WHO.

Further Reading

Asian Development Bank (1999) *Health Sector Reform in Asia and the Pacific: Options for Developing Countries*. Manila, Philippines: Asian Development Bank.

Block MAG (1997) Comparative research and analysis methods for shared learning from health system reforms. *Health Policy* 42: 187–209.

Lee RP (1982) Comparative studies of health-care system. *Social Science and Medicine* 16: 629–642.

Liman TJ and Robins L (1971) Comparative analysis of health-care systems: Socio-political approach. *Social Science and Medicine* 5: 573–581.

Mills AJ and Ranson MK (2001) The design of health systems. In: Merson M, Black R, and Mills AJ (eds.) *International Public Health: Diseases, Programs, Systems, and Policies*. Gaithersburg, MD: Aspen.

Raffel MW (1985) *Comparative Health Systems: Descriptive Analysis of Fourteen National Health Systems*. University Park, PA: Pennsylvania State University Press.

Seedhouse D (1995) *Reforming Health Care: The Philosophy and Practice of International Health Reform*. West Sussex, UK: Wiley.

World Bank (1993) *World Development Report 1993: Investing in Health: World Development Indicators*. New York: Oxford University Press.

Thai KV, Wimberley ET, and McManus SM (2002) *Handbook of International Health Care Systems*. New York: Marcel Dekker.

Twaddle AC (1996) Health system reforms: Toward a framework for international comparisons. *Social Science and Medicine* 43(5): 637–653.

World Bank (1993) *World Development Report 1993: Investing in Health*. New York: Oxford University Press.

The Health Care of Indigenous Peoples/Nations

G Bodeker, University of Oxford, Oxford, UK; Columbia University, New York, NY, USA

© 2008 Elsevier Inc. All rights reserved.

Background

Indigenous peoples have suffered from historic injustices as a result of, *inter alia*, their colonization and dispossession of their lands, territories and resources, thus preventing them from exercising, in particular, their right to development in accordance with their own needs and interests.

Indigenous peoples have the right to their traditional medicines and to maintain their health practices, including the conservation of their vital medicinal plants, animals and minerals. Indigenous individuals also have the right to access, without any discrimination, to all social and health services.

Indigenous individuals have an equal right to the enjoyment of the highest attainable standard of physical and mental health. States shall take the necessary steps with a view to achieving progressively the full realization of this right.

(Draft UN Declaration on the Rights of Indigenous Peoples, 2007)

The term 'indigenous peoples' is widely used to characterize a reported 300–350 million people worldwide (WHO, 2007) – from the Arctic to the South Pacific, from the Kalahari Desert in southern Africa to Tierra Del Fuego at the southernmost tip of the Americas. With ancient roots in their local areas, these peoples are among the world's most marginalized populations – politically, economically and territorially – and suffer the highest burden of health challenges.

In 1990, the United Nations proclaimed the International Decade of the World's Indigenous People, starting on 10 December 1994 (resolution 48/163). By the end of the Decade, the health of indigenous peoples was widely seen as of global concern and, in one instance – Australia – of proportions of a national emergency.

Who Are Indigenous Peoples?

Asia, according to the International Work Group for Indigenous Affairs (IGWIA), is home to the vast majority (70%)

of the world's indigenous peoples. In India alone, there are 68 million Advasis, or indigenous peoples. The Orang Asli, the Mon-Khmer-speaking peoples of the Malaysian peninsula, by contrast, have a population of 150 000 and claim continuous presence in the world's most ancient rainforests. In East Asia, Taiwanese aboriginal groups are held to be the source of the Austronesian language family, which is now found throughout Oceania. And indigenous peoples in West Asia include the Bakhtiari, Laks, Lurs, and Qashqai of Iran, and Assyrian peoples of Iran, Iraq, and Turkey.

Despite this large population that self-identifies as indigenous, the term 'indigenous' has been contested, as almost all Asians and Africans consider themselves indigenous.

In Africa, the term 'indigenous' has come to refer to nomadic peoples, such as the Tuareg of the Sahara and Sahel, hunter gatherers such as the San people of the Kalahari, and pastoralists, including the Masai of East Africa. Their claim to indigenous status has been endorsed by the African Union's African Commission on Human and Peoples Rights, which has noted their status of underrepresentation in government and the need for affirmative action to ensure their survival.

In North and South America, where every nation has indigenous peoples, violence, marginalization, and isolation on native reservations and in remote locations reduced access to traditional food supplies and increased susceptibility to disease. From the seventeenth century to the early twentieth century there were a reported 93 waves of epidemics that devastated native populations with diseases such as typhoid, malaria, smallpox, measles, cholera, a range of sexually transmitted infections, pneumonia, and yellow fever, resulting in population declines of up to 90–95% (Encarta, n.d.).

In the United States, census data indicate that there are approximately 2 million Native Americans. And in Canada, where Aboriginal people, including the Inuit of the Arctic region, have been designated as members of First Nations, the population is approximately 1 million.

In South America, indigenous populations now range from Bolivia with up to 70% of the nation to approximately half of the nation in Peru and Guatemala to a reported 8% in Uruguay (The World Factbook, 1997).

In Greenland, also home to the Inuit, indigenous people comprise 85% of the population. Other indigenous European groups include the Kumandin Peoples of Russia and the Sami of northern Scandinavia.

Oceania, which includes Australia, New Zealand, Papua New Guinea, and approximately 25 000 Pacific Islands, including the Marshall Islands, is home to indigenous groups from Polynesian, Melanesian, and Micronesian origins, as well as to Torres Straits Islanders.

It is also home to indigenous Australians, who have at least 40 000–50 000, and potentially up to 70 000 years presence on the continent, with genetic linkages to the peoples of Papua New Guinea. Indigenous Australians now represent approximately 2.5% of Australia's population of 20.3 million. Appropriation of land and water and the introduction of disease were two early features of colonial presence in Australia. Introduction of alcohol, opium, and tobacco began a problem of substance abuse that has continued in epidemic proportions. In New Zealand, there were similar patterns of conflict between British settlers and the Maori, as well as the introduction of new diseases. There were however, formal treaties covering land acquisition and ownership (The World Factbook, 2007).

The lives of the majority of the world's 300 million indigenous peoples are characterized by extreme conditions of social and environmental risk, and historical injustice. Through remoteness, poverty, landlessness, and political marginalization, they have minimal access to health care.

Public Health Status

Low levels of identification of indigenous people in national vital statistics and administrative data collections constitute a global barrier to the development of accurate indigenous health information. This in turn hinders a public health response. In the absence of comprehensive global data, a case example from Australia will illustrate the health issues and profile characteristic of some indigenous groups.

The health status of indigenous Australians has been in world news in mid-2007. The Australian Government, mobilized by a report highlighting high levels of child sexual abuse and violence in indigenous communities (Northern Territory Government, 2007), declared a state of emergency in the Northern Territory, banning alcohol in indigenous communities and mobilizing police and armed forces to enter indigenous communities to seize computers and other sources of pornography held to be the source of child sexual abuse. Part of a sequenced strategy, this was designed to be followed by teams of doctors to examine children and for possible referral for placement in foster care outside their communities. Such a drastic response led to strong condemnation by indigenous leaders, while others supported the action as overdue and needed in the face of endemic abuse (http://news.bbc.co.uk/2/hi/asia-pacific/6229708.stm). A change in federal government led to a review of this policy and, in February 2008, to a national apology to indigenous Australians for past injustices (http://www.aph.gov.au/house/news/news_stories/news_sorry.htm).

Reiterating themes found across the literature on indigenous health, the Overview of Australian Indigenous Health (Thomson et al., 2006) notes that in Australia,

> The current health status of Indigenous people is only explicable in terms of their extreme social disadvantage. This social disadvantage, directly related to dispossession

and characterised by poverty and powerlessness, is reflected in measures of their education, employment, income and housing. (p. 10)

Indigenous infant mortality rates varied by state, ranging from a third higher to more than double the rate for non-indigenous infants. Newborns of indigenous women were more than twice as likely to be of low birth weight than those born to non-indigenous women; the lowest average birth weights for infants were those whose mothers used marijuana with tobacco or with both tobacco and alcohol. Overall, life expectancy was lower by 17 years for indigenous women and men.

The leading cause of death among males and females in most states was cardiovascular disease (CVD), with rates up to 30% higher than the non-indigenous population. The next leading cause of death for indigenous males was injuries. These included automobile accidents, intentional self-harm and assault (3.0 times that of the total male population), cancer (1.3), respiratory diseases (3.9), and endocrine, nutritional, and metabolic disorders (primarily diabetes) (7.3). The most frequent causes of death for indigenous women, after CVD, were cancer (1.6 times the total female population), endocrine, nutritional, and metabolic disorders (11.7), injuries (2.9), and respiratory diseases (3.6). Lung cancer is among the leading forms of cancer for indigenous males and females, and cervical cancer is an important cause of death for indigenous women; the death rate in several states is more than seven times that of non-indigenous women.

Leading communicable diseases among indigenous peoples are tuberculosis, hepatitis A, B, and C, sexually transmitted infections, HIV/AIDS, hemophilus influenza type b (Hib), pneumococcal disease, and meningococcal disease. Poverty, overcrowding, malnutrition, smoking, alcohol, and drug abuse rank high as key risk factors for this constellation of communicable diseases. The incidence of tuberculosis, for example, is 15 times higher than that of the wider Australian-born population.

Diarrheal disease, eye and ear problems, and skin infections are also significantly higher among indigenous people and especially so among young children. Levels of disability and handicap are estimated to be at least double that of the general population.

Despite uncertainty over definitions of mental health/illness and inadequate data on mental health problems, indigenous people have high levels of mental health challenges and stress. A prominent manifestation of this is the rate of suicide. Based on sex-specific rates for the Australian population, suicide rates are more than 2.8 times that expected for indigenous males and 1.9 times more than expected for indigenous females. Thomson et al. (2006) note that these rates mask a very high youth suicide rate: indigenous to non-indigenous ratios are 3.4 for males and 6.1 for females in the 15–24 age groups.

Health risk factors include high tobacco, alcohol and other drug use, poor nutrition, low income, limited education, high unemployment, high levels of stress, social marginalization, inadequate working conditions and housing, and gender-related challenges. These in turn interact with cultural and traditional factors to influence behavior, health status, and health outcomes.

Intervention Programs

A key theme in communities is that self-management, self-policing, and culturally based solutions offer the most viable means of tackling socially based health problems.

As noted in the report from Australia, substance abuse and violence rank high among health concerns of many indigenous communities (Thomson et al., 2006). In the early 1990s Yuendumu, a remote Aboriginal township on the edge of the Tanami Desert, was gripped by an epidemic of petrol sniffing among young people.

This northern Australian indigenous community adopted a 'zero tolerance' policy when violence and property damage fueled by petrol sniffing was destabilizing the community. With up to 70 regular 'sniffers' in a community of 400, elders sent young petrol sniffers to Mt. Theo, an outstation 160 km from their remote township of Yuendumu and 50 km from the nearest road. A program of recovery from addiction and instruction in traditional culture, matched by a comprehensive youth program in Yuendumu offering alternatives to petrol sniffing, succeeded in breaking the cycle of addiction and violence. Within a decade there were no petrol sniffers in Yuendumu and the Mt. Theo program is now viewed as a model for other communities afflicted by petrol sniffing (Australians for Native Title and Reconciliation, 2007).

Native North American communities have been incorporating traditional forms of treatment into health programs for some years. In the United States, Indian Health Service (IHS) alcohol rehabilitation programs include traditional approaches to the treatment of alcoholism. An early analysis of 190 IHS contract programs revealed that 50% of these programs offered a traditional sweat lodge at their site or encouraged the use of sweat lodges. Treatment outcomes improved when a sweat lodge was available (Hall, 1986). Often these sweat lodges include the presence of medicine men or healers, and the presence of a traditional healer greatly improved the outcome when used in combination with the sweat lodge.

Although reliable data on indigenous mental health are scarce, the World Health Organization has highlighted the inevitable mental health consequences of trauma and grief resulting from invasion, dislocation, and, not infrequently, genocide (Cohen, 1999). Generational experience of these and associated trauma such as family separations, Aboriginal deaths in custody, and high levels of imprisonment are linked with the high levels of substance abuse in many indigenous communities (Thomson et al., 2006). Culturally sensitive research methodology is essential in studying indigenous mental health issues. An ethnographic and participatory approach is basic in ensuring that meaningful data are generated (Kirmayer et al., 2000). A Canadian study on indigenous mental health used a participatory research design to survey causes of sadness and happiness. It found that children and adolescents (ages 7–18) judged school and victimization as sources of sadness more frequently than did other age groups and cited alcohol less frequently. Women cited death and relatives as sources of sadness whereas males cited boredom (Bopp, 1985). The Arctic Climate Impact Assessment has also highlighted that alterations of the physical environment can lead to rapid and long-term cultural changes and loss of traditional culture. This in turn can create psychological distress and mental health challenges in indigenous communities (Berner et al., 2004).

Environmental Factors

Biodiversity and Human Health

The environmental impact of landscape changes on health is now gaining attention in both public health and conservation arenas, where it is recognized that environmental disturbance affects the ecological balance of the hosts of diseases as well as of disease-causing pathogens and parasites. The World Health Organization has recorded over 36 new emerging infectious diseases since 1976, many of which, particularly malaria and dengue, are the direct result of landscape influencing the ecology of disease (Taylor et al., 2001). As has been noted by the Harvard Project on Biodiversity and Health, human health, biodiversity, and poverty reduction represent a nexus of interrelated issues that lie at the center of human development; biodiversity, in turn, is dependent upon human health, as undernourished communities and those weak with disease will draw heavily on their surroundings for wild food resources and fuelwood (Epstein et al., 2003).

A program in India involving indigenous (so-called 'tribal') communities and landless and marginal farmers promoted the concept of home herbal gardens (HHG) as a means of decreasing family health problems and reducing high expenditures on health care (Hariramamurthi et al., 2007). This was part of a wider program to promote medicinal plant conservation and the forests that are their home (see Relevant Websites).

Medicinal plants were selected to address such common ailments as cold, cough, fever, diarrhea, dysentery, cuts and wounds, irregular menstruation and other menstrual conditions, joint pain, insect bites, indigestion and gastric complaints, mouth ulcer, and urinary infections and disorders. In each setting, a village resource person was trained in how to grow and use the medicinal plants, and she in turn trained the households.

An independent evaluation showed that the HHG program was adopted by the poorest of the poor, namely landless (33%), marginal landholding (37%), and small landholding (21%) farmers; 86% of adopters belonged to socially deprived communities, particularly indigenous communities.

HHGs benefited mainly women and children in poor communities as a first response to common conditions such as cold, cough and fever. HHG participants reported economic benefits in the form of savings from PHC-related expenses by use of home remedies. Health expenditures by non-HHG households was approximately 5 times greater than for HHG households.

Climate Change and Indigenous Health

The Arctic Climate Impact Assessment (ACIA) has evaluated Arctic climate change and its impact for the region and the world (Berner et al., 2004). Indigenous people make up approximately 10% of the total Arctic population, which includes populations from Norway, Sweden, Finland, Denmark, Iceland, Canada, Russia, and the Untied States. ACIA argues that changing weather conditions, resulting in increased storms, reduced sea ice, and thawing ground, and the accompanying reduction in species' ranges and availability, will affect human health and food security and possibly the survival of some indigenous cultures. Changes in climate are occurring faster than traditional knowledge is able to adapt. Across the Arctic indigenous people are reporting changes in climate and in the fish and animal and bird populations on which they depend for food. Melting ice makes travel to traditional hunting areas difficult and reduction in summer sea ice makes ringed seals harder to find. Elevated ultraviolet (UV) light levels will lead to UV exposure of young people by more than 30%, thus increasing the risk of skin cancers, cataracts, and immune system disorders.

Drought and associated desertification are also risks of climate change and threats to the health and livelihoods of indigenous communities. In western Arnhem Land in northern Australia, indigenous people are reviving traditional landscape burning patterns, begun soon after the rains, to reduce combustible material that can cause far larger, damaging fires and to regenerate useful plants and animals.

Supported by a gas refinery, required by environmental law to reduce its greenhouse emissions, a unique carbon trading agreement has been forged with government and indigenous communities. The agreement recognizes that if, in one year, indigenous people could reduce the area burned in wildfires by just 7%, they would create the equivalent of at least 100 000 tonnes in greenhouse gas savings. Starting in 2007, the refinery owner, Conoco-Phillips, has contracted to pay a $1 million a year for 17 years to employ Arnhem Land people and support their fire management. The money will be used to support community health and education programs. Enhanced self-sufficiency in health care has been won through a revival of traditional practices, also contributing to reduced carbon emissions, improved global health, and environmental security – surely a sound contemporary model for integrated indigenous health development (BBC, 2007b).

Conclusion

The health of indigenous people is typically influenced by histories of social injustice, loss of territorial rights, marginal social status, and limited employment and income opportunities.

Overall, the intractability of indigenous health determinants and health status warrants a comprehensive global strategy, based on a human rights approach, with local action by governments in partnerships with indigenous organizations. The challenge by several governments – with significant indigenous populations – to the eventual passage on September 13, 2007, of the UN Declaration on the Rights of Indigenous Peoples through the UN General Assembly underscores the obstacles ahead in any such global strategy. Another challenge is the need for comprehensive local, national, and regional data collection, inclusive of indigenous peoples and their health conditions, as an epidemiological framework for action.

Despite repeated challenges from indigenous peoples for stronger action, the World Heath Organization, through a number of World Health Assembly (WHA) resolutions, is mandated to accord special attention to the health of indigenous peoples. There is also commitment to convene partners and catalyze action to improve indigenous peoples' health and human rights. The Pan American Health Organization of WHO has been the most active in addressing these issues and in identifying successful models of change (Alderete, 1999).

As for the basic prerequisites for improvement and development, Health Unlimited has outlined priorities for indigenous health development:

1. Train local people to provide basic health services in remote areas.
2. Ensure that traditional practitioners are involved and that their views are appreciated, so new ideas about health are more likely to be taken on board in isolated, indigenous communities.
3. Provide safe water and improve sanitation.
4. Provide information regarding indigenous peoples' rights and entitlement to health care (see World Directory of Minorities and Indigeneous Peoples: www.minorityrights.org/?lid=3).
5. Work with state health providers to ensure indigenous peoples are not discriminated against when it comes to accessing health services (www.healthunlimited.org).

As the global rural–urban drift continues and indigenous peoples join marginal groups living in urban poverty, the future would seem to hold a mix of trends: continued intractability in the determinants of poor health, accompanied by isolated models of success. Where solutions do present themselves, success would seem to be based on self-sufficiency, recourse to traditional cultural practices, and equitable partnerships with agencies receptive to new models of work.

See also: Human Rights, Approach to Public Health Policy.

Citations

Alderete E (1999) *The Health of Indigenous Peoples*. Washington, D.C: PAHO.

Australians for Native Title and Reconciliation (2007) *Success Stories in Indigenous Health*. Rozelle, NSW, Australia: ANTR.

BBC (2007a) http://news.bbc.co.uk/2/hi/asia-pacific/6229708.stm (accessed December 2007).

BBC (2007b) http://news.bbc.co.uk/2/hi/asia-pacific/6726059.stm (accessed December 2007).

Berner J, Furgal C, Bjerregaard P, et al. (2004) Human health. In: ACIA (eds.) *Impacts of a Warming Arctic: Arctic Climate Impact Assessment*, ch. 15. Cambridge, UK: Cambridge University Press.

Bopp M (1985) *Developing Healthy Communities: Fundamental Strategies for Health Promotion*. Lethbridge, UK: Four Worlds Development Project: University of Lethbridge.

Cohen A (1999) *The Mental Health of Indigenous Peoples: An International Overview*. Geneva, Switzerland: Department of Mental Health, World Health Organization.

Encarta (n.d.) http://encarta.msn.com/text_761570777___2/Native_Americans_of_North_America.html (accessed December 2007).

Epstein PR, Chivian E, and Frith K (2003) Emerging diseases threaten conservation. *Environmental Health Perspectives* 111(10): A506–A507.

Hall RL (1986) Alcohol treatment in American Indian communities: An indigenous treatment modality compared with traditional approaches. *Annals of the New York Academy of Science* 472: 168–178.

Hariramamurthi G, Venkatasubramanian P, Unnikrishnan PM, and Shankar D (2007) Kitchen herbal gardens: Biodiversity conservation and health care at the local level. In: Bodeker G and Burford G (eds.) *Traditional, Complementary and Alternative Medicine: Policy and Public Health Perspectives*. London: Imperial College Press.

Kirmayer LJ, Macdonald ME, and Brass GM (2000) The mental health of indigenous peoples. *Proceedings of the Advanced Study Institute, the Mental Health of Indigenous Peoples*. McGill Summer Program in Social and Cultural Psychiatry and the Aboriginal Mental Health Research Team May 29 – May 31, Montreal, Quebec. Montreal: Culture and Mental Health Research Unit Report No. 10.

Northern Territory Government (2007) *Report of the Northern Territory Board of Inquiry into the Protection of Aboriginal Children from Sexual Abuse*. Darwin, Australia: Northern Territory Government.

Taylor LH, Latham SM, and Woolhouse ME (2001) Risk factors for human disease emergence. *Philosophical Transactions of the Royal Society, London* 356: 983–989.

Thomson N, Burns J, Burrow S, and Kirov E (2006) *Overview of Australian Indigenous Health 2006*. http://www.healthinfonet.ecu.edu.au/html/html_overviews/overview.pdf (accessed December 2007).

UN (2007) Declaration on the Rights of Indigenous Peoples: http://www.un.org/esa/socdev/unpfi/en/deciuration.html (accessed January 25, 2008).

World Factbook (1997) Central Intelligence Agency. Washington, DC. http://www.odci.gov/cia/publications/factbook/ (accessed 25 January 2008).

World Factbook (2007) CENIMAR, Troy studios, Loomis, California. http://www.seminar.com/factbook/index.jsp (accessed 25 January 2008).

Pan American Health Organization (PAHO) (n.d.) *Health of Indigenous Peoples* http://www.paho.org/english/ad/ths/os/Indig-home.htm (accessed December 2007).

UN (2003) *Risks Posed By Substance Abuse, Environmental Pollutants, Lack of Health Services*. http://www.un.org/news/Press/docs/2003/hr4668.doc.htm (accessed December 2007).

WHO (n.d.) *The Health and Human Rights of Indigenous Peoples* http://www.who.int/hhr/activities/indigenous/en/ (accessed December 2007).

WHO (1999) *The Mental Health of Indigenous Peoples: An International Overview*. Geneva, Switzerland: WHO.

WHO (2001) *WHO's Contribution to the World Conference Against Racism, Racial Discrimination, Xenophobia and Related Intolerance: Health and Freedom from Discrimination*. Health and Human Rights Publication Series no. 2. Geneva, Switzerland: WHO.

WHO (2001) *Global Compendium of Indigenous Health Research Institutions*. Geneva, Switzerland: WHO.

WHO (2003) *Indigenous Peoples and Participatory Health Research: Planning and Management/Preparing Research Agreements*. Geneva, Switzerland: WHO, CINE.

Further Reading

Bodeker G (2007) Traditional medicine. In: Cook G and Zumla A (eds.) *Manson's Tropical Diseases*, 22nd edn. London: WB Saunders, Elsevier Health Sciences.

Bodeker G and Burford G (eds.) (2007) *Public Health and Policy Perspectives on Traditional, Complementary and Alternative Medicine*. London: Imperial College Press.

Bodeker G, Ong C-K, Burford G, Grundy C, and Shein K (eds.) (2005) *World Health Organization Global Atlas on Traditional and Complementary Medicine*, 2 vols. Geneva, Switzerland: World Health Organization.

London School of Hygiene and Tropical Medicine (2003) *UN Decade of Awareness Fails to Advance Indigenous Peoples' Health or Rights*. http://www.lshtm.ac.uk/news/2003/indigenous.html (accessed December 2007).

Relevant Websites

http://www.hc-sc.gc.ca/ahc-asc/activit/strateg/fnih-spni/ahhri-irrhs_e.html – Aboriginal Health Human Resources Initiative – Canada.

http://www.healthinfonet.ecu.edu.au/ – Australian Indigenous Health InfoNet.

http://www.frlht.org – Foundation for Revitalization of Local Health Traditions.

http://www.iphrc.ca/ – Indigenous People's Health Research Centre, Canada.

http://www.lshtm.ac.uk/news/2003/indigenous.html – London School of Hygiene and Tropical Medicine.

http://www.oxfam.org.au/campaigns/indigenous/health.php – Oxfam: Close the Gap: Indigenous Health in Crisis.

http://www.un.org/esa/socdev/pfii/index.htmlwww.unesco.org/culture/indigenous/index.shtmlwww.who.int/gb/EB WHA/PDF/WHA55/EA5535.pdf – UN Decade of Indigenous Peoples.

SUBJECT INDEX

Cross-reference terms in italics are general cross-references, or refer to subentry terms within the main entry (the main entry is not repeated to save space). Readers are also advised to refer to the end of each article for additional cross-references - not all of these cross-references have been included in the index cross-references.

Subentries (or subsubentries) to a specific index entry having the same page number, have been included to indicate the breadth of the discussion (as opposed to just the location), as additional assistance to the reader.

The index is arranged in set-out style with a maximum of three levels of heading. Major discussion of a subject is indicated by bold page numbers. Page numbers suffixed by T and F refer to Tables and Figures respectively. vs. indicates a comparison.

This index is in letter-by -letter order, whereby hyphens and spaces within index headings are ignored in the alphabetization. Prefixes and terms in parentheses are excluded from the initial alphabetization.

A

Aboriginal peoples *see* Indigenous peoples
'Accountability for reasonableness,' meso-level resource allocation 183, 184, 184*t*
Acquired immune deficiency syndrome (AIDS) *see* HIV/AIDS
Action Program on Essential Drugs 287
Activities of daily living (ADLs)
  long-term care assessment 355*t*, 358–359
Acute care hospitals
  functions 402–403
  home care substitution *see* Home care
Advocacy
  evidence-based public health policy 34*t*
Africa
  community health insurance 238, 238*t*, 240
  health-care financing 201
  Middle East and North *see* Middle East and North Africa (MENA)
  Millennium Development Goals 82–83
  pharmaceutical expenditure 178–179
  social health insurance 237–238
  sub-Saharan *see* sub-Saharan Africa
Agreement on Trade-Related Aspects of Intellectual Property Rights (TRIPS) *see* Trade-related Aspects of Intellectual Property Rights (TRIPS) agreement
AIDS *see* HIV/AIDS
Albania
  private health-care provision 306*t*
Alcohol rehabilitation programs
  Indian Health Service, USA 424
Alma-Ata Declaration (1978) *see* Declaration of Alma-Ata
Alternative medicine *see* Traditional, complementary, and alternative medicine (TCAM)
American Medical Association (AMA) 10
Antiretroviral therapy (ART)
  HIV/AIDS
    access issues 344
Arctic Climate Impact Assessment (ACIA) 424–425
Argentina
  health-care financing, risk pooling 400
  health insurance, transition to universal coverage 217
  health sector corruption prevention 142*t*, 143
  private health-care provision 306*t*, 307*f*, 308*f*
Aristotle
  justice principle conceptions 98
Armenia, health-care system
  private health-care provision 306*t*
Asia
  community health insurance 240
  South *see* South Asia
  South-East *see* South-East Asia
Assistive living, long-term care provision 353
Association of the British Pharmaceutical Industry (ABPI), interest group status 117

Asthma
  provider performance-based payment systems 327
Atkinson's index, health-care financing equity 198
Australia
  health insurance, transition to universal coverage 216
  health promotion financing 263, 264*t*, 268*t*
  indigenous peoples 423
    health status 423
  mortality rates
    infant 424
  private health-care provision 306*t*
  provider payment methods 326–327
Australian National Public Health Partnership 58
Austria
  health insurance, transition to universal coverage 215
  health promotion financing 265, 268*t*
  long-term care provision 354
  private health-care provision 306*t*
Autonomy ethical principle
  health inequalities 90–91
Average variable cost 336
  economic hospital behavior models 338
Azerbaijan
  private health-care provision 306*t*
  see also Former Soviet Union (FSU)

B

Balanced Budget Act (1997), US 333
Bamako Initiative 399
Bangkok Charter for Health Promotion 259
Bangladesh
  community health worker programs 387
  health insurance, transition to universal coverage 214, 214*t*, 219, 221, 222
  private health-care provision 306, 306*t*
'Barefoot doctor' concept 381
Behavioral therapy
  health-care demand 249
Belgium
  health-care provision
    private 306*t*
Beneficence ethical principle
  health inequalities 90–91
Bermuda, private health-care provision 306*t*
Beverage, William 52
Beveridge model, health-care system *see* National Health Services (Beveridge) model of health-care
Bill and Melinda Gates Foundation (BMGF) 18–19
Billboard Utilising Graffitists Against Unhealthy Promotions (BUGA UP) 117–118
Biological weapons (BW)
  ethical issues 102–103
Bismarck model, social health insurance 215, 237–238, 275–276, 279, 282

features 215, 419*t*
innovations 281*t*
reform 13
strengths 281*t*
sustainability 283
weaknesses 281*t*
Bolivia
  health sector corruption prevention 142*t*
  private health-care provision 307*f*, 308*f*
Brazil
  health insurance, transition to universal coverage 218
  private health-care provision 306*t*, 307*f*, 308*f*
Breast cancer
  health inequalities 95
  interventions, decision analytic modeling 192–193, 193*t*
British Public Health Act (1848) 52
Brundtland, Gro 68
Bryant, John 66–67
Budget constraints, health-care demand 245
Buenos Aires 30/15 International Conference 74, 78
BUGA UP (Billboard Utilising Graffitists Against Unhealthy Promotions) 117–118
Bureaucratic model, public health 53
Burkina Faso
  community health insurance schemes 238*t*, 239
  private health-care provision 306*t*

C

Cabinet Office Social Exclusion Task Force 57
Cambodia
  community health insurance 242, 243*t*
  health sector corruption prevention 142*t*
  private health-care provision 306
Cameroon, private health-care provision 306*t*
Campbell Collaboration 36
Canada
  health-care, public-private partnerships 318
  health-care expenditure
    pharmaceuticals 178*f*, 179*f*
  health insurance, transition to universal coverage 216
  long-term care provision 253, 353–354
    Compassionate Care Benefit 253
Cancer United 122
Capitation, managed care 330
Cardiac surgery, Urgency Rating Scores 184
Cardiovascular disease (CVD)
  indigenous peoples 424
Caregivers
  burden, long-term care assessment 355*t*
  'expert,' UK investment 394
  home care, acute hospital substitution 353
  informal 252, 352
Carers *see* Caregivers

Subject Index

Caribbean
　health-care expenditure, pharmaceuticals 178–179
Cayman Islands, private health-care provision 306t
Certificate of Need (CON) laws, hospital competition 311
Cervical cancer screening
　performance-based payment systems 327
Chan, Margaret 74, 76
CHFplus project, Tanzania 240
Childhood diarrhea
　mortality 286–287
Child mortality
　governance indicator 208, 209f, 210t
　Millennium Development Goals 82t, 83t, 85t
　parental educational attainment impact
　　see Educational attainment
Child Survival Revolution, UNICEF 289
Chile
　health insurance, transition to universal coverage 214t, 217
　health sector corruption, prevention 142t
China
　community health insurance 240–241
　community health worker program 381
　health-care system
　　historical aspects 280
　health insurance
　　transition to universal coverage 220, 222
　primary health care 290
　private health-care provision 306t
CHOICE project see Choosing Health Interventions that are Cost-Effective (CHOICE) project, WHO
Choosing Health Interventions that are Cost-Effective (CHOICE) project, WHO
　cost-effectiveness analysis 188
　objective 183
Christian Medical Commission (CMC)
　composition 60
　Declaration of Alma-Ata, history 60
　establishment 60
　joint working with WHO 61
Chronic disease(s)
　health promotion, global goals 260
Citizen participation, public health policy/research see Public/consumer participation
Civil service, public health policy 55
Civil society, definition 116–117
Civil Society Initiative (CSI), WHO 126–127
Civil society organizations see Interest groups
Classification of individual consumption by purpose (COICOP) 165f
Classification of the functions of government (COFOG) 165f
Climate change
　health impacts
　　indigenous peoples 425
Close-to-the-client (CTC) systems 72
Cochrane Collaboration 33–34, 36
Cognition
　long-term care assessment 355t
Columbia
　health-care financing, risk pooling 400, 400t
　health sector corruption prevention 143
　public health policy reform 27–28
Commercial health insurance
　scheme characteristics 237, 237t
　voluntary 212
Commission on Health Research and Development 179
Commission on Macroeconomics and Health 72, 73, 174, 179
Commission on the Social Determinants of Health (CSDH), UN 73, 75
Commonwealth, public health role 56
Communicable disease(s) see Infectious disease(s)
Community Based Health Financing (CBHF) conference, Kenya 240
Community-based health promotion
　primary health care development 291

Community/communities
　empowerment 372, 373f
　public health policy 119
Community health insurance (CHI)
　classification 236–237
　definition 211
　developing countries 236–245
　　advantages 243
　　challenges associated 243
　　disadvantages 243
　　Indian subcontinent 236, 241, 242t
　nongovernmental organizations 241
　origins 236
　scheme characteristics 212, 236, 237t
　scope 236
Community health workers (CHWs) 381–390
　definition 381, 383
　effectiveness 383, 385
　history 381
　primary health care implementation 293, 381
　program sustainability 387
　role 383, 388
　training/support needs 384
Community prepayment schemes, health-care financing 151
Comparative health systems see Health-care systems
Compassionate Care Benefit, Canada 253
Complementary medicine see Traditional, complementary, and alternative medicine (TCAM)
Computed tomography (CT)
　health-care expenditure impact 178
Concentration index (CI), health-care financing equity 197–198, 197f
Condoms/condom use
　HIV/AIDS prevention 84–85
Consumption see Tuberculosis
Continence, long-term care assessment 358
Convention on the Elimination of All Forms of Discrimination Against Women, UN 107
Convention on the Rights of the Child, UN 107
Corruption, health sector 137–145
　causes 141
　cultural issues 138
　definition 138
　health-care financing 139t, 205, 211
　health consequences 138, 208, 209f
　health reform and 144
　perceptions of 207, 207f
　pharmaceutical sector 347
　prevention 142, 142t, 144
　　accountability 143
　　discretion 143
　　research directions 144
　　transparency 142
　types 139t, 140f, 140t
Costa Rica
　health sector corruption, prevention 143
　primary health care 290
　private health-care provision 306t
Cost-effectiveness analysis (CEA) 186–190
　CHOICE project, WHO 188
　decision analysis see Decision analytic modeling
　ex ante vs. ex post 188
　focus 186
　incremental 187
　interventions, interactions between 187
　resource efficiency 187
　scales 187
　sectoral 186
　technical efficiency studies 186
　unit costs 187
Cost-influenced treatment decisions see Health-care financing
Cost sharing 322
　see also Provider payment methods
Critical care studies, resource allocation 184
Croatia
　health sector corruption, prevention 142t
Cromwell's model, hospital economic behavior 339
CT see Computed tomography (CT)

Cuba
　health-care system 280
Cultural rights, health inequalities 92
Culture
　corruption, health sector 138
　traditional, complementary, and alternative medicine see also Indigenous therapeutics
Cyprus, private health-care provision 306t
Czech Republic
　health-care expenditure, pharmaceuticals 178f, 179f
　private health-care provision 306t

D

Daniels, Norman
　justice principle conceptions 99
Decision analytic modeling 190–195
　expected value concept 190
　Monte Carlo simulation 194
　sensitivity analysis 193, 194f
　strategy comparison 190, 191f, 192f
　strengths 195
　types 191
　　Markov models 191, 193f, 193t
　　simple decision trees 191, 191f
Decision trees, decision analytic modeling 191, 191f
Declaration of Alma-Ata 59–81
　addendum to 74
　Commission on Macroeconomics and Health 72, 73, 174, 179
　Commission on the Social Determinants of Health see Commission on the Social Determinants of Health (CSDH), UN
　Director's letter 70
　Executive Summary 70
　health definition 63–64
　health planning influence 42
　history 60
　primary health care 63, 64
　　aims/focus 107, 284, 286
　　Americas 70
　　criticisms 65
　　David Sanders 68
　　global review 69
　　Gro Brundtland 68
　　Pan American Health Organization role 70–71
　　principles 63, 123
　　prologue 74
　　public health 53
　　reflections/remarks 78
　　　David Tejada 62
　　　Dmitry Venediktov 67
　　　historical 66
　　　Margaret Chan 74
Declaration on the Rights of Indigenous Peoples, United Nations 426
Declaration on the TRIPS Agreement and Public Health 313
Defensive medicine, health-care expenditure impact 177
Demand, health-care see Health-care provision
Demand curve, definition 336
Demographic transition
　definition 174–176
　long-term care 251, 251t, 252t
Demography
　urban health/health-care trends 408, 409f
Denmark
　health-care expenditure, pharmaceuticals 178f, 179f
　health-care financing
　　private health insurance 399t
　health insurance, transition to universal coverage 216
　private health-care provision 306t
Developing countries
　community health insurance see Community health insurance (CHI)
　essential drugs expenditure 342
　managed care history 334
　social health insurance 237–238

Diabetes Empowerment Scale 373, 374t
Diabetes mellitus
  provider performance-based payment systems 327
Diagnostic Related Grouping system see Provider payment methods
Diphtheria vaccination
  shortages 286
Directly observed treatment - short-course (DOTS) see DOTS
Disability-adjusted life expectations (DALEs) 98
Disability-adjusted life years (DALYs)
  concepts underlying
    utilitarianism 98
  definition 17
  health planning 46–47
  see also Quality-adjusted life years (QALYs)
Disasters
  resource allocation, justice principle 100–101, 102, 104
Discrimination
  health inequalities and 91–92
  public health policy 111
Disease Control Priorities in Developing Countries project 183
Disease prevention/preventive medicine
  tertiary 402–403
  see also Health promotion
Doha Declaration on Trade-Related Property Rights and Public Health 313
Dominican Republic
  health-care expenditure, pharmaceuticals 178–179
  private health-care provision 306t, 307f, 308f
  public health policy reform 28
DOTS
  control strategy, community health worker programs 387
  effectiveness, evidence 287
Drop the Debt campaign, Jubilee 2000 121
Drug(s)
  essential 287
    policy see Essential drugs policy/legislation
  expenditure 178, 178f, 179f
    developing countries 342
  generic, competition 313
  international development agencies 343
  latent functions 342
  marketing
    corruption issues 139t, 141
  see also Pharmaceutical industry

E

Eco-health see Ecosystem health
Ecological framework/approach (to health) see Ecosystem health
Economics/financial issues
  health-care see Health-care financing
  health inequalities 92
  hospital behavior models see Hospitals/hospital services
Ecosystem health
  urban research 413
Ecuador
  health-care expenditure, pharmaceuticals 178–179
  private health-care provision 306t, 307f, 308f
Educational attainment
  Millennium Development Goals 83–84
Egypt
  health-care expenditure
    health insurance effects 176
    household income effects 176
    pharmaceuticals 178–179
  health insurance
    health-care expenditure and 176
    transition to universal coverage 214t
Elderly
  health-care resources 115
El Salvador
  health-care expenditure, pharmaceuticals 178–179

Emergency Medical Services (EMS)
  resource allocation, justice principle 100–101, 102, 104
Emergency planning 43
  resource allocation see Resource allocation
Employee Retirement Income Security Act (1974), USA 312
Empowerment 370–381
  applications 370–371, 371f
  communities 372, 373f
  definition/conceptualization 371, 373f
  families 372, 373f
  nurses 370–371, 371f
  organizations 370–371, 371f
  patients see Patient empowerment
  physicians 370–371, 371f
  principles 370
  theory 371
Endogenous variable, definition 336
Entropy measures, health-care financing equity 198
Environment
  health-care systems impact 282
  physical, urban health determinants 412
  social see Social environment
Environmental sanitation see Sanitation
Epidemiological transition
  definition 173
Equity ethical principle see Justice/equity ethical principle
Essential care packages (ECPs), strategic health-care purchasing 401
Essential drugs policy/legislation 342–351
  assessment 347
  components 346t
  corruption and 347
  development
    actors in 343
    concepts 345
    monitoring 349
    strategies/process 348
  enforcement 349
  goals 342
  literature 343
  regulatory agencies 343
  WHO perspectives 345
  World Bank perspectives 343–344, 346
Estonia, health promotion financing 264, 268t
Ethics/ethical issues
  biological weapons 102–103
  health inequalities 90
  health promotion see Health promotion
  immunization see Immunization/immunization programs
  infectious disease control see Infectious disease
  principles
    autonomy see Autonomy ethical principle
    beneficence see Beneficence ethical principle
    equity see Justice/equity ethical principle
    justice see Justice/equity ethical principle
    resource allocation see Resource allocation
    utility see Utility ethical principle/utilitarianism
Ethiopia
  health-care expenditure, pharmaceuticals 178–179
  private health-care provision 306t
European Medicines Agency (EMEA) 343
Evidence-based medicine (EBM)
  definition 30
  public health policy see Public health policy
  systematic reviews' contribution 33–34
Executive-benefit-maximization model, hospital economic behavior 340
Exogenous variable, definition 336
Expected value concept, decision analytic modeling 190
Expenditure
  health-care see Health-care expenditure
  household 196
'Expert carers,' UK investment 394

F

Fairness in financial contribution (FFC) index, health-care financing 198
Family Empowerment Questionnaire 373, 374t
Family/families
  empowerment 372, 373f
Federal systems, public health 55
Fee-for-service (FFS) payments
  physician competition 323
  provider payment methods 323, 325, 420t
Feldstein's model, hospital economic behavior 339
Fight for Herceptin Campaign 122
Financial issues see Economics/financial issues
Finland
  health-care expenditure 172
    pharmaceuticals 178f, 179f
  health insurance, transition to universal coverage 216
  private health-care provision 306t
Fixed cost, definition 336
Flexner Report (1910), USA 310
Focus groups
  urban health research 413
Folic acid supplementation
  decision analytic modeling 193
Former Soviet Union (FSU)
  health insurance, universal coverage 218
  see also Russian Federation
France
  health-care expenditure, pharmaceuticals 178, 178f, 179f
  health-care financing
    private health insurance 397, 399t
    social health insurance 394, 397, 398f
  health-care provision
    private 306t
  health-care system, stewardship 405
  health insurance, transition to universal coverage 215
Fred Hollows Foundation 118–119
Free market model of health-care 160, 275–276, 278
  strengths 281t
  weaknesses 281t
Functionalism, health policy 5–7

G

Game theory, health-care expenditure 176–177
Gantt charts, health planning implementation/monitoring 48
Garcia, Gines Gonzalez 74
GAVI Alliance 128–129, 131, 135t, 347
Gay rights movement 121–122
Gender see Gender/gender considerations
Gender/gender considerations
  life expectancy 94
  Millennium Development Goals 83–84
  see also Women/women's health
General Agreement on Trade in Services (GATS)
  public-private partnerships 317
General practitioners see Primary health care (PHC)
Generic drugs, competition 313
German Green Party 116
Germany
  consumer choice, health plans 231
  health-care expenditure 172
    pharmaceuticals 178f, 179f
  health-care financing 394
    private health insurance 399t
  health-care provision
    disease management programs 403
  health insurance, transition to universal coverage 215
  long-term care provision 354, 355
  private health-care provision 306t
  sickness funds, health-care services provision 232, 397
Ghana
  community health insurance schemes 238t, 239
  health information systems 292

Subject Index

Ghana (*continued*)
  health insurance, transition to universal coverage 219
Global Alliance on Vaccines and Immunization (GAVI) *see* GAVI Alliance
Global Forum for Health Research 17
Global Fund to Fight AIDS, Tuberculosis and Malaria (GFATM) 128, 131, 133, 135*t*
Global Health Initiatives (GHIs) **128–137**
  coordinated development assistance mechanisms 130
  definition 128
  governance mechanisms 131
  health-care systems 285
  organizational types 130*f*, 130*t*
  policy making effects 133, 134*f*, 135*t*
  Public Private Partnership for Health 129, 129*t*
Global Health Partnerships (GHPs) 131, 132*f*
  definition 154–155
  health-care systems 285
Globalization
  health sector reform 12, 13
  primary health care policy context 285
Global People's Health Charter 124
Global Public Private Partnership for Health 129, 129*t*, 130*t*, 131, 132*f*
Global warming *see* Climate change
Goldfarb–Hornbrook–Rafferty's model, hospital economic behavior 340
Governance
  child mortality as indicator 208, 209*f*, 210*t*
  definition 4
  health-care expenditure determination 171
  health-care financing *see* Health-care financing
  health promotion financing, Thailand 269
  interest groups 115
  nongovernmental organizations *see* Nongovernmental organizations (NGOs)
Grameen bank model of credit extension 249
Grant, James 65
Greece
  health-care expenditure, pharmaceuticals 178*f*, 179*f*
  health-care provision
    private 306*t*
Greenpeace 118
Gross domestic product, global health expenditure 166, 168*f*, 168*t*, 169*f*
Gross income, health-care financing equity 196
Growth monitoring, oral rehydration techniques, breastfeeding, and immunizations (GOBI) interventions 286
  Declaration of Alma-Ata 65
Guinea
  community health insurance schemes 238*t*, 239

H

Haiti
  community health worker programs 386
  nongovernmental organizations 328
Harvard Project on Biodiversity and Health 425
Health
  behaviors *see* Health behavior(s)
  definitions/concepts 3
    Alma-Ata 63–64
    ecological *see* Ecosystem health
    rights-based *see* Human rights
    WHO *see* World Health Organization (WHO)
  determinants *see* Health determinants
  epidemiological transition *see* Epidemiological transition
  gender considerations *see* Gender/gender considerations
  influences 92
  mental *see* Mental health
  see also Public health
Health accounting framework, health-care expenditure 164, 165, 165*f*
Health Care Commission, UK 405

Health-care competition **309–314**
  health insurance 225, 312
  hospital services 311
  pharmaceutical industry 312
  physician services 310, 323
  principles 309
Health-care delivery *see* Health-care provision
Health-care demand **245–250**
  behavioral change 249
  budget constraints 245
  consumer preferences 245
  discrete choice 248
  extensions 247
  future research perspectives 249
  information imperfections and 248
  maximization hypothesis 245–246
  own-price effect 247
  reduced-form models 247
  refinements 247
  self-control and 249
  time cost 249
  traditional healers 248
  unified model 245, 246, 249
Health-care expenditure **164–171**, 419*t*
  challenges 186
  cost-effectiveness analysis *see* Cost-effectiveness analysis (CEA)
  definition 164
  determinants **171–180**
    analysis framework 171, 172*f*
    governance and 171
    health-care system organization 171
    health insurance effect 176
    household income 174, 175*f*, 176*t*
    physician behavior 176
    population health needs 173
    technology role 177
  distribution by financing agent 168, 169*f*
  estimation 165
  global 166, 171, 261*t*
    gross domestic product 166, 168*f*, 168*t*, 169*f*
  health accounting framework 164, 165, 165*f*
  health outcomes correlation 168, 170*f*
  health policy influence 169
  indicators 166, 167*t*
  long-term care *see* Long-term care
  low-income countries 277
  middle-income countries 277
  national 164, 169–170
  pharmaceuticals 178, 178*f*, 179*f*
  population aging impact 173
  priority setting *see* Resource allocation
  reporting 165, 166*f*
    conventions 166
  resource consumption 164
  revenue collection method comparisons 202
Health-care financing **149–164**, 204, 212
  agencies 416
  archetypal systems 149
    performance evaluation 158
  community prepayment schemes 151
  cost-effectiveness analysis *see* Cost-effectiveness analysis (CEA)
  cost-influenced treatment decisions *see* Cost-effectiveness analysis (CEA)
  developmental aid partners' funding 154
  donations 399
  efficiency 156
  equity 156, **195–204**
    cross-country comparisons 199, 200*t*, 201*t*
    definition 195
    global 199, 199*f*
    improvement measures 203
    measurement, household expenditure and 196, 197
    measurement methodologies 196
    policy implications 201
    societal perceptions 196
    within-country differences 200
  evaluation 155, 159*t*
    frameworks 157, 158

free market systems *see* Free market model of health-care
functions 394
global review 260, 261*t*
governance **204–211**
  challenges 207
  corruption *see* Corruption, health sector
  funding 205, 205*f*
  health outcomes and 208, 209*f*
  as international issue 209
  measurement 207
  problems associated 206
Grameen bank model of credit extension 249
grants 399
health insurance *see* Health insurance
health promotion initiatives *see* Health promotion
high-income countries 160*t*
human resource planning *see* Human resource planning/management
informal fees 153
justice/equity ethical principle 156
loans 399
medical savings accounts 152
mixed systems 160
nongovernmental organizations' funding 154, 155
options 11
out-of-pocket systems 153, 153*t*, 154*f*, 160
  features 399
  long-term care 255
  risks 394–395
payment methods and incentives
  demand side 322
  supply side *see* Provider payment methods
priority setting *see* Resource allocation
private health insurance *see* Private health insurance (PHI)
process 172
reform 207
  see also Health sector reform (HSR)
resource pooling 400, 400*t*
revenue collection methods 394
risk pooling 400, 400*t*
social health insurance *see* Social health insurance (SHI)
solidarity-based systems 150
  definition 212
sources 205, 205*f*, 394, 395*f*, 419*t*
stages 205
sustainability 157
taxation 150, 395
Victorian Health Promotion Foundation 259, 260–261, 264*t*
World Health Report (2000) 195–196, 199, 199*f*
Health Care Modernization Act (2004) 333
Health-care planning **39–51**
  actors involved 49
  approaches 43, 44*t*
  capacity required 49
  challenges 49
  conceptual framework 40, 41*f*
  context 42
  definition 39
  emergencies 43
  evaluation/monitoring 48
  features 40
  financial 49
  historical roots 40
  human resources *see* Human resource planning/management
  implementation 48
  infrastructure 49
  inputs, specific 48
  levels 45*t*
  option appraisal 47
  priority setting 46, 48*f*
  programing 47
  public health policy relationship 39
  public-private mix 42
  purpose 39
  questions, health system components 40, 41*t*
  resource allocation 46, 48*f*

Subject Index

situational analysis 46
stages 45, 47f
technical issues 43, 44t
transitional countries 43
types 43, 45t
values 40
Health-care policy *see* Health policy
Health-care provision
  corruption *see* Corruption, health sector
  expenditure *see* Health-care expenditure
  financing *see* Health-care financing
  models 394f, 402
  private sector role **303–309**
    government policy interaction areas 305t
    high-income countries 305, 305t, 306t
    low-income countries 305, 306t, 307f, 308f
    primary care 305, 305t, 307
    profit orientation 304, 307
    tertiary care 306, 307f, 308f
  systems *see* Health-care systems
Health-care purchasing 394f, 400
  diagnosis-related groups 401
  process 401
  prospective funding 401
  strategic 401
Health-care systems **275–284, 393–408**
  accountability 204–205, 206
    see also Governance
  capacity, declining 285
  characteristics 275
  comparative analysis **415–422**
    definition 415–416
    methods 416, 418t
    problems associated 420
    variation 275, 417
  corruption *see* Corruption, health sector
  definition 275, 393, 416
  development 288
  environment, impact of society 282
  evaluation 155
    effectiveness criteria 405, 406t
    framework 158
    quality dimensions 393, 394t
  expenditure *see* Health-care expenditure
  financing *see* Health-care financing
  formal *vs.* lay care 393
  functions 204, 393
  future developments 282
  goals, measurement indicators 417, 418t
  innovations 280, 281t
  models 278, 281t
    free market *see* Free market model of health-care
    health-care expenditure determination 171
    new, emerging 403
    NHS *see* National Health Services (Beveridge) model of health-care
    public-private partnerships *see* Public-private partnerships (PPPs)
    social insurance *see* Social health insurance (SHI)
    socialist *see* Socialist model of health-care
  patient empowerment antecedent 378
  primary health care *see* Primary health care (PHC)
  private sector role *see* Health-care provision
  reform *see* Health sector reform (HSR)
  regulation/stewardship 393, 405, 420, 421t
  research 288, 292–293
  resource allocation 183
  structural components 416, 416f, 420f
  structure 393, 394f
  sustainability 183
  transitional perspective 276, 276f
  World Bank *see* World Bank
Health determinants
  broad 124
  urban context *see* Urban health
Health disparities *see* Health inequalities
Health economics/finance *see* Economics/financial issues
Health Education Authority for England 54
Health expenditure *see* Health-care expenditure
Health facilities construction, corruption issues 139t

Health financing *see* Health-care financing
Health for All by the Year 2000 62, 65, 107
  feasibility 65
  progress 68
Health for All Now! 123
Health for All program 54
Health governance *see* Governance
Health Impact Assessment (HIA) 112
Health inequalities **89–97**
  avoidability 93
  cultural rights 92
  definition 89, 92, 95
  discrimination and 91–92
  economic issues 92
    see also Economics/financial issues
  ethical issues 90
  gender-related *see* Gender/gender considerations
  human rights 91
  indigenous peoples *see* Indigenous peoples
  inequity *vs.* 93
  measurement 93
  resource allocation, implications 94
  social rights 92
Health information
  Internet-based
    essential drugs policy discussion forum 344
Health initiatives, global *see* Global health initiatives
Health insurance
  definition 212
  health-care expenditure determination 176
  industry, essential drugs policy development 344
  plans/programs *see* Health insurance plans/programs
  risk pooling 212
  risk rating, definition 212
  types/systems 237t
    commercial *see* Commercial health insurance
    community *see* Community health insurance (CHI)
    direct payment 212
    explicit 212
    implicit 212
    indirect payment 212
    mutual health organizations *see* Community health insurance (CHI)
    private *see* Private health insurance (PHI)
    social *see* Social health insurance (SHI)
    tax-based 202
    voluntary commercial 212
  universal coverage, definition 213
  universal coverage, transition to **211–223**
    degree of pooling 214, 214t
    developing countries 217
    OECD countries 214
    patterns 219
    technical concerns 213
  see also Health-care financing
Health insurance plans/programs **223–236**
  benefits package 211
  competition 225, 312
  design 224, 233–234
    adverse selection 225, 226–227, 233–234
  health outcomes and 233
  implementation challenges 206–207, 206t, 232
  low-income countries 232
  middle-income countries 232
  premium calculation 226, 226t
  revenue collection 232
  risk spreading 224–225
  universal coverage, transition to 213
  value 224, 224f
  moral hazard 176, 225
Health Insurance Portability and Accountability Act (1996), USA 358
Health maintenance organizations (HMOs) 323, 329
  aims 173
  demise 398–399
  group models 330
  staff models 330
Health management information systems (HMIS)
  health planning monitoring 48

Health outcomes
  health expenditure correlation 168, 170f
  health insurance programs and 233
Health Plan Employer Data Information Sheet (HEDIS) 331
Health planning *see* Health-care planning
Health policy **3–17**
  analysis 12
  definition 3, 30
  financing options 11
  global 9
  health expenditure influence 169
  implementation framework 8
  objectives 149
  outcomes 12
  political economy and 5–7
  politics 12
  power issues 5–7
  practice 9
  public participation *see* Public/consumer participation
  resource allocation, justice principle *see* Resource allocation
  socioeconomic factors 5–7
  terminology 4–5
  typologies 7, 7t
  see also Public health policy
Health promotion
  chronic disease, global goals 260
  community-based *see* Community-based health promotion
  definition 259
  effectiveness 32
  financing **259–272**, 262f
    conventional 271t
    funding sources 269t
    global 261t
    innovative 263, 268t, 271t
    recommendations 271
    ThaiHealth *see* ThaiHealth
  mental health *see* Mental health promotion
  Ottawa Charter 65, 66
  see also Disease prevention/preventive medicine
Health sector reform (HSR)
  anticorruption 144
    see also Corruption, health sector
  capitalist state and 14
  debate associated 12
  globalization 12, 13
  resistance 378
Health systems *see* Health-care systems
Health Systems Research Institute (HSRI), Thailand 267
Healthway (Western Australia Health Promotion Foundation) 263
Helen Keller International 314–315
High-income countries
  health-care systems 275–276, 277, 278, 283
  health problems 275
  health worker population ratios 297t
High Level Forum, Millennium Development Goals 88
Highly Indebted Poor Country (HIPC) Initiative 131
HIV/AIDS
  community health worker programs 385, 386
  human rights 108
  Millennium Development Goals 82, 82t, 84–85, 85t
  mortality 287
  pandemic 66–67
  services, interest groups promotion role 118, 121–122
HMO act 332
Holistic medicine *see* Traditional, complementary, and alternative medicine (TCAM)
Home care
  long-term provision 254
Home herbal gardens (HHG), indigenous therapeutics 425
Honduras, private health-care provision 306t
Hospitals/hospital services 402–403
  acute care *see* Acute care hospitals

Hospitals/hospital services (continued)
  competition 311
  economic models of behavior **336–342**
    application 340
    executive-benefit-maximization 340
    profit-maximizing 337, 338f
    quantity-maximizing 338, 338f
    research directions 341
    revenue-maximizing 339
    utility-maximizing 339
Household expenditure, health-care financing 196
Household income
  health-care financing, equity measurement 197
Human immunodeficiency virus (HIV) see HIV/AIDS
Human resource planning/management 49, **296–303**
  corruption 139t
  health worker absenteeism 207, 208f
  health worker demand 297
    adjustment policies 300
    definition 297
    determinants 299
    factors influencing 297, 298t
  health worker need 296–297
    definition 298
    overmet 298
    unmet 298
  health worker population ratios 296, 297t
  health worker shortages 298, 301
  health worker supply 297
    adjustment policies 300
    definition 298
    determinants 299, 300f
  health worker surplus 298
  primary health care 289, 293
  skill mix issues 301
  see also Health-care planning; Resource allocation
Human rights
  frameworks/approaches
    health attainment 106, 106t
    health inequalities 91
    HIV/AIDS 108
  public health policy see Public health policy
Hungary
  health insurance, transition to universal
    coverage 215
  private health-care provision 306t
Hurricane Katrina
  resource allocation following, justice principle
    97–98, 101, 103, 104
Hypertension
  prevention
    community health worker program 383

I

Iceland, health insurance 216
Ideologies
  health policy and 5–7
Immunization/immunization programs
  community health workers 386
  measles, as governance indicator 208,
    209f, 210t
  provider performance-based payment
    systems 327–328
Incentives, provider payment methods see Provider
  payment methods
Income see Household income
Independent practice associations (IPAs) 329
In-depth interviews, urban health research 413
India
  community health insurance 236, 241, 242t
  primary health care 290
  private health-care provision 306t, 307f, 308f
  public health policy reform 26
  Rural Health Mission 382
  tuberculosis control, public-private
    partnerships 318
Indian Health Service (IHS), USA, alcohol
  rehabilitation programs 424
Indifference curve, definition 336

Indigenous peoples **422–427**
  definition 422
  health status 423
    cardiovascular disease 424
    climate change impact 425
    environmental factors 425
    infectious diseases 424
    intervention programs 424
    mental health 424–425
Indigenous therapeutics
  home herbal gardens 425
  see also Traditional, complementary, and alternative
    medicine (TCAM)
Indonesia
  community health insurance 242
  private health-care provision 306–307, 306t,
    307f, 308f
Infant mortality
  population structure impact 174–176
Infection(s) see Infectious disease(s)
Infectious disease(s)
  indigenous peoples 424
Influenza vaccine/vaccination
  cost-effectiveness, decision analytic modeling 190,
    191f, 192f, 194, 194f
  resource allocation, post-Hurricane Katrina 97–98,
    101, 103, 104
Informal care, long-term 252, 352
Institutional care, long-term provision 253
Instrumental activities of daily living (IADLs),
  long-term care assessment 355t, 358–359
Interest groups **115–123**
  business 115, 120
  civil society organizations 115, 116f
    global activity 120
    public health policy impact 120
    public health policy reform 28
  definition 116
  governance 115
  HIV/AIDS services promotion 118, 121–122
  'insider' 117
  issue networks 119
  'outsider' 117
  policy communities 119
  public health policy contribution 26, 118,
    121t, 122
  representative bodies 115–116
  resources 117
  types 115–116
International Conference on Harmonization of
  Technical Requirements for Registration of
  Pharmaceuticals for Human Use (ICH), United
  Nations 343
International Conference on Population and
  Development (ICPD), UN 21
International Covenant on Civil and Political Rights
  (ICCPR), UN 105–106
  history 108
International Covenant on Economic,
  Social and Cultural Rights (ICESCR), UN
    105–106, 106t
International Department of the Belgian Christian
  Mutalities 238
International Financial Institutions (IFIs) 73
International Health Regulations (IHR)
  revision process 110
International Labour Organization (ILO), UN
  Social Security Convention (1952) 213–214
International People's Health University 126
Interviews/interviewing
  in-depth, urban health research 413
Iran
  community health worker programs 384, 384f
Ireland
  health-care expenditure, pharmaceuticals 178,
    178f, 179f
'Iron triangles' 119
Israel
  long-term care provision 354
  private health-care provision 306t
Issue networks, interest groups 119

Italy
  health-care expenditure, pharmaceuticals
    178f, 179f
  health insurance, transition to universal
    coverage 216
  private health-care provision 306t

J

Jakarta Declaration on Health Promotion 259
Japan
  long-term care financing 256
  long-term care provision 353–354
Joint Learning Initiative (JLI), primary health care 293
Jordan
  health-care expenditure
    health insurance impact 176
    household income effects 176
    pharmaceuticals 178–179
    population aging impact 173–174
Jubilee 2000: Drop the Debt campaign 121
Justice/equity ethical principle
  definition/conceptions 98
    equality of opportunity 99
    prioritarianism 99
    utilitarianism 98
  health-care financing see Health-care financing
  long-term care financing 256–257
  resource allocation see Resource allocation

K

Kaiser Family Foundation 28
Kaiser Health Plan 332
Kaiser Permanente Medical Care Program, USA
  disease management model 403–404
'Kaiser Triangle' disease management model 403–404
Kakwani index (KI), health-care financing 197–198,
  197f, 199
Kazakhstan
  private health-care provision 306t
Kenya
  community health insurance schemes 240
  community health worker program 383
  health-care expenditure
    household income effects 176
  health insurance, transition to universal
    coverage 219
  health sector corruption, prevention 142t
  private health-care provision 306t
Kerala People's Campaign for Decentralized Planning
  (1996-2001) 58
King's evil see Tuberculosis
Knowledge
  provision, Millennium Development Goals 87
  transfer, evidence-based public health policy 35, 36t
Korea, Republic of
  health-care expenditure 171
  health-care financing, risk pooling 400t
  health-care, public-private partnerships 317
  health insurance, transition to universal
    coverage 219
  health promotion financing 264, 268t
  provider payment methods 326

L

Labor organizations, public health policy reform 28
Lambourne, Robert 60
Latin America
  community health insurance 243
  health-care expenditure, pharmaceuticals 178–179
  health financing equity 201
  social health insurance, mixed model 394–395
Latvia, private health-care provision 306t
Lay participation, public health policy/research
  see Public/consumer participation
Leadership 75

Lebanon
  health-care expenditure
    pharmaceuticals 178–179
    technology impact 178
Lee's model, hospital economic behavior 339
Life expectancy
  factors affecting
    gender 94
    per capita income 278, 278f
Lithuania, private health-care provision 306t
Logframe, health planning 45t, 47
Long-term care (LTC) 351–357, 357–370
  aims 351–352
  assessment 354, 358–359
    activities of daily living *see* Activities of daily living (ADLs)
    instruments 355t
  community-based 365, 365t, 366t, 367t, 368t
  definition 250, 351
  demographics 362, 362t, 363t, 364t
  demographic transition 251, 251t, 252t
  disability estimates 359, 360t, 361t
  declines 368, 369t
  entitlement 352
  financing 250–259, 357, 352
    expenditure levels 257, 257t
    Health Insurance Portability and Accountability Act, provision 358
    method comparisons 256
    out-of-pocket payments 255
    self-directed services 257
    social insurance 256
    system differences 257
    tax-based 256
    voluntary insurance 255
  home-based 365, 365t
  mixed economy 252
  organization 250–259, 352
  Personal Social Services Research Unit model 251
  provision 253
    ambulatory settings 353
    assistive living 353
    coordination 254
    home 353
    home-based 253
    informal 252, 352
    institutional 254, 353
    issues 352
    pluralism 254
    quality 255
    service-enriched housing 353
    service integration 354
    sheltered housing 353
    target population 351, 352
  social work theory 257–258
  surveys 357
    National Long-Term Care, US *see* National Long-Term Care Surveys (NLTCS), US
Low birth weight (LBW)
  health inequalities, racial/ethnic 94
  see also Premature birth
Low-income countries
  health-care expenditure 277
  health-care systems 277, 282, 283
  health insurance, transition to universal coverage 219
  health insurance plans/programs 232
  health problems 275
  health worker population ratios 297t
  see also Developing countries
Lung cancer
  epidemiology
    historical aspects 287

M

Magnetic resonance imaging (MRI)
  health-care expenditure impact 178
Mahler, Halfdan 59, 60, 66–67, 75

Malaria
  eradication/eradication programs
    governance issues 210–211
    Millennium Development Goals 82t, 83t, 85t
    mortality associated 287
    prevention *see* Malaria prevention
Malaria prevention
  community health worker programs 386
Malawi
  private health-care provision 306t, 307f, 308f
Mali
  community health insurance schemes 238t, 239
Malnutrition
  Millennium Development Goals 82–83, 82t, 83t, 84–85, 85t
Managed care 329–336
  capitation 330
  carve out models 332
  case management 331
  disease management 331
  effects 334
    quality 335
    selection 334
    spillover effects 335
    utilization 334
  elements 330
    behavioral care 331
    monitoring service utilization 331
    paying providers 330
    pharmaceutical benefits 331
    preventative benefits 331
    provider organization 330
    provider selection 330
    quality monitoring 331
  fee-for service 330
  gatekeeper arrangements 331
  history 332
    developing world 334
    Europe 333
    Latin America 333
    United States 332
  pay for performance 330
  pharmacy benefits management 332
  private health insurance, health-care services provision 229, 233, 283
  public health 335
  vertically integrated plans 330
Manila Declaration on Governance (1999) 57
Marginal budgeting for bottlenecks (MBB), health planning 45
Marginal cost
  definition 336
  hospital economic behavior models 337–338
Marginal revenue, definition 336
Marginal utility, definition 336
Markets, provider payment methods 325
Markov models
  decision analysis 191, 193f, 193t
Marmot, Michael 75
Maternal death *see* Maternal mortality
Maternal mortality
  developing *vs.* developed countries 286
  Millennium Development Goals 82, 82t, 83t, 84, 85t
Maximization hypothesis, health-care demand 245–246
Mean logarithmic deviation (MLD), health-care financing equity 198
Measles vaccine/vaccination
  rates, governance indicator 208, 209f, 210t
Médecins Sans Frontières (MSF)
  as civil society 314–315
Media coverage/campaigns
  public health 55
  policy reform 28
Medicaid Program
  eligibility 318–319
  fiscal sustainability 401
  funding 318–319
  long-term care 353, 354
Medical arms race, hospital competition 311

Medical research
  corruption issues 139t
  see also Research and development (R&D)
Medicare Program
  coverage gaps 319
  eligibility 318–319
  fiscal sustainability 401
  HMO's 332–333
  long-term care 354
  provider compensation 326
Medium-Term Expenditure Frameworks, health planning 45, 49
Mental disorders
  indigenous peoples 424–425
  primary health care 287
Mental health
  indigenous peoples 424–425
  patient empowerment 372
  promotion *see* Mental health promotion
Mental health disorders *see* Mental disorders
Mental health promotion
  patient empowerment 372
Mexico
  health insurance
    transition to universal coverage 218
  private health-care provision 306t
Middle East *see* Middle East and North Africa (MENA)
Middle East and North Africa (MENA)
  health-care expenditure
    pharmaceuticals 178–179
Middle-income countries
  health-care expenditure 277
  health-care systems 282, 283
  health insurance plans/programs 232
  health worker population ratios 297t
Millennium Declaration, UN 72
Millennium Development Goals (MDGs)
  agenda 69, 182
  attainment
    shortfalls 186
  education 83–84
  gender considerations 83–84
  health-related 82–88
    child mortality 82t, 83t, 85t
    development assistance 88
    goals 82t, 83t
    health planning influence 42
    HIV/AIDS 82, 82t, 83t, 84–85, 85t
    indicators 82, 83t
    interventions 84, 85t
    knowledge provision 87
    malnutrition 82–83, 82t, 83t, 84–85, 85t
    maternal mortality 82, 82t, 83t, 84, 85t
    outcomes 112
    policy improvement 86
    progress acceleration 84, 85
    service delivery issues 87
    targeting 86
  High Level Forum 88
  history 72
  intersectoral synergies 87
  limitations 82, 84
  primary health care contribution 76
Minimal Data Set (MDS), long-term care assessment 354
Mixed economy of care, long-term care planning 252
Moldova
  private health-care provision 306t
Monopolies
  definition 336
  health-care competition 309–310
Monopsony power, health insurance competition 312
Monte Carlo simulation
  decision analytic modeling 194
Moral hazard, health insurance 176, 225
  universal coverage transition 213
Moral model, health sector corruption 142
Morocco
  health-care expenditure, pharmaceuticals 178–179

Mozambique
  private health-care provision 306t
MRI see Magnetic resonance imaging (MRI)
Multi-Country AIDS Program (MAP), World Bank 128
Multilevel analysis
  urban health research 414
Mutual health organizations see Community health insurance (CHI)

N

Nanny statist 52
Narayan, Ravi 76
The National Committee for Quality Assurance (NCQA) 331
National Health Accounts (NHAs) 165, 261
  see also Health-care expenditure
National Health Interview Survey (NHIS), USA 357
  Aging Supplement 357
National Health Service (NHS), UK
  creation/establishment 52
  managed care history 333–334
  stewardship 405
National Health Services (Beveridge) model of health-care 275–276, 279
  health insurance 215, 237–238
  innovations 281t
  strengths 281t
  sustainability 283
  weaknesses 281t
  see also National Health Service (NHS), UK
National health systems see Health-care systems
National Long-Term Care Surveys (NLTCS), US 358
  protocol bias 359–360
  purpose 358
  sampling 357, 358
National Medical Care Expenditure Survey, USA 176–177
National Medical Expenditure Survey (NMES), USA 357
National Nursing Home Survey (NNHS), USA 357
Netherlands
  consumer choice, health plans 231
  health-care expenditure, pharmaceuticals 178f, 179f
  health-care financing
    private health insurance 399t
  long-term care provision 353–354
  private health-care provision 306t
  provider payment methods 326
Net income 196
Network theory
  health policy 5–7
  public health policy reform analysis 25
Nevis, private health-care provision 306t
New public management (NPM) 54
  state role 57
New social movements (NSMs)
  emergence 119
  features 119
  see also Interest groups
New Zealand
  health insurance, transition to universal coverage 216
  private health-care provision 306t
NGO Committee on Primary Health Care 61–62
Nicaragua
  health-care expenditure, pharmaceuticals 178–179
Nigeria
  private health-care provision 306t
911 see World Trade Center, terrorist attack
Noncommunicable disease(s)
  burden 287
Non-democratic regimes 53
Nongovernmental organizations (NGOs)
  community health insurance schemes, developing countries 241
  community health worker program support 381–382, 386, 387
  see also Community health workers (CHWs)

definition 117
essential drugs policy development 344
provider performance-based payment systems 328
role 108
tertiary care provision, low-income countries 306
see also Interest groups
Nonmalfeasance ethical principle, health inequalities 90–91
North Africa see Middle East and North Africa (MENA)
Norway
  health insurance, transition to universal coverage 216
  private health-care provision 306t
Nurse(s)
  empowerment 370–371, 371f
Nutrition
  elderly see Elderly
  HIV see HIV/AIDS
  Millennium Development Goals 82–83, 82t, 83t, 85t
  see also Malnutrition
Nutritional deficiencies see Malnutrition

O

Obesity
  health-care expenditure, impact on 174
Objective function, definition 336
Obstetric mortality see Maternal mortality
Older persons see Elderly
Oligopolies
  definition 336
  economic hospital behavior models 339
  health-care competition 309–310, 312
Onchocerciasis
  eradication, governance issues 209–210
Ordinary least squares (OLS), health-care demand 247
Organization for Economic Co-operation and Development (OECD)
  universal coverage transition 214
Ottawa Charter for Health Promotion 65
  approach/strategies 259
  principles 107–108
  reflections 66
  see also Health promotion
Out-of-pocket systems, health-care financing see Health-care financing
Own-price effect, health-care demand 247
Oxfam 118–119

P

PACE program, long-term care provision 355
Pakistan
  community health worker programs 386
  health insurance, transition to universal coverage 219
Panama, private health-care provision 306t, 307f, 308f
Pan American Health Organization (PAHO)
  primary health care review 70–71
Participant observation 413
Partisan model, public health policy reform analysis 24
Partners for Health Reform Plus (PHRplus) 173–174
Patient Activation Measure (PAM) 373, 374t
Patient decision aids 376
Patient empowerment 372
  antecedents 377, 378
  barriers to 377, 378
  definition 372
  holistic model 373, 375f
  measurement 373
  mental health promotion 372
  outcomes 377, 379
  processes 375
    decision-making 376
    information-sharing 375
    physician-patient communication 376
  self-care 376

self-help movement 376
types 372, 373f
Patient Empowerment Scale (PES) 374t
Patient organizations, essential drugs policy development 344
Patient outcomes
  empowerment 377
Patient participation, public health policy/research see Public/consumer participation
Pay for performance (P4P) payment systems 172–173, 327
People's Charter for Health 124, 126
People's Health Assembly 123, 125, 126
People's Health for All Movement 76, 123–127
  aims 124–125
  gains 125
  World Health Organization, relationship with 126–127
Performance-based payment systems 327
Periago, Mirta Roses 77
Personal Social Services Research Unit (PSSRU) model, long-term care 251
Peru
  private health-care provision 306t
Pharmaceutical industry
  competition 312
  global resource allocation 181, 181t
  international 344
Pharmaceutical Inspection Cooperation Scheme (PIC/S) 343
Pharmaceuticals policy see Essential drugs policy/legislation
Philippines
  community health insurance 242
  health-care expenditure, population aging impact 173–174
Physical environment, urban health determinants 412
Physician(s)
  behavior
    health-care expenditure determinants 176
    health-care expenditure effects 176–177
  competition 310, 323
  conflicts of interest 141
  see also Corruption, health sector
  empowerment 370–371, 371f
Physician-patient communication 376
Planning spiral model, health planning 45, 47f
Pluralist model 24
Poland
  private health-care provision 306t
Political economy, health policy and 5–7
Political factions model 24
Political survival model 24
Political will model 24, 24t
Poor Law (1834), UK 215
Population(s)
  aging see Population aging
  epidemiological profiles 417
  epidemiological transition see Epidemiological transition
  health needs, health-care expenditure determination 173
  urban see Urban health
Population aging
  challenges associated 251
Portugal
  health insurance, transition to universal coverage 216
  private health-care provision 306t
Poverty Reduction Strategy Plans (PRSPs) 131
  health planning 45t
Power issues, health policy 5–7
P4P (pay for performance) payment systems 172–173, 327
Preferred provider organizations (PPOs) 329
Premature birth
  health inequalities, racial/ethnic 94
  see also Low birth weight
President's Emergency Plan for AIDS Relief (PEPFAR) 128, 133–134
Pressure groups see Interest groups
Price elasticity of demand, definition 337

Price taker, definition 337
Primary health care (PHC) **284–296**
   Declaration of Alma Ata *see* Declaration of Alma-Ata
   definition 285
   development 291
      community-based programs 291
      human resources 289, 293
      needs identification 69
   equity monitoring 293
   evidence issues 69
   history 284
   human resources 289, 293
   implementation 285, 286, 292, 419–420
      community health worker programs 293, 381
      system building 72
   interpretations 285
   Millennium Development Goals, contribution to 76
   policy context 285
   principles 284
   rationale 402–403
   revitalization 290
   system composition 71–72
   values 381, 383
   WHO approach 60, 61
Primary prevention *see* Disease prevention/preventive medicine
Primordial prevention *see* Disease prevention/preventive medicine
Priority setting/prioritarianism, justice principle 99
   see also Resource allocation
Private health insurance (PHI) 151, 152*f*, 227
   access 229, 234
   equity 203
   features 397, 419*t*, 421*t*
   functions 227
   health-care services provision 229
      managed care 229, 233, 283
   high-income countries 305
   low-income countries 305, 397
   profit orientation 304, 307
   regulation 227–228, 234
   supplementary 228
   see also Health-care provision
Private-public partnerships, health-care systems *see* Public-private partnerships (PPPs)
Profit-maximizing model, hospital economic behavior 337, 338*f*
Provider payment methods **322–329**, 418, 420*t*
   breadth 322, 324, 324*f*
   coarseness 322, 324, 324*f*
   competition 325
   definition 172–173, 418–419
   delivery structure 325
   Diagnostic Related Grouping system 323–324, 401
      'creep' 326
      incentives created 325
      post-discharge services 324
   dimensions 322
   fee-for-service 323, 325, 420*t*
   fineness 324, 324*f*, 326
   future trends 328
   generosity 322, 324
   hospital behavior models *see* Hospitals/hospital services
   incentives 172–173, 325, 418–419, 419*t*
      capitation 325
      eligibility 327
      fixed budgets 325
      mixed payment systems 326
      salaries 325
   information types 322, 322*f*
   markets 325
   performance-based 327
   types 401, 402*t*
Public accountability *see* Governance
Public/consumer participation
   preferences
      health-care demand 245
      social health insurance 231
      public health policy reform 27

Public health
   definition 3
   functions 404, 405*t*
   policy *see* Public health policy
   public participation *see* Public/consumer participation
   state role in **51–59**
      behavior promotion 54
      bureaucratic model 53
      cross-cutting work 57
      delayed administrations 56
      evaluation 58
      evolution 51
      feedback loops 58
      government tools 53
      health campaigns 54
      implementation 58
      inclusive policymaking 58
      industrial revolution 52
      issue handling 56
      Marxist ideologies 52
      middle ages 51–52
      ministries of health 54
      national health system establishment 52
      policy, process of making 55
      public-private partnerships 54
      socialist ideologies 52
      taxation 54
      Totalitarian regimes 52
      treaties 56
Public health policy
   agenda setting **17–23**
      actors 18, 18*t*
      definition 17
      future research 22
      international influences 21
      models 19, 19*t*, 20
      social constructionism 18
   civil society organizations impact 120
   'communities' 119
   cycle 32, 33*f*
   definition 17
   discrimination and 111
   evidence-based **30–39**
      advocacy 34*t*
      definition 30
      generation process 32, 33*f*, 34*t*
      improvement mechanisms 35, 36*t*
      influences 34, 35*t*
      knowledge transfer 35, 36*t*
      popularity 30
      requirements 31
      research focus 31, 32*t*, 33*t*
      Sicily Statement 31
   formulation, 'iron triangles' 119
   global health initiatives *see* Global health initiatives
   health planning relationship 39
   human rights approach **105–114**
      concepts 110
      context 112
      discrimination issues 111
      governmental obligations 105, 106*t*
      history 107
      HIV/AIDS 108
      impact 113
      limitations 110
      outcomes 113
      process 113
   implementation 55
   'issue networks' 119
   networks 21
   planning *see* Health-care planning
   public participation *see* Public/consumer participation
   reform **23–29**
      champions 27
      context 26
      feasibility 28
      institutions 26
      interest groups' participation 24*t*, 26, 28
      models 23, 24*t*

      players 28
      public participation 27
      theoretical analysis 23, 25
      timing 27
      tobacco use 34
      transfer 21
   see also Health policy
Public Investment Programme (PIP) 49
Public policy 5
   definition 3, 4, 115
   terminology 4
   see also Health policy; Public health policy
Public-private partnerships (PPPs) **314–321**
   definition 314, 316
   features 316, 421*t*
   framing 321
   preventive services 317*t*
   problems associated 320
   theme 314
Public sector organizations 28
Puerto Rico
   private health-care provision 306*t*
Punctuated equilibrium model 24, 25

Q

Quality-adjusted life years (QALYs)
   concepts underlying
      utilitarianism 98
   decision analytic modeling 190
   see also Cost-effectiveness analysis (CEA)
Quality of life (QOL)
   long-term care assessment 355*t*
Quangos 54
Quantity-maximizing model, hospital economics 338, 338*f*

R

Rand Insurance Experiment 225
   results 176, 225*t*, 233, 234
Rational choice model, health sector corruption 141
Rawls, John 98
Redistributive effect (RE) 197–198, 197*f*
Reduced-form models, health-care demand 247
Research and development (R&D)
   evidence-based public health policy 31, 32*t*, 33*t*
   health-care expenditure impact 177
   resource allocation, justice principle 100
   systematic reviews *see* Systematic reviews
   urban health *see* Urban health
Resource allocation **180–186**
   definition 180–181
   health-care planning 46, 48*f*
   implications, health inequalities 94
   justice principle **97–105**, 102*t*, 181
      medical emergencies/disasters 100–101, 102, 104
      prioritarianism 99
      public health challenges 99
      public health research 100
      utilitarianism 98
   macro-level, health-care systems 183
   mega-level (global) 181
      pharmaceutical industry 181, 181*t*
   meso-level, institutions 183
      'accountability for reasonableness' 183, 184, 184*t*
   see also Human resource planning/management
Respiratory disease(s)
   mortality associated 286–287
Respite care 252–253
Retrenchment 52
Revenue-maximizing model, hospital economics 339
Reviewing Primary Health Care in the Americas 70
Rockefeller Foundation 60
   community health worker program 381
Roll Back Malaria 128–129, 131
Rosko's model, hospital economic behavior 340
Rural Cooperative Medical System (RCMS), China 240–241

Russian Federation
　health insurance, transition to universal coverage 216
　see also Former Soviet Union (FSU)
Rwanda
　community health insurance schemes 240
　private health-care provision 306t

S

Sanders, David 68
Sanitation
　access 286
Scale invariance, definition 198
Science see Science/technology
Science/technology
　health-care expenditure determination 177
　public health 55
Scrofula see Tuberculosis
Secondary care see Hospitals/hospital services
Secondary prevention see Disease prevention/preventive medicine
Sector-Wide Approach (SWAp)
　health planning 45t, 50
　public health policy 131
Self-care 376
Self-directed services 257
Self-help movement
　patient empowerment 376
Senegal, community health insurance schemes 238t, 239
Sensitivity analysis, decision analytic modeling 193, 194f
Service-enriched housing, long-term care 353
Sheltered housing 353
Sicily Statement, evidence-based public health policy 31
Simple decision trees, decision analytic modeling 191, 191f
SIPA (system of integrated care for older persons) 355
Situational analysis, health-care planning 46
SKY scheme 242, 243t
Sloan–Steinwald's model, hospital economic behavior 340
Social constructivist theory/social constructionism
　public health policy, agenda setting 18
Social environment
　urban health determinants 411
Social Exclusion Unit 57
Social health insurance (SHI) 150, 229, 397
　advantages 397
　Beveridge model 215, 237–238
　Bismarck model see Bismarck model, social health insurance
　consumer choice 231
　definition 212, 397
　developing countries 237–238
　health-care expenditure determination 172
　health-care services provision 231
　long-term care financing 256
　mandatory 232
　principles 150
　public prepayment 202
　risk adjustment 230
　scheme characteristics 212, 237, 237t
　typology 229, 230t
Social Health Insurance Networking and Empowerment (SHINE), Philippines 242
Social Insurance and Allied Services, Beverage 52
Socialist model of health-care 275–276, 280
　innovations 281t
　strengths 281t
　weaknesses 281t
Social rights, health inequalities 92
Social Security Convention (1952) 213–214
Social security model of health-care see Social health insurance (SHI)
Social work theory 257–258
Sociocultural context/perspective
　medical science/technology see Science/technology

Socioeconomic status (SES)
　health policy and 5–7
South Africa
　health-care expenditure, pharmaceuticals 178–179
South Asia
　Millennium Development Goals 84–85
South-East Asia
　private health-care provision 306
South Korea see Korea, Republic of
Spain
　health-care provision 403
　health insurance, transition to universal coverage 216
　private health-care provision 306t
Sri Lanka
　primary health care 290
St. Kitts, private health-care provision 306t
St. Vincent, private health-care provision 306t
Stagist model 24–25
State Children's Health Insurance Program (SCHIP), USA 318–319
Stop TB Partnership 128–129, 131
Structural adjustment programs (SAPs)
　primary health care policy context 285
　principles 73
sub-Saharan Africa
　health-care financing 394–395
　health-care systems
　　private provision 306
Suicide
　rates
　　indigenous peoples 424
Sustainable Health Financing, Universal Coverage, and Social Health Insurance, World Health Assembly 203
Sweden
　health-care expenditure 171
　health-care financing 394, 395–397, 396f
　　private health insurance 399t
　health-care system 395–397
　health insurance, transition to universal coverage 216
　long-term care provision 353
　private health-care provision 306t
Switzerland
　consumer choice, health plans 231
　health-care expenditure, pharmaceuticals 178f, 179f
　health insurance, transition to universal coverage 215
　health promotion financing 265, 268t
　private health-care provision 306t
　sickness funds, health-care services provision 232
Systematic reviews
　evidence-based medicine, contribution to 33–34
System of integrated care for older persons (SIPA) 355

T

Taiwan
　health-care system
　　provider payment methods 326
Tanzania
　community health insurance schemes 240
　private health-care provision 306t
Tanzania Network of Community Health Funds (TNCHF) 240
Technical efficiency studies, cost-effectiveness analysis 186
Technical Union of Community Health Insurance Schemes 239
Technocratic model, public health policy reform analysis 24, 24t
Technology see Science/technology
Tejada, David 62
Tertiary prevention see Disease prevention/preventive medicine
ThaiHealth 270–271
　financial profile 269
　governance 269
　history 267

　mission 267
　performance 269
　population impact 270
　priorities 267
　project funding 269, 270f
　recommendations 271
Thailand
　health insurance, transition to universal coverage 219, 220, 221
　health promotion financing 270f
　　innovative 267, 268t
　see also ThaiHealth
Therapeutic Alliance Scale, patient empowerment 373, 374t
3-by-5 initiative 42
Thresholder groups 118
Time cost, health-care demand 249
Tobacco Control Act (1991), Australia 263
Tobacco policy/control
　public health policy 34
　Thai health promotion initiative 270
Totalitarian regimes 52
Trade-related Aspects of Intellectual Property Rights (TRIPS) agreement 112
　essential drugs policy 345
Traditional, complementary, and alternative medicine (TCAM)
　health-care demand 248
　patient empowerment 373, 375f
　see also Indigenous therapeutics
Traditional medicine/healing see Traditional, complementary, and alternative medicine (TCAM)
Transdisciplinarity see Ecosystem health
Transnational corporations, regulation 120
Triage
　definition 100
　ethical issues 100–101, 102
Tuberculosis (TB)
　control
　　community health worker programs 387
　　Directly Observed Therapy see DOTS
　　public-private partnerships, India 318
　Millennium Development Goals 85t
　mortality 287
　treatment
　　strategy decisions 195
Turkey
　private health-care provision 307f, 308f
Two-stage least squares (TSLS), health-care demand 247

U

Uganda
　community health insurance schemes 240
　health sector corruption, prevention 142t
　private health-care provision 306t
Ugandan Participatory Poverty Assessment Project 58
UK see United Kingdom (UK)
Ungovernable state 52
UNICEF see United Nations Children's Fund (UNICEF)
Unified model, health-care demand 245, 246, 249
Union Technique de la Mutualité Malienne (UTM) 239
Unitary states, public health 55
United Kingdom (UK)
　'expert carers' investment 394
　health-care financing 394
　　private health insurance 399t
　health-care system
　　private provision 306t
　　see also National Health Service (NHS), UK
　health insurance, transition to universal coverage 214, 214t, 215
　long-term care provision 353
United Nations (UN)
　Commission on the Social Determinants of Health see Commission on the Social Determinants of Health (CSDH), UN

Convention on the Elimination of All Forms of Discrimination against Women *see* Convention on the Elimination of All Forms of Discrimination Against Women, UN
Convention on the Rights of the Child *see* Convention on the Rights of the Child, UN
Declaration on the Rights of Indigenous Peoples 426
International Conference on Harmonization of Technical Requirements for Registration of Pharmaceuticals for Human Use (ICH) 343
International Conference on Population and Development *see* International Conference on Population and Development (ICPD), UN
International Covenant on Civil and Political Rights *see* International Covenant on Civil and Political Rights (ICCPR), UN
International Covenant on Economic, Social and Cultural Rights *see* International Covenant on Economic, Social and Cultural Rights (ICESCR), UN
International Labour Organization *see* International Labour Organization (ILO), UN
Millennium Declaration 72
Millennium Development Goals *see* Millennium Development Goals (MDGs)
Universal Declaration of Human Rights *see* Universal Declaration of Human Rights, United Nations
United Nations Children's Fund (UNICEF)
Child Survival Revolution 289
United States (US) *see* United States of America (USA)
United States of America (USA)
health-care, public-private partnerships 318
health-care expenditure 171
defensive medicine effects 177
determination, technology effects 177–178
health insurance effects 176
pharmaceuticals 178, 178f, 179f
health-care financing, private health insurance 398–399, 399t
health-care system
private provision 306t
health promotion financing 265, 266t, 268t
health sector corruption, prevention 142t
Indian Health Service, alcohol rehabilitation programs 424
local health departments 319–320
long-term care provision 353, 354, 355
public health privatization 319
Universal Declaration of Human Rights, United Nations 182
history 105–106
Urban health **408–415**
definition 409, 411
determinants 410
physical environment 412
resource infrastructure 412

social environment 411
history 408
measurement 411
research 410, 413
interurban 411
intraurban 411
qualitative 413
quantitative 413
urban *vs.* rural studies 410
trends
demographic 408, 409f
municipal, national and global 412
Urgency Rating Scores, cardiac surgery prioritization 184
US *see* United States of America (USA)
USA *see* United States of America (USA)
Utility, definition 337
Utility ethical principle/utilitarianism
resource allocation 98
Utility function, definition 337
Utility-maximizing model, hospital economic behavior 339

V

Variable cost, definition 337
Venediktov, Dmitry 67
Venezuela
private health-care provision 306t
Victorian Health Promotion Foundation (VicHealth) 263, 264t
Vietnam
health insurance, transition to universal coverage 221
Voluntary insurance 255

W

Wasting (slim) disease *see* HIV/AIDS
Welfare reforms 52
Western Australia Health Promotion Foundation (Healthway) 263
Whitehall studies 75–76
White plague *see* Tuberculosis
WHO *see* World Health Organization (WHO)
Women/women's health
life expectancy 94
World Bank
essential drugs policy development 343–344, 346
global health role 18–19
health sector reform approach 13
Multi-Country AIDS Program 128
World Council of Churches 60
World Development Report (1993) 131
World Health Assembly (WHA) 61

International Health Regulations *see* International Health Regulations (IHR)
Sustainable Health Financing, Universal Coverage, and Social Health Insurance 203
see also World Health Organization (WHO)
World Health Organization (WHO)
aims/objectives 37
Choosing Health Interventions that are Cost-Effective project *see* Choosing Health Interventions that are Cost-Effective (CHOICE) project, WHO
Civil Society Initiative 126–127
constitution 92
Declaration of Alma-Ata *see* Declaration of Alma-Ata
Declaration on the Health and Survival of Indigenous Peoples 426
essential drugs policy perspectives 345
health sector reform approach 13
International Health Regulations *see* International Health Regulations (IHR)
joint working with Christian Medical Commission 61
People's Health Movement, relationship with 126–127
primary health care
approach 60, 61
World Health Report (2000) 406
health-care financing 195–196, 199, 199f, 260–261
health-care system performance evaluation 195–196, 199, 199f
health inequalities 93
World Health Survey (WHS) 306–307
World Trade Center, terrorist attack
resource allocation following 97–98, 100, 103, 104
World Trade Organization (WTO)
essential drugs policy 345
General Agreement on Trade in Services *see* General Agreement on Trade in Services (GATS)
Trade-related Aspects of Intellectual Property Rights *see* Trade-related Aspects of Intellectual Property Rights (TRIPS) agreement
WTO *see* World Trade Organization (WTO)

Y

Yemen
health-care expenditure
pharmaceuticals 178–179

Z

Zambia
health-care financing, risk pooling 400, 400t

Printed in the United States
By Bookmasters